PHARMACEUTICAL
DOSAGE FORMS

PHARMACEUTICAL DOSAGE FORMS

Disperse Systems

In Three Volumes
VOLUME 2
Second Edition, Revised and Expanded

EDITED BY

Herbert A. Lieberman

H. H. Lieberman Associates, Inc.
Livingston, New Jersey

Martin M. Rieger

M. & A. Rieger Associates
Morris Plains, New Jersey

Gilbert S. Banker

University of Iowa
Iowa City, Iowa

Marcel Dekker, Inc.   New York • Basel • Hong Kong

ISBN: 0-8247-9713-2

The publisher offers discounts on this book when ordered in bulk quantities. For more information, write to Special Sales/Professional Marketing at the address below.

This book is printed on acid-free paper.

Marcel Dekker, Inc.
270 Madison Avenue, New York, New York 10016

Current printing (last digit):
10 9 8 7 6 5 4 3 2 1

PRINTED IN THE UNITED STATES OF AMERICA

Preface to the Second Edition

For this second volume of *Pharmaceutical Dosage Forms: Disperse Systems*, comprehensive coverage of the topic required the addition of new material (about 25%) and the inclusion of several new chapters. As in Volume 1 of the Second Edition, the text has been significantly updated and the references expanded. This volume concentrates on specific types of disperse system dosage forms and presents practical examples of their formulations and stability test procedures. The contents have been reorganized such that several chapters from the second volume of the first edition now appear in Volumes 1, 2, and 3 of this edition.

The revised chapter on pharmaceutical suspensions covers both the theoretical and practical aspects. Additional practical experiences are described for the formulation, manufacture, and testing procedures for pharmaceutical suspensions. A detailed checklist for appraising suspension performance and testing is provided, together with a procedure for the dissolution testing of active ingredients.

One important change in this volume was the combination of the chapter on pharmaceutical emulsions with that on emulsions and microemulsions to form one single, enhanced chapter on pharmaceutical emulsions and microemulsions. The new chapter addresses a significant number of the theoretical and practical issues required for the development of stable and effective emulsion-type products. The chapter is a comprehensive, up-to-date review of the literature on pharmaceutical emulsions, offering more than 250 references. It includes discussions of formulations, reviews of patents, and studies covering diverse drugs. The editors gratefully acknowledge Dr. Bernard Idson's contributions to the topic as it appeared in the first edition.

The chapter on antacids and clay products has been considerably modified. Several new figures have been added to help the reader better understand the intricacies of dealing with these types of disperse systems. The concept of "point of zero charge" is introduced, and its utility for developing stable formulations is described. Information on mixing and homogenizing equipment is presented, and procedures for testing and evaluating antacid suspensions are included.

The chapter on reconstitutable suspensions covers an important dosage form, as documented by the continuing increase during recent years in the number of monographs on such preparations in the *United States Pharmacopeia*. The most significant addition to this chapter is up-to-date information on stability evaluation of reconstituted antibiotic oral suspensions. This includes determination of shelf-life at various temperatures, the effect of repackaging, and the impact of elevated temperatures on the mechanism of drug degradation. In addition, the listing of manufacturers of typical antibiotic, reconstitutable, oral suspensions has been updated.

The chapter on topical suspensions includes significant updates and changes to guide and assist formulators. The chapter provides details on all processes from laboratory to scale-up to pilot plant to production, offering solutions to problems at each of these intermediate stages. The section on stability has been greatly expanded by including the guidelines of the International Conference on Harmonization (ICH) and the Food and Drug Administration (FDA).

The chapter on oral aqueous suspensions contains many new references and also includes more detailed descriptions of several topics. For the sake of clarity, coverage of sedimentation, particle size reduction, thixotropy, suspending and wetting agents, sweeteners, bioavailability, and physical stability testing procedures has been expanded. As in the first edition, this chapter includes several formulations that illustrate the use of different ingredients and compounding methods for preparing stable oral aqueous suspensions.

The chapter on injectable emulsions and suspensions reflects recent advances in parenteral medications, including excipient selection and compatibilities, as well as methods for meeting current regulatory requirements. The importance of physicochemical properties, processing constraints, and physiological considerations in formulation development and drug release is emphasized, accompanied by several illustrative case studies. The effect of microfluidization on particle size and on size distribution is described, with emphasis on dosage form stability and aseptic filtration. Modified stability protocols are provided based on the proposed recommendations of the ICH.

The intended replacement of all CFC-type propellants with HFC products required revision of the chapter on aerosol suspensions and emulsions. Substitute formulation approaches for products, such as antiasthmatics, are described. Additional information addresses the use of the bag-in-can or other barrier systems that are finding increased use in pharmaceutical products. The section on emulsions has been expanded to reflect the use of foam systems for topical, rectal, and vaginal applications.

In the updated chapter on ophthalmic ointments and suspensions, the authors have included novel approaches relating to the use of microparticles, liposomes, absorbable gelatin sponges, collagen shields, and in situ gels and inserts. The section dealing with product safety considerations, including sterility and preservation, has undergone major revision. A new section has been added, describing the packaging aspects of ophthalmic ointments and suspensions.

The chapter on gels was rewritten to conform to current terminology. The section on gel-forming compounds has been updated and expanded, and information on applications and requirements has been added. This chapter includes an overview of compounds utilized in bioadhesives and hydrogels, and their mechanisms of action. This is followed by a brief discussion of hydrogels, and ophthalmic and topical formulations.

The chapter on toothpastes was revised to include information reflecting developments in the marketplace since the publication of the first edition. Formulations are tabulated to provide easier comparisons, and case histories show the sequential changes required to reach an acceptable final formula. The use of new ingredients, such as sodium bicarbonate, is illustrated, and the section on stability testing is expanded.

The final chapter, on suppository development and production, has been susbstantially updated, with some portions entirely rewritten to reflect the most recent information describing the use and selection of suppository bases. The chapter now features a broad overview of the technical and theoretical considerations germane to formulation and manufacture. Critical aspects of production, including controls, compounding, and alternative filling methods, are described. The chapter includes broadened coverage of quality control issues and suggestions for troubleshooting problems that occur during manufacture.

The chapter authors were chosen because of their expertise in their respective topics. We are particularly grateful for their cooperation in modifying and adding material to their chapters based on our suggestions. The editorial staff at Marcel Dekker, Inc., is due recognition for its help in bringing this volume to publication.

We hope that these volumes will prove invaluable in teaching and providing information to a broad range of industrial pharmacists and to others in related industries, academia, and government.

Herbert A. Lieberman
Martin M. Rieger
Gilbert S. Banker

Preface to the First Edition

Volume 2 of *Disperse Systems* completes the seven-volume series *Pharmaceutical Dosage Forms*. In addition to two volumes on disperse systems, the series includes three volumes on tablets (now in its second edition) and two volumes on parenterals.

The ten chapters that make up Volume 1 on disperse systems were selected to provide the reader with basic information and theory for the various dosage forms and with some of the major characteristics of disperse system products. By contrast, in Volume 2 the editors have tried to emphasize the dosage form as well as describe some of the attributes of such applied aspects as scale-up, production, quality control, and formulation of specific products of two or more phases.

As a result of describing the preparation of a particular drug in one dosage form, the product formulator may then find it can be adapted for use with a different drug—either in the same dosage form or, conceivably, for use with a different but related dosage form. At times, excipients may be a common denominator for a type of disperse system product, even when made up of entirely different drugs. Preservatives and antioxidants that have been found useful in one type of drug product may be useful in an unrelated drug product. Information on processing equipment may be useful in manufacturing a wide variety of dispersed products. Quality assurance details are applicable to all of these dosage forms. Thus, technologists who read this book are likely to find clues to immediate applications even in a foreign class of formulations.

Product formulators are encouraged not to review just one or two chapters in this volume but to devote time to gaining insight into products and procedures that they may not feel have an immediate apparent relationship to the formulation problem they are trying to solve. The editors also urge readers to re-examine Volume 1 for its more theoretical information, even if their primary problem is covered specifically in one or more of the chapters in Volume 2, which are devoted to specific formulations.

The editors hope that the two volumes on disperse systems will prove to be useful sources of information on both the theory and practice of drug formulation. These volumes can be utilized as basic teaching and reference texts in colleges, research institutions, government agencies, and pharmaceutical and related industries.

The contributing authors represent a cross-section of scholars and highly knowledgeable and experienced formulators of particular types of disperse products. These experts have labored hard to provide our readers with information and insight concerning the particular products and product characteristics they cover in their valuable contributions. The contributing authors deserve the thanks not only of the editors but of our readers for their devotion to the task of creating the many pedagogic chapters in this text. By sharing their knowledge and experience with us and by warning of potential formulation pitfalls, the authors have rendered an invaluable service to the profession.

The tasks of the editors and of the authors are now completed. Our hope is that all who work in the broad field of pharmaceutical sciences will find our efforts worthwhile and an ever-ready source of helpful information.

Herbert A. Lieberman
Martin M. Rieger
Gilbert S. Banker

Contents

Contributors

Krishna M. Bapatla, Ph.D.   Director, Pharmaceutical Technical Affairs, Research & Development, Alcon Laboratories, Inc., Fort Worth, Texas

Hridaya N. Bhargava, Ph.D.   Professor, Department of Pharmaceutical Sciences, Massachusetts College of Pharmacy and Allied Health Sciences, Boston, Massachusetts

Lawrence H. Block, Ph.D.   Professor and Chair, Department of Pharmaceutical Chemistry and Pharmaceutics, Mylan School of Pharmacy, Duquesne University, Pittsburgh, Pennsylvania

Alison Green Floyd, Ph.D.   Research Investigator, Department of Pharmaceutics, Glaxo Wellcome, Inc., Greenville, North Carolina

David Garlen   Founding Partner, Cosmetech Laboratories, Inc., Fairfield, New Jersey

Marion Gold   Director, Corporate Development and Planning, Centerchem, Inc., Stamford, Connecticut

Richard J. Harwood, Ph.D.   Private Formulations, Inc., Edison, New Jersey

Gerald Hecht, Ph.D.   Senior Director, Department of Ophthalmology, Alcon Laboratories, Inc., Fort Worth, Texas

Sunil Jain, Ph.D.   Senior Scientist, Department of Pharmaceutics, Glaxo Wellcome, Inc., Greenville, North Carolina

Gregory P. Kushla, Ph.D.   Research Investigator, Product Development Department, Knoll Pharmaceutical Company, Whippany, New Jersey

Joseph R. Luber, B.Sc.   Johnson & Johnson Merck Consumer Products Co., Fort Washington, Pennsylvania

Robert A. Nash, Ph.D.   Associate Professor, Department of Pharmaceutics, St. John's University, Jamaica, New York

Daniel W. Nicolai, B.S., MBA   President, Stiefel Research Institute, Inc., Oak Hill, New York

Clyde M. Ofner III, Ph.D.   Associate Professor, Department of Pharmaceutics, Philadelphia College of Pharmacy and Science, Philadelphia, Pennsylvania

Bharat J. Oza, Ph.D.   Oza Enterprises, Summit, New Jersey

Roger L. Schnaare, Ph.D.   Professor, Department of Pharmaceutics, Philadelphia College of Pharmacy and Science, Philadelphia, Pennsylvania

Joseph B. Schwartz, Ph.D.   Professor, Department of Pharmaceutics, Philadelphia College of Pharmacy and Science, Philadelphia, Pennsylvania

John J. Sciarra, Ph.D.   Sciarra Laboratories, Inc., Hicksville, New York

Edward W. Sunbery, B.Sc., R.Ph.   Senior Scientist, Department of Pharmaceutical Engineering and Technical Services, Merck & Co., Inc., West Point, Pennsylvania

Murit VePuri   CEO, Able Labs, South Plainfield, New Jersey

Joel L. Zatz, Ph.D.   Professor and Chair, Department of Pharmaceutics, Rutgers College of Pharmacy, Rutgers—The State University of New Jersey, Piscataway, New Jersey

Contents of Pharmaceutical Dosage Forms: Disperse Systems, Second Edition, Revised and Expanded, Volumes 1 and 3

edited by Herbert A. Lieberman, Martin M. Rieger, and Gilbert S. Banker

VOLUME 1

VOLUME 3

Contents of Pharmaceutical Dosage Forms: Tablets, Second Edition, Revised and Expanded, Volumes 1–3

edited by Herbert A. Lieberman, Leon Lachman, and Joseph B. Schwartz

Contents of Pharmaceutical Dosage Forms: Parenteral Medications, Second Edition, Revised and Expanded, Volumes 1–3

edited by Kenneth E. Avis, Herbert A. Lieberman, and Leon Lachman

VOLUME 1

VOLUME 2

VOLUME 3

1

Pharmaceutical Suspensions

Robert A. Nash

St. John's University, Jamaica, New York

I. INTRODUCTION

Since the publication of *Pharmaceutical Suspension* in 1965–1966 [1], several updated reviews of the subject have appeared in the literature [2–7]. Any useful discussion of the topic must also take into account the importance of suspensions to both food and cosmetic formulations. In addition, much is owed to the paint industry for our current understanding of the formulation and manufacture of physically stable suspensions. At the start, a working definition of the term "suspension" will be provided in connection with the more general term *dispersion*, or *dispersed system*.

A suspension is a particular class or type of dispersion or dispersed system in which the internal or suspended phase is dispersed uniformly with mechanical agitation throughout the external phase, called the suspending medium or vehicle. The internal phase, consisting of a homogeneous or heterogeneous distribution of solid particles having a specific range of sizes, is maintained uniformly in time throughout the suspending vehicle with the aid of a single or a particular combination of suspending agent(s). In addition, unlike a solution, the suspended particles exhibit a minimum degree of solubility in the external phase. When the suspended solids are less than about 1 μm in size, the system is referred to as a *colloidal suspension*. When the particles are greater than about 1 μm in diameter the system is called a *coarse suspension*. The practical upper limit for individual suspendable solid particles in coarse suspensions is approximately 50 to 75 μm [8]. When one or more of the type of solid particles that constitute the internal phase are pharmaceutically useful and/or physiologically active, the system is known as a pharmaceutical suspension.

When the particles of the internal phase are spherical or liquid droplets and are dispersed throughout a liquid external phase, the system is called an emulsion. Even though the particles may be liquid only at elevated temperatures (say 50–80°C) and are semisolid or rigid at room temperature, as long as they appear spherical upon careful microscopic examination they are generally considered to be emulsified rather than suspended. Thus, a clue to the presence of a suspended particle is its lack of sphericity or its definitive lattice structure. The exceptions to this general rule are spherical microspheres (Estapor, Rhône-Poulenc) and related spherical solid microparticles.

The wide range of suspensions, as a particular class or type of dispersion or dispersed system, is classified in Table 1 based on the physical states of matter (i.e., gas, liquid, solid) for both the internal and external phase of dispersed systems.

II. THE PHARMACEUTICAL SUSPENSION

Martin and Bustamente [9] listed three general classes of pharmaceutical suspensions: orally administered suspensions (sometimes referred to as mixtures), externally applied suspensions (topical lotions), and injectable (parenteral) suspensions.

A. Oral Suspensions

The solids content of an oral suspension may vary considerably. For example, antibiotic preparations may contain 125 to 500 mg of active solid material per 5 ml (teaspoonful) dose, while the drop concentrate may provide the same amount of insoluble drug in a 1 or 2 ml dose. Antacids and radiopaque suspensions also typically contain relatively high amounts of suspended material for oral administration. The vehicle may be a syrup, sorbitol solution, or gum-thickened water with added artificial sweeteners, since, in addition to safety of ingredients, taste and mouth feel are important formulating considerations. In cases of limited "shelf life" (i.e., chemical stability of the insoluble drug is limited) the dosage form may be prepared as a dry granulation or powder mixture that is reconstituted with water prior to use. In the case of dry granulations and powders for reconstitution, the inert ingredients are often similar to preconstituted systems. Formulating emphasis, however, is often placed on powder flow without segregation and efficient wettability (water understood) to build rapid suspendability with minimal externally applied agitation.

B. Topical Suspensions

Historically, the externally applied "shake lotion" is the oldest example of a pharmaceutical suspension. Calamine lotion USP, as well as other dermatological preparations, are closely associated with the technical development of the pharmaceutical suspension

Table 1 Classification of Dispersions

Internal phase	External phase	Example
Gas	Gas	Mixture (air)
Gas	Liquid	Foam
Gas	Solid	Adsorbate
Liquid	Gas	Wet spray (fog)
Liquid	Liquid	Emulsion
Liquid	Solid	Absorbate
Solid	Gas	Dry spray (smoke)
Solid	Liquid	Suspension
Solid	Solid	Mixture (powders and granules)

[10–13]. Because safety and toxicity are most readily dealt with in terms of dermatological acceptability, many useful new suspending agents were first introduced in topical formulations [14–16]. In addition, the protective action and cosmetic properties of topical lotions usually require the use of high concentrations of dispersed phase (in excess of 20%). Therefore, topical lotions represent the best example of suspensions that exhibit hindered settling rates [17]. A variety of pharmaceutical vehicles has been used in the preparation of topical lotions. A list of such vehicles would include diluted oil-in-water emulsions bases, diluted water-in-oil emulsion bases, determatological pastes, magmas, and clay suspensions.

C. Parenteral Suspensions

The solids content of parenteral suspensions is usually between 0.5% and 5.0%, with the exception of insoluble forms of penicillin in which concentrations of the antibiotic may exceed 30%. These sterile preparations are designed for intramuscular, intradermal, intralesional, intraarticular, or subcutaneous administration. The viscosity of a parenteral suspension should be low enough to facilitate injection. Syringeability, a factor that is discussed later in this chapter, depends on the preparation of a low-viscosity suspension. Common vehicles for parenteral suspensions include preserved sodium chloride injection or a parenterally acceptable vegetable oil. The primary factor governing the selection of injectable ingredients must include safety. Ophthalmic suspensions that are instilled into the eye must also be prepared in a sterile manner. The vehicles employed arc cssentially isotonic and aqueous in composition. The special techniques required for the preparation of sterile ophthalmic suspensions have been described by Portnoff, Cohen, and Henley [18].

D. Utility of Suspensions

The suspension is often selected as a pharmaceutical dosage form when the drug is insoluble in water and aqueous fluids at the dosage required for administration, and when attempts to solubilize the drug through the use of cosolvents, nonionic surface active agents (surfactants), and other complexing and solubilizing agents would compromise the stability or the safety and, in the case of oral administration, the taste properties of the dosage form. The taste of a bitter or unpleasant drug can often be improved by the selection of an insoluble form of the active drug moiety.

An aqueous suspension is a useful oral dosage form for administering insoluble or poorly soluble drugs. The large surface area of dispersed drug may help ensure a high degree of availability for absorption. Unlike tablets or capsules, the dissolution of drug particles in suspension and subsequent absorption commence upon dilution in gastrointestinal fluids. According to Wagner [19], finely divided particles dissolve at a greater rate and have higher relative solubilities than similar macroparticles. When the particle size is greater than about 10 μm, the rate of dissolution is directly proportional to the surface area. Hence, surface area, not particle size, is a prime factor in controlling dissolution rate. However, when particles below 10 μm are considered, the particle radius, and not the surface area, may become more important. Rheinhold et al. [20] showed that fine particles of suspended sulfadiazine gave more rapid absorption with higher maximum serum levels and greater area under the serum level versus time curve than a similar suspension containing somewhat larger particles of the drug.

The bioavailability of a drug is assumed to increase in the following order: solutions > suspensions > capsules > compressed tablets > coated tablets. However, many other factors beside particle size can affect the rate and extent of drug absorption, and this order of relative bioavailability does not always hold. For example, Hirst and Kaye [21] showed that the same dose of thioridazine given either dissolved in a syrup formulation or prepared as an oral suspension gave significantly lower serum levels of the drug when formulated in solution. Either some ingredient in the syrup inhibited absorption or an ingredient in the suspension facilitated drug uptake.

Mullins and Macek [22] showed that the active amorphous form of novobiocin changes to the inactive crystalline form in aqueous suspension and that such changes in crystalline habit affect the drug's bioavailability.

The parenteral suspension is an ideal dosage form for prolonged therapy. Administration of a drug as an aqueous or oleaginous suspension into subcutaneous or muscular tissue results in the formation of a depot at the injection site. The depot acts as a drug reservoir, slowly releasing drug molecules at a rate related to both the intrinsic aqueous solubility of the drug form and the type of suspending vehicle used, either aqueous or oil for the purpose of maintaining systemic absorption of drug from the injection site. A number of injectable depot suspension products—for example, penicillin G procaine, B_{12}–zinc tannate, medroxyprogesterone acetate, ACTH–zinc tannate, desoxycorticosterone pivalate, triamcinolone acetonide (diacetate or hexacetonide), progesterone, testosterone, and zinc-insulin—are currently available for this purpose. The suspension form of the drug frequently provides more prolonged release from the injection site than a comparable solution of the same drug in a suitable injectable oil. Chien [23] pointed out in his extensive review of the subject that the depot form for parenteral administration often results in reduced drug dose, decreased side effects, and/or improved drug utilization.

The importance of the solubility of drugs to their pharmacological effect following depot injection of parenteral suspensions is illustrated by data presented in Table 2 for five anti-inflammatory coritcosteroids. With respect to the data reported, a significant negative correlation ($r = -0.78$) was found to exist between steroid solubility in water and duration of the anti-inflammatory effect at the tissue site.

Table 2 Relationship Between the Aqueous Solubility of Five Depot Corticosteroids and Their Duration of Effect Following Intrasynovial Injection of Similarly Constituted Suspension Formulations

Corticosteroid	Solubility in water at 25°C ($mg\ mL^{-1}$)	Average duration of Anti-inflammatory effect (days)
Hydrocortisone acetate	0.01	6.0
Methylprednisolone acetate	0.016	8.2
Triamcinolone diacetate	0.0056	10.0
Triamcinolone acetonide	0.004	14.2
Triamcinolone hexacetonide	0.0016	21.2

Source: Data reported by I. L. Hollander, Intrasynovial corticosteroid therapy. In: *Arthritis and Allied Conditions*, 7th ed. Lea & Febiger, Philadelphia, 1966, pp. 381–398.

III. BASIC CONCEPTS OF PHARMACEUTICAL SUSPENSIONS

A. Internal Phase

Insoluble solids, regardless of particle size, that have a relatively low interfacial tension and are readily wetted by water are called *hydrophilic solids*. These include clays (bentonite, kaolin, talc, magnesium aluminum silicate), bismuth salts, barium sulfate, carbonates, hydroxides or oxides of calcium, magnesium, zinc, and aluminum, and titanium dioxide. The hydrophilicity of a powder surface can be judged by performing moisture adsorption study where the solid particles are exposed to various relative humidities. Materials that adsorb moisture below relative humidities of 70% to 80% at room temperature are said to be hydrophilic solids. Fine, insoluble solids that are not easily wetted by water and have a relatively high interfacial tension are referred to as *hydrophobic solids*. These include a large number of relatively low density organic materials and pharmaceutical substances, such as charcoal and sulfur. The hydrophobic nature of the latter group is accentuated by entrapped air adsorbed on the surface of these particles. Materials that are hydrophobic may be wetted by oils and semipolar liquids and thus are called *lipophilic solids*; conversely, hydrophilic materials behave like *lipophobic solids* in oils. A listing of common water-insoluble pharmaceutical hydrophilic and hydrophobic solids is presented in Table 3.

Hydrophilic solids can be suspended easily in water without the aid of a water-dispersible surfactant or wetting agent, and conversely hydrophobic solids can be suspended in oils and nonpolar vehicles with the use of lipid-soluble surfactants.

B. Particle Size Considerations

The mean particle diameter and the particle size distributions of suspended insoluble drugs are important considerations in formulating physically stable pharmaceutical suspensions. Hiestand [8] defined the lower limit of coarse suspensions as particles larger than 0.1 μm. Except for a number of clays, oxides, charcoal, and pigments, the average particle size of drugs and pharmaceutical excipients rarely falls below 1 μm. While most submicrometer inorganic excipients appear to behave like hydrophilic solids, the preponderance of insoluble drugs and pharmaceutical materials are usually soft, organic, essentially crystalline, hydrophobic solids ranging in particle size from several micrometers to several hundred or more.

Drug particle size is an important factor influencing product appearance, settling rates, drug solubility, in vivo absorption, resuspendability, and overall stability of pharmaceutical suspensions.

Insoluble drug particles are seldom uniform spheres or cubes even after size reduction and classification. Goodarznia and Sutherland [24] have shown that small deviations from spherical shape (e.g., grains of sand) and small deviations from size uniformity have only minor effects on the packing density of suspensions of cubes and spheroids. Packing density is defined by them as the weight to volume ratio of the sediment at equilibrium. They also showed that wide distributions in particle size often lead to high density suspensions and that systems with widely differing particle shapes (plates, needles, filaments, and prisms) often produce low density slurries. The authors also reported that the degree of particle aggregation, irrespective of particle shape and size, showed a marked effect on the porosity of suspensions at equilibrium.

Crystal growth over time of unprotected slightly soluble drug solids and changes in their particle size distribution in suspension have been reviewed separately by

Table 3 Classification of Some Insoluble
Pharmaceutical Solids According to Their Wettability

Solids	Crystal density (g cm^{-3})
Hydrophilic	
aluminum oxide	4.0
bentonite	2.2
bismuth subcarbonate	6.9
bismuth subnitrate	4.9
calcium carbonate	2.6
calcium oxide	3.3
calcium phosphate, dibasic	2.3
calcium sulfate, hydrate	2.4
ferric oxide	5.3
kaolin	2.4
magnesium aluminum silicate	2.0
magnesium carbonate	3.0
magnesium oxide	2.8
magnesium oxide, heavy	3.6
silicon dioxide	1.5
talc	2.7
titanium dioxide	4.3
zinc oxide	5.5
Hydrophobic	
aspirin	1.4
benzoic acid	1.3
boric acid, powder	1.4
calcium stearate	1.0
cellulose, microcrystalline	1.5
charcoal	2.2
griseofulvin	1.4
magnesium stearate	0.9
paraffin	0.9
phenobarbital	1.3
prednisolone acetate	1.1
progesterone	1.1
starch	1.4
stearic acid	1.0
sulfadiazine	1.5
sulfathiazole	1.5
sulfur, precipitated	2.0
testosterone	1.1

Frederick [25], Higuchi [26], and Matthews [27]. According to these authors crystal growth is usually attributed to one or more of the following mechanisms:

1. "Ostwalt ripening" is the growth of large particles at the expense of small ones, owing to a difference in solubility rates of different size particles. The effect may be expressed by the following simple relationship:

$$\log\left(\frac{S}{S_o}\right) = \frac{k}{2.303r}$$

where S is the initial solubility rate of small particles, S_o is the solubility rate of large particles at equilibrium, r is particle radius in (cm), and $k = 1.21 \times 10^{-6}$, a constant that includes surface tension, temperature, molar volume, and thermodynamic terms. Thus, the increase in solubility rate of a 0.2 μm particle is 13%; it is 1% for a 2 μm particle and negligible for particles of 20 μm and larger.

2. Crystal growth due to temperature fluctuations on storage is of minor importance, unless suspensions are subjected to temperature cycling of a difference of 20°C or more.

3. Change from one polymorphic form to another more stable crystalline form or changes in crystal habit may be related to the degree of solvation or hydration of the drug. Such changes have been observed to occur during the manufacture and storage of some steroid suspensions [28]. For example, when steroid powders are subjected to dry heat sterilization, subsequent rehydration of the anhydrous steroid in the presence of the aqueous suspending vehicle will result in the formation of large, needlelike crystals. A similar effect may be produced by subjecting finished suspensions to moist heat sterilization in an autoclave.

Higuchi [26] showed that crystal growth may also arise when the more energetic amorphous or glassy forms of a drug exhibit significantly greater initial solubility in water than their corresponding crystalline forms. In addition, size reduction by crushing and grinding can produce particles whose different surfaces exhibit high or low solubility rates, and this effect can be correlated to differences in the free surface energy introduced during comminution. However, crystal growth and changes in particle size distribution can be largely controlled by employing one or more of the following procedures and techniques.

1. Selection of particles with a narrower range of particle sizes, such as the use of microcrystals between 1 and 10 μm.
2. Selection of a more stable crystalline form of the drug, which usually exhibits decreased solubility in water. The most physically stable crystalline form of the drug will usually have the highest melting point.
3. Avoidance, if possible, of the use of high energy milling during particle size reduction. This may be accomplished by forming microcrystals by controlled precipitation techniques.
4. Use of a wetting agent (water-dispersible surfactant) in formulating to dissipate free surface energy of particles by reducing the interfacial tension between the solid and suspending vehicle.
5. Use of a protective colloid, such as gelatin, gums, or cellulosic derivatives, to form a film barrier around the particle, thus inhibiting dissolution and subsequent crystal growth.
6. Increase the viscosity of the vehicle to retard particle dissolution and subsequent crystal growth.
7. Avoidance of temperature extremes during product storage, such as the exposure to freeze-thaw conditioning.

Most drugs vary in particle size and sometimes in particle shape. Both properties can influence the physical stability, appearance, bioavailability, and potency of pharmaceutical suspensions. Haleblian [29] has listed the following factors that may affect crystal habit.

1. As supersaturation is increased, the crystals formed tend to change from prismatic to needlelike shapes. Since needlelike crystals are undesireable for suspension use, the degree of supersaturation during the crystallization procedures should be minimized.
2. Rapid cooling and high agitation result in relatively thin, small crystals. When the drug is slowly crystallized by evaporation, it yields more compact crystals. The rate of cooling is effective in altering crystal habits because of its influence on the degree of supersaturation.
3. The nature of the crystallizing solvent influences differences in crystal size and shape. This is often related to the tendency of a solvating liquid to be absorbed on certain faces of the crystal and thus to inhibit the growth of those particular crystal faces.
4. The presence of cosolutes, cosolvents, and adsorbable foreign substances may result in crystal habit modification and variation in the physical stability of finished suspensions. For example, the presence of adsorbed foreign lipids from crystallizing liquids will influence the aggregation potential of many drug particles.
5. The constancy of conditions (i.e., the replication of the habit of growing crystals) requires that the crystallization be carried out under identical processing conditions. Batch-to-batch variation in crystal size and shape is often associated with the inability to control processing and crystallization procedures.

In addition, preparation of amorphous solids, single-entity polymorphic forms, and solvates is often related to the five basic factors listed previously with respect to simple crystal formation.

Because of batch-to-batch variation in particle size and shape, reduction of particle size has a beneficial effect on the physical stability of pharmaceutical suspensions especially in the range of fine particle suspensions (1–20 μm) [30]. Variations in assay results can often be avoided by preparation of homogeneous, well-mixed, or nonsettling fine particle suspensions. Particle size reduction also produces slow, more uniform settling rates. The bioavailability of drugs is often improved by reducing the size of suspension particles [31]. Finally, drug particles below 20 μm produce less pain and tissue irritation when injected parenterally [32]. Lees [33], however, has reported that the production of fine particles may have a deleterious effect on chemical stability because of the increased dissolution rate of small particles.

C. Particle Size Reduction

According to Smith [34] drug solids are comparatively easy to grind. Reduction to a size range of about 50 to 75 μm usually produces a powder that is in general free flowing. As a rule, most solids tend to exhibit aggregation or agglomeration in the dry state when the individual particles are smaller. Furthermore, below about 10 to 50 μm increased free surface energy—as evidenced by cohesion of small particles—becomes a factor interfering with further size reduction. The powder may become damp, especially if there is a tendency to attract moisture. Material may "ball up," and this will suggest that the particles are agglomerated and larger than their actual individual size. As the pores between powder particles become smaller with decreasing particle size, the increase of surface area may become more accessible to liquid penetration. Aggregates often behave like hydrophobic solids, entrapping air and becoming difficult to wet.

The most efficient method of producing fine particles is by dry milling prior to suspension manufacture. In contrast, dispersion equipment, such as colloid mills and homogenizers are normally used to wet-mill finished suspensions in order to break up poorly wetted fine particle aggregates or agglomerates. Among the several methods of producing small, reasonably uniform drug particles are micropulverization, fluid energy grinding, controlled precipitation, and spray-drying.

Figure 1 illustrates the four basic types of size reduction equipment used in the pharmaceutical industry to produce fine powder particles.

1. *Micropulverization*

Micropulverization is one of the most rapid, convenient, and inexpensive methods of producing fine drug powders. The milling equipment includes hammer mills, micropulverizers, universal mills, end-runner mills, and ball mills. Micropulverizers are high speed attrition or impact mills especially adapted for fine grinding. Some mills are fitted with classifiers to facilitate particle separation by centrifugation. Because ultrafine particles below 10 μm are infrequently produced, buildup of electrostatic charge on the surface of milled powder is encountered only occasionally. The main disadvantage of micropulverization is the large distribution of particle sizes produced, normally in the range of 10 to 50 μm or more. Nevertheless, micropulverized powder is satisfactory for the preparation of most oral and topical suspensions.

The operational ranges for initial feed size and resulting product size of mills are given in Table 4.

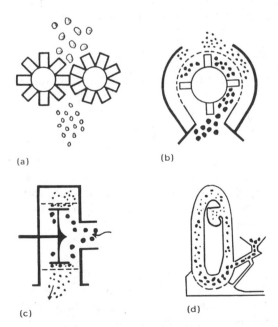

(a)

(b)

(c)

(d)

Fig. 1 The four basic types of size reduction equipment used to produce fine solid particles: (a) crushers and shredders, (b) hammer mills, (c) colloid mills, and (d) fluid energy mills.

Table 4 Size Reduction Equipment for Medium-Hard to Soft
Pharmaceutical Materials

Mills	Size of feed (mm)	Size of product (mm)

Low speed, without classifiers
  roller mill
  end-runner mill
  ball mill
  universal mill
  hammer mill
	1–10	0.1–1

High speed, with classifiers
  hammer mill
  vibratory mill
  stud mill
	1–10	0.01–0.1

Fluid energy	0.1–10	0.001–0.01

2. *Fluid Energy Grinding*

The process of fluid energy grinding, sometimes referred to as jet milling or micronizing, is the most effective method for reducing particles below 10 μm. The ultrafine particles are produced by the shearing action of high velocity streams of compressed air on particles in a confined space. The chief disadvantage of fluid energy grinding is the high electrostatic charge built up on the surfaces of the milled powder, which makes powder classification and collection exceedingly difficult. However, since it is important that a majority of drug particles in parenteral suspensions fall below 10 μm, fluid energy grinding is the most convenient method used for their production.

Table 5 summarizes grinding data determined using a laboratory-size energy mill, at 100 psig air pressure, for 20 drug substances and pharmaceutical excipients. The efficiency of the fluid energy milling process, at a constant air velocity, appears to be related to both the feed rate and the difference between the average initial feed size and the resulting size of the micronized powder produced. The most efficiently milled materials, according to the data reported in Table 5, appear to be caffeine, zinc oxide, aspirin, sugar, aluminum oxide, and sodium chloride. The least efficiently milled materials listed are zinc stearate, carnauba wax, kaolin, calcium sulfate, and benzoic acid. Milling efficiency appears to be related to the hardness of the material and the initial feed size but not to the hydrophilic or hydrophobic character of the material. These data indicate that harder, more brittle, and larger materials are more efficiently milled than smaller, softer, more plastic or waxy substances.

3. *Controlled Crystallization*

A solvent that dissolves a solid very readily at room temperature may serve as a cystallizing medium when mixed with another miscible solvent in which the compound is only sparingly soluble. A solution that is nearly saturated at a temperature about 10°C below the boiling point of the solvent combination is prepared in a temperature range between 60 and 150°C. Separation of microcrystals from such hot concentrated solutions is commonly induced by cooling and stirring. However, when supersaturation is

Table 5 Typical Grinding Data for 20 Pharmaceutical Substances Using a Small Fluid Energy Mill at 100 psig Air Pressure

Substance	Feed rate (g min^{-1})[a]	Mean feed size (µm)	Mean product size (µm)
Caffeine	75.7	840	1.0
Zinc oxide	454.0	75	0.6
Aspirin	60.5	840	1.0
Sugar	151.0	700	2.5
Aluminum oxide	90.8	175	0.7
Sodium chloride	75.7	840	2.9
Niacinamide	30.3	840	2.0
Magnesium oxide	15.1	180	0.3
Calcium phosphate	37.8	840	5.0
Potassium chloride	75.7	840	12.4
Sorbic acid	151.0	250	7.5
Phenacetin	60.5	75	1.0
Zinc stearate	75.7	150	2.5
Carnauba wax	22.7	840	5.0
Terramycin[b]	15.1	350	2.0
Kaolin	30.3	10	0.7
Penicillin[b]	15.1	75	3.7
Procaine penicillin[b]	22.7	10	2.0
Barium sulfate	15.1	3	0.5
Benzoic acid	15.1	10	3.3

[a]Feed rate depends on mill size.
[b]Air jet milling was conducted at reduced air pressure to minimize degradation.
Source: Frost Air Mill Department, Plastomer Corp., Newton, PA.

obtained by agitation and shock cooling of the hot solution and through the rapid introduction of another cold miscible solvent in which the drug is only sparingly soluble, formation of minute crystalline particles (nucleates) proceeds without appreciable crystal growth and uniform microcrystals of the drug are thus obtained. Microcrystals can also be conveniently produced by bubbling liquid nitrogen through saturated solution of a solute prior to solvent freezing.

In addition, ultrasonic insonation techniques have also been used during shock cooling procedures to promote the formation of steroid microcrystals [35]. Shock cooling methods used in the production of crystals offer a possible solution to the electrostatic charge problems associated with ultra-fine dry particle milling.

4. *Spray Drying*

Particles of microcrystalline size can also be obtained by the use of spray drying procedures. The process reviewed by Riegelman et al. [36] produces a porous, free-flowing, easily wetted, essentially monodispersed powder. Control of process variables results in the production of spherical particles that may be coated with wetting and suspending agents to aid suspension or promote stability. However, the process is not normally considered for the preparation of ultrafine powders for suspension purposes because of the expense involved in operating the process for small-scale manufacture.

IV. STABILIZATION OF SUSPENSIONS

A. Chemical Stability

Waltersson and Lundgren [37] pointed out that the potency a chemical stability of a drug in suspension is controlled by the fact that the rate of degradation is related to the concentration of drug in solution, rather than to the total concentration of drug in the product. Generally a suspended drug decomposes only in solution as the solid phase gradually dissolves; thus, a solution concentration equal to the solubility of the drug is maintained. Drug degradation in a suspension usually follows zero-order kinetics with the rate constant being dependent on the equilibrium solubility of the drug. Decreasing the solubility of the drug in the suspending vehicle decreases the rate of degradation of the suspended drug. Improved potency stability may be accomplished either by selecting a pH value or range where the drug is least soluble or by replacing the drug with a more vehicle-insoluble derivative or salt. Examples of drug suspensions that follow such a zero-order rate of decomposition are procaine penicillin, ampicillin, chloramphenicol, hydrocortisone, and aspirin. In the case of tetracycline suspensions, the kinetics of the reaction is complicated by the fact that the inactive steric isomer formed in solution is less soluble than the decomposing tetracycline; thus, the parent tetracycline degrades by non-zero-order kinetics [38]. Decomposition may also be described by a diffusion-controlled process or by catalysis initiated by environmental factors, such as oxygen, light, and trace metals.

B. Physical Stability

As a rule, the problem of stability of suspensions is complicated by the fact that the physical stability of pharmaceutical suspensions and the factors affecting such stability are equal to or more important than chemical stability. This is based on the fact that since a suspension exists in more than one state (liquid and solid), there are more different ways in which the system can undergo either chemical or physical change. Higuchi [26] and Weiner [39] have each, in separate discussions, touched on some of the difficulties inherent in predicting the stability of suspension formulations from a physical and chemical viewpoint.

C. Physical Factors

Some of the more obvious difficulties involved in making stability predictions are based on the fact that simple hydrostatic relationships (Stokes' law, etc.) used to define settling rates assume a spherical, deflocculated, free-falling particle, which is uncomplicated by particle-particle or particle-vehicle interactions. Most pharmaceutical suspensions do not conform to such simple assumptions. Suspensions that exhibit non-Newtonian flow are also difficult to define in terms of the basic expressions. In addition, suspensions that are described in terms of a single representative particle do not reflect the influence of the entire particle size distribution. A number of modifications of the basic equations have been reported that take some of these factors into account [8].

D. Chemical Factors

Chemical stability predictions are sometimes complicated by the difficulty of determining the pH of suspensions, which often change the liquid junction potential of the measuring electrode. Part of this results from "pH drift" associated with surface coating of electrodes, and partly from the disparity in pH value between bulk suspension and supernatant vehicle. If two glass electrodes are used, one in the supernate and one in the sediment, each electrode will show the same pH value in both portions of the suspension.

In addition, slow attainment of saturation often complicates steady state treatment of rate data. Finally, accelerated, elevated temperature stability testing will often have a pronounced and adverse effect on suspension viscosity, particle solubility, and size distribution.

E. Stable Colloidal Suspensions

The empirical method of producing pharmaceutical suspensions is based on an attempt to prepare a colloidally stable dispersion of a drug in a potentially suitable suspension vehicle. In the past, a series of suspensions was often prepared using different concentrations of suspending agents to identify the formulation that would produce the most homogeneous-looking and stable suspension. The finished preparation at that time was usually passed through a homogenizer or colloid mill to improve the dispersion. A list of commonly used suspending agents for this purpose is presented in Table 6, and some of these agents are also listed in a paper by Gerding and Sperandio [40].

Oral suspensions of sulfa drugs, which were frequently used in the 1940s and 1950s were formulated as dispersions with one or more of the suspending agents listed in Table 6. Smooth-looking viscous suspensions were produced but, upon standing on the shelf, the drug particles settled slowly, forming a tightly packed sediment that was almost impossible to resuspend even with vigorous shaking. Primary particles or small aggregates, reaching the bottom of the container during sedimentation, slipped past each other and produced compact, solid layers. The interparticle interaction in such compact sediments is relatively high because the interparticle distances are small and because the weak van der Waals forces of attraction, which decrease exponentially with distance, are appreciable. Such conditions frequently lead to the undesirable phenomenon of "caking or claying," which requires extensive agitation for resuspension [41]. The particles in these preparations were not completely dispersed, nor were they in the size range normally associated with colloids.

The physical instability of these early sulfa suspensions led many companies in the pharmaceutical industry to resort to other methods of producing physically stable pharmaceutical suspensions. In such method, the density of the vehicle was made to equal or approach the density of the suspended drug particles. If the drug particles are small enough and the vehicle sufficiently viscous, the particles will remain suspended indefinitely according to Stokes' law [42]. Because the crystal density of most organic drug particles lies between 1.1 and 1.5 g cm^{-3}, the only liquid vehicles for oral use with densities at 25°C high enough to be considered are sorbitol solution USP (1.29 g cm^{-3}), syrup USP (1.31 g cm^{-3}), and high fructose corn syrup (1.41 g cm^{-3}). In practice, however, it is extremely difficult to prepare oral suspensions by the matched density technique alone, since dilution with water and other liquids will decrease vehicle density appreciably. Nevertheless, the use of high density liquids as suspending vehicles will often have a beneficial effect on physical stability.

Table 6 Pharmaceutically Useful Suspending Agents

Suspending agent	pH range for maximum stability	Common incompatibilities
Gums		
acacia	3–9	Insoluble in alcohol over 10%
agar	4–10	Calcium and aluminum ions, borax, and alcohol over 10%
carrageenan	4–10	Calcium and magnesium ions and alcohol over 10%
guar	3–9	Calcium and aluminum ions, borax, alcohol, and glycerin over 10%
karaya	3–7	Insoluble in alcohol over 10%
locust bean	3–9	Borax, insoluble in alcohol and glycerin over 10%
pectin	2–9	Zinc oxide and alcohol over 10%
propylene glycol alginate	3–7	Calcium and magnesium ions and alcohol over 10%
sodium alginate	4–10	Calcium ions and alcohol over 10%
tragacanth	3–9	Bismuth salts and alcohol over 40%
xanthan	4–10	Borax and cationic surfactants
Cellulosics		
carboxymethyl methyl-cellulose, sodium	3–10	Tannins, cationic surfactants, and concentrated salt solutions
microcrystalline cellulose and carboxymethyl-cellulose, sodium	3–10	Tannins, cationic surfactants, and concentrated salt solutions
hydroxyethylcellulose	2–10	Insoluble in alcohol over 10%
hydroxypropylcellulose	2–10	—
hydroxypropylmethyl-cellulose	2–10	—
Clays		
bentonite (colloidal aluminum silicate)	3–10	Calcium ions and polyvalent cations—increase viscosity
colloidal magnesium aluminum silicate (hectorite)	3–10	Calcium ions—increase viscosity
colloidal magnesium aluminum silicate (attapulgite)	3–10	Calcium ions—increase viscosity
magnesium silicate (sepiolite)	3–10	Calcium ions—increase viscosity
Miscellaneous		
carbomer	6–10	Acids
gelatin (Pharmagels A and B)	5–8	Acids, bases, and aldehydes
polyethylene glycols (3350, 8000)	3–10	Phenols
lecithin	5–8	Insoluble in water
povidone (K30)	3–10	Oils and lecithin

The settling velocities for various average size, nonflocculated particles were determined in the range of 0.2 to 200 µm at density differences between the solid particles and the suspending liquid of 0.2 and 2.0 g cm^{-3}, respectively, when the absolute viscosity of the suspending liquid varied between 1 and 1000 centipoise (cP). Terminal settling rates were calculated by a method described by Carpenter [43] for two concentrations of suspended solids, namely, less than 2% and 20% v/v, respectively.

According to the data presented in Table 7, permanent-type suspensions, which exhibit a settling velocity of less than 0.14 cm per year at 25°C, can be obtained when the suspending liquid approaches a viscosity of 1000 cP and the average particle size of the suspended solid is 0.2 μm or less.

Colloidally stable dispersions are systems in which particles are completely deflocculated or peptized. As a rule, since the distribution of particles sizes is generally greater than 1 μm, deflocculated or peptized systems will settle very slowly in stages, with larger particles settling more rapidly than smaller ones. Ultimately when they do settle, they form a tight, dense sediment that is difficlut to resuspend. When viewed under a microscope, the dispersed suspension consists of individual particles, each in random (Brownian) motion, showing no apparent association among particles. An excellent example of a colloidally dispersed system is a stable, well-formulated oil-in-water emulsion. In this system the oil globules, which are usually smaller than 1 μm, are well distributed, and little or no association (creaming or coalescence) is observed.

There are three general methods of producing colloidally stable dispersions:

1. *Mutual repulsion due to a large zeta potential.* This is best achieved by the adsorption of an ionic electrolyte (KCl) or polyelectrolyte dispersant (sodium hexametaphosphate) on the suspended particles to create a strong mutual repulsion between the microsize particles. For example, moderate physical stability is achieved when the zeta potential is between ±30 and ±60 mV and good to excellent physical stability is achieved when the zeta potential is between ±60 and ±100 mV. As the size and density of the suspended particles increase beyond 1 μm and densities greater than 1.0 g cm^{-3}, the effect of zeta potential becomes less important. Zeta potential is discussed later in this chapter, and in other chapters of this text and is illustrated in Fig. 2 of this chapter.

2. *Adsorption of a smaller hydrophilic or lyophilic (solvent or vehicle loving) colloid on larger suspended particles.* When a strongly hydrated hydrophilic protective colloid, such as gelatin, is adsorbed on the surface of the suspended particles, the affinity for water exceeds the mutual attraction of adjacent particles for each other. Essentially the protective colloid and hydrogen-bonded water molecules form a protective hydration layer around each suspended particle.

3. *Steric hindrance due to adsorption of an oriented nonionic surfactant or polyelectrolyte.* Adsorption of a nonionic polymer (gum or cellulosic) or surfactant (polysorbate 80) of sufficient chain length creates steric hindrance and prevents adjacent suspended particles from coming close enough to join. This method is widely employed in emulsification. Steric stabilzation has one major advantage over electrostatic stabilization in that it is relatively insensitive to the presence of added electrolyte.

The best approach to producing a colloidally stable, dispersed system is to determine the region of maximum dispersion by use of instruments capable of measuring the zeta potential of the suspended particles. When fine hydrophobic drug particles are suspended in aqueous solution, adsorption of ions from solution takes place, imparting a surface charge to the particle. If the molecules making up the structure of the particle contain ionizable groups, adsorption of ions from solution may take place to a lesser or greater degree, depending on the number of such ionizable groups on the surface of the particle and the pH value of the surrounding liquid. The charge in either case is referred to as being fixed to the surface of the particle. Because the surface charge of most drug

Table 7 Terminal Settling Rates (cm sec^{-1}) at 25°C of Nonflocculated Suspended Particles

Average particle diameter (μm)	Absolute viscosity (cP)	Density difference Δρ = 0.2 g cm^{-3}		Density difference Δρ = 2.0 g cm^{-3}	
		Solids content < 2%	Solids content = 20% v/v	Solids content < 2%	Solids content = 20% v/v
0.2	1	4.36E-7[a]	1.54E-7	4.36E-6	1.54E-6
	10	4.36E-8	1.54E-8	4.36E-7	1.54E-7
	100	4.36E-9	1.54E-9	4.36E-8	1.54E-8
	1000	4.36E-10[b]	1.54E-10[b]	4.36E-9	1.54E-9
2	1	4.36E-5	1.54E-5	4.36E-4	1.54E-4
	10	4.36E-6	1.54E-6	4.36E-5	1.54E-5
	100	4.36E-7	1.54E-7	4.36E-6	1.54E-6
	1000	4.36E-8	1.54E-8	4.36E-7	1.54E-7
20	1	2.83E-3	1.22E-3	1.46E-2	7.08E-3
	10	2.83E-4	1.22E-4	1.46E-3	7.08E-4
	100	2.83E-5	1.22E-5	1.46E-4	7.08E-5
	1000	2.83E-6	1.22E-6	1.46E-5	7.08E-6
200	1	3.45E-2	1.99E-2	1.09E-1	6.48E-2
	10	3.45E-3	1.99E-3	1.09E-2	6.48E-3
	100	3.45E-4	1.99E-4	1.09E-3	6.48E-4
	1000	3.54E-5	1.99E-5	1.09E-4	6.48E-5

[a]4.36E-7 = 4.36 × 10^{-7}.
[b]Essentially a permanent suspension (settling rate < 0.19 cm per year at 25°C).

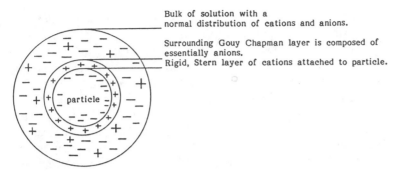

Bulk of solution with a
normal distribution of cations and anions.

Surrounding Gouy Chapman layer is composed of
essentially anions.
Rigid, Stern layer of cations attached to particle.

Fig. 2 Zeta potential represents the potential gradient across the diffuse Helmholtz double layer surrounding the particle, that is, the Stern layer plus the Gouy-Chapman layer.

particles in suspension is negative, the particle will attract from solution a layer of oppositely charged, positive ions, which are held more loosely than the primary adsorbed ions. These oppositely charge ions form the so-called Stern layer (see Fig. 2). The remaining counterions, which are farther away but still within the immediate vicinity of the particle, form the so-called diffuse or outer portion of the double layer, which is referred to as the Gouy-Chapman layer. This condition of a fixed surface charge surrounded by more loosely held counter ions is known as the electrical or Helmholtz double layer (see Fig. 2).

Drugs may bond with water, as is the case with hydrophilic particles. If more water molecules are bound to the surface of the particle, less ion adsorption will take place. In this case, the composition of adsorbed ions and water molecules surrounding the particle may be referred to as the *hydration layer*. The zeta potential, which may be calculated from microelectrophoretic mobility measurement of the charged particles in an electrical field, represents the difference between the total intrinsic charge of the particle or its Nernst potential and the charges neutralized by the Stern layer. In other words, the zeta potential represents the net effective charge on the surface of the particle or the potential across the diffuse layer of counterions surrounding the particle. A theoretical diagram of the zeta potential of an idealized particle is presented in Fig. 2.

When a liquid containing such charged particles is placed in an electrical field, the negatively charged particles are attracted to the anode (+) and the counterions to the cathode (–). The attraction increases with the charge on the particle. Friction between particle and surrounding liquid containing the diffuse double layer tends to slow the resulting motion toward the electrode. The more the double layer is extended, the smaller are the zeta potential and the frictional resistance created by the moving particle. The velocity of the particle in a given electrical field increases with the zeta potential of the particle. The larger the zeta potential the greater is the charge density and the greater is the force of mutual repulsion that keeps particles apart. If these particles are driven together by thermal agitation or mechanically induced motion from high shear agitators, they will again separate rather than flocculate in spite of the van der Waals short-range forces of mutual attraction between the particles.

The addition of a dispersing agent to a suspension, which increases the charge density of the electrical layer surrounding the suspended particles, is primarily related to the physical adsorption process [43]. Particles that achieve a maximum zeta potential reach a point of maximum stability with respect to dispersion, thermodynamically speaking [44]. If in addition the viscosity of the vehicle can be increased sufficiently to aid suspension without altering the zeta potential that has been established for the system, a physically stable suspension of the drug is possible. The particle size, however, should be about 1 μm or less, and the density of the vehicle and the particle should be approximately equal in order to produce systems in which the suspended particles are in a state of so-called permanent suspension. As has been noted, these two conditions are difficult to achieve for many insoluble drugs. Many pharmaceutical suspensions are not capable of achieving a state of complete electrostatic repulsion and thus the method of producing a colloidally stable suspension has been thought to be unworkable by many investigators [8, 44–46]. The application of zeta potential in accordance with Derjaguin, Landau, Verwey, and Overbeek's theory, which governs the preparation of colloidally stable suspensions, has been extensively reviewed by Schneider et al. [42].

F. Flocculated Suspensions

Haines and Martin [44], Hiestand [46], and Ecanow and coworkers [47–51] are generally credited with establishing the "structured particle" concept or flocculated pharmaceutical suspension. The following definitions should prove useful in avoiding confusion among three closely related terms: flocculation, agglomeration, and coagulation. *Flocculation* refers to the formation of a loose aggregation of discrete particles held together in a networklike structure either by physical adsorption of macromolecules, bridging during chemical interaction (precipitation), or when the longer range van der Waals forces of attraction exceed the shorter range forces of repulsion. The floccule referred to as a "stable floc" usually contains varying amounts of entrapped liquid medium or vehicle within the networklike structure.

In *agglomeration*, a large number or mass of particles are closely bound together as aggregates either in a dry (air) or liquid state. *Coagulation* or severe overflocculation refers to the massing of particles in a liquid state alone and sometimes in the form of a fluid gel structure.

According to Ecanow [46], the aggregated particles of overflocculated systems including adsorbed surface films are in surface contact with each other and each mass or *coagula* acts as a unit. The particles of such coagulated systems are held together by strong film-film bonds. Coagulated suspensions, like colloid dispersion and unlike flocculated suspension, tend to "cake" on standing.

Soon after milling and suspension, unless steps are taken to prevent it, micrometer-size particles tend to grow with time. Since the solubility rate of unprotected, nucleated particles relates to Ostwald ripening (see previous discussion in this chapter) and is greater than that of the large crystals, dissolution of smaller particles creates a temporary or metastable state of saturation, which causes eventual growth from solution onto the proper crystal edge of the large particles until a new, more thermodynamically stable distribution of particle sizes is achieved. This phenomenon tends to promote "caking or cementing" together of particles.

The creation of a protective coat or boundary layer with a hydrophilic colloid about such particles offers the best protection to crystal growth. Since protective barriers may or may not flocculate the substrate particles, the sign (positive or negative) and the charge potential on the particle surface will govern the choice between flocculation or dispersion. The processes involved in the formation of suspensions are depicted in Fig. 3.

According to Fig. 3, the flocculated stable state (C) may be reached either directly by wetting and dispersing hydrophobic particles (A) with a suitable flocculating surfac-

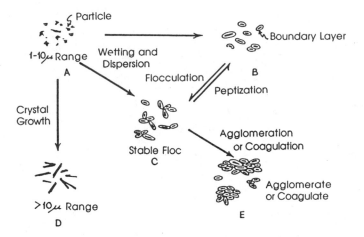

Fig. 3 Processes involved in the formation of suspended particles.

tant, or indirectly by first wetting and dispersing to produce a dispersed or peptized particle (B) with a suitable surfactant and then flocculating with a suitable agent such as a hydrophilic colloid or polyelectrolyte.

In contrast to peptized or deflocculated particles, flocculated suspensions (C), which are considered pharmaceutically stable—although colloidally unstable—can always be resuspended with gentle agitation, while severe overflocculation caused by the addition of too much flocculating agent or by prolonged exposure to extreme thermal conditions (freezing-thawing cycles or storage at elevated temperatures will tend to produce agglomerated or coagulated systems (E). Such suspensions, which are both pharmaceutically and colloidally unstable, are irreversible. The term "plaque" (platelike) is used to describe essentially flat agglomerates, while "coagula" (clumplike) is reserved for thicker, more three-dimensional particle masses. Finally, in the absence of a protective colloid, the process of crystal growth is illustrated in Fig. 3 by the arrow connecting A to D.

Good pharmaceutical suspensions, according to Martin and Bustamente [9] and Hiestand [46] are best achieved through the formation of a stable floc, which resists the tendency toward either deflocculation or agglomeration. Michaels and Bolger [52], in an excellent review of the topic, preferred to use the term "partially flocculated" to describe this state. Stable flocs consist of rigid particles of suspended material, which tend to cluster together in weak aggregates with a minimum of contact points. The greater the number of particle-to-particle contact points in the cluster, the greater is the degree of flocculation.

The chief advantages of the stable floc are as follows:

1. The aggregates tend to break up easily under the application of small amounts of shear stress, such as gentle agitation of a bottle or vial, or by the flow through a small orifice (hypodermic needle and/or syringe), and reform an extended network of particles after the force is removed. Flocculation, therefore, imparts a structure to the suspension with virtually no increase in viscosity.
2. In contrast to peptized or deflocculated systems, the stable floc will settle rapidly, usually to a high sediment volume, and may be easily resuspended even after standing for prolonged periods of storage (see Fig. 4).

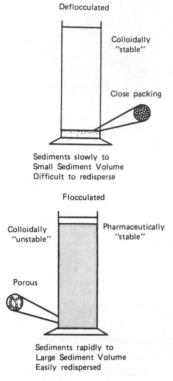

Fig. 4   Characteristics of flocculated and deflocculated suspensions. (From Ref. 8.)

State	Rate of settling	Sediment volume	Nature
Flocculated	Fast	High	Porous, easy to redisperse
Deflocculated	Slow	Low	Compact, difficult to redisperse

3.   The stable floc can be produced if required by employing aseptic techniques using vehicle components that are safe for intramuscular injection.

There are several methods of producing flocculated pharmaceutical suspensions. The
choice of method depends on the properties of the drug and the class of suspension
desired.

The following example illustrates how suspensions may be prepared by controlled
flocculation procedures:

1.   The wetting agent, polysorbate 80 (nor more than 0.1–0.2% w/v of the final
concentration), is dissolved thoroughly in approximately half the final volume of aqueous vehicle. An anionic surfactant, such as docusate sodium USP, may also be used as
a wetting agent. The latter, however, is more sensitive to pH and electrolyte concentration. In the case of hydrophilic solids, a wetting agent is usually not required.

2.   Ultrafine particles of the drug at the desired final concentration are uniformly and carefully spread over the surface of the vehicle and the drug is permitted to wet undisturbed for as much as 16 hr (overnight).

3.   The wetted slurry is passed through a very fine wire mesh screen (120 mesh size or larger) to remove poorly wetted powder. Alternately, a single pass through a colloid mill can be used to achieve the same result.

4.   The slurry concentrate of the drug is agitated gently using an impeller-type mixer.

5.   Small amounts of a 10% w/v solution of aluminum chloride hexahydrate are then added dropwise to the drug slurry from a buret or dropping pipette until the flocculation end point is reached (zero zeta potential). To judge the end point, small samples of the slurry are withdrawn individually and transferred to a graduated cylinder, an equal amount of vehicle is added to each, and the cylinders are gently shaken, then permitted to stand undisturbed. The sample with the highest ratio of sediment to total suspension volume exhibiting a clear supernate and good drainage characteristics is considered to be at the appropriate end point. Usually not more than about 0.1% to 0.2% aluminum chloride hexahydrate should be required to achieve the flocculation end point. Alternately, a 10% solution of calcium chloride dihydrate may be used as the flocculating agent. In this case, as much as 1% to 2% of the calcium salt may be required to achieve "stable floc" formation. If the drug fails to flocculate in the presence of either polyvalent aluminum or calcium ion, the water-insoluble drug particles are considered to be positively charged and the procedure is repeated, this time using a polyvalent anionic flocculating agent, such as 10% w/v sodium hexametaphosphate or 10% trisodium citrate.

6.   After the flocculation end point has been established and verified, the rest of the suspension components (preservative, colorant, flavor, buffer, etc.) dissolved in the liquid vehicle are added, and the slurry is brought to final volume with liquid vehicle.

Another popular method of preparing an oral suspension consists of suspending the drug in a solution of a hydrophilic colloid (gelatin or gum) or a dilute magma of bentonite, attapulgite, or colloidal magnesium aluminum silicate. The concentration of flocculating agent usually required to flocculate *most* drugs suspended in water, or sorbitol or syrup solution, is between 0.1% and 1%. If some degree of overflocculation is produced, it may be reversed by the careful addition of small amounts of suitable surfactant or polyvalent deflocculating agent [54]. Since clays cannot be used in injectable products, two other practical methods of producing flocculated suspensions will be mentioned.

One method, especially useful for the preparation of physically stable "noncaking" suspensions, consists of titrating concentrated aqueous solutions of soluble salt forms of either acidic or basic drugs with a corresponding solution of either a strong acid or a strong base, to precipitate the water insoluble free acid or base at the pH of minimum solubility of the precipitated drug. In this procedure the concentrations of reacting solutions and the order of addition may be varied to produce an acceptable stable floc. If required, the electrolyte thus formed during precipitation may then be reduced through slurry decantation or filtration to adjust tonicity and/or maintain physical and chemical stability. Such procedures can also be carried out using aseptic processing techniques.

Finally, stable floc formation may be produced by dispersing insoluble particles in a turbid or hazy vehicle consisting of finely dispersed or emulsified semipolar, liquid droplets, which will cause the droplets to be adsorbed on the surface of the insoluble drug particles and result in stable floc formation [52]. Turbid aqueous vehicles have been prepared through the interaction of polysorbates and preservatives, such as benzyl alcohol or methyl and propyl parabens. The concentration of surfactant and preservative required for hazy formation may be reduced by the addition of small amounts of sorbitol. Occasionally, this technique will fail to produce physically stable suspensions, as in cases involving nonpolar, water-insoluble polypeptides, such as cyclosporins.

G. Structured Vehicle

The final approach to the preparation of a stable suspension is based on the concept of the "structured vehicle," in which the viscosity of the preparation, under static conditions of very low shear on storage, approaches infinity. The vehicle is said to behave like a "false body," which is able to maintain the suspended particle in a state of more or less permanent suspension.

Structured vehicles are not normally considered for the preparation of parenteral suspensions: because of their high viscosity, such systems lack sufficient syringeability for ease of use.

1. *Bingham-Type Plastic Flow*

Vehicles that exhibit the unusual property of Bingham-type plastic rheological flow are distinguished by the need to overcome a finite yield stress before flow is initiated. Calculations made by Meyer and Cohen [55] and by Chong [56] indicate that permanent suspension of most pharmaceutical systems requires yield-stress values of at least 20 to 50 dynes cm^{-2}. Meyer and Cohen also showed that Bingham plastic flow is rarely produced by solutions of most pharmaceutical gums and hydrophillic colloids. Moreover, in their investigation of such systems, only the use of carbomer NF as a suspending agent (see Table 6) was found to exhibit a sufficient yield value at low solution concentration and low viscosity to produce permanent suspension. Carbomer, however, requires a pH value between 6 and 10 for maximum suspension performance. The polymer is also incompatible with cationic resins, certain polyvalent ions, and high concentrations of electrolytes.

2. *Thixotropic Flow*

Another rheological property that develops yield stress on standing is thixotropy. Thixotropic flow is defined as a reversible, time-dependent, isothermal gel-sol transition. Thixotropic systems exhibit easy flow at relatively high shear rates, but when the shear stress is removed the system is slowly reformed into a structured vehicle. The usual property of thixotropy results from the breakdown and buildup of floccules under stress. A small amount of particle settling will take place until the system develops a sufficient yield value. Procaine penicillin G parenteral suspensions in concentrations above 40% exhibit thixotropic flow. However, most examples of thixotropic suspensions have been prepared for oral or topical use with bentonite [57], colloidal magnesium aluminum silicate [58], trihydroxystearin, and calcium and magnesium ion–tragacanth combinations [59]. The primary advantage of thixotropy is pourability, high viscosity, and a sufficient yield stress. Formulas 1 and 2 represent examples of suspensions prepared with thixotropic clays.*

---

*In these and other formulas "qs" (quantum suffict) means "as much as is needed"; where necessary to indicate "to make to," the word "ad" is used.

Formula 1 Colloidal Magnesium Aluminum Silicate Premix (5% fully hydrated magma)

Colloidal magnesium aluminum silicate	5.0% w/v
Methyl paraben	0.12% w/v
Propyl paraben	0.03% w/v
Purified Water, qs ad	100%

Procedure

1. The parabens are dissolved in approximately 60% of the purified water at 90°C.
2. The colloidal magnesium aluminum silicate is slowly added to step 1 and maintained at 90°C for one hour with gentle agitation.
3. The premix is cooled to 40°C and passed through a colloid mill or homogenizer (2500 psi) rinsing through with fresh purified water.
4. The premix is brought to final volume with purified water and agitation.
5. The premix may be stored in suitable containers at room temperature for several months or more.

Formula 2 Sulfa Drug Oral Suspension

Sulfa drug, microcrystals	5.13 % w/v
Colloidal magnesium aluminum silicate premix (5%; formula 1)	20.0% w/v
Poloxamer 331	0.05% w/v
Glycerin	10.0% w/v
Potassium sorbate	0.2% w/v
Sodium benzoate	0.1% w/v
Colorant	qs
Flavor	qs
Liquid sugar (SpG = 1.33)	65.0% w/v
Citric acid or sodium hydroxide to pH 5.5	qs
Purified water, qs ad	100%

Procedure

1. Dissolve potassium sorbate, sodium benzoate, colorant in aqueous glycerin.
2. Add liquid sugar, colloidal magnesium aluminum silicate premix, and half the poloxamer 331 to step 1 with agitation.
3. Disperse the rest of the poloxamer 331 and sulfa drug in step 2 with agitation.
4. Add flavor to step 3 and pass the suspension through a colloid mill or homogenizer rinsing through with purified water.
5. Adjust pH to 5.5 with either citric acid or sodium hydroxide solution.
6. Add purified water to final volume.

3. *Pseudoplastic–Clay*

Another interesting approach to the preparation of a suspension with a structured vehicle was reported by Samyn [60]. The system consists of a pseudoplastic (sodium carboxymethylcellulose) in combination with a clay (hydrated colloidal magnesium aluminum silicate). To select desirable flow and suspension characteristics, concentrations of each agent are evaluated in combination with the drug to be suspended. The combination recommended by Samyn appears to possess some thixotropic flow characteristics, probably related to the flocculating properties of the clay and the viscosity of the pseudoplastic. A chief disadvantage of such a system is that suspension depends on complete compatibility among clay, polymer, and drug to maintain physical stability. This is sometimes difficult to achieve with combinations of agents. Replacement with other pseudoplastics, such as hydroxyethylcellulose, may be required to overcome possible incompatibilities with sodium carboxymethylcellulose. Formulas 3 and 4 represent examples of suspensions with a pseudoplastic and a clay.

4. *Emulsion Base*

A final system worth mentioning is the use of an emulsion base or a waxy-type emulsifier to develop structure or "false body" in suspension. The use of an emulsion system is not often considered for this purpose, because of the complexities involved in mixing emulsion and suspension systems. The concept of a "three-dimensional creamed or flocculated" emulsion to build structure, was first advanced by Riegelman [61]. For this purpose, the use of fatty glycerol esters, polyethylene glycol fatty esters, and emulsifying wax, NF, should prove extremely valuable in the preparation of smooth-looking, nonsettling suspensions. The drug particles are dispersed in the primary emulsion prior to dilution with other vehicle components. In addition, emulsifiers that exhibit plastic or thixotropic flow characteristics could be added to aid suspension. Formula 5 represents an example of suspension prepared with an emulsifying agent. Formula 6 represents an example of a suspension prepared with a combination of an emulsifier and thixotropic agent.

Formula 3   Kaolin-Pectin Oral Suspension

Kaolin	17.5% w/v
Pectin	0.5% w/v
Colloidal magnesium aluminum silicate premix (5%, formula 1)	17.5% w/v
Carboxymethylcellulose, sodium	0.2% w/v
Glycerin	2.0% w/v
Saccharin, sodium	0.1% w/v
Flavor	qs
Preservative	qs
Purified water, qs ad	100%

Procedure

1. Slurry pectin and carboxymethylcellulose, sodium (medium viscosity grade), in glycerin and dissolve in sufficient purified water with high shear agitation.
2. Add colloidal magnesium aluminum silicate premix to step 1 with agitation.
3. Disperse kaolin in step 2 with agitation.
4. Dissolve saccharin, sodium, and preservative in sufficient purified water and add to step 3.
5. Add flavor and pass suspension through a colloid mill or homogenizer, rinsing through with purified water.
6. Bring the suspension to final volume with purified water.

Formula 4   Antacid Oral Suspension

Aluminum hydroxide–magnesium trisilicate Co-dried gel	7.0% w/v
Magnesium hydroxide	3.0% w/v
Simethicone 30% emulsion	1.75% w/v
Colloidal magnesium aluminum silicate (5%, formula 1)	10.0% w/v
Xanthan gum	0.2% w/v
Saccharin, sodium	qs
Flavor	qs
Preservative blend	qs
Sorbitol solution (70% w/w)	20.0% w/v
Purified water, qs ad	100%

Procedure

1. Dissolve preservative blend and saccharin, sodium in sufficient purified water.
2. Dissolve xanthan gum in sufficient purified water with high shear agitation and add to step 1.
3. Add colloidal magnesium aluminum silicate premix to step 2 with agitation.
4. Mix separately aluminum hydroxide–magnesium trisilicate Co-dried gel, magnesium hydroxide, and simethicone in sorbitol solution until uniformly dispersed and added to step 3 with agitation.
5. Add flavor and pass suspension through a colloidal mill or homogenizer, rinsing through with purified water.
6. Bring suspension to final volume with purified water.

Formula 5   Calamine Topical Suspension

Calamine	3.0% w/v
Zinc oxide	1.0% w/v
Camphor	0.1% w/v
Menthol	0.1% w/v
Squalane	1.5% w/v
Glycerin	2.0% w/v
Emulsifying wax NF[a]	2.0% w/v
Colorant (iron oxide)	qs
Fragrance	qs
Preservative	qs
Purified water, qs ad	100%

[a]Combination of cetostearyl alcohols and ceteareth emulsifiers.

Procedure

1. Dissolve squalane in fused emulsifying wax NF and add sufficient purified water to form a thin, but stable oil-in-water emulsion.
2. Dissolve separately camphor and menthol in glycerin and add to step 1 with agitation.

3. Dissolve preservative in sufficient purified water and slowly add to step 1 with agitation.
4. Mix calamine, zinc oxide, and colorant together and suspend in step 1 with agitation.
5. Add fragrance and pass suspension through a colloid mill or homogenizer rinsing through with purified water.
6. Bring suspension to final volume with purified water.

Formula 6   Barium Sulfate Oral Suspension

Barium sulfate, microcrystals	35.0% w/v
Docusate, sodium	0.16% w/v
Colloidal microcrystalline cellulose	1.5% w/v
Emulsifying wax NF	2.0% w/v
Preservative blend	qs
Flavor	qs
Saccharin, sodium	qs
High fructose corn syrup (SpG = 1.41)	20.0% w/v
Purified water, qs ad	100%

Procedure

1. Dissolve docusate, sodium, in a portion of purified water and thoroughly wet barium sulfate overnight.
2. Dissolve preservative blend and saccharin, sodium, in a separate portion of purified water.
3. Disperse colloidal microcrystalline cellulose and emulsifying wax in step 2 with agitation.
4. Add the barium sulfate slurry (step 1) to step 3 with agitation.
5. Add flavor and high fructose corn syrup to step 4.
6. Pass suspension through a colloidal mill or homogenizer, rinsing through with purified water.
7. Add purified water to final volume.

V. FORMULATION OF SUSPENSIONS

During the preparation of physically stable pharmaceutical suspensions, a number of formulation components are employed to help keep the solid particles in a state of suspension (suspending agents), whereas other components are merely part of the liquid vehicle itself. These formulation components are classified as follows:

1. Components of the suspending system
   a. Wetting agents
   b. Dispersants or deflocculation agents
   c. Flocculating agents
   d. Thickeners
2. Components of the suspending vehicle or external phase
   e. pH control agents and buffers
   f. Osmotic agents

g. Coloring agents, flavors and fragances
h. Preservatives to control microbial growth
i. Liquid vehicles

Not all of the components listed above are required in each of the three types of pharmaceutical suspensions: oral, topical, and parenteral.

A. Wetting Agents

According to Idson and Scheer [62], certain solids are readily wet by liquids, whereas others are not. The degree of wettability depends on the affinity of drugs for water, and whether the solids are hydrophilic or hydrophobic. Hydrophilic solids are easily wetted by water and can increase the viscosity of aqueous suspensions. Hydrophobic solids repel water but can be wetted by nonpolar liquids. When properly wetted, the latter usually do not alter the viscosity of aqueous suspensions. Hydrophilic solids usually can be incorporated into suspensions without the use of wetting agents. The majority of drugs in aqueous suspension are, however, hydrophobic. These are extremely difficult to suspend and frequently float on the surface of water and polar liquids due to entrapped air and poor wetting.

Wetting agents are surfactants that lower the interfacial tension and contact angle between solid particles and liquid vehicle. If, according to Hiestand [8], a wetting agent is present when the powder is added to the liquid vehicle, penetration of the liquid phase into powder will be sufficiently rapid to permit air to escape from the particles and the resulting wetted particles will either sink en masse or separate with low shear agitation. According to hydrophile-lipophile balance (HLB) theory [9], the best range for wetting and spreading by nonionic surfactants lies between 7 and 10.

A number of surfactants that may be used as pharmaceutical wetting agents are listed in Table 8. Note that the 7–10 HLB values listed in the table for optimum wetting are greater than the range normally recommended. The usual concentration of surfactant varies from 0.05% to 0.5% and depends on the solids content intended for suspension.

The use of surfactants as wetting agents will also retard crystal growth in the range of 0.05% to 0.5%. On the other hand, employing surfactants at concentrations less than about 0.05% can result in incomplete wetting. Concentrations greater than 0.5% surfactant may solubilize ultrafine particles and lead eventually to changes in particle size distribution and crystal growth.

The high HLB surfactants are also foaming agents; however, foaming is an undesirable property during wetting of a suspension formulation. In addition, the ionic types, even though claimed to be more effective at the preferred concentration range than nonionic types, are considered pH sensitive and incompatible with many excipients.

Most of the surfactants, except poloxamers, have a bitter taste that often rules against their use in oral suspensions. Nevertheless, polysorbate 80 is still the most widely used surfactant for suspension formulation because of its lack of toxicity and compatibility with most formulation ingredients. Steric stabilization of suspensions with poloxamers was reviewed by Rawlins and Kayes [63]. Nonoxynols and poloxamers were also found to be effective agents below their critical micelle concentration.

The rate of wetting is often determined by placing a measured amount of powder on the undisturbed surface of water containing a given concentration of surfactant and measuring the time required to completely wet and sink the powder. For example, Carino and Mollet [64] found the most rapid sinking time for a hydrophobic solid (SpG > 1)

Table 8 Surfactants Used as Pharmaceutical Wetting Agents

Surfactant	HLB[a] value	Surface tension (dynes cm^{-1} at 0.1% w/v in water)	Comment
Anionic type			
docusate sodium	>24	41	Bitter taste, foaming agent
sodium lauryl sulfate	40	43	Bitter taste, foaming agent
Nonionic type			
polysorbate 65	10.5	33	Bitter taste
octoxynol-9	12.2	30	Bitter taste
nonoxynol-10	13.2	29	Bitter taste
polysorbate 60	14.9	44	Bitter taste
polysorbate 80	15.0	42	Most widely used, bitter taste
polysorbate 40	15.6	41	Low toxicity, bitter taste
poloxamer 235	16	42	Low toxicity, good taste
polysorbate 20	16.7	37	Bitter taste
polyoxamer 188	29	50	Foaming agent

[a]Term introduced by W. Griffin to describe the hydrophilic-lipophilic balance or properties of nonionic surfactants; it has a numerical value between 1 and 20.

was at a concentration of 0.018% docusate sodium USP in water, which is above the critical micelle concentration of the surfactant. The authors also showed that wetting proceeds via liquid penetration into powder pores followed by spreading of wetted powder aggregates prior to sinking.

The addition of smaller amounts of neutral electrolyte, such as potassium chloride, has been found [65] to lower the critical micelle concentration and the interfacial tension of surfactant solutions and thus improve wetting. The resultant suspensions, however, are more susceptible to aggregate or floc formation.

Two simple tests have been devised by the paint industry for wetting agent evaluation.

1. The *wet point* method, which measures the amount of suspending vehicle required to just wet all of the powder. The reduction of the wet point by an additive, such as a wetting agent at a particular concentration, is a practical test of wettability.
2. The *flow point* method measures the amount of suspending vehicle used to achieve *pourability*, i.e., rheologic flow beyond the yield-stress value. The extent to which the flow point of a powder-vehicle system is reduced by a particular concentration of wetting agent is related to the wetting agent's ability to deflocculate the system or its ability to inhibit the buildup of networklike structures (agglomerates).

Both these test methods are best designed for high solids containing topical suspensions.

B. Deflocculants or True Dispersing Agents

Mitsui and Takada [66] showed that the dispersibility of a powder in water depends largely on the magnitude of its surface charge and particle density, whether the powder was forcibly dispersed by applying mechanical shear or not. Deflocculating agents are polymerized organic salts of sulfonic acid of both alkyl-aryl or aryl-alkyl types that can alter the surface charge of particles through physical adsorption. These special polyelectrolytes are marketed under the following trade names: Daxad (Dewey and Almay Chemical Co., Cambridge, MA), Darvan (R. T. Vanderbilt Co., New York, NY), Marasperse (Marathon Corp., Rothschild, WI), and Orzan (Crown Zellerbach, Camas, WA). Their mechanism of action is not completely understood, but they appear to function by producing a negatively charged particle or increasing the negative charge already present in order to aid dispersibility. The reduction of cohesive forces between primary particles through the repulsion of like charge helps break up flocs and agglomerates and also aids dispersion.

Unlike surfactants, these agents do not appreciably lower surface and interfacial tension; hence they have little or no tendency to create foam or wet particles. Most deflocculants, however are *not* generally considered safe for internal use and, as a result, the only acceptable dispersant for internal products is lecithin (a naturally occurring mixture of phosphatides and phospholipids), which is related in activity to the deflocculants listed above. Because lecithins are natural-occurring substances and vary in their water solubility and dispersibility characteristics, in order to obtain reproducible results, proper raw material specifications of lecithins must be rigidly controlled.

C. Flocculating Agents

Simple neutral (1:1) and cation to anion (2:1 or 3:1) electrolytes in solution that are capable of reducing the zeta potential of suspended charged particles to zero are considered to be primary flocculating agents. The mechanism of their activity in stable floc formation has been described previously in this chapter. Small concentrations (0.01–1%) of neutral electrolytes, such as sodium chloride or potassium chloride, are often sufficient to induce flocculation of weakly charged, water-insoluble, organic nonelectrolytes, such as steroids. In the case of more highly charged, insoluble polymers and polyelectrolytes species, similar concentrations (0.01–1%) of water-soluble divalent or trivalent ions, such as calcium salts and alums or sulfates, citrates, and phosphates, are usually required to achieve floc formation depending on particle charge, positive or negative. Often these salts can be used jointly in formulations as pH buffers and flocculating agents.

D. Thickeners and Protective Colloids

Protective or hydrophilic colloids, such as gelatin, natural gums (tragacanth, xanthan, etc.) and cellulose derivatives (sodium carboxymethylcellulose, hydroxypropylcellulose, and hydroxypropylmethylcellulose), which are adsorbed, increase the strength of the hydration layer formed around suspended particles through hydrogen bonding and molecular interaction. Since these agents do not reduce surface and interfacial tension greatly, they function best in the presence of a surfactant. Many of these agents are protective colloids in low concentrations (<0.1%) and viscosity builders in relatively high concentrations (>0.1%).

E. pH Control Agents and Buffers

A properly formulated pharmaceutical suspension should exhibit excellent physical stability over a wide range of pH values. On the other hand, if a specific pH value is found necessary to provide for optimum stability and/or to minimize solubility in the suspending vehicle, the system can be maintained at this desired pH value by the use of a specified concentration of a pharmaceutically acceptable buffer. This is especially important for drugs that possess ionizable acidic or basic groups; then the pH of the vehicle often influences drug stability and/or solubility. Careless or indiscriminate use of salts and buffers however, should be avoided, because small changes in electrolyte concentration will often alter the surface charge of suspended particles. Such effects can influence the nature and stability of flocculated suspensions. This is especially noticeable when polyvalent ions, such as citrates and phosphates, are used in buffering systems. Suspensions of stable, neutral drugs, which possess no formal charge, such as corticosteroids, are usually insensitive to pH change. The control of pH by buffering of these particular suspensions is normally required as a quality control procedure for maintaining a desired pH specification. Again, buffering components and their concentrations are often selected on an experimental basis so as not to adversely affect the physical stability of the final suspension.

F. Osmotic Agents and Stabilizers

The previous discussion also applies to the use of osmotic agents (sodium chloride, etc.) and stabilizers (disodium edetate, etc.), many of which are electrolytes or potential electrolytes in suspension products. Substituting organic nonelectrolytes, such as dextrose, mannitol, or sorbitol, for inorganic salts and electrolytes to adust osmolarity or tonicity in an ophthalmic or injectable suspension will often reduce batch variation with respect to physical stability when these materials are used as osmotic agents and stabilizers.

G. Colorants, Flavors, and Fragrances

Organoleptic agents, such as colorants, flavors, or fragrances, should not normally affect the physical stability of topical or oral suspensions as long as the formulator realizes that cationic materials will interact with negatively charged suspension particles and thereby adversely affect physical stability.

On the other hand, since many flavoring agents and fragrances are water-insoluble, oily liquids that are usually added to the batch in the final phase after the primary physical stability of the suspension has been established, the formulator should be alert to the possibility that these oily materials may be adsorbed on the surface of suspended particles and thereby influence the physical stability of the final suspension.

H. Preservatives to Control Microbial Growth

Preservation against microbial growth is an important consideration, not only in terms of its effect on the chemical stability of the ingredients and the safety and acceptability of the products but also on the physical integrity of the system. Riddick [67] indicated that many colloidal dispersed systems were judged unstable because they agglomerated in time. The effect apparently was not due to aging but to continued microbial activity, which gradually decreased the zeta potential of the system. If such systems had been properly preserved, they would not have agglomerated but would have remained in a colloidal state of dispersion. The same may be said of systems that are prepared initially by controlled flocculation procedure and later deflocculate in the absence of adequate preservation. Adequacy of preservation is a particularly troublesome problem in antacid suspensions where pH values greater than 6 or 7 often compromise the effectiveness of commonly used, orally accepted preservatives, such as parabens, benzoates, and sorbates.

Sweeteners, nonionic surfactants, and suspending agents, such as clays, gelatin, lecithin, natural gums, and cellulose derivatives, are particularly susceptible to microbial growth. The use of cationic antimicrobial agents, such as benzalkonium chloride, is usually contraindicated, because cationic agents may be inactivated by formulation components or they may alter the charge of the suspended particles.

A well-preserved oral or topical suspension does not have to be sterile to prevent microbial growth. The use of small amounts of propylene glycol (5–15%) disodium edetate (about 0.1%) or a decrease of pH all have been used to increase the efficiency of preservative systems without adversely affecting physical stability of pharmaceutical suspensions [68]. A list of commonly used antimicrobial preservatives in pharmaceutical suspensions is presented in Table 9.

I. External Phase

The suspending vehicle chosen also governs the selection of the suspending agent(s) to be employed. For example, in the case of nonpolar liquids, such as aliphatic or halogenated hydrocarbons, fatty esters, and oils, the best suspending agents are low HLB surfactants, stearalkonium hectorite, water-insoluble resins, and water-insoluble film-formers. On the other hand, in the case of polar liquids such as water, alcohols, polyols, and glycols, the higher HLB surfactants, clays, silicates, gums, and cellulose derivatives are usually preferred. The physically most stable systems are designed to wet particles and then to disperse them in a gelled liquid formed by the interaction between suspending agent(s) and vehicle component(s). Liquid vehicles are selected based on safety, density, viscosity, taste, and stability considerations.

J. Sterile Suspensions

In most reviews of pharmaceutical suspensions very little space is devoted to a discussion of sterile suspensions. Yet there are factors peculiar to this dosage form, which are not commonly shared by other suspension systems. Some of these are sterility, syringeability, ease of resuspension, slow settling after shaking, and drainage, as well as absence of pyrogens and foreign particulate matter. Akers et al. presented an excellent review of the topic [69].

Preparation of a sterile parenteral suspension is a very difficult procedure. It requires complete attention to detail during the following broad phases of manufacture:

Final recrystallization of the drug
Size reduction of the drug
Sterilization of the drug
Sterilization of the vehicle
Aseptic wetting of the powder with a portion of the sterile vehicle
Aseptic dispersion and milling of the bulk suspension
Aseptic filling of the finished suspension into sterile containers

Alternate procedures for the manufacture of sterile suspensions have been reported separately by Akers et al. [69], Grimes [70], and Portnoff [71]. At the present time, there is no pharmaceutically acceptable chemical agent that can be added to the finished

Table 9 List of Preservatives Used in Pharmaceutical Suspensions[a]

Agent	Concentration (%)	Comments
Parabens (Me, Et, Pr, Bu)	0.2	Potential sensitizer, poor activity above pH 7, inactivated by high concentration of surfactants, poor solubility in water, active against molds and yeasts, slow kill time, poor taste properties
Sorbic acid	0.2	Low sensitizing potential, poor activity above pH 6, unstable in polyethylene containers, soluble in water, compatible with surfactants, good taste properties
Thimerosal	0.01	Potential sensitizer, good activity above pH 7, inactivated by EDTA and sulfites, slow kill time, used in injectables
Quaternary ammonium salts	0.01	Potential sensitizer, active at neutral pH, inactivated by anionic surfactants and polymers, will affect negatively charged particles, soluble in water, activity potentiated by EDTA, rapid kill time, ophthalmic preservative
Benzyl alcohol	1.0	Low sensitizing potential, active at neutral pH, use in large-volume parenterals is restricted, soluble in water, inactivated by high concentrations of surfactants, injectable and topical preservative
Benzoic acid	0.2	Poor activity above pH 5, soluble in water, good taste properties
Chlorhexidine gluconate	0.01	Active above pH 7, soluble in water, incompatible with borates, rapid kill time, ophthalmic preservative
Phenylethanol	1.0	Potentiates activity of parabens, quaternary ammonium salts, and chlorhexidine, soluble in water, topical and ophthalmic preservative

[a]The preservatives phenol, chlorocresol, phenylmercuric acetate, and chlorobutanol are rarely used in present-day pharmaceutical formulations.

suspension to render it both sterile and safe. Therefore, an elaborate program of sterility checks at critical phases of the operation is required. There is no simple way to prepare sterile parenteral suspensions other than reliance on sound parenteral techniques and aseptic practices.

Special facilities to handle the preparation of sterile powders for parenteral suspensions should be made available for this purpose. Pharmaceuticals that are handled in this manner include antibiotics, biological materials, and steroids. The final workup and purification steps of such drugs are conducted in sterile rooms. Aseptic techniques and sterile or particle-free solvents are used for the purpose of performing final recrystallizations.

There are several advantages in establishing such a program. The foreign matter content of sterile powders for parenteral use is greatly reduced through the extra care involved in such an operation. The chance of preparing pyrogenic materials or contaminating with pyrogens is greatly reduced. Sterile powder can be provided for the manufacture of parenteral products, thereby greatly simplifying the subsequent sterilization operations.

1. *Selection of Milling Equipment*

Some type of mechanical dispersion equipment is often required to break up agglomerates of poorly wetted, hydrophobic particles shortly after a primary slurry is formed between the sterile powder and a portion of the sterile suspending vehicle. For most efficient handling in production, a one-pass dispersion step is desirable through the use of a colloidal mill that can be sterilized prior to use, with either ethylene oxide gas or live steam. The principal advantage of this particular mill is that the head, which is composed entirely of stainless steel, can be detached from the motor housing and sterilized in an autoclave. The hopper of the mill is removed, and a stainless steel plate and baffle are inserted in its place for parenteral operation. Mill heads are relatively inexpensive, and, therefore, several units can be purchased to provide continuous trouble-free operation. Piston-type homogenizers have also been used for the preparation of parenteral dispersions [72]. These units, however, lack the flexibility of a colloid mill and are more difficult to sterilize. Ultrasonic devices [73] and high speed mixers [68] have been used experimentally for the same purpose.

2. *Syringeability*

One of the most important properties of a good parenteral suspension is syringeability, the ability of a parenteral solution or suspension to pass easily through a hypodermic needle, especially during the transfer of product from vial to hypodermic syringe prior to injection. Increases in the following characteristics tend to reduce syringeability or make material transfer through the needle more difficult:

The viscosity of the vehicle
The density of the vehicle
The size of suspended particulate matter
The concentration of suspended drug

Probably the most important of these factors is viscosity. Fortunately, with parenteral suspensions, viscosity is perhaps the easiest parameter for the formulator to control. The preparation of a stable floc contributes little to the overall viscosity of the system and hence does not adversely influence syringeability. Even though the individual suspension particles are loosely held together in large multiple aggregates, they are easily broken up and reformed during their passage from vial to syringe, and from syringe to injection site.

To give the physician flexibility in selecting hypodermic needles for various routes of parenteral injection, the following standard for syringeability can be established: the entire contents of a parenteral suspension is expected to pass through a 25 gauge needle without difficulty where the needle's internal diameter is 0.3 mm and no individual particle size is greater than about one-third the needle's internal diameter. The needle size of such a specification can be extended to 27, 28, and 30 gauge only when extreme care is exercised by the physician. Making routine injections with very fine bore hypodermic needles (>25 gauge), however, is not normally recommended.

3. *Drainage*

The ability of the suspension to break cleanly away from the inner walls of the primary container-closure system is another important characteristic of a well-formulated parenteral suspension. Completely peptized to flocculated systems show this property, while overflocculated systems exhibit some degree of poor drainage. Poor drainage is further characterized by the use of the term "buttermilk appearance," an expression that aptly describes this unsightly condition. The effect is produced by the rapid drainback of vehicle through channels created by the residual adhering flocculant.

The process of silicone coating of containers, vials, and plugs with dimethicone makes good suspensions drain better and helps reverse the tendency toward poor drainage by slightly overflocculated systems [74].

4. *Resuspendability*

Resuspendability is defined as the ability to resuspend settled particles with a minimum amount of shaking after a suspension has stood for some time. The difficulty lies in estimating how much effort will be required to resuspend the solids in a suspension after reading a "shake well" label. Unless a suspension can be prepared in which the suspended particles do not settle—in other words, the "permanent suspension"—the best answer to the problem is preparation of a physically stable, flocculated suspension. This is especially important in the case of parenteral suspensions, for which the structured vehicle approach cannot be considered because of the poor syringeability of such systems. Preparation of a stable floc offers the formulator a convenient method of overcoming this problem. Stable, flocculated parenteral suspensions that have stood undisturbed for prolonged periods of storage are therefore the easiest systems to resuspend.

5. *Compatibility with Diluents and Other Injectable Products*

Unlike other pharmaceutical suspensions, dilution of parenteral suspensions prior to use is often necessary, especially if only small concentrations of drug are required. Often times, parenteral suspensions are mixed and injected with solutions of a local anesthetic agent, such as Lidocaine Hydrochloride Injection USP, to diminish the pain associated with administration. For this reason some sort of compatibility testing is extremely useful.

Dilution of the suspension with water or normal saline will often cause the system to deflocculate. This is not necessarily detrimental, since dilutions are often made prior to administration, long before "caking and cementing" can take place. On the other hand, if dilution or mixing with other injectable preparations causes the suspension to agglomerate or coagulate, this will result in a more serious incompatibility. Therefore, some basic compatibility testing is recommended with common injectable diluents during the development of a parenteral suspension. Increasing the solids content of suspensions 10-fold (from, say, 0.5% to 5%) will often increase the physical stability of the system itself as well as its compatibility with diluents and other injectable products.

K. Cosmetic Suspensions

There are basically two types of cosmetic suspension system used at the present time. The first are the pigmented products that are suspended in aqueous vehicles (such as liquid makeups, eyeliners, mascaras, and blushers). These products feature high solids content, high density, impalpable powders, and pigments permanently suspended in either a primary oil-in-water, emulsion type base or a complex system of hydrophilic cellulosic derivatives, clays, and/or polymeric film-formers, in which the gelling and suspending properties of the vehicle often are reinforced by the presence of a small amount of a Bingham-type plastic, such as carbomer [75].

The second type of cosmetic suspension consists of the pigment-containing nail enamels. The coloring tints, pigments, pearls, and lakes in the latter system are suspended with the aid of organophilic, thixotropic gellant, such as stearalkonium hectorite (Bentone 38: trademark of NL Industries, Inc., Hightstown, NJ), in a nonaqueous vehicle consisting of a mixture of butyl acetate, ethyl acetate, and isopropyl alcohol solvents in which the primary plasticized nitrocellulose and toluene sulfonamide–formaldehyde resin film-formers are dissolved. Patents covering such products have been reviewed separately by Markland [76] and Kahn and Eichhorn [77].

Examples of cosmetic-type suspensions are given in Tables 10 through 13.

L. Manufacturing Guidelines

Technical guidelines with respect to the formulation, manufacture, and testing of pharmaceutical suspensions have been published separately by Scheer [78] and Idson and

Table 10 Typical Aqueous Cream Makeup Formula

Ingredients	% w/w	Function
Stearic acid	10	Gelling agent/suspending agent
Glyceryl monostearate	2	Emulsifier/suspending agent
Cetyl alcohol	2	Thickener/suspending agent
Isopropyl myristate	2	Emollient
Polyethylene glycol 400 monostearate	1	Emulsifier/suspending agent
Propylene glycol	12	Dispersant and humectant
Titanium dioxide	2	
Talc	8	Suspensoid mixture
Pigment blend	1	
Preservative	qs	
Fragrance	qs	
Water	60	Primary vehicle
	100	

Table 11 Typical Nonaqueous Nail Enamel Formula

Ingredients	% w/w	Function
Nitrocellulose	12	Film-former
Toluene sulfonamide–formaldehyde resin	6	Film-former
Camphor	2	Plasticizer
Pigment blend	3	Colorant (suspensoid)
Ethyl acetate	8	Cosolvent
Butyl acetate	25	Cosolvent
Isopropyl alcohol	8	Coupler
Toluene	35	Primary vehicle
Stearalkonium hectorite	1	Suspending agent
	100	

Scheer [62]. Especially useful in their reviews is a listing of potential suspension problems, their probable cause, and suggested practical remedies for their successful resolution.

Following is another list of practical suggestions that the formulator may find useful in connection with the preparation of physically stable pharmaceutical suspensions.

1. In addition to dry grinding of insoluble particles for suspension to the smallest and most uniform size that is practical, it is important to maintain absolute control of the crystallographic form of the drug during bulk chemical manufacture and to make sure that solid surfaces are free of adsorbed impurities and lipid films, to prevent variation in the physical stability of finished suspensions.

Table 12 Water-Resistant Sport Tint

Ingredients	% w/w	Function
Magnesium aluminum silicate	1.60	Suspending agent
Xanthan gum	0.40	Suspending agent
Propylene glycol	5.00	Dispersant and humectant
Water	70.40	Primary vehicle
Iron oxides	0.67	Pigment
Manganese violet	0.10	Pigment
Talc	4.27	Whitener
Titanium dioxide	6.96	Whitener and sunblock
Isocetyl alcohol	3.00	Thickener
Octyl methoxycinnamate	3.00	Chemical sunscreen
Mineral oil	1.00	Dispersant
Lanolin alcohol	1.00	Emulsifier
Oleth-3 phosphate	2.20	Emulsifier
Povidone	0.40	Suspending agent
Preservative	qs	
Fragrance	qs	
	100.00	

Table 13 Waterproof Mechanical Sunblock

Ingredients	% w/w	Function
Isocetyl alcohol	8.00	Thickener
C12–15 Alcohols Benzoate	2.00	Dispersant
Stearic acid	2.00	Gelling agent/emulsifier
PEG-40 stearate	2.00	Emulsifier
Dimethicone copolyol	1.00	Waterproofing agent
Glyceryl stearate	0.50	Emulsifier
Dimethyl steramine	2.00	Emulsifier
Acrylates/octylacrylamide	2.00	Film-former
Titanium dioxide, microfine	10.00	Mechanical sunblock
Water	59.30	Primary vehicle
Carbomer (2% solution)	10.00	Suspending agent
Trolamine	0.80	Neutralizer/emulsifier
Preservative	qs	
Fragrance	qs	
	100.00	

2. Where practical, the solids to be suspended should first be allowed to wet out completely (usually overnight) without agitation in a small portion of the aqueous component of the suspending vehicle, which contains a proper amount of wetting agent in order to release entrapped air slowly and to reduce the number of non-wetted agglomerates that may remain during subsequent processing.
3. The suspending agent should be dissolved or dispersed in the main portion of the liquid vehicle (external phase). Sufficient time and appropriate dispersion equipment should be employed to permit complete hydration and the attainment of proper viscosity. Each suspending agent used should have a specific function in the formula, and the temptation to overformulate should be avoided.
4. The slurry concentrate of wetted particles should be slowly added with the aid of low shear agitation (anchor or gate type) to the main portion of the suspending agent(s), and not the other way round.
5. Electrolyte additions, such as pH adjustments with acids, bases, and buffers, or tonicity adjustments with salts and electrolytes, should be carefully controlled to prevent variations in particle charge.
6. Colloid mills, homogenizers, ultrasonic devices, or pumps should be used only after all additions and adjustments have been completed as a finishing procedure during the final transfer of the suspension to holding tanks or filling lines, to reduce the size of poorly wetted, agglomerated particles.
7. All finished aqueous suspensions must be carefully preserved against microbial growth.
8. Finally, the concentration of strong electrolytes used in the formula should be reduced, if possible, through the selection of weaker monovalent acids and bases for pH and buffer control and use of nonelectrolytes (sorbitol, dextrose, etc.) for tonicity adjustment.

Factors to be considered in the scale-up of pharmaceutical suspensions were discussed by Hem at the 1993 AAPS workshop jointly sponsored by the FDA and the USP (reported in *Pharm. Res. 11*, 1140, 1994).

M.   Test Methods for Pharmaceutical Suspensions

Tingstad [79] reviewed test methods available for determining the physical stability of pharmaceutical suspensions. The procedures outlined were designed to determine whether a given formula is flocculated. Since there is more than one method of preparing stable suspensions, the following tests were found useful for determining the stability of both flocculated and dispersed systems.

1.   *Photomicroscopic Techniques*

One of the oldest and most useful techniques for measuring the properties and stability of a suspension is microscopy. The microscope can be used to estimate and detect changes in particle size distribution and crystal form. Its usefulness can be enhanced through the use of a Polaroid camera attached to the eyepiece of a monocular microscope to permit the rapid processing of photomicrographs. Photomicrographs, similar to those shown in Fig. 5, can be used, for example, to distinguish between flocculated and nonflocculated particles and to determine changes in the physical properties and stability of such systems conveniently with time.

2.   *The Coulter Counter*

The Coulter Multisizer II (an electrical sensing zone instrument, Coulter-Scientific Instruments Hialean, FL) is an electronic particle counter and sizer that measures the change of resistance caused by the presence of a particle in an electrolyte [80]. The suspension flows through a small orifice with electrodes on either side of the opening. Particles pass through the aperture substantially one at a time. The size range of the counter is 0.2 to 1200 μm. Each particle passing through the orifice displaces electro-

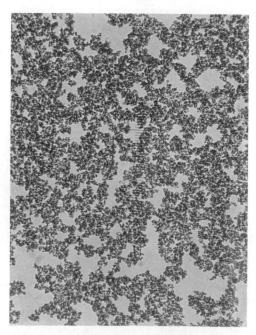

Fig. 5   Flocculated steroid particles. (From Ref. 65.)

lytes within the aperture, thus momentarily changing the resistance between the electrodes and producing a voltage pulse of a magnitude proportional to the particle volume. The resulting series of pulses is electronically amplified, scaled, and counted. The instrument has proved extremely valuable in determining the particle size distribution of hydrophobic particles, such as steroids and some antibiotics. Suspensions must be diluted, however, with electrolyte and surfactant to produce monodispersed samples prior to particle size analysis. Therefore the Coulter counting technique cannot be used to determine the physical stability and properties of particle aggregates. Similar instrumentation (ELZONE 280 Pc system) is also available from Particle Data, Inc., Elmhurst, IL.

Since the electrical sensing impulse of the instrument is proportional to particle volume, particle diameter is calculated by taking the cube root of the particle volume. For the data to be meaningful, particles must approach a sphere or cube in shape. Particle size distribution of needlelike microcrystalline prisms was found to be inaccurate by this method, especially when comparisons were made to data obtained for other particle shapes [81]. The use of the technique is usually restricted to oil-in-water emulsions and deflocculated aqueous suspensions. The various techniques for measuring both the macro- and micro-particle size distributions were reviewed recently by Pietsch (82) (see Fig. 6).

4. *Graduated Cylinders*

Simple, inexpensive, graduated cylinders (100–1000 ml) are quite useful for determining the physical stability of suspensions. They can be used, for example, to determine the settling rates of flocculated and nonflocculated suspensions, by making periodic measurement of sedimentation height without disturbing the system. Tingstad [79] indicated that a flocculated suspension, which settles to a level that is 90% of the initial or total suspension height and no further, is probably satisfactory. Such a standard may be too demanding for parenteral suspensions, where systems with sedimentation heights of only 30% to 60% are often encountered.

Volumetric graduated cylinders have also been used to determine the F or flocculation ratio, a value that has been described by Haines and Martin [44] and Hiestand [8]. The F value, which is the ratio of the sediment volume to the original suspension volume at a given time, is used to measure the relative degree of flocculation and physical sta-

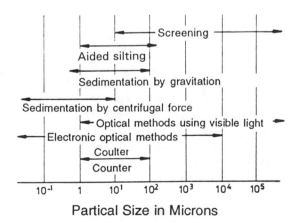

Fig. 6 General methods for particle size analysis. (From Ref. 82.)

bility of certain suspensions. Great care must be exercised in the use of graduated cylinders because decreases in the diameter of small containers produce a "wall effect," which can often affect the settling rate or ultimate sedimentation height of flocculated suspensions. Such small vessels have a tendency to hold up suspensions due to the adhesive forces acting between the inner surface of the container and the suspended particles.

5. *Brookfield Viscometer with Helipath Attachment*

The Helipath attachment used with a Brookfield viscometer is a valuable piece of rheological equipment for measuring the settling behavior and structure of pharmaceutical suspensions. A description of the apparatus was presented in the paper by Tingstad [79]. The instrument consists of a slowly rotating T-bar spindle, which while descending slowly into suspensions encounters new, essentially undisturbed material as it rotates. The dial reading of the viscometer measures resistance to flow that the spindle encounters from the structure at various levels in the sediment. Taking rheograms at various time intervals, under standard conditions of sample preparation, gives a description of the suspension and its physical stability. The technique is most useful for viscous suspensions high in solids, that develop sufficient shear stress for measurement. The instrument is also excellent for characterizing flocculated systems.

6. *Specific Gravity Measurement with Hydrometers*

The use of series of short-range precision hydrometers provides a quick, accurate, and inexpensive method of determining the specific gravity or density of pharmaceutical suspensions. Such measurements provide qualitative information on the amount of air entrapped by a suspension during manufacture. This type of data is predictive of the unhappy experience of having aerated flocs floating on the surface of suspensions and also provides better control during production.

7. *Aging Tests*

Subjecting suspensions to cyclic temperature testing—that is, to conditions of repeated freezing and thawing—or exposing them to elevated temperatures ($>40°C$) for short periods of shortage to test for physical stability is considered drastic. The value of such aging test procedures may be open to question, since exposure of suspensions to storage at elevated temperatures causes significant amounts of drug to go into solution, and subsequent cooling induces excess drug in solution to reprecipitate. Most suspension systems contain surfactants and protective colloids to prevent particle growth. Thus, inducing crystal growth during age testing may be of limited value. The use of stressful aging tests, however, has one advantage. If a given suspension is able to withstand exposure to extremes in temperature, it is safe to assume that the preparation will have good physical stability during prolonged storage at ambient temperature. On the other hand, failure of suspensions to meet such stringent testing procedures should not be considered a bar to further testing, because many marketed pharmaceutical suspensions would have been rejected from further consideration on this basis alone.

8. *Zeta Potential*

The determination of the zeta potential of particles in a suspension provides useful information concerning the sign and magnitude of the charge and its effect on the physical stability of the system with time. At the present time, there are a number of instruments that can be used for this purpose. Among them are the electrophoretic mass transport analyzer (Zeta Potential Analyzer by Micrometrics Instrument Corp., Norcross, GA), the streaming current detector (Hydroscan by Leeds and Northrup Co., No. Wales, PA), and electrokinetic sonic amplitude device (by Matec Instruments, Inc., Warick, RI), plus three additional instruments that determine zeta potential by measuring the electrophoretic mobility of the suspended particles in a charged field (Zeta-Reader by Komline-Sanderson, Peapack, NJ), a semiautomatic instrument (the laser Zee Meter Model 400 by Pen Kem Inc., Bedford Hills, NY), and a microelectrophoretic mobility apparatus (Zeta-Meter, Inc., Long Island City, NY). The first three devices are suitable for determining the average zeta potential of coarse suspensions in high-solids systems; while the latter three instruments are more useful for measurement of colloidal particles in low-solids systems. Several new instruments are currently available that take advantage of light-scattering technology (Delsa 440 by Coulter, Hialeah, FL) or simplify electrophoretic mobility measurement (Zeta-Plus, Brookhaven Instruments, Holtsville, NY; Zeta-Sizer, Malvern Instruments, Southborough, MA; and Mobility Meter, Paper Chemistry Lab, Inc., Carmel, NY). These devices are expensive, and their use in the study of flocculated suspensions is limited by the fact that flocculated as well as agglomerated particles have a zero zeta potential. The use of zeta potential to measure the physical stability of pharmaceutical suspensions has been extensively reviewed by Cardwell [83], Ross and Long [84], Kaye [85], and Akers [86].

9. *Aggregation Kinetics*

Much has been made of the term "rate of aggregate formation" (either described as flocculation rate and/or coagulation rate) when applied both to colloidal and coarse suspensions [3]. The decrease in the concentration of deflocculated particles as the direct result of aggregate formation appears in most cases to follow first-order kinetics.

In most pharmaceutical suspensions this thermodynamically driven phenomenon is essentially completed within not less than several days is not more than several months and is dependent upon particle size, particle concentration, the viscosity of the suspending vehicle and the presence or absence of suitable steric stabilizers (polymers, surfactants, and electrolytes).

The following factors, which influence the physical stability and performance of pharmaceutical suspensions, are more appropriate candidates for testing and evaluation than are rates of aggregate formation or deformation.

10. *Checklist for Suspension Performance and Stability Testing*

1. *Appearance* (macro) as viewed through a graduated glass cylinder or transparent container:
   At equilibrium, is the color and appearance of the sediment uniform?
   At equilibrium, are there breaks or air-pockets in the sediment?
   Is the residual drainage above the sediment uniform and minimal or is there coagulated material adhering to the inside walls of the container?
2. *Sedimentation Rate*.
   Using a suitable graduated cylinder, is the initial settling rate (the falling height of interface vs. time) of the suspension similar when sedimentation rate test is repeated during shelf-life storage?

3. *Sedimentation Volume and Redispersibility.*
   Is the volume of sediment at equilibrium sufficiently large to support uniform resuspension when gentle agitation is applied?
   Is the volume of sediment similar and reproducible batch after batch?
4. *Viscosity.*
   Is the apparent viscosity of the suspension at equilibrium, as measured at a given temperature with a suitable calibrated viscometer or rheologic instrument, reproducible with time? Apparent viscosity like pH is an exponential term and therefore *log apparent viscosity* is an appropriate way to report viscosity results.
5. *pH Value.*
   The pH value of aqueous suspensions should be taken at a given temperature and only after equilibrium settling has been achieved to minimize "pH drift" and electrode surface coating with suspended particles. Electrolyte should not be added to the external phase of the suspension to stabilize the pH for reading, because the addition of neutral electrolyte will disturb the physical stability of the suspension.
6. *Density or Specific Gravity.*
   The apparent density of the suspension is an important parameter for measurement. A decrease in density often indicates the presence of entrapped air within the structure of the suspension. Density measurements should be made at a given temperature using well-mixed, uniform-looking suspensions. The use of precision hydrometers facilitates such measurements.
7. *Aspect* (color, odor and taste).
   Color, odor and taste are especially important considerations with respect to orally administered suspensions. Variation in color often indicates poor multi-ingredient distribution and/or differences in particle size. Differences in taste (especially of actives) can often be attributed to changes in particle size, crystal habit and subsequent particle *dissolution.* Changes in color, odor and taste can also indicate chemical instability.
8. *Microscopic Examination.*
   Microscopic examination is the single most important method used to characterize the physical stability of suspensions. Are the individual particles flocculated or not? Sufficient fields and samples should be examined to make such a determination. Dilutions taken for microscopic examination should be made with supernatant external phase rather than purified water. Individual particle sizes can be estimated here but are more accurately determined using electronic instrumentation—i.e., Coulter Multisizer II or Elzone 280 PC system.
9. *Drug Content Uniformity.*
   This important testing procedure for drug potent uniformity is best performed using either "unit of use" volume (i.e., 5 ml of oral liquid or a spray actuation of a oral inhalation product) or sampling from the dispensing container (i.e., from the top, middle, and bottom). In either case, the dispensing container should be well mixed prior to sampling for assay, because most pharmaceutical suspensions are not permanent.
10. *Freeze-Thaw Cycling.*
    Although freeze-thaw cycling is a useful guide to physical stability of suspensions, the most reliable information is normally obtained from testing at room temperature (26–30°C). Relative humidity conditions are not relevant here. If freeze-thaw

cycling or elevated temperature exposures are chosen for physical stability testing, companion samples of a closely related marketed product should be included in the testing protocol for comparative purposes, because pharmaceutical suspensions are not normally designed to withstand temperature extremes during shelf storage.

11. *Miscellaneous Testing.*

Assay for potency, preservative effectiveness, compatibility with container/closure system, off-torque, simulated-use testing can be handled in a manner similar to that used for conventional liquid solutions with the provision that the container is well mixed prior to testing.

Dissolution testing of suspension products is still evolving. The best approach at present appears to be to place a small, but known amount of oral or injectable aqueous suspension inside a secure Durapore (polyvinylidene fluoride) membrane (Millipore Products Div., Bedford, MA) pouch of a suitable porosity and submerge and suspend it "tea bag" fashion in a suitable dissolution medium using the USP Method I paddle apparatus. Optimization of experimental conditions will be required to achieve reproducible results.

REFERENCES

1. R. A. Nash, *Drug Cosmet. Ind.,* 97:843 (1965); 98:40 (1966).
2. N. K. Patel, L. Kennon, and R. S. Levinson, Pharmaceutical suspensions. In: *Theory and Practice of Industrial Pharmacy* (L. Lachman, H. A. Lieberman, J. L. Kanig, eds.), Lea & Febiger, Philadelphia, 1986, pp. 479–501.
3. C. T. Rhodes. Dispersed Systems in *Modern Pharmaceutics,* 2nd Edition, Revised and Expanded, Marcel Dekker, Inc., New York, 1989, pp. 339–353.
4. A. Arancibia, Formulation considerations of pharmaceutical suspensions (in Spanish), *Farmaco, Ed. Prat.,* 26:721 (1971).
5. J. C. Boylan, The development of semi-solid dosage forms: An overview, *Drug Dev. Commun.,* 2:320 (1976).
6. G. Zografi, J. Swarbrick and H. Schott, Dispersed Systems In: *Remington's Pharmaceutical Sciences* (A. R. Gennaro, ed.), Mack Publishing Co., Easton, PA, 1990, pp. 257–309.
7. B. Ecanow, Liquid medications, In: *Dispensing Pharmacy* (R. E. King, ed.), 9th ed., Mack Publishing Co., Easton, PA, 1984, pp. 117–124.
8. E. N. Hiestand, Theory of coarse suspension formulation, *J. Pharm. Sci.,* 53:1–18 (1964).
9. A. Martin, and P. Bustamante, Coarse dispersions. In: *Physical Pharmacy*, 4th ed., Lea & Febiger, Philadelphia, 1993, p. 477.
10. A. D. Marcus and H. G. DeKay, A study of calamine lotion, *J. Am. Pharm. Assoc., Pract. Ed.,* 11:227–229 (1950).
11. F. B. Gable, H. B. Kostenbauder, and A. N. Martin, The calamine lotion problem, *J. Am. Pharm. Assoc., Pract. Ed.,* 14:287–289 (1953).
12. R. S. Escabi and H. G. DeKay, New developments in calamine lotion, *J. Am. Pharm. Assoc., Pract. Ed.,* 17:30–33, 47–49 (1956).
13. L. W. Willits and E. A. Holstius, Calamine lotion–suggested improvements, *J. Am. Pharm. Assoc., Pract. Ed.,* 17:108–109 (1956).
14. S. W. Goldstein, New formulas for calamine lotion, *J. Am. Pharm. Assoc., Pract. Ed.,* 13:250–251, 278–280 (1952).
15. P. J. Pantle et al., A proposed formula for calamine lotion, *J. Am. Pharm. Assoc., Pract. Ed.,* 15:418–419, 448 (1954).

16. J. E. Haberle and W. B. Swafford, *Am. J. Pharm.* 133:58–62 (1961).
17. M. J. Robinson, Third Annual National Industrial Pharmaceutical Research Conference, Land O'Lakes, WI, 1961.
18. J. P. Portnoff, E. M. Cohen, and M. W. Henley, Development of parenteral and sterile ophthalmic suspensions, *Bull. Parenter. Drug Assoc.,* 31:136–143 (1977).
19. J. G. Wagner, Biopharmaceutics: Absorption aspects, *J. Pharm. Sci.,* 50:359–387 (1961).
20. J. G. Rheinhold, et al., Comparison of the behavior of microcrystalline sulfadiazine with that of ordinary sulfadiazine in man, *Am. J. Med. Sci.,* 210:141–147 (1945).
21. C. A. Hirst and R. C. Kaye, Effect of pharmaceutical formulation of thioridazine absorption; *J. Pharm. Pharmacol.,* 23:2465 (1971).
22. J. D. Mullins and T. J. Macek, Some pharmaceutical properties of novobiocin, *J. Am. Pharm. Assoc., Sci. Ed.,* 49:245–248 (1960).
23. Y. W. Chien, Long-acting parenteral drug formulations, *J. Parenter. Sci. Technol.,* 35:106–139 (1981).
24. I. Goodarznia and D. N. Sutherland, Floc simulation: Effects of particle size and shape, *Chem. Eng. Sci.,* 30:407–412 (1975).
25. K. J. Frederick, Performance and problems of pharmaceutical suspensions, *J. Pharm. Sci.,* 50:531–535 (1961).
26. T. Higuchi, Some physical chemical aspects of suspension formulation, *J. Am. Pharm. Assoc., Sci. Ed.,* 47:657–660 (1958).
27. B. A. Matthews, The use of the Coulter Counter in emulsion and suspension studies, *Can. J. Pharm. Sci.,* 6:29–34 (1971).
28. J. E. Carless, et al., Dissolution and crystal growth in aqueous suspension of cortisone acetate, *J. Pharm. Pharmacol.,* 10:630–639 (1968).
29. J. K. Haleblian, Characterization of habits and crystalline modification of solids and their pharmaceutical applications, *J. Pharm. Sci.,* 64:1269–1288 (1975).
30. F. H. Buckwalter and H. L. Dickison, *J. Am. Pharm. Assoc., Sci. Ed.,* 47:661–665 (1958).
31. R. M. Atkinson et al., *Nature,* 193:588–589 (1962).
32. R. E. Collard, *Pharm. J.,* 132:113–117 (1961).
33. K. A. Lees, Fine particles in pharmaceutical practice, *J. Pharm. Pharmacol.,* 15:43t–55t (1963).
34. E. A. Smith, Particle size reduction to micron size, *Manuf. Chem. & Aerosol News,* July:31–36 (1967).
35. R. M. Cohn and D. M. Skauen, Controlled crystallization of hydrocortisone by ultrasonic irradiation, *J. Pharm. Sci.,* 53:1040–1045 (1964).
36. S. Riegelman et al., Application of spray-drying techniques to pharmaceutical powders, *J. Am. Pharm. Assoc., Sci. Ed.,* 39:444–450 (1950).
37. J. Waltersson and P. Lundgren, Nonthermal kinetics applied to drugs in pharmaceutical suspensions, *Acta Pharm. Suec.,* 20:145–154 (1983).
38. R. A. Nash, Unpublished data.
39. N. Weiner, Strategies for formulation and evaluation of emulsions and suspensions, *Drug Dev. Ind. Pharm.* 12:933–951 (1986).
40. P. W. Gerding and G. J. Sperandio, Factors affecting the choice of suspending agents in pharmaceuticals, *J. Am. Pharm. Assoc. Pract. Ed.,* 15:356–359 (1954).
41. B. T. Crowl, The theory and practice of dispersion, *J. Oil Colour Chem. Assoc.,* 55:388–420 (1972).
42. W. Schneider, S. Starchansky, and A. N. Martin, Pharmaceutical suspensions and DLVO theory, *Am. J. Pharm. Ed.,* 42:280–289 (1978).
43. C. R. Carpenter, Calculate settling velocities for unrestricted particles on hindered settling, *Chem. Eng.,* Nov. 14, 1983.
44. B. A. Haines and A. N. Martin, Interfacial properties of powdered material, *J. Pharm. Sci.,* 50:228–232, 753–759 (1961).

45. B. A. Matthews, and C. T. Rhodes, Use of DLVO theory to interpret pharmaceutical suspension stability, *J. Pharm. Sci.*, 59:521–525 (1970).

46. E. N. Hiestand, Physical properties of coarse suspensions, *J. Pharm. Sci.*, 61:268–272 (1972).

47. B. Ecanow, R. Grundman, and R. G. Wilson, Flocculation and coagulation, *Am. J. Hosp. Pharm.*, 23:404 (1966).

48. R. G. Wilson and B. Ecanow, Powdered particle interactions: Suspension flocculation and caking, *J. Pharm. Sci.*, 52:757–762, 1031–1038 (1963).

49. B. Ecanow, B. Gold, and C. Ecanow, Newer aspects of suspension theory, *Am. Perfum. Cosmet.*, 84: Nov. 27–31 (1969).

50. B. Ecanow and H. Takruri, Flocculation theory and polysorbate 80 sulfaguanidine suspensions, *J. Pharm. Sci.*, 59:1848–1849 (1970).

51. B. Ecanow, J. Webster, and M. I. Blake, Conductivity studies of suspension systems in different states of aggregation, *J. Pharm. Sci.*, 71:456–457 (1982).

52. A. S. Michaels and J. C. Bolger, The plastic flow behavior of flocculated kaolin suspension, *Ind. Eng. Chem. Fundam.*, 1:153–162 (1962).

53. R. A. Nash and B. A. Haeger, Stable syringeable suspensions of parenteral drugs in complex floc form, U.S. Patent 3,457,548, July 22, 1969.

54. J. L. Zatz, Physical stability of suspensions, *J. Soc. Cosmet. Chem.*, 36:393–441 (1985).

55. R. J. Meyer and L. Cohen, Rheology of natural and synethetic hydrophilic polymer solutions and related to suspending ability, *J. Soc. Cosmet. Chem.*, 10: May, 1–11 (1959).

56. C. W. Chong, Factors influencing the selection of suspending agents, *J. Soc. Cosmet. Chem.*, 14:123–133 (1963).

57. H. Bernstein and M. Barr, *J. Am. Pharm. Assoc. Sci. Ed.*, 44:375–377 (1955).

58. T. H. Simon, H. G. DeKay, and G. S. Banker, Effects of processing on the rheology of thixotropic suspensions, *J. Pharm. Sci.*, 50:880–885 (1961).

59. H. J. Schneiderwirth, U.S. Patent 2,487,600, Nov. 8, 1949, assigned to Sharp & Dohme.

60. J. C. Samyn, An industrial approach to suspension formulation, *J. Pharm. Sci.*, 50:517–522 (1961).

61. S. Riegelman, Third Annual National Industrial Pharmaceutical Research Conference, Land O'Lakes, WI, 1961.

62. B. J. Idson and A. J. Scheer, Suspensions. Technical bulletin, FMC Corporation, Philadelphia, PA 19103.

63. D. A. Rawlins and J. B. Kayes, Steric stabilization of suspensions. *Drug Dev. Ind. Pharm.*, 6:427–440 (1980).

64. L. Carino and H. Mollet, Wetting of a powder by aqueous solutions of surface active agents, *Powder Technol.*, 11:189–194 (1975).

65. R. A. Nash and B. E. Haeger, Zeta potential in the development of pharmaceutical suspensions, *J. Pharm. Sci.*, 55:829–837 (1966).

66. T. Mitsui and S. Takada, On factors influencing dispersibility and wettability of powder in water, *J. Soc. Cosmet. Chem.*, 20:335–351 (1969).

67. T. M. Riddick, *Control of Colloid Stability Through Zeta Potential*. Livingston Publishing Co., Wynnewood, PA, 1967.

68. J. L. Zatz and R. Lue, Effect of polyols on physical stability of suspensions containing nonionic surfactants, *J. Soc. Cosmet. Chem.*, 33:149–155 (1982).

69. M. J. Akers, A. L. Fites, and R. L. Robinson. Formulation design and development of parenteral suspensions. J. Parenter. Sci. Technol., 41:88–96 (1987).

70. T. L. Grimes, Scaleup and manufacture of sterile suspensions. American Pharmaceutical Association, 133rd Annual Meeting, San Francisco, March 19, 1986.

71. J. B. Portnoff, The development of sterile suspensions—Case Studies American Pharmaceutical Association, 133rd Annual Meeting, San Francisco, March 19, 1986.

72. R. A. Nash, Parenteral suspensions, *Bull. Parenter. Drug. Assoc.*, 26:91–95 (1972).

73. B. Misek and D. M. Skauen, Study of dispersion with ultrasound, *J. Am. Pharm. Assoc., Sci. Ed.,* 47:32–36 (1958).
74. U.S. Patents 2,504,482, Apr. 18, 1050; and 2,622,598, Dec. 23, 1952, assigned to Premo Pharmaceutical Laboratories.
75. T. C. Patton, Pigment suspension in paint vehicles, *J. Paint Technol.,* 38:387–397 (1966).
76. W. R. Markland, Pigment suspending in nail polish, *Norda Briefs,* No. 468, July–August, 1975, Norda, Inc., New York.
77. C. Kahn and C. J. R. Eichhorn, Organically modified clay mastergels, a new approach to cosmetic formulating, *Cosmet. Perfum.,* 89: Dec., 31–35 (1974).
78. A. J. Scheer, Practical guidelines for suspension formulation, *Drug. Cosmet. Ind.,* 129: April–June, 1981.
79. J. E. Tingstad, Physical stability testing of pharmaceuticals, *J. Pharm. Sci.,* 53:955–962 (1964).
80. B. A. Matthews and C. T. Rhodes, Coulter Counter for investigating mixed monodisperse particulate systems, *J. Colloid Interface Sci.,* 28:71–81 (1968).
81. B. A. Matthews and C. T. Rhodes, Coulter Counter Model B in coagulation studies, *J. Colloid Interface Sci.,* 32:339–348 (1970).
82. W. Pietsch, *Size Enlargement by Agglomeration,* J. Wiley & Sons, New York, NY, 1991.
83. P. H. Cardwell, Adsorption studies using a streaming current detector, *J. Colloid Interface Sci.,* 22:430–437 (1960).
84. S. Ross and R. P. Long, Electrophoresis as method of investigating electric double layer, *Ind. Eng. Chem.,* 61: October 58–71 (1969).
85. J. B. Kayes, Pharmaceutical suspensions: Microelectrophoretic properties, *J. Pharm. Pharmacol.,* 29:163–168, 199–204 (1977).
86. R. J. Akers, Zeta potential and the use of the electrophoretic mass transport analyzer, *Am. Lab.,* June 1972, 41–53.

2

Pharmaceutical Emulsions and Microemulsions

Lawrence H. Block

Duquesne University, Pittsburgh, Pennsylvania

I. EMULSION AND MICROEMULSION CHARACTERISTICS AND ATTRIBUTES

A. Emulsions

In classical terms, emulsions are colloidal dispersions comprising two immiscible liquids (e.g., oil and water), one of which (the internal or discontinuous phase) is dispersed as droplets within the other (the external or continuous phase). The droplets of the dispersed phase are polydisperse spherical particles formed by subjecting the emulsion components to a milling or comminution process. Given the free energy associated with the interface between two immiscible liquids, the concomitant substantial increase in interfacial area results in a thermodynamically unstable system that tends to revert back to the original two-phase system with its minimum interfacial area. Amphiphilic molecules added to the system migrate preferentially to the interface between the liquids. Their interfacial adsorption is accompanied by a lowering of interfacial tension and a rise in interfacial viscosity. The net effect is a marked increase in the stability of the emulsion.

The classical definition of emulsions also embraces systems that are extensions of two-phase emulsions in which the discontinuous, or internal, phases themselves comprise emulsified systems. Each internal phase, in turn, may be polydisperse; in this manner, tertiary, quaternary, and even higher order emulsions, with more than one discontinuous phase, may be possible [1]. Thus, double and multiple emulsions (e.g., oil-in-water-in-oil, O/W/O; water-in-oil-in-water, W/O/W; three-phase systems with multiple drop formation) correspond to the classical definition. In actuality, if the nature of the stabilizing moiety and the structure of the system are considered, an even broader array of emulsion types exists than that encompassed by the historic definition of emulsions as two-liquid systems. Thus, two-liquid systems stabilized by a third nonliquid phase (e.g., solid particles or lyotropic liquid crystals) and three-liquid systems are also appropriately described as emulsion systems [1–4]. The potential complex-

47

ity of emulsion systems is exemplified by Bevacqua et al. [1], who describe a five-phase emulsion containing liquid crystals, an aqueous gel phase, a perfluorinated oil phase, and water dispersed within a continuous silicone fluid.

Stable emulsions represent an effective formulation approach for the resolution of problems in drug and cosmetic agent delivery. Rieger [5] cites patient (consumer) acceptance as the most important reason for the popularity of emulsions for oral and topical formulations: disagreeable taste or mouth feel of a drug can be dealt with by placing the drug in the internal phase of an emulsion surrounded by an inert, external phase. The interjection of an inert phase between the drug and the biosurface eliminates or minimizes the likelihood of detection of objectionable tastes or sensations. Interestingly, Gardner [6] links the relative bitterness of compounds to their lipophilicity: Thus, the very compounds that may be most unpalatable may be most readily administered via the internal phase of an emulsion system. Topically applied formulations may be more acceptable to patients as emulsions than as single-phase systems because components that have poor skin feel or spreadability or that may stain clothing can be placed in the internal phase of the emulsion. Ease of administration may also play a role in the acceptability of emulsions. For oral or topical use, for example, emulsion systems may be easier to administer or apply than other disperse systems such as suspensions. The water-washability of topically applied emulsions may be advantageous to the user. Finally, where efficacy is not adversely affected by dilution, emulsions may be economically advantageous to the manufacturer and consumer by permitting the use of lower concentrations of relatively expensive water-immiscible components.

Increased efficacy may also result from emulsification: gastrointestinal absorption of poorly absorbed species such as markedly lipophilic compounds, poorly water-soluble compounds, peptides, proteins, or polymers can often be enhanced by presentation in the form of an emulsion [7–9]. Increased peroral bioavailability of a compound administered in an emulsion formulation may stem from an increase in the concentration or amount of the absorbable (molecularly dispersed) species relative to the total, from a formulation component (e.g., fatty acid)–induced decrease in gastrointestinal motility, or from increased endocytotic uptake. There are limited data that suggest that emulsions may also offer an alternative to liposomal formulations as vehicles that allow preferential drug uptake by the reticuloendothelial system and by inflammatory cells [10,11]. Lymphatic uptake or targeting of drugs can be enhanced by the use of emulsion systems [9,11–13].

Administration of poorly water-soluble drugs in solution is often not practical, because of the large solution volume required to deliver an effective dose. Even when water-miscible cosolvents are used to formulate solutions with higher solute concentrations, drug precipitation often occurs upon solution addition to other fluids or, in the case of intravenous formulations, infusion into blood. Emulsion formulation may overcome this problem of limited solubility and miscibility [11,14]. Emulsification has made intravenous administration of lipid nutrients practical for malnourished or stressed patients [15].

Gases such as oxygen, nitrogen, and carbon dioxide have solubilities in water-immiscible perfluorocarbons (e.g., perfluorodecalin, perfluorotripropylamine, and perfluorotributylamine) that are an order of magnitude greater than those in water or plasma [16]. Accordingly, emulsified perfluorocarbon formulations have been considered for use as oxygen-transport fluids or blood substitutes [17].

Release of an active species from an emulsion system, prior to its appearance at the absorption site, may also be prolonged due to either the necessity for partitioning of the species in the emulsion system or decreased diffusivity resulting from species interaction with formulation components, increased inter- or intraphase microscopic viscosity, or the lengthening of the species' diffusion path length due to obstruction by the dispersed phase. Thus, emulsion formulations have also been employed parenterally (intramuscularly) to retard drug release and provide a prolonged effect not obtainable with other formulations [12,18–20].

B. Microemulsions

The concept of microemulsions was first introduced by Schulman in 1943 [21] and applied to systems prepared by first dispersing an oil in an aqueous surfactant solution and then adding a sufficient amount of a fourth component, generally an intermediate chain length alcohol, to form a transparent system. Although a vast literature on these systems has developed since Schulman's initial efforts [22–24], there has been and continues to be substantial controversy as to the exact nature of these systems and the appropriateness of the terminology [25]. Terms such as transparent emulsions, micellar solutions, solubilized systems, and swollen micelles have all been applied to the same or similar systems. As Hiemenz [25] notes, the confusion in the literature is a reflection of the differences in perspective among those in the field. According to some, microemulsions are liquid-liquid disperse systems; others view them as micellar systems. Nonetheless, emulsions and microemulsions may be differentiated on the basis of particle size: microemulsions contain particles at least an order of magnitude smaller (i.e., 10–100 nm) than those in conventional emulsions that contain particles at the upper end of the colloidal size range (100–100,000 nm). Thus, conventional emulsions are termed *coarse emulsions* or *macroemulsions* when contrasted with *microemulsions*. More recently, the phrase *submicron emulsion* has been applied to emulsions that possess a dispersed phase mean droplet diameter under 1 μm (i.e., < 1000 nm) [26].

The small particle size of microemulsions corresponds to a very large interfacial area and a correspondingly large free energy contribution from the liquid-liquid interfacial tension, $\gamma_{o/w}$. Ruckenstein and Chi [27] have shown theoretically that the thermodynamic stability of microemulsions results from the entropic changes brought about when $\gamma_{o/w}$ is sufficiently small (typically, $\gamma_{o/w} \leq 0.01$ dynes/cm). Nonetheless, the physical stability of microemulsions and the spontaneity of their formation are hard to reconcile with the concept of microemulsions as disperse systems. Thus, microemulsions are more aptly described in terms of the degree of solubilization attained [25], with surfactant micelles at one end of the spectrum, emulsion droplets at the other end, and micelles with varying degrees of solubilization in between. There is also some indication in the literature that the kinetics of solubilization are dependent upon the degree of solubilization and consistent with a micelle-emulsion droplet transition [28]. Given the current inability to determine the point at which the micellar core is indistinguishable from a bulk oil phase, Attwood [29] considers the definition proposed by Danielsson and Lindman to be most appropriate: a microemulsion is "a system of water, oil and amphiphile which is a single optically isotropic and thermodynamically stable liquid." For the formulator, the inference to be drawn is that phase diagrams, relating composition and temperature, are the most appropriate link to understanding system behavior [25,30–34].

Microemulsion technology has been extensively and successfully applied in areas as diverse as microencapsulation, polymer synthesis by emulsion polymerization, and tertiary oil recovery from natural reservoirs (oil fields). Nonetheless, there is growing recognition of the potential utility of microemulsions for cosmetic and pharmaceutical applications [33,34] as a result of the distinct differences between macro- and micro-emulsions. Ritschel [35] has described the formulation and evaluation of microemulsion-based gastrointestinal delivery systems for cyclosporine, insulin, and vasopressin.

C. Distinctions between Macroemulsions and Microemulsions

Schulman's early studies of microemulsions emphasized the light transmission characteristics of microemulsions. Whereas macroemulsions were ordinarily opaque, micro-emulsions were transparent or translucent (opalescent), a reflection of their much smaller particle size (generally, less than one-quarter the wavelength of light). More recent studies have emphasized the relative stability and ease of formation of microemulsions rather than their transparency. Macroemulsions, though they may have some physical stability, ultimately will coalesce. Microemulsions, in contrast, are generally considered to be thermodynamically stable, although examples of unstable microemulsions can be found [23,24]. Macroemulsion formation generally requires vigorous mixing or comminution, whereas microemulsions tend to form spontaneously. Safran [36] regards this spontaneity of solubilization of water in oil or oil in water via the surfactant as the distinguishing feature of microemulsions. Furthermore, microemulsions can also accommodate substantial proportions of the dispersed phase (ca. 20–40%), often without corresponding increases in viscosity [37]; there is some evidence for shear thinning at high internal phase volume ratios [38]. Thus, microemulsions ought to be considered as viable alternatives to classical macroemulsions for both cosmetic and pharmaceutical applications.

II. FORMULATION COMPONENTS

A wide variety of natural and synthetic ingredients have been employed in emulsion formulations. The lack of an all-inclusive, nonempirical approach to emulsion formulation to date is a reflection of the chemical and physicochemical diversity of the components of pharmaceutical and cosmetic emulsions.

A. Immiscible Phases

Table 1 lists a number of immiscible phase components, apart from emulsifiers and emulsion stabilizers, preservatives, antioxidants, and other functional ingredients, that can be a part of a pharmaceutical or cosmetic emulsion system. Clearly, the concept of emulsions as systems composed of two immiscible liquids is an anachronism. Dispersions containing three (or more) mutually insoluble fluids can be prepared: Bader et al. [39] have advocated the use of perfluoropolyethers as water- and oil-insoluble components for cosmetic and pharmaceutical products; some immiscible silicone oils may require formulation as multiphase emulsions. Just as emulsions are not restricted to systems composed of only two immiscible liquids, there is no requirement that the polar immiscible phase be water or that phase components be liquid. The limited cosmetic and pharmaceutical literature on nonaqueous emulsion technology is evidence of the bias of formulators toward aqueous systems. Nonetheless, other polar immiscible liquids such

Table 1 Some Immiscible Phase Components

Polar ingredients
  Polyols
    Butylene glycol
    Glycerin
    Polyethylene glycols
    Propylene glycol
  Water
Nonpolar ingredients
  Esters
    Fats
    Lanolin
    Synthetics (e.g., isopropyl myristate, isopropyl
      palmitate, glyceryl monostearate)
    Vegetable oils
  Ethers
    Perfluoropolyethers
    Polyoxypropylenes
  Fatty acids
  Fatty alcohols
  Hydrocarbons
    Butane, propane
    Microcrystalline waxes
    Mineral oils
    Petrolatum
    Squalene
  Miscellaneous
    Halohydrocarbons (e.g., perfluorocarbons;
      chlorofluorocarbons)
    Waxes, plant and animal
    Silicone fluids

as various glycols (e.g., propylene glycol, glycerin, polyethylene glycol) can, in fact, be effectively employed in emulsion systems. Petersen and Hamill [40] have formulated a variety of glycol–olive oil emulsions with anionic, cationic, and nonionic surfactants: glycerin–olive oil emulsions were more stable than propylene glycol– or polyethylene glycol 400–olive oil emulsions. Potential advantages of nonaqueous emulsions, vis-a-vis aqueous emulsions, include increased viscosity, improved emulsion stability, greater stability of emulsion components subject to degradation involving a polar transition state, and increased system solubility of less polar solutes. Finally, many emulsion system components incorporated as fluids at elevated temperatures congeal as the temperature is lowered, forming solid-liquid dispersions. Yet, the notion persists that an emulsion is a two-phase system made up of incompletely miscible liquids.

B. Emulsifiers/Emulsion Stabilizers

Macroemulsion formation results from two competing processes: disruption of the interface(s) between bulk, immiscible phases and stabilization of the dispersed phase(s) once formed [41]. Dispersal of one immiscible phase within another can be accomplished through mechanical means (e.g., by agitation). Emulsifiers decrease the energy required to disrupt phase continuity and achieve complete phase dispersal by lowering interfacial tension. In the absence of an emulsion stabilizer, however, droplets of the dispersed phase will subsequently either flocculate (i.e., associate reversibly with one another) or coalesce (i.e., merge to form larger droplets).

1. *Emulsifiers*

The reduction of interfacial tension by emulsifiers is a direct result of their adsorption at the interface. It has long been held that the affinity of such surface-active agents (surfactants) for the interfacial region facilitates the formation of a relatively rigid film of the emulsifier at the interface that acts as a mechanical barrier to droplet adhesion and coalescence. Thus, as a generalization (not always borne out by the data), emulsion stability will increase as the surface viscosity and yield value of the film increase [42]. There is mounting evidence for emulsion stabilization by liquid crystal formation in the interphase (the interfacial region) and in the vicinity of adjacent droplets of the disperse phase [23,43].

An additional consideration is the effect of the surfactant phase on the efficiency of emulsification. Pasternacki-Surian et al. [44] investigated the efficiency of perfluorocarbon emulsification by polyoxyethylene oleyl ether surfactants and found that, in general, emulsions prepared at temperatures where the surfactant was in a lamellar-to-isotropic surfactant solution transition were more efficiently emulsified—that is, had less perfluorocarbon separation upon emulsion centrifugation at 25°C. Their findings corroborate other data in the literature regarding surfactant phase–influenced efficiency of emulsification and the isotropic surfactant solution phase (designated L_3), in particular [45]: solubilization capacity tends to be maximal at temperatures favoring the L_3 phase; the composite interfacial tensions among system components reach a minimum; and the interphase becomes more flexible compared to that formed by a rigid lamellar surfactant phase.

The nature and intensity of the interactive electrical forces between emulsion droplets may also be influenced by surfactants (especially ionic ones) with a concomitant effect on emulsion stability. The classification of surfactant types provided in Table 2 is based on the ionic charge of the surfactant [46,47]. The diverse, multifunctional character of surfactants in emulsion systems renders their selection for emulsion systems difficult and empirical at best. In 1913, Bancroft recognized the impact of emulsifier solubility on the type of emulsion formed: the phase in which the emulsifying agent is most soluble tends to form the continuous phase of the emulsion [48]. Not until Griffin's [49] introduction of the HLB (hydrophile-lipophile balance) concept in 1949 and his subsequent development of it in the 1950s [50] was the formulator provided with a means of characterizing surfactants in a manner that was relevant to emulsion formulation. The HLB system provided a scale of surfactant hydrophilicity (0–20) that simplified emulsifier selection and blending. Surfactants with a low HLB (≤ 6) tended to provide stable water-in-oil (W/O) emulsions; those with a high HLB (≥ 8) tended to stabilize O/W emulsions. The admixture of surfactants of known HLB to provide a blend with an HLB appropriate to the emulsification of the water-immiscible phase was but a matter of alligation or algebraic manipulation; if a and b are the HLBs of surfactants A and B, respectively, and the desired HLB is c, then the proportional parts required of surfactants A and B are x and y, respectively:

$$\frac{x}{y} = \frac{(c-a)}{(a-c)} \qquad\qquad (1a)$$

or

Table 2 Surfactant Classification

Type	Examples[a]
Anionic	Alcohol ether sulfates
	Alkyl sulfates (30–40)
	Soaps (12–20)
	Sulfosuccinates
Cationic	Quaternary ammonium compounds (30)
Zwitterionic	Alkyl betaine derivatives
Amphoteric	Fatty amine sulfates
	Difatty alkyl triethanolamine derivatives (16–17)
Nonionic	Lanolin alcohols (1)
	Polyoxyethylated (POE) alkyl phenols (12–13)
	POE fatty amide
	POE fatty alcohol ether
	POE fatty amine
	POE fatty ester
	Poloxamers (7–19)
	POE glycol monoethers (13–16)
	Polysorbates (10–17)
	Sorbitan esters (2–9)

[a]The HLB number or range of HLB numbers encompassed by a surfactant type is given in parentheses, where available.

$$HLB_{blend} = fHLB_A + (1 - f) HLB_B \qquad (1b)$$

where f is the fraction of surfactant A in the surfactant blend.

The HLB system is simple and easily implemented. Approximations of the HLB for those surfactants not described by Griffin can be made either from the characterization of their water dispersibility [51] (Table 3) or from an experimental estimation of their HLBs: blends of the unknown emulsifier in varying ratios with an emulsifier of known HLB are used to emulsify an oil of known "required" HLB. The blend that performs best is assumed to have an HLB value approximately equal to the "required" HLB of the oil. Davies and Rideal [52] suggested an empirical calculation of HLB based upon the positive or negative contribution of various functional groups to the overall hydrophilicity of a surfactant. These "group numbers" (Table 4) are employed in the calculation of HLB from the following equation:

Table 3 HLB Estimation of Surfactants Based on Water Dispersibility

HLB range	Water dispersibility
1–4	Not dispersible
3–6	Poor dispersion
6–8	Milky dispersion only after vigorous agitation
8–10	Stable milky dispersion
10–13	Translucent to clear dispersion
≥ 13	Clear solution

Source: Ref. 50.

$$\text{HLB} = \sum(\text{hydrophilic group numbers}) - \sum(\text{lipophilic group numbers}) + 7 \quad (2)$$

Griffin's HLB system, based upon the percentage weight of the hydrophilic component of the amphiphilic compound, is no panacea. The HLB is influenced by the nature of the immiscible phase, other adjuvants, emulsifier concentration, phase volume, temperature, and processing method [53]. The rheological behavior of the emulsion system and its effect on emulsion stability are not accounted for by the HLB relationship. In fact, emulsion stability may be unrelated to HLB value: stable O/W emulsions can be prepared throughout the range of HLB values from ≤ 2 to ≥ 17 [54]. Direct calculation of HLB values is not applicable to poloxamers (e.g., polyoxyethylene-polyoxypropylene block polymers), ionic surfactants, or nitrogen- or sulfur-containing surfactants. Finally, in spite of the long-accepted view that the HLBs of mixtures of surfactants could be calculated on the basis of algebraic additivity, Becher and Birkmeier [55] have indicated that the actual HLB of surfactant blends may diverge from calculated values. Nonetheless, in spite of these shortcomings, the HLB system has been widely adopted by formulators for emulsifier selection and blending and continues to find acceptance among technologists. There is a growing recognition that the principal drawback to HLB numbers is that they are not indicative of emulsion behavior or stability because they are a reflection of the isolated surfactant molecule rather than of the emulsion system. In contrast, the phase inversion temperature (PIT) concept introduced by Shinoda [56] is a characteristic of the emulsion system, not of the surfactant alone—at least for systems employing nonionic surfactants. The PIT, defined as the temperature at which the emulsion inverts (i.e., from W/O to O/W or vice versa), can be related to the same factors

Table 4 HLB Group Numbers[a]

Group		Group no.
Hydrophilic moieties:	$-SO_4^=Na^+$	38.7
	$-COO\text{-}K^+$	21.1
	$-COO\text{-}Na^+$	19.1
	$-SO_3\text{-}Na^+$	11.0
	R_3N	9.4
	Ester (sorbitan ring)	6.8
	Ester (free)	2.4
	$-COOH$	2.1
	$-OH$ (free)	1.9
	$-O-$	1.3
	$-OH$ (sorbitan ring)	0.5
	$-(OCH_2CH_2)-$	0.33
	$-(OCH_2CH)-$	0.15
Lipophilic moieties:	$-CH-, -CH_2-, -CH_3, =CH-$	0.475
	$-CF_2-, -CF_3$	0.870

[a]The sum of the lipophilic moiety HLB group numbers of a surfactant subtracted from the sum of the hydrophilic moiety group numbers should provide an estimate of the HLB of the amphiphile. The more hydrophilic the surfactant, the larger the HLB.
Source: Ref. 52.

as can HLB number: hydrophilic-lipophilic character of the surfactant, type of oil phase, emulsion type, and other emulsion components. However, although the PIT can be related to emulsifier concentration and phase volume, the HLB number dependency of these latter factors is problematical.

It must be emphasized that HLB numbers and PITs (also termed HLB temperatures) are of value, principally, for nonionic surfactants. As Shinoda and Kunieda [56] pointed out, ionic and nonionic emulsifiers of the same HLB number do not behave similarly. Furthermore, PIT is usually not observed for ionic surfactants, as the temperature-dependence of their HLB number is minimal. Thus, the application of these concepts to ionic surfactants is less appropriate. If, however, phase composition is altered (e.g., electrolyte concentrations or counterions are changed) or cosurfactants are added, the HLB number may vary and a distinct PIT may become discernible.

Given the dependency of HLB number or PIT on a wide variety of factors, surfactant selection on the basis of these parameters alone, especially HLB, remains highly empirical. A more appropriate approach to surfactant selection involves the use of optimization techniques where initial consideration is given to the PIT or the required HLB number for various immiscible phase components followed by preliminary formulation work.

Alternatively, the "maximum solubilization" method proposed by Lin [57,58] for O/W emulsion formulation may be of value. This method is based upon the inverse correlation between the maximum amount of the aqueous phase that can be solubilized in the oil phase containing the surfactant and the average droplet size of the O/W *macro*emulsion subsequently formed when the W/O *micro*emulsion is inverted by additional aqueous phase (Fig. 1). Experimentally, the surfactant or surfactant blend is dissolved in the oil phase and the aqueous phase then added dropwise with agitation until turbidity persists. In effect, maximal solubilization corresponds to lower interfacial tension and correspondingly greater efficiency of emulsification. This method is potentially useful even for mixtures of ionic and nonionic surfactants.

Blends of surfactants are often employed as the emulsifier in formulations rather than single surfactants as the resultant emulsions tend to be more stable. Multiple surfactant systems that have been studied include mixtures of amphiphilic compounds, such as fatty alcohols, with anionic, cationic, or nonionic surfactants. Such amphiphilic compounds, though relatively weak emulsifying agents, can provide increased emulsion stability and better control of consistency. These mixed surfactant effects have been attributed to increased density or closer packing of surfactant molecules at the oil-water interface [59]. However, surfactant concentrations are far in excess of that required to form a close-packed interfacial film [60]. Furthermore, oil-water interfacial viscosity for mixed surfactant systems does not appear to be markedly elevated [61]. It is the substantially more viscoelastic character of the mixed-surfactant emulsion system that is most likely responsible for the improvements noted [61,62].

2. *Emulsion Stabilizers*

Following emulsification, emulsion stabilization can be achieved through interference with creaming, droplet flocculation or coalescence. Thus, stability can be conferred by equalizing phase densities, increasing the viscosity of the continuous phase, or by ad-

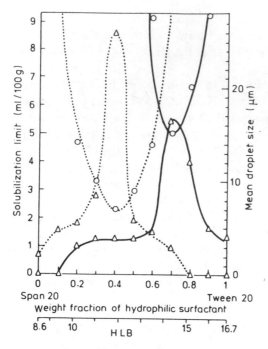

Fig. 1 Shift of optimum emulsification peak by addition of lauryl alcohol: emulsions contain 30% oil phase, 65% deionized water, and 5% surfactant mixtures. Surfactant mixtures consist of hydrophilic Tween 20 and lipophilic Span 20 at ratios and corresponding HLB values indicated by abscissa. Dotted lines (·····) represent data for pure mineral oil systems; solid lines (——) represent data for oil mixture consisting of eight parts mineral oil and two parts lauryl alcohol. Circles (○) and triangles (Δ) show mean droplet size and solubilization limit, respectively. (From Ref. 54.)

sorbing stabilizing substances at the oil-water interface. These interventions can be described in terms of Stokes' equation (for sedimentation or creaming):

$$\frac{dh}{dt} = \frac{2(\rho_1 - \rho_2)r^2 g}{9\eta} \tag{3}$$

and Einstein's equation (for diffusion):

$$D = \frac{kT}{6\pi\eta r} \tag{4}$$

where dh/dt is the change in height with time, ρ_1 and ρ_2 are the densities of phases 1 and 2, respectively, η is the Newtonian viscosity, r is the radius of the emulsion droplet, g is gravitational acceleration, D is the diffusivity of the emulsion droplet, k is the Boltzmann constant, and T is temperature (°K). When sedimentation or creaming is hindered by interparticulate interaction—e.g., when the internal phase or drop volume fraction ϕ exceeds 0.005–0.02—Stokes' equation is not strictly applicable. T. Higuchi [63] likened the problem to the flow or movement of the continuous phase through a bed of packed particles and proposed the use of a modification of the Kozeny equation for such "concentrated" dispersions:

$$\frac{dV}{dt} = \frac{(\rho_1 - \rho_2)g}{K\eta A^2}\left[\frac{\varepsilon^2}{1-\varepsilon}\right] \tag{5}$$

where V is the volume of the continuous phase, K is the Kozeny constant, A is the specific surface area, and ε is the "bed" porosity. As particle size and particle size distribution are not an explicit part of this relationship, this modified Kozeny equation is more appropriate for the relatively concentrated polydisperse systems encountered in pharmaceutical and cosmetic products. In any event, whether one invokes the Stokes or the Kozeny equation, the rate of emulsion droplet translocation decreases as the difference in density between the immiscible phases decreases. Phase density equalization— or density matching—minimizes the rate of approach of droplets to one another, thus decreasing the rate of flocculation. Some adjuvants employed to effect phase density equalization include polyols (e.g., glycerin or propylene glycol) for the polar phase and brominated vegetable oils or perfluoropolyethers for the nonpolar phase. The most serious limitation to density matching as a means of stabilizing emulsion systems is the temperature dependency of $(\rho_1 - \rho_2)$, which is a reflection of the thermal expansion coefficients for the respective phases.

The formulator should also appreciate the fact that Stokes' equation was derived for Newtonian systems in which the rate of shear D is proportional to the shearing stress τ, i.e., $\tau = \eta D$, where the proportionality constant η is the coefficient of Newtonian viscosity. As many pharmaceutical and cosmetic emulsions exhibit non-Newtonian behavior in which η is a complex function of τ or D, Eqs. (3)-(5) are unlikely to provide a direct correspondence between the rate of creaming and equation parameters such as the difference in phase density or the apparent fluidity of the dispersion medium. In fact, for pseudoplastic or shear-thinning systems, for which the viscosity can often be described in terms of a power function of the form $\tau = \eta D^n$ [64,65], where n is a constant ranging between 0 and 1, the likelihood is that sedimenation rates will be more appropriately described by

$$\frac{dh}{dt} \propto (\rho_1 - \rho_2)^{1/n} \tag{6}$$

rather than the direct proportionality predicted by Stokes' equation [66].

If the particle size is small enough, thermal agitation can overcome settling or creaming. Such Brownian motion, dependent only upon the viscosity of the dispersion medium, results in particulate displacement that is proportional to $t^{1/2}$. Increasing the viscosity of the continuous phase with lyophilic colloids (e.g., carbomers, clays, polysaccharides) decreases the rate of creaming or flocculation as Eqs. (3)-(5) suggest, but as noted above for the relationship of dh/dt to the difference in phase density, the relationship is likely to be complex.

Colloidal particles in a dispersion are also subject to forces stemming from attraction (arising from London–van der Waals forces) and electrostatic repulsion (between the electrical double layers surrounding charged droplets). While attractive forces predominate at short and long distances, electrostatic repulsion predominates at intermediate distances between particles [67–69]. Accordingly, interfacial adsorption of some emulsion system components may stabilize emulsions against flocculation or coalescence. In some instances, the adsorbate stabilizes the emulsion system by preventing contact between adjacent droplets, i.e. electrostatic repulsion is enhanced. In other instances, when contact between emulsion droplets is not prevented, adsorbates stabilize emulsion droplets by preventing coalescence—i.e., by preventing or minimizing thinning and subsequent rupturing of the contiguous thin liquid film that forms between droplets upon contact.

London–van der Waals forces of attraction and electrostatic (diffuse double layer) repulsion that affect lyophobic colloid stability—generally described in terms of the DLVO (Derjaguin and Landau–Verwey and Overbeek) theory—may be supplemented by other phenomena [68,69]. These non-DLVO effects include attractive forces involving electrostatic interaction of oppositely charged particles or surfaces (mutual flocculation) or macromolecular or polymeric adsorption on more than one particle is simultaneously (steric stabilization), which can also contribute to the stabilization of a dispersion. In addition, entropic repulsion due to the loss of entropy resulting from the restriction of movement of long-chain molecules adsorbed at the droplet interface may also affect emulsion stability when particles approach one another at distances less than the sum of the lengths of the chains adsorbed on each particle. Feigin and Napper [70] proposed the existence of "depletion stabilization" wherein the concentration of segments of free polymer in solution, lowered in the vicinity of the particulate phase, can effect either flocculation or stabilization. Other interparticle effects have been described that are related to cybotaxis (i.e., ordering in the dispersion medium in the vicinity of the dispersed phase) and that become important when particles are separated by distances of less than 5 nm [69].

The potential gradient of the diffuse double layer surrounding droplets of the internal phase will be affected by changes in the ionic strength of the formulation. Thus, the stability of the product will be altered by the addition or deletion of non–surface active electrolytes as well as ionic surfactants. Rheological characteristics of emulsions may also be affected by the ionic strength of the dispersion medium: electroviscous effects have been described wherein viscosity is increased at low shear rates with the addition of electrolyte due to increased mutual repulsion of interacting diffuse double layers [71,72]. Given the potential effect of electrolytes on emulsion stability, the formulator should take note of the equations derived by Niebergall [73] which permit buffers of known pH and ionic strength to be prepared in a relatively straightforward manner.

Table 5 constitutes a partial listing of emulsion stabilizers that have been employed in pharmaceutical or cosmetic products. Natural polymers or macromolecules (e.g., hydrophilic gums; proteins) have effectively stabilized emulsions via interfacial adsorption and the subsequent formation of condensed films of high tensile strength that resist droplet coalescence [74]. A dramatic example of this has been published for emulsions stabilized with acacia [75]. Many other hydrocolloids such as the cellulose ethers (e.g., sodium carboxymethyl cellulose; methylcellulose) [76] and the carbomer resins [77] have long been employed as emulsion stabilizers though they primarily serve to increase the viscosity of the dispersion medium. Oza and Frank [78] have employed microcrystalline cellulose, in conjunction with various surfactants, to stabilize W/O/W emulsions.

Any discussion of emulsion stabilization is incomplete without a consideration of the interface and the associated interphase(s). During the emulsification process, the interfacial area increases as the radius of the dispersed phase droplets decrease. Thus, an emulsion containing 10^{12} dispersed phase droplets, each with a diameter of 2.0 μm, has an aggregate interfacial area of about 12.6 m^2; when the dispersed phase droplets are reduced to 0.2 μm in diameter, the number of droplets increases to 10^{15} and the corresponding interfacial area to 126 m^2 [79]. Thermodynamically, the work done to reduce droplet size and increase the interfacial area, ΔF, is proportional to $\gamma \Delta A$, as a first

Table 5 Miscellaneous Emulsion Stabilizers

Lyophilic colloids:		
Polysaccharides	Amphoterics	Synthetic or semisynthetic polymers
Acacia	Gelatin	Carbomer resins
Agar		Cellulose ethers
Alginic acid		Carboxymethyl chitin
Carrageenan		PEG-n (ethylene oxide
Guar gum		polymer
Karaya gum		$\approx H(OCH_2CH_2)_nOH$)
Tragacanth		
Xanthan gum		

Finely divided solids:
    Clays (attapulgite; bentonite; hectorite; kaolin; magnesium aluminum silicate; montmorillonite)
    Microcrystalline cellulose
    Oxides and hydroxides (aluminum hydroxide; magnesium hydroxide; silica (pyrogenic or
        fumed))
Cybotactic promoters, gellants:
    Amino acids; peptides; proteins (e.g. casein; β-lactoglobulin)
    Lecithin and other phospholipids
    Poloxamers

approximation, where γ is the interfacial tension and ΔA is the increase in the interfacial area. A substantial increase in the interfacial area, then, as in the above example, entails a substantial increase in surface free energy and in system instability that can be offset by adsorption at the interface and a decrease in γ. It is this potential for adsorption—accompanying the reduction in particle size—that is responsible, in large measure, for the marked effect of variations in adjuvant source on the stability of these disperse systems. Source variations may involve ingredient composition (e.g. presence of surface-active impurities, molecular weight distribution, degree of substitution) or physical properties (e.g., surface area, porosity, density, etc.)

Various thermodynamic treatments of adsorption phenomena have attempted to facilitate modeling by characterizing the region between one phase and another as an infinitely thin *boundary* rather than the *inhomogeneous region* that it is [80,81]. Nonetheless, this inhomogeneous interfacial region or interphase (also termed the mesophase by Groves [82,83]) defines the physical properties and stability of an emulsion and justifies further attention of researchers and formulators. One representation of the interphase is depicted in Fig. 2 [84].

Though formulators may rarely employ finely divided solids as emulsion stabilizers per se, they should be aware that pharmaceutical and cosmetic emulsions often include solid particles. Even when no solid is knowingly added, Adamson [85] hypothesizes that emulsion stabilization by solids at the liquid-liquid interface may be involved: whenever the surface film is sufficiently rigid or in sufficiently slow equilibrium with the bulk phases, film material may be ejected as a solid or gel phase as a result of droplet coalescence or mechanically induced distortions in droplet shapes. Finely divided solids (preferably in the colloidal size range), wetted to some extent both by water and by oil, tend to accumulate at the oil-water interface, thereby serving as emulsion stabiliz-

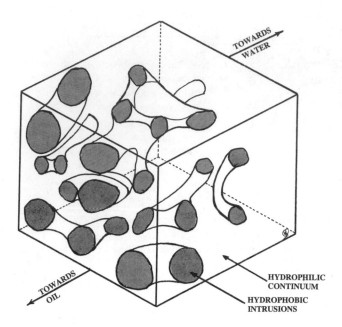

Fig. 2 A plausible schematic representation of a segment of an anisotropic interphase (mesophase) structure comprising a "bicontinuous gyroid with channels from one side to the other." The hydrophobic intrusions become more substantial in the vicinity of the oil phase. (From Ref. 84.)

ers [2,86–88]. Clays, in particular, may become very effective emulsifiers or emulsion stabilizers, especially when an organic compound is adsorbed on their surface. Due to the difference in polarity of charge on edge and face surfaces of clay particles (platelets), one can expect that organic cations will be adsorbed at the negative faces and organic anions at the positive edges, while polar unionized organic species will be adsorbed on both hydrophilic surfaces. Thus, for clay-organic cation complexes, the face surfaces of the clay become oleophilic, whereas the edge surfaces remain hydrophilic, because no adsorption of the organic cation occurs on these surfaces [88]. Ciullo and Braun [89] have used combinations of magnesium aluminum silicates and various carbomers to effectively stabilize O/W emulsions, presumably due to synergistic rheological interactions in the *external* phase.

Solids may modify emulsion stability by altering the rheological behavior of the interfacial film. According to van Olphen [90], optimum emulsifying ability of an equivalent-exchange complex of a clay and an organic cation appears to be due in part to a substantial increase in viscosity of the interphase. Another way that solids may affect the stability of an emulsion is by modifying the rheological behavior of the *external* phase. If sufficient solid is present in the external phase to alter its rheology, the properties of the final product are likely to change. Furthermore, if the solids content increases the density or effective radius of the *dispersed* phase droplets, there can be a concomitant loss in stability.

Lissant [91] notes that knowledge of the interactions among immiscible liquids and solids—wetting phenomena—can facilitate the preparation of stable dispersions because solid particle localization at the liquid-liquid interface tends to stabilize emulsions by preventing coalescence. If the solid particles are larger than the dispersed liquid droplets and the latter have a tendency to engulf the solid, the solid particles, acting as scavengers for the dispersed liquid, will facilitate coalescence. Thus, Friberg and coworkers [3] advocate the use of solid particles, as emulsion stabilizers, which are small in comparison to the emulsion droplets and which preferentially adsorb at the interface. The incremental addition of surfactant to modify and optimize solid-liquid interactions, as recommended by Friberg et al. [3], may improve stability with smaller amounts of surfactant than would be required in the absence of the finely divided solids.

Wetting phenomena, which involve the replacement of air on the surface of a solid by a liquid, can be described in terms of contact angles and spreading coefficients. Traditionally, the contact angle θ between a solid particle and a liquid has been related to the surface and interfacial energies by means of the Young and Dupre equation:

$$\cos \theta = \frac{\gamma_{SL_1} - \gamma_{SL_2}}{\lambda_{L_1L_2}} \tag{7}$$

where γ is the interfacial free energy at the interfaces denoted by the subscripts SL_1, SL_2, and L_1L_2, which refer to the interfaces between the solid and the first liquid, the solid and the second liquid, and to both liquids, respectively. An alternative relationship between θ and molecular forces acting at the interfaces has been derived by Bikerman [92]. When $\theta > 90°$, wetting does not take place. When θ is $0°$, the solid is wetted by the liquid. The relationship between the two liquids, L_1 and L_2, and the solid is shown schematically in Fig. 3. For intermediate contact angles or degrees of wetting, where $0° < \theta < 90°$, the driving force for spreading of the liquids on the solid surface can be defined in terms of a wetting or spreading coefficient S for each of the phases in accordance with the derivation by Torza and Mason [94]:

$$S_S = \gamma_{L_1L_2} - [\gamma_{SL_1} + \gamma_{SL_2}] \tag{8}$$

$$S_{L_1} = \gamma_{SL_2} - [\gamma_{SL_1} + \gamma_{L_1L_2}] \tag{9}$$

$$S_{L_2} = \gamma_{SL_1} - [\gamma_{SL_2} + \gamma_{L_1L_2}] \tag{10}$$

Three arrays of the spreading coefficients for the respective phases can be postulated:

S_S	S_{L_1}	S_{L_2}
< 0	< 0	> 0
< 0	< 0	< 0
< 0	> 0	< 0

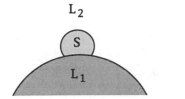
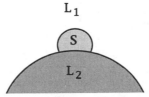

Fig. 3 Schematic representation of a solid particle, S, in the interface between two liquids, L_1 and L_2: (a) $\theta SL_1 > \theta SL_2$; (b) $\theta SL_2 > \theta SL_1$ (Adapted from Ref. 93.)

The first row of the S array corresponds to the complete engulfment of the solid by L_2; the second row, to the partial wetting of the solid by each of the liquids; and, the third row, to the complete engulfment of the solid by L_1. The addition of enough surfactant to the phase with $\theta > 90°$ in order to reduce θ to $\sim 90°$ can effect stabilization of the emulsion by the solid particles [3]. The addition of less polar cosolvents to the polar phase can have a similar effect. Given the ubiquity of solids in pharmaceutical and cosmetic emulsions, it is evident that the emulsion technologist should be conversant with contact angles and spreading coefficients and their estimation from interfacial free energies. Shanahan et al. [95] derived the following general condition that must be satisfied if either liquid is to displace the other from the solid surface, depending on which liquid makes the initial contact with the solid:

$$\left| \gamma_{SL_1} - \gamma_{SL_2} \right| < \gamma_{L_1L_2} \neq 0 \tag{11}$$

Although contact angles have been measured for a wide variety of drugs and excipients [96,97], more work remains to be done. Nonetheless, the complexity of solid–multiple liquid interactions has discouraged research in this area [91]. Factors such as the particle size of the solid relative to that of the dispersed liquid droplets, the shape of the solid particles, the volume fraction and relative density of each of the phases, and the rheological behavior of the components all affect the stability of the formulation.

Although intraphase molecular interactions in emulsion systems have been extensively studied [98], the intentional employment of solutes to alter phase structure is not routine among emulsion formulators. Various promoters of cybotaxis have been evaluated as emulsion stabilizers. Amino acids have been used along with certain *lipophilic* emulsifiers to prepare exceptionally stable w/o emulsion [99]. The effect of the amino acids involves their interaction with and immobilization of water. Successful amino acid–water–emulsifier combinations display highly ordered lamellar structures that persist in the emulsion systems prepared with them. Although a wide range of amino acids and their salts—including D- and DL-stereoisomers as well as the L-isomers—apparently function satisfactorily as W/O emulsion stabilizers in these formulations, only a limited number of emulsifiers appear to be acceptable. The latter include glyceryl oleate, glyceryl isostearate, and sorbitan sesquioleate; of these Kumano et al. [99] used glyceryl oleate extensively.

Groves et al. [82,83] have reported the effect of various amino acids, dextrose, and urea on bulk water structure through the determination of the conductivity, Λ, and viscosity, η, of aqueous solutions. The interrelationship of these properties, termed the Walden Product, is defined by Eq. (12),

$$\textit{Walden Product} = \Lambda_0\eta_0 \Rightarrow \Lambda_0\eta_c \tag{12}$$

where Λ_0 is the conductivity of a solution at infinite dilution, and η_0 is the viscosity of the solvent or continuous phase through which the ions migrate. The use of η_c—the *slope* of the viscosity-concentration curve—instead of η_0 is advantageous because it appears to be unique to the solute and is relatively unaffected by experimental error [82]. Based on their modified Walden Product, most amino acids appear to have marginal water-structure-*breaking* activity. However, L-lysine, L-glutamic acid, and L-aspartic acid, and their respective salts, all showed relatively higher activity. Dextrose, on the other hand, exhibited water-structure-*making* activity, which was shown to progressively inhibit the effect of L-lysine [82]. The effects of these solutes on water structure and on emulsion stability need to be further elucidated.

Liquid crystalline phase formation in emulsions is not uncommon when formulations include cybotactic promoters or certain mixed surfactant systems (e.g., sodium lauryl sulfate–cetyl alcohol [62]; cetearyl alcohol with various sodium *n*-alkyl sulfates [100]; cetearyl alcohol and cetrimonium bromide [101]). Indirect evidence has been provided by rheological studies [62], which have demonstrated the presence of a viscoelastic network in the continuous phase of some emulsion systems; or by thermogravimetry [100], which differentiates between bulk water and interlamellar water. Still other studies have provided more direct evidence via optical microscopy, using either polarized light [102] or differential interference contrast techniques [103]. Freeze fracture or electron microscopy techniques have proved to be useful in the structural evaluation of emulsions [104]. More recently, cryogenic scanning electron microscopy [101] has made it possible to achieve high resolution in a more direct, less time-consuming manner. Observation, direct or indirect, may not always disclose cybotaxis or structuring in emulsion systems. Friberg and Solyom [105] demonstrated that certain emulsion systems may form liquid crystalline phases under shear. Thus, for a water–*p*-xylene system emulsified with nonylphenol diethylene glycol ether, no liquid crystal phase was evident by polarized light microscopy at the outset. After shearing at a constant shear rate of 1000 sec^{-1} for several minutes, emulsion droplets were found to have increased in size and an optically anisotropic phase was now evident. Aside from their serendipitous formation in emulsion systems, liquid crystals may also be incorporated intentionally in emulsions to promote system stability and to provide a matrix for delivery of emulsion ingredients. Bevacqua and coworkers [1] have described the incorporation of thermotropic liquid crystals in multiple emulsions intended for cosmetic application. They suggest that lipophilic active ingredients can be accommodated within the liquid crystal phase while hydrophilic active ingredients can be dissolved in another of the aqueous phases, thus providing for both short- and long-term effects.

Gel polymerization of either the inner or outer aqueous phase of W/O/W multiple emulsions has been reported by Florence and Whitehill as a means of improving stability [106]. They achieved gelation of either aqueous phase by incorporating acrylamide and an appropriate crosslinking agent (*N*,*N*′-methylene-bis-acrylamide) in the phase and subsequently subjecting it to γ-irradiation to form a poly(acrylamide) gel. As residual acrylamide monomer could pose problems with regard to toxicity, it would be advantageous to use relatively nontoxic poloxamer surfactants (with an ethylene oxide content less than 70%) that could also be irradiated to form gels in the continuous aqueous phase. A principal disadvantage to the method, irrespective of the gellant, is exposure of formulation components to γ-irradiation.

C. Preservatives and Antioxidants

1. *Preservatives*

Every emulsion system is subject to microbial contamination and degradation [107]. Certainly, the safety of contaminated products must be the primary concern of the formulator. Parker [108] has discussed the clinical or pathologic significance of the microbial contamination of pharmaceutical and cosmetic products. The consequences of microbial contamination have implications for the formulation itself and may be confused with faulty product development. The product may become discolored or malodorous; instability may occur arising from emulsifier or emulsion stabilizer breakdown; product consistency may change dramatically. Esthetically, visible bacterial or fungal growth is unacceptable.

Contamination sources include raw materials, processing equipment and facilities, manufacturing personnel, and the consumer. The inclusion of an antimicrobial agent may be necessary—even when sterile components are specified and processed under aseptic conditions by the manufacturer—if the product's integrity is to be maintained during storage and use. Obviously, selection of an appropriate preservative requires consideration of the probable microbial contaminants and the spectrum of activity of the available preservatives.

The most common bacterial contaminants include *Enterobacter aerogenes*, *Bacillus subtilis*, *Flavobacterium* spp., *Klebsiella* spp., *Proteus* spp., *Pseudomonas* spp., *Salmonella* spp., and *Staphylococcus aureus*, among others; common fungal contaminants include *Penicillium* spp., *Aspergillus niger*, *Rhizopus* spp., *Candida albicans*, *Monilia*, *Torula* spp., and *Zygosaccharomyces* [107–109].

A substantial number of preservatives are available for use in pharmaceutical and cosmetic products [107,110]. However, selecting the optimal preservative or combination of preservatives for a given formulation, based solely on delinearting likely contaminants and selecting those antimicrobial agents with corresponding activity, is insufficient. Additional factors that may negate one's initial choices must be considered. These include susceptibility of the product to microbial contamination and growth, preservative compatibility with formulation components and packaging, esthetic effects (e.g., on color, taste, or odor), and safety.

Emulsion formulations prone to microbial contamination include those packaged in wide-mouthed containers or in flexible bottles or tubes that draw air back into them following use [107]. Difficulties with collapsible containers, particularly those with narrow orifices, may stem from incomplete cleaning prior to filling. Furthermore, because most emulsions employ an aqueous polar phase, these products tend to encourage or support microbial growth. The notions that the oil or nonpolar phase is hostile to bacteria or fungi and that W/O emulsions—because of the continuous oil phase—do not facilitate microbial survival or growth are incorrect [107,111]: spores of *B. subtilis* have been known to survive even in completely anhydrous vegetable oils. The preservation efficacy of "self-preserving" or "problem-free" W/O emulsions, with no antimicrobial preservative, when tested in accordance with pharmacopeial methods, has been shown to be inconsistent or unsatisfactory [111].

Microbial growth in emulsion systems may be inhibited by components that have some inherent preservative activity [112]. Typical ingredients (and the concentrations required for "self-preservation") include ethanol ($\geq$20%), sugars such as sucrose ($\approx$67%), and polyols such as propylene or hexylene glycol ($>$10%) and glycerin or sorbitol (40–50%). Below these concentrations, such components are potential nutrients that facilitate microbial growth. Loss of the self-preserving component resulting from container or closure inadequacies, temperature cycling of products during storage, or interaction with the container or with other ingredients can lead to inadequate antimicrobial activity.

In general, proteins, carbohydrates, and sterols—metabolized by bacteria and fungi—support the growth of microorganisms. Natural hydrocolloids, including cellulose derivatives, are often heavily contaminated and are also subject to microbial metabolism, as are anionic and nonionic surfactants. Cationic surfactants, on the other hand, often inhibit microbial growth. Essential oils, at high concentrations, are growth inhibitors.

Interaction of antimicrobial preservatives with formulation components can involve complexion, solubilization, partitioning, adsorption, or precipitation phenomena. Thus, preservative efficacy may also be affected by the pH of the aqueous phase or its ionic strength. Garrett and Woods [113] recognized, early on, the pH-dependent efficacy of organic acids as preservatives. They also studied the effect of partitioning of the preservative species between the oil and water phases in conjunction with the volume fraction of the phases. Horn et al. [114] demonstrated that profound adsorption of preservatives by solids could occur and result in a loss of preservative activity. Tilbury [115] and Bean et al. [116] examined preservative-surfactant interactions in emulsion systems. Though numerous workers have addressed these issues, Bean [112] and Garrett [117] have developed models that allow the formulator to estimate preservative concentration or action in emulsion systems wherein binding, solubilization, and partitioning occur. Thus, the concentration of *free* preservative C_{free} in an aqueous phase can be shown to be a function of the oil:water ratio, ϕ; the total concentration of preservative in the system, C_{tot}; the preservative's oil-water partition coefficient, $K_{o/w}$; the surfactant concentration, S; and a constant, K [112]:

$$C_{free} = \frac{C_{tot}(\phi + 1)}{K_{o/w}\phi + (SK + 1)} \tag{13}$$

It can also be shown that C_{tot} can be related to the minimum inhibitory concentration of a specific preservative species (e.g., the free acid) at a given pH for any specific (known) binding or complexing phenomena involving macromolecules or surfactants [117]. The use of these models should be tempered by the knowledge that preservative efficacy may vary with the microbial species. Thus, Yamaguchi and coworkers [118] found that butylparaben activity, in surfactant solutions, vis-a-vis *Candida albicans* was related to the free or non-solubilized acid whereas activity against *Ps. aeruginosa* was a function of the total butylparaben concentration. The emulsion formulator may also find that differences in antimicrobial preservative stability, solubility, and so on, may necessitate a different preservative for each phase.

Bean [112] notes that antimicrobial preservatives ought to be biocidal rather than biostatic although lethality of a given agent may only be a reflection of its contact time with the microorganism. In the final analysis, as antimicrobial preservatives are subject to complex interactions that may alter their effectiveness, it behooves the formulator to test the efficacy of the preservative in situ. Standardized tests of antimicrobial preservative efficacy, described in the United States Pharmacopeia and British Pharmacopoeia, should be considered part of the development phase of a formulation rather than as final tests before a product is released for distribution [111,119]. If such tests of preservative efficacy by microbiological challenge are augmented by analysis of preservative content in the aqueous phase of emulsions (following partial phase separation by ultrafiltration or ultracentrifugation) [120], empirical product development insofar as antimicrobial preservation is concerned can be minimized.

A more detailed discussion of the preservation of emulsions can be found in Chapter 9, Volume 1, of this treatise.

2. Antioxidants

The inclusion of an antioxidant in an emulsion formulation may be necessary to protect not only an active ingredient but also formulation components (e.g., unsaturated lipids) that are oxygen-labile. Oxidation occurring spontaneously under mild conditions generally involves free radical reactions [121]. Olefinic bonds can readily undergo fragmentation to produce volatile and nonvolatile aldehydes, acids, and alcohols as well as multiple radicals that can propagate the reaction. Qualitatively, oxidative degradation is often preceded by a lag phase corresponding to the gradual increase of free radicals via an initiation reaction. Unless the resultant radicals are stable, radical propagation ensues (generally in accordance with first-order kinetics). If chain branching occurs, reaction kinetics will tend to be more complex. The termination of this oxidative sequence involves the interaction of free radicals with one another to form stable or metastable products. Ultraviolet light can initiate this free radical chain process of oxidative degradation as well as a second class of photooxidation reactions involving dye-sensitized photooxygenation.

Kinetic measurements of fat oxidation in O/W emulsions indicate that the rate of oxidation is dependent upon the rate of oxygen diffusion in the system as well as upon oxygen pressure or content [122]. Trace amounts of metals such as copper, manganese, or iron may also initiate or catalyze oxidative reactions. Thus, the use of chelating agents in a formulation may markedly improve product stability.

Some oxidative degradation is pH-dependent as pH affects the degree of ionization of the labile compound and its corresponding susceptibility to oxidation—the charged and uncharged species are not necessarily equally reactive [121]. The pH-stability profiles of the active ingredients and of prospective formulations should be established during product development. Antioxidants are often added to emulsion systems by formulators a priori, without considering the specific kinetic mechanism involved. Some antioxidants function as retardants, in that they decrease the rate of oxidation, while others function as inhibitors, which induce or prolong a lag period prior to the onset of oxidation. Combinations of retardants and inhibitors may act synergistically; for example, used together, chelating agents and chain terminators are more effective than either agent alone.

Various antioxidants are listed in Table 6. As for preservatives, so too for antioxidants: each phase of an emulsion system may require a different antioxidant. Ascorbyl palmitate, one of the most commonly used antioxidants, has a solubility limit of about 1% in vegetable oils. Most chelating agents have limited nonaqueous solubility. Fat-soluble derivatives of hydroxy acids are available that may be useful in combination with phenolic antioxidants such as BHA, BHT, or propyl gallate.

With the development of a coulometric oxygen assay suitable for use with emulsions and oily solutions [123], the content of dissolved oxygen in the system can be determined readily. The amount of antioxidant required can be estimated from knowledge of the stoichiometry of the reaction between oxygen and the antioxidant and the oxygen content of the system, including the headspace [121]. Hermetically sealed systems (e.g., ampules), tight containers, or single-use packages could be expected to require less antioxidant than "open" systems or multiple-use packages. The selection of an antioxidant will depend not only on its solubility but also on its safety, stability, and other characteristics. For example, sulfites have been associated with allergic reactions and are apt to yield acid sulfates upon oxidation, which lower aqueous-phase pH. They also can react with some constituents to form addition compounds, among others. Minimizing oxidation warrants a consideration of other measures as well as prudent selection of an antioxidant. The formulator may wish to consider the use of liquids that have

Table 6 Selected Antioxidants for Emulsion Systems

Chelating agents:	Citric acid
	EDTA
	Phenylalanine
	Phosphoric acid
	Tartaric acid
	Tryptophane
Preferentially oxidized compounds:	Ascorbic acid
	Sodium bisulfite
	Sodium sulfite
Chain terminators:	*Water-soluble*
	Thiols (e.g., cysteine HCl, thioglycerol, thioglycolic acid, thiosorbitol)
	Lipid-soluble
	Alkyl gallates (octyl, propyl, dodecyl)
	Ascorbyl palmitate
	t-Butyl hydroquinone (TBHQ)
	Butylated hydroxyanisole (BHA)
	Butylated hydroxytoluene (BHT)
	Hydroquinone
	Nordihdyroguaiaretic acid (NDGA)
	α-Tocopherol

been deaerated as by sparging (i.e., bubbling nitrogen gas through the liquid to remove dissolved air or oxygen), boiling before use, or exposure to vacuum during ultrasonic agitation. The headspace above the container could also be flushed with nitrogen just before sealing. Again, as some oxidative degradation is light-initiated [121], the use of opaque or light-resistant containers, wraparound labeling or cartons, or the addition of ultraviolet light–absorbing compounds (e.g., benzophenones) can negate the problem.

III. PHARMACEUTICAL APPLICATIONS

Virtually all administration routes have been employed for emulsion-based drug delivery systems [11], including topical, oral, parenteral, pulmonary [124], and ophthalmic [125] routes. Emulsion systems have also been widely utilized by pharmacists as vehicles or matrices for extemporaneous compounding, particularly for dermatological formulations for which their ease of application and innocuous character tend to ensure patient acceptability. An annotated alphabetical listing of drugs incorporated in macro- and microemulsions is provided in Appendix I.

A. Emulsions for Topical Use

Topical formulations, reviewed by Block [126] in some detail, have been employed per se to alter skin structure and functionality and as vehicles for drugs in order to effect local, regional, or systemic drug delivery. Historically, virtually all topical products, including dermatologicals, were developed empirically, based on principles of esthetics rather than of efficacy. Today, it is realized that topical systems provide the astute formulator with unique opportunities for efficacious formulation [126–128].

Insofar as skin structure and functionality are concerned, water has been the principal concern of formulators and clinicians alike for decades [129,130]. As Warner and Lilly [131] note:

> The importance of water to the proper functioning of the SC [stratum corneum] is so well recognized and so often stated that it has become a cliché, obscuring our nearly complete ignorance of the quantity and distribution of water in this tissue and its relevance to pathological or physiological states. . . . For instance, it is not known by direct experimental measurements whether the water content of "dry" skin induced chemically by surfactants differs from that induced by environmental factors, or whether the water content of good skin differs substantially from that of skin afflicted with any pathological condition.

Nonetheless, skin softness and pliability *are* directly related to the water content of the stratum corneum; the retention of moisture by the skin helps prevent the development of dry, chapped skin. Since evaporative moisture loss from the skin surface (transepidermal water loss or TEWL) can be minimized by surface occlusion, the topical application of an occlusive water-impermeable film can facilitate rehydration of dry skin and a return to near-normal functionality. Nevertheless, the use of hydrocarbons (e.g., petrolatum, paraffins) and hydrophobic oils as efficient occlusive moisturizers is thwarted by their inelegance. Formulators would prefer to develop a product that rubs into the skin to leave a residue that is undetectable to the eye and is neither tacky nor greasy. Furthermore, products with a high yield value may be difficult to rub into the skin or to apply as an even film; application to damaged skin may be painful. On the other hand, emulsions—whether W/O or O/W—can be formulated to provide the requisite occlusivity and reduction in TEWL while meeting criteria for esthetic appearance, ease of removal from the container, ease of application, and adherence to the treated area without tackiness or difficulty in removal.

Insofar as occlusivity is concerned, W/O emulsions are somewhat less occlusive than "greases." Substances in the vehicle, such as humectants, that have a high affinity for water may under certain circumstances dehydrate the stratum corneum and decrease penetration. Similarly, powders increase the surface area and increase the rate of evaporation of water, and so decrease the extent of hydration. Wepierre and Adrangui [132] evaluated the occlusivity of O/W emulsions using hydrated gelatin as a model substrate upon which test emulsions were spread. Water loss from the gelatin substrate was determined gravimetrically. Whatever the nature of the oil (dielectric constants ranged from 2.08 to 3.78), increased occlusivity was associated with increased oil/surfactant ratios and with HLB values at which the formation of an isotropic "oily" phase, upon evaporation of the emulsion water, was maximal.

The evaluation of topical emulsion formulations necessitates their physicochemical characterization—rheological properties, phase composition, apparent pH, particle size and particle size distribution of the dispersed phase, and so on—*and* an evaluation of their physical and chemical stability. Recent studies by Flynn and coworkers [133] pinpoint an additional concern for the physicochemical stability of topical emulsions *post-application*. Because most topical formulations are left open to the air after application, evaporation and loss of volatile formulation components such as water or ethanol post-application can be expected to affect topical emulsion system composition and performance. However, even presumably nonvolatile excipients (e.g., propylene glycol) evaporate after topical application. Skin permeation by excipients may also occur after application, leading to further compositional changes in the applied film on the skin surface. The impact of this evaporative and absorptive loss of adjuvants on formulation composition, skin effects, and drug delivery capabilities of real vehicles increases as the volume of the topical formulation applied is reduced.

The efficiency of vehicles of various types in aiding skin penetration by a drug molecule can be predicted by the way in which the vehicle alters the activity of water in the stratum corneum and influences the drug's stratum corneum/vehicle partition coefficient. Rougier [134] has demonstrated that the two principal markers of the integrity of the skin barrier, percutaneous absorption and TEWL, are directly linked. Increased occlusivity leads to increased hydration of the stratum corneum and a correspondingly lower diffusional resistance to permeating solutes. Furthermore, decreased TEWL results in a slight elevation in skin temperature in the occluded area, and increased solute flux in the affected cutaneous environment.

Although the mathematical characterization of drug release from emulsion systems has been developed to some extent [135,136], the thermodynamic instability of macroemulsions, their potential for compositional changes after application, and the anisotropic nature of the biological barriers that constitute the skin preclude a rigorous solution of the problem of predicting drug release and bioavailability at this time. Furthermore, the bioavailability of topically applied compounds may be significantly affected by epidermal biotransformation, but the relative level of skin metabolism of compounds is likely to be inversely proportional to the transepithelial flux in accordance with Michaelis-Menten kinetics.

Emulsions may facilitate drug permeation into and through the skin by their occlusiveness or by virtue of their penetration-enhancing components, which may either have a direct effect on skin permeability by affecting barrier (i.e., stratum corneum) integrity—e.g., surfactants, urea, terpenes and sesquiterpenes—or may increase the thermodynamic activity or solubility of the penetrant—e.g., glycerin, propylene glycol [126].

B. Emulsions for Systemic Use

As noted at the outset, emulsions may not only *facilitate* the systemic absorption of poorly water soluble drugs but may also *prolong* drug release from the administration site. Whether the *rate* or *extent* of drug release from an emulsion delivery system is increased or decreased depends on the interfacial area of the emulsion system, the agitation intensity in each of the phases, the efficiency of drug partitioning from one phase to another, the drug's thermodynamic activity and diffusivity in each of the phases, the volume fractions of the dispersed phase and the continuous phase, and the drug's apparent absorption rate constant. Early efforts by Kakemi and coworkers [137,138], who examined the intestinal absorption of drugs from O/W emulsions and oil solutions, and by W. I. Higuchi et al. [139–143], who modeled transport phenomena in emulsion systems, have provided us with a more comprehensive but still incomplete view of drug delivery from emulsions. Additional factors to consider include drug-adjuvant interactions, the effect of the interphase on drug transport from one phase to the other, the stability of the emulsion at the administration site and in the biological milieu, and the residence time of drug at the absorbing surface. Inability to assess these latter factors quantitatively hampers our ability to fully characterize and design emulsion-based drug delivery systems.

Figure 4 depicts the sequential transfer of drug from the dispersed phase of an emulsion 1 through the interphase into the continuous phase of the emulsion 2 into the

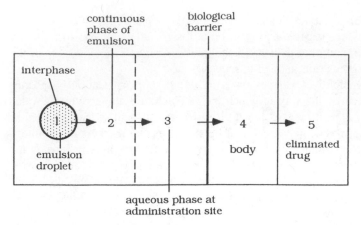

Fig. 4 Schematic diagram depicting the sequence of events governing drug absorption from an emulsion-based drug delivery system: phase 1 is the emulsion droplet, phase 2 is the continuous phase of the emulsion, phase 3 is the aqueous phase at the site of administration, phase 4 is composed of body fluids and tissues, and phase 5 consists of drug eliminated from the body either unchanged, in the excreta, or as metabolites. The dashed line between phase 2 and phase 3 indicates the presence of an interface when the continuous phase of the emulsion is immiscible with the aqueous phase at the administration site.

aqueous fluids at the site of administration 3 to the absorbing surface or biological barrier. Absorption processes provide for subsequent drug uptake into body fluids and tissues 4 from which drug is ultimately eliminated 5. For an O/W emulsion, the continuous (external) phase of the emulsion commingles with the aqueous fluid at the administration site so that the external phase volume ultimately corresponds to that of the aqueous fluids at the administration site. For W/O emulsions, the external phase remains relatively discrete at the administration site so that the external phase volume is approximately the same as that in the administered dose. In addition, Fig. 4 conveys the thermodynamic openness of the biological milieu in which drug delivery systems operate: the emulsion environment is not a closed system but an open one. Hence, drug transport processes—governed by drug delivery system residence time—tend to proceed to completion rather than to some equilibrium. The implications for drug delivery are substantial.

   Interfacial area effects. As the total surface area of the dispersed phase in an emulsion system is extremely large, the efficiency of transfer from the dispersed phase to the continuous phase could be substantial as well [143], unless other factors—such as the barrier effect of the interphase or the affinity of the drug for the dispersed phase—intervene. Thus, for O/W emulsions in which the aqueous phase behaves as a perfect sink, a drug dissolved in the oil droplets will transfer rapidly to the aqueous phase and the aqueous fluids in the lumen of the gut, thus assuring bioavailability and decreasing the possibility of prolonged or sustained drug absorption. On the other hand, the interfacial area of an oil solution or a W/O emulsion vis-a-vis aqueous fluids in the gut lumen would tend to be much smaller, resulting in a substantially decreased efficiency of transfer into the aqueous phase in the gut lumen and correspondingly less efficient systemic absorption.

1. Peroral Emulsions

Perorally administered emulsions are almost exclusively O/W or W/O/W systems, although the use of multiple emulsions of the O/W/O type has been reported [144]. This is more than likely a matter of esthetics and consumer acceptance (see Rieger [5]). On the other hand, the choice of an O/W emulsion system allows the internal phase droplets to be dispersed in the aqueous milieu of the gastrointestinal tract. This large aqueous volume accommodates a large amount of drug, thus providing a substantial gradient for systemic absorption.

The immunosuppressant cyclosporine has been available for some time in the form of a solution in olive oil containing polyethoxylated oleic glycerides. This solution, diluted with milk or orange juice just before peroral dosing, forms a *macro*emulsion that provides for gastrointestinal absorption. Nonetheless, considerable inter- and intraindividual variability in cyclosporine pharmacokinetics has been observed with the use of the olive oil formulation. The recent development of a peroral microemulsion "preconcentrate" of cyclosporine—which forms a microemulsion in the aqueous fluids of the gastrointestinal tract akin to a mixed micellar phase—permits more rapid and complete absorption of cyclosporine with considerably less variability than that provided by the olive oil dispersion [145].

Although multiple emulsions have been recommended as matrices for drug delivery for labile drugs (e.g., drugs susceptible to enzymatic, chemical, or physical degradation), they are not a cure-all for problematic drugs. For example, in spite of preliminary reports on the efficacy of multiple emulsion formulations in promoting the intestinal absorption of insulin in rats and rabbits [146,147], subsequent research was abandoned because of the lability of the insulin and the need for excessive doses (250 U kg^{-1} three times a day) to maintain glucose homeostasis [148]. Nonetheless, the innermost phase of multiple emulsions—if properly formulated—can provide advantages not attainable with simpler emulsion systems by (a) protecting substances incorporated therein from the environment, (b) prolonging their partitioning, diffusion, and release into the continuous phase, (c) allowing the incorporation of incompatible substances in different phases of the same system, or (d) providing for different release profiles for substances incorporated in the various phases of the multiple emulsion system [128,149].

Self-emulsifying drug delivery systems (SEDDSs). These complex systems are composed of isotropic oil-surfactant mixtures that undergo "spontaneous" emulsification on mixing with water (e.g., the aqueous contents of the stomach). The spontaneity of emulsion formation is arguable (from a thermodynamic point of view) but emulsification typically occurs within a matter of seconds after mixing and requires minimal energy input. Following early fundamental studies by Groves and coworkers [150,151], much effort in recent years has been devoted to the formulation of SEDDSs to enhance the peroral bioavailability of poorly soluble drugs as well as to minimze gastrointestinal irritation [152]. Charman et al. [152] developed a SEDDS for an investigational lipophilic compound that substantially improved the reproducibility of the maximum plasma drug concentration, C_{max}, and the time to reach the maximum concentration, t_{max}, after peroral dosing. Craig [153] has extensively reviewed the theory and applications of SEDDSs.

2. Parenteral Emulsions

Parenteral (i.e., injectable) emulsions are employed for a wide variety of reasons. For more than three decades, phospholipid-stabilized lipid emulsions have been used parenterally as a source of energy (ca. 9 kcal per gram of fat) and as a source of essential fatty acids in nutritionally debilitated patients [154]. Within the last decade or so, these phospholipid-stabilized lipid emulsions have been viewed also as vehicles for drug delivery, especially for those drugs with limited water solubility or stability, and, increasingly, for controlled drug release and the targeting of drugs to specific sites in the body [11,155].

It is desirable that the fat particles in an aritificial lipid emulsion undergo transport, distribution, and clearance in much the same way as the natural lipids in the body. Following a meal, fatty acids and cholesterol are absorbed by intestinal cells and then esterified to form triglycerides and cholesteryl esters, which are subsequently incorporated into the core of small droplets called chylomicrons. These chylomicrons are 0.08 to 0.50 μm spheres consisting of a central core of triglycerides and an outer layer of phospholipids containing some apolipoproteins. Lymph channels provide the chylomicrons with access to the venous circulation. Subsequently, chylomicron core triglycerides are hydrolyzed—in a matter of minutes—by lipoprotein lipase in the capillaries with the concomitant release of free fatty acids. During this lipolytic process, the chylomicron shrinks; its remnants are removed rapidly from the plasma by the liver [156]. The preferential clearance of such particles by the liver, adipose tissue, heart muscle, and lactating mammary gland, and the close association between individual fat droplets and the endothelium, provides a rationale for the use of artificial lipid emulsions as drug delivery systems, provided that the drug is very lipid soluble or that barriers to retard drug diffusion and transfer can be created at the O/W interface. Thus, the similarity between the fat droplets of lipid emulsions and the body's lipid transport system is of some consequence.

Systemic clearance of an emulsion is determined largely by its interaction with the reticuloendothelial system, as is the case for suspensions, radiodiagnostic agents, and liposomes (phospholipid vesicles). Emulsion particle size and surface charge are critical factors affecting clearance. In general, fine particle size emulsions are cleared more slowly than coarse particle size emulsions; negatively charged and positively charged particles are cleared more quickly than neutral particles; emulsions stabilized by low molecular weight emulsifiers are cleared more rapidly than those stabilized by high molecular weight emulsifiers. The potential interaction between drug-loaded emulsion droplets and plasma proteins could result in opsonization and rapid phagocytotic uptake by the reticuloendothelial system. Emulsion droplet instability, due to migration of surfactant, cosolvent, or other adjuvants after administration, could result in precipitation of insoluble drug or droplet flocculation and an increased likelihood of pulmonary embolism or reticuloendothelial system uptake [157–159].

Both oil-in-water (O/W) and water-in-oil (W/O) emulsions are used as parenteral drug delivery systems as are their corresponding multiple emulsions (W/O/W and O/W/O). The type of emulsion employed is usually determined by the drug, the intended route of administration, and the anticipated role of the emulsion vehicle. For example, W/O, O/W/O, and W/O/W emulsions are often used as depot formulations to provide a sustained or controlled release of a drug following intramuscular administration. In contrast, only O/W emulsions are normally given by the intravenous route as drug carriers or as medicinal or nutritional agents in their own right. The suitability of W/O/W emulsions and microemulsions for intravenous administration is unclear at this time.

In the past, the relative paucity of parenteral emulsions was due, ostensibly, to the difficulty in achieving stable, sterile dispersions with droplets smaller than 1 μm in diameter. These constraints—on stability, sterility, and particle size—are necessary if emboli and sepsis are to be avoided. Accordingly, the use of high-shear emulsification equipment (e.g., multistage homogenizers, ultrasonic homogenizers, microfluidizers) is mandated in conjunction with appropriate sterilization methods. In recent years, increasing attention has been focused on submicron emulsions. Benita and Levy [160] have provided a comprehensive review of submicron emulsions (for intravenous use) that examines formulation design, excipient selection, manufacturing options, physicochemical characterization, stability assessment, and in vitro release kinetics. Sterile emulsion processing has become somewhat less problematic as submicron emulsion manufacturing has become more facile. Lidgate et al. [161] were able to employ sterile membrane (cartridge) filtration of an O/W emulsion after subjecting the product to multiple passes through a microfluidizer, operating at pressures greater than 16,000 psi, and achieving a narrow droplet size distribution, with all droplets' diameters < 0.22 μm (220 nm).

Nonetheless, conventional sterilization methods (e.g., terminal autoclaving at high temperature) may still be applicable, but the formulator should be aware that these methods must still yield acceptable emulsions after the heating/cooling cycle. The widespread use of triglycerides and phospholipids in parenteral emulsion formulations compounds the problem because of their potential instability at elevated temperatures [162,163]. Fortuitously, the thermal stress of autoclaving (heat sterilization) results in *enhanced* stability of phospholipid-stabilized emulsions, apparently because of a rapid, irreversible redistribution of phospholipid from the aqueous phase to the oil phase. This redistribution occurs in conjunction with the formation—in the interphase—of cubic liquid crystalline phospholipid phases that convert to stable lamellar phases upon cooling [163].

Beyond issues of viable and nonviable particulate contamination, parenteral emulsion formulation is further complicated by the need to avoid hemolysis—a problem inherent with most surfactants—and toxicity related to the solubilization of components of packaging and administration sets. Isotonicity, pH, nonpyrogenicity, and biodegradability requirements, as well as pharmacopeial standards, must also be met [160].

Excipient selection. The selection of appropriate lipids or oils and emulsion stabilizers is critical to the functionality of parenteral emulsion systems, whether they are used as a part of parenteral nutrition or as vehicles for drug delivery. Intravenous fat emulsions usually contain 10% oil (typically soybean or safflower oil), although the lipid level may range up to 20%. The increased utilization of medium chain triglycerides (MCTs), obtained by coconut oil hydrolysis and fractionation, alone or in combination with long chain triglycerides (LCTs) is more commonplace now in parenteral lipid emulsions. Parenteral use of these oils and lipid fractions requires processing to remove waxy components and hydrogenated or saturated fatty materials that could present difficulties later on [160]. Peroxidation of unsaturated fatty acids (e.g., linoleic acid) to hydroperoxides can lead to altered arachidonic acid metabolism or the formation of organic free radicals and a consequent cascade of damage to endogenous lipids [164]. The principal emulsion stabilizers employed in parenteral formulations are egg yolk or soybean phospholipids, poloxamers, acetylated monoglycerides, fatty acid esters of sorbitans, and polyoxyethylene sorbitans. Given the complexity and variability of the phospholipid products available commercially—in terms of composition and concentration—the importance of proper emulsifier selection and modification cannot be stressed enough. Rydhag [165] investigated the effect of phase behavior of phospholipids on emulsion stability and found that both the degree of dispersion and emulsion stability could be optimized by the addition of negatively charged lipids to neutral phospholipids or by selecting lecithin/phospholipid products with adequate amounts of negatively charged phospholipids. In addition to such emulsion stabilization (e.g., oleic, cholic, or deoxycholic acids and their respective salts), other excipients for parenteral emulsions include adjuvants for pH control (often achieved through the use of aqueous solutions of sodium hydroxide or hydrochloric acid) and isotonicity (glycerin). Relevant standards and requirements for all of these excipients are to be found not only in the various national and multinational pharmacopeias but also in specialized monographs and publications such as the *Handbook of Excipients* [166].

IV. FORMULATION AND PROCESSING OF EMULSIONS

A. Formulation Optimization

Emulsion formulation is still at an empiric level. As Lissant [91] notes:

> Starting in the late 1890s, many careful studies were made of emulsion systems, and several excellent books were written on the subject . . . In spite of all this work, we still do not have good predictive methods to apply in making . . . emulsions. If faced with the problem of making a stable emulsion from two new liquid phases, we do not have an effective way of calculating what emulsifier to use or what technique of emulsification to employ to obtain the best results . . . Most new emulsion systems are ultimately perfected by trial and error.

The inability of emulsion theory to predict the composition of appropriate emulsion systems is mitigated to some extent by the development of optimization techniques that facilitate product development. The formulation of any product, even by a trial-and-error approach, involves an optimization process: goals are defined, evaluation procedures are selected, initial compositions are defined, products are prepared and evaluated appropriately, and the prospective formulation then modified until acceptable data are obtained. Presumably, a series of logical steps is taken by the experimenter who controls the variables until a satisfactory product results. Nonetheless, in the absence of a mathematically or statistically rigorous approach to optimization, this satisfactory product is but a provisionally satisfactory product; it is not necessarily the optimal formulation. Subsequent experience with the less than optimal formulation during scale-up or processing or in the marketplace often demonstrates the formulation's suboptimal character whether by instability, poor performance, or lack of acceptance by the consumer. The utilization of mathematical optimization techniques can circumvent this problem for the emulsion technologist. These various approaches to optimization, which can be adapted readily by the emulsion formulator, are described at length by Bolton [167].

Principal component analysis, a multivariate statistical procedure, was used by Bohidar et al. [168]. This method determines the interrelationships and covariances among the measurements employed to evaluate the adequacy of a formulation. That is, it identifies the variables that best distinguish one formulation from another and which should be the criteria used in product development. Schwartz and coworkers [169,170] employed factorial designs along with computer techniques to optimize formulations.

Phase diagrams delineating the behavior of multiple components have been extensively utilized in formulation optimization in spite of the large amount of data that must be obtained if adequate diagrams are to be prepared. Without the use of phase diagrams, the characterization of emulsion component behavior in multiphase systems is somewhat unpredictable. (For example, docusate sodium—an ionic surfactant—has greater solubility in oil than in water but produces stables O/W emulsions [171].) During the course of experimentation, emulsions, gels or solids as well as fluid phases of either low or high viscosity may be encountered. Liquid crystal formation may be evident. Most studies have involved ternary or three-component systems—a polar phase, a nonpolar phase, and an amphiphile—so that data are represented by triangular graphs. Additional components can be accommodated within the confines of a triangular graph by keeping the ratios of two components (e.g., water and propylene glycol) constant or by making the concentration of a component constant. The phase equilibria depicted are based upon data obtained under isothermal (and isobaric) conditions. Ternary diagrams are also useful in plotting information pertaining to system behavior including viscosity, stability, clarity, and emulsion type. When the formulator wants to portray phase diagrams, and array them as a function of temperature, this can be facilitated by computer graphics programs that allow one to stack the isotherms prismatically [172]. Phase diagrams are described extensively by Lissant [91] and triangular diagrams, in particular, by Swarbrick [26], Mackay [173], and Francis and Smith [174]. Variants of these geometric representations include the simplex lattice procedure that has been employed to determine the optimal composition of a formulation with respect to certain variables or to a specific outcome. Shek et al. [175] applied the simplex method to the optimization of a capsule formulation.

The use of glyphs—symbols that convey meaning nonverbally—has been advocated by Everitt [176] and Lissant [177] as a means of coping with data in multivariant systems. Processing variables, stability, and subjective evaluations can all be represented in glyph plots, which are far easier to understand and assimilate than the corresponding tables of data.

Although optimization techniques involving statistical or graphical analysis of data have been available for some time, their mathematical or physicochemical bases are not universally recognized or appreciated. As a result, some formulators are loath to employ optimization techniques even though these can minimize the number of experimental runs needed to develop a suitable product. (See Chapter 10, Volume 1, of this treatise.)

B. Emulsion Processing

In processing emulsions, the initial location of the emulsifiers (i.e., whether in one bulk phase or another), the method of incorporation of the phases, the rates of addition, the temperature of each phase, and the rate of cooling after mixing of the phases have considerable effect on the droplet size distribution, viscosity, and stability of the final emulsion. (While the aforementioned process variables are generally given full attention by emulsion technologists, the effects of *post-emulsification* processing on emulsion characteristics are often ignored at the outset. For example, the continuous rotation of an auger in the hopper of the filling machine may cause a cream to liquefy. The replacement of the auger by another, gentler feeding device may be a better alternative than reformulating the product.)

The usual practice in preparing emulsions is to add the internal phase to the external phase—while subjecting the system to shear or fracture—so that the internal phase is dispersed within the external phase. For example, in the preparation of O/W emulsions, the internal phase—the oil phase—is usually added to the water phase. However, many technologists prefer the *phase inversion* technique, wherein the aqueous phase is initially added to the oil phase, resulting in the formation of a W/O emulsion. At the inversion point, the addition of more water results in the inversion of the emulsion system and the formation of an O/W emulsion. The phase inversion method allows the formation of small droplets with minimal mechanical action and attendant heat [178]. Nonetheless, the use of the phase inversion method is often difficult in commercial production. For production-size batches (e.g., 1000 kg), two large kettles would be required to hold the oil and water phases separately. In many O/W formulations, the oil phase represents a small fraction of the total volume and may not be effectively processed by the equipment at hand (e.g., the oil phase may barely reach the agitator blades in a large processing kettle). In addition, as more of the internal phase is added to the emulsion (up to $\phi \approx 0.6$ to 0.7), an increasingly greater attenuation of the external phase occurs, resulting in an increasingly greater viscosity of the emulsion system. This viscosity increase, pre-inversion, may pose a problem if available equipment is unable to content with altered rheological behavior and provide adequate mixing and dispersal. Subsequent addition of the internal phase results in phase inversion and the formation of a less viscous emulsion system. Occasionally, inversion of the W/O emulsion takes place at $\phi \leq 0.6$ to 0.7. When this occurs, the viscosity of the inverted emulsion is higher but because the external phase is aqueous, the further addition and incorporation of water is less problematic.

When preparing water-in-oil emulsions, the water phase is generally added slowly to the oil phase with constant stirring. Usually these emulsions are homogenized or milled to further subdivide the particles in the internal phase, which increases the stability and improves the gloss of the emulsion.

The common practice in formulating emulsions is to dissolve or disperse lyophilic components in the corresponding phases before emulsification is initiated. Thus, oil-soluble or dispersible ingredients are incorporated in the oil phase and water-soluble or dispersible ingredients in the water phase. A classic exception to the rule—which is particularly effective—involves the use of the phase inversion technique when hydrophilic colloids are a part of the formulation. The preliminary dispersion of the hydrocolloid in the oil phase, without wetting, (the so-called *dry gum* technique) tends to be more rapid and complete than can be achieved at higher shear or impact were the hydrocolloid dispersed in the aqueous phase at the outset. Ordinarily, if a gum or hydrocolloid is employed it should be completely hydrated or dissolved in the aqueous phase before the emulsification step, unless the dry gum method described above is employed. If a heat-sensitive component is used, it may be necessary to incorporate it (in solution, if appropriate) after the emulsion has been formed. The use of anionic and cationic emulsifiers or emulsion stabilizers in about equimolar quantities rarely yield satisfactory emulsions.

Often, the various phases are heated, prior to emulsification, to temperatures about 5 to 10°C above the melting point of the highest melting ingredient (e.g., waxes or fats). The elevated temperatures are then maintained as the phases are combined. This practice minimizes the likelihood of premature or inappropriate solidification or crystallization of high melting point components during admixture of the phases. It also facilitates processing due to the lower viscosities at higher temperatures. Care must be taken not to heat the phases excessively because degradation of temperature-sensitive components may result (e.g., hydrolysis of emulsifiers, decomposition of preservatives, or discoloration of amine soaps such as TEA stearate).

After the emulsion has formed at an elevated temperature, the rate of cooling is extremely important in determining the final texture and consistency of the emulsion. A laboratory beaker containing a hot emulsion cools fairly rapidly to room temperature, but in production a tank filled with hundreds of kilograms of hot material cools more slowly unless external means of cooling are employed. This is one reason the simple transfer of laboratory process to production requires extensive studies of the cooling and agitation schedule. It is also advisable to utilize jacketed equipment for the large-scale preparation of emulsions, so that the heating and cooling cycles can be carefully controlled.

Following the addition of the phases, the rate of cooling is generally slow, to allow for adequate mixing while the emulsion is still fluid. The temperature of the cooling medium in the kettle jacket should be decreased gradually and at a rate consistent with the mixing of the emulsion and scraping of the kettle walls to prevent formation of congealed masses of the emulsion system, especially when the semisolid contains a large percentage of high melting substances. The drug is added in solution form, if not already incorporated, or as crystals, provided it is soluble in the external phase. An insoluble powder should be dispersed in the continuous phase prior to removing the semisolid from the kettle for further processing (e.g., homogenization) and/or storage.

Adjustment of the final water content of a water-in-oil emulsion is not easy once the emulsion has been formed. Several batch runs help to determine the amount of water lost on heating in the particular process, and this lost water should be added to the required amount at the start of manufacture. The oil surrounding each emulsified water droplet in a water-in-oil emulsion tends to retard evaporation, so that water loss is not excessive following this type of emulsification.

Aeration or entrainment of air in the emulsion can occur during the mixing, homogenizing, or milling stage, during the transfer of the product to storage and/or filling equipment, and during the filling or packaging operation. It may lead to emulsion instability and variation in density within a batch, resulting in weight variation of the emulsion in its container. Aeration may be prevented at the primary emulsion step if one phase is introduced into the other in such a manner that splashing and streaming are avoided. The incoming liquid should enter the mixing kettle below the surface of the other liquid. Vortexing and splashing are overcome by careful adjustment of the mixing conditions and liquid flow pattern. In most cases, use of a side sweep agitator is highly recommended. When an auger device or a worm drive is used in a hopper to deliver the material to a tube or jar at the filling outlet, the hopper must be kept full of product, or the rotation of the auger will drive air into the emulsion. More positive protection can be obtained by processing in an enclosed tank under vacuum.

If these approaches fail to eliminate or reduce foaming, it is sometimes necessary to add foam suppressants (antifoams). The most effective defoamers are long chain alcohols and commercially available silicone derivatives, both of which spread over the air-water interface as insoluble films. However, if at all possible, their use should be avoided, because they represent a potential source of incompatibility.

1. *Emulsification Equipment*

Various types of equipment are available to effect droplet dispersion and emulsification either in the laboratory or in production. The choice of emulsification equipment is usually dictated by the application of the resulting emulsions and by the throughput required. This equipment, whether simple or complex, serves to break up or disperse the internal phase into the external phase so that the droplet size of the resulting emulsion is sufficiently small to prevent coalescence and resulting instability. Scott [179] has ably reviewed the equipment used in emulsion processing.

Emulsion processing methods generally involve either *shear* or *fracture* to achieve phase attenuation or droplet dispersion in the continuous phase, although turbulence and cavitation forces may also be a part of the process [180]. High shear forces are achieved through the use of narrow gaps and/or high flow rates; fracture is achieved by impact, often involving substantially higher energy.

The emulsion technologist must remember that product consistency and stability are affected by equipment choice and operation. Variations in the number of passes of product through the emulsification equipment and in operating conditions (e.g., the rotational speeds, applied pressures or frequencies used for processing, the clearance between a rotor and stator, etc.) can markedly influence the outcome. Temperature increases in emulsions during processing can be substantial, especially if energy-intensive processes are involved (e.g., homogenizers, colloid mills, microfluidizers) and no provisions are made for temperature modulation. The resultant thermally induced degradation or alteration of the product can be disastrous!

C. The Influence of Processing on Emulsion Stability and Characteristics

Trial-and-error methodology is rampant in emulsion formulation because—all too often—the expected results are not obtained. The difficulty experienced by formulators is not entirely a reflection of the complex physicochemical interactions of the emulsion components. Emulsion processing also exerts considerable influence on the outcome. It is not surprising that the formulation and manufacture of emulsions continues to be conducted *secundem artem.*

The primary focus of most references on the processing technology of emulsions is on mixing [181,182], although other unit operations such as deaeration, heat transfer, and pumping are integral parts of emulsion processing as well. The emulsion technologist must also have some familiarity with still other processing issues that take precedence over the unit operations already noted. Thus, the physical state and characteristics of the components and their admixtures, the method of preparation (order and rate of combination of ingredients; type of equipment), the duration of processing, and the rheological character of the formulation markedly influence the outcome.

One indication of the difficulty to be encountered by emulsion formulators is provided by experiences with microemulsion formulation [183]. Transparent O/W microemulsions were formed whether water with dissolved sodium lauryl sulfate was admixed with pentanol and then with *p*-xylene or the more traditional approach was used in which the cosurfactant (pentanol) was added last. The former microemulsion was more stable than the latter, which separated in one to two weeks. Different methods of addition may provide products that differ in their stability.

Initially, most methods of emulsification mechanically induce deformation of the liquid-liquid interface such that droplets are formed. These droplets are then disrupted and dispersed further. The greater the number of droplets formed, the greater the likelihood of droplet collision and coalescence. Obviously, the number of droplets of a given size that can be formed per unit time is a function of the phase volume ratio, ϕ, and of the mechanical factors associated with the specific type of emulsification equipment employed and whether laminar flow, turbulent flow, or cavitation is involved [184]. Davies and Rideal [185] applied the von Smoluchowski relationship to emulsion formation. Presumably, droplets of both phases form during emulsification. Their persistence with respect to time is related to their size and diffusivity, D:

$$\frac{1}{n} = \frac{1}{n_o} = 4\pi DRt \tag{14}$$

where n and n_o are the number of droplets per cm^3 at time t and at zero time, respectively, and R is the collision diameter ($= 2r$). The coalescence rates of the oil and water phases are described by the following equations:

$$Rate_o = \frac{d\bar{V}}{dt} = \left[\frac{4\phi kT}{3\eta_w}\right]e^{-W_o/kT} \tag{15}$$

$$Rate_w = \frac{d\bar{V}}{dt} = \left[\frac{4(1-\phi)kT}{3\eta_o}\right]e^{-W_w/kT} \tag{16}$$

The subscripts o and w refer to the oil and water phase, respectively, and $\bar{V}$, is the mean volume of the droplets. The exponential terms in the rate equations, W_o and W_w, are the interfacial energy barriers to coalescence. Whether an O/W or W/O emulsion forms depends on whether the water or the oil droplets coalesce more rapidly to form the continuous phase. Though Eqs. (15) and (16) are somewhat simplistic, the implications are that phase volume ratios and phase viscosities play a substantial role in emulsion formation [186]. The order of mixing and the rate and extent of mixing—for example, the slow addition of one phase to another during processing—may ensure the predominance of droplets of one phase over those of another and the nature of the final emulsion.

As Zografi [171] pointed out, Eqs. (15) and (16) err to the extent that they do not take flocculation into account. Flocculation is a particularly important phenomenon insofar as W/O emulsion formation and stabilization are concerned, because repulsive forces for water droplets are not substantial. Fox and Shangraw [187] demonstrated the marked stabilizing effect of electrolytes added to the internal aqueous phase of water/light mineral oil emulsions stabilized with mannide mono-oleate.

Davies [188] notes that when oil and water are forced between shearing plates—as is the case in many emulsification devices or emulsators—the wettability of the plates exerts a marked influence on the emulsion type: oil-wetted plates favor W/O emulsions. As wettability of the emulsator surfaces can be altered by surfactants, their inclusion in one phase or the other, or both, will affect the results.

Duration of processing can affect emulsion stability. Becher [189], using an emulsator similar to that of Fox and Shangraw [187], showed that the number of passes of product through the device affected the mean particle size and the particle size distribution. Repeated processing or cycling resulted in a decrease in average particle size and in narrowing of the particle size distribution followed by an increase in mean particle size and in the standard deviation as processing continued. In effect, it is possible to overprocess an emulsion.

The rheological behavior of an emulsion system is a principal factor contributing to its acceptability by the consumer. During processing, it is a major determinant of the uniformity of mixing, the degree of dispersion achieved, the energy requirements for manufacture, the stability of the product, and the ease of packaging. Rheologically, dilute emulsion systems behave as Newtonian fluids. One can define the viscosity of the dispersion in terms of the viscosity of the continuous phase, η_o, and the internal phase volume ratio, ϕ:

$$\eta = \eta_o (1 + 2.5\ \phi) \tag{17}$$

This relationship, proposed by Einstein [190], accounts for the increase in viscosity due to the inclusion of particles that dissipate energy and modify the flow pattern in their vicinity. When the viscosity of the internal phase, η_i, is not very much different from that of the dispersion medium, when fluid circulation occurs within the droplets, and when the flow pattern around the droplets is less disturbed, Eq. (17) becomes [191]:

$$\eta = \eta_o \left(1 + 2.5 \left[\frac{\eta_i + \frac{2}{5}\eta_o}{\eta_i + \eta_o} \right] \phi \right) \tag{18}$$

Thus, for dilute emulsions, η increases linearly with an increase in ϕ.

For more concentrated emulsions, rheological behavior may be demonstrably non-Newtonian (pseudoplastic, plastic, or viscoelastic) and its dependence on ϕ more marked (see [192]). Emulsions with high internal phase ratios ($\phi \geq 0.70$) tend to exhibit anomalous rheological properties owing to drop deformation and particle interaction [193].

The rheological properties of microemulsions run the gamut from Newtonian to non-Newtonian behavior depending on the shape of the microemulsion particles. The more nearly spherical the particles, the more Newtonian the behavior [194].

The mixing process specified in a formulation protocol is often a high agitation intensity procedure. Individual droplets of the phases collide continuously with one another as they are formed, disrupted, and dispersed. Most droplets rebound elastically rather than coalesce, owing to the elastic properties of their interfacial film and the liquid between the droplets. If agitation intensity is high enough, coalescence can be prevented by local pressure and velocity fluctuations in the fluid and shear forces in the vicinity of the impeller and the wall [195]. As a result, emulsion samples taken from the top of a tank, far from the impeller zone, would tend to yield a larger mean droplet diameter than samples taken at or near the impeller zone [196]. Sampling protocols that do not consider the location of a sampling probe to be an important variable may well provide misleading data to the formulator.

Although emulsion production equipment is not limited to mixing tanks fitted with rotating turbine, propeller, or paddle impellers [184], much of the definitive literature [181,182] deals with these systems rather than with non-impeller-type or high-shear equipment. Optimization of the manufacturing process must consider the degree of shear required to produce a product with the appropriate particle size distribution. The formulator should keep in mind that it is possible to adjust mixing equipment to satisfy product specifications, although it may be at the cost of increased energy requirements, lengthier processing time, or poorer performance [181].

The amount of energy expended in conventional emulsion processing is far greater than the amount theoretically required. In many instances, thermal energy must be supplied to heat the ingredients in addition to the mechanical energy required for actual mixing and emulsification. Additional energy is expended to cool the product. According to Subramanyam and Gopal [197], the power used by commercial emulsators, spent mainly in fluid motion, increases with Q^2, Q being the amount of the bulk phase dispersed per unit time. In recent years, there has been an increased emphasis on low-energy processing of emulsions. Multiple emulsions, in particular, may be adversely affected by the use of high energy processing equipment because droplet distortion and subsequent instability are more likely to occur.

Lin [198] advocates a low-energy method that involves a considerable reduction in energy requirements by heating only some of a batch's formulation components, which are combined to form a concentrated emulsion to be diluted with the remaining ingredients. The time saved by such a low-energy technique can also be substantial. One limitation of the method is that the viscosity of the emulsion concentrate may be too high, even at an elevated temperature, to assure complete mixing. Second, the emulsion formed by dilution of the concentrate may not have the requisite characteristics of the product prepared in the more conventional manner. Reng [199] has also described a variety of low-energy processes that could be adapted for batch or continuous maufacture of emulsions. Savings are not limited to time and energy, as equipment requirements—and capital expenditures—may also be reduced: for example, small jacketed kettles, instead of large ones, may suffice for production.

D. Scale-Up Considerations

Emulsion manufacture can be either intermittent—in batches—or continuous. Continuous processes, though generally easier to control and far more economical, may not be practical when production requirements are minimal [200]. The major factors affecting scale-up from laboratory bench to manufacturing plant are size of the production batch and kind of processing equipment and its efficiency [200,201]. The lack of temperature uniformity (i.e., the presence of hot or cold spots), deviations in the rate of cooling or heating, differences in holding time (of components prior to emulsification, of admixture during emulsification, and of product after emulsification), and variations in agitation intensity are among the significant contributors to problems in scale-up [202].

Bench-scale experiments generally involve 1 to 5 kg of formulation. Pilot plant facilities may accommodate 10 to 100 kg quantities and production facilities may involve 1000 kg or more. The pilot plant stage is sometimes omitted for economic reasons or when a new product is similar to one with an established process. This omission, though a calculated risk, may be acceptable if processing is monitored and the product is evaluated. Another alternative to the pilot plant stage involves computer simulation of the manufacturing process [203] in accordance with data gathered during bench-scale experimental studies [204].

The transition from the laboratory to commercial production should be gradual, not abrupt. For each product scale-up problem, the emulsion technologist should identify the factors that affect product quality. Lin [204] stresses the need for experimentation under carefully controlled conditions that duplicate those in full-scale production. If at all possible, bench-scale equipment should be employed that is comparable, geometrically and mechanically, to production-scale equipment. If not, experimental results for small batches or quantities may not be translatable to large batches or quantities. Laboratory formulations prepared by multiple passes through a colloid mill, or by prolonged exposure to an immersion homogenzier, exhibit a degree of dispersion or homogenization that is often difficult to duplicate with large batches using standard production equipment. The use of bench-scale mixing, emulsification, and heat exchange equipment in conjunction with dynamometer attachments or other devices to measure power input or energy use can facilitate the scale-up process considerably [204]. The prudent formulator should evaluate the droplet size distribution and rheological behavior of the product prepared in scale-up experiments and compare the data with those for the original formulation [201].

E. Representative Formulations

A number of formulae are presented below along with comments regarding their composition and method of preparation. The author makes no claims for safety, stability, or regulatory compliance of these formulations, which have been taken from the literature and adapted for illustrative purposes only.

Moisturizing Lotion [205]

PART A	Deionized water	88.1
	Glycerin	5.0
	Propylene glycol	0.8
	Disodium EDTA	0.1
	Carbomer 1342	0.4 (B. F. Goodrich)
PART B	Mineral oil, 100 cs	4.0
	Cetyl alcohol	0.2
	Dimethicone	0.5
PART C	Triethanolamine	0.3
PART D	Preservative	0.3
	Fragrance	0.3

The disodium EDTA is dissolved in an admixture of the water, glycerin, and propylene glycol heated to 70°C. The carbomer resin is then sprinkled into the rapidly agitated solution to form a uniform dispersion. The cetyl alcohol is separately melted and blended with the mineral oil at 70°C. The oil phase components (Part B) are then added to Part A with moderate agitation followed by the addition of triethanolamine (Part C) to neutralize the resin. The remaining components are subsequently added with agitation during the cooling phase. This unusual formulation has been reported to be stable to flocculation and coalescence on storage for at least one year as evidenced by a negligible change in viscosity during that time. Nonetheless, when spreading the emulsion on the skin surface, contact of the dispersion with a small amount of electrolyte (from perspiration) is sufficient to destabilize the emulsion quickly resulting in the rapid coalescence and spreading of the occlusive oil phase on the skin surface. This type of formulation can provide a beneficial moisturizing effect due to the formation of a continuous oil film on the skin surface. The emulsion's sensitivity to electrolyte is the result of carbomer 1342 resin (Carbopol® 1342), an atypical carbomer resin in that it is an amphipathic substance that can serve as the primary emulsifier [206]. As with any carbomer resin, excessive shear and exposure to light should be avoided during processing to avoid polymer breakdown.

Emollient Lotion [207]

PART A	Water	83.8
	Tromethamine magnesium aluminum silicate	1.5 (R. T. Vanderbilt)
PART B	Glycerin	3.5
	Triethanolamine	0.1

PART C	Mineral oil	3.6
	Petrolatum	0.4
	Stearic acid	1.6
	Cetyl alcohol	1.5
	Glyceryl stearate SE	1.4
	Cetyl acetate (and) acetylated lanolin alcohol	2.0 (Amerchol)
	Dimethicone	0.6
	Preservative	q.s.

This medium-viscosity emollient lotion exemplifies the use of particulate solids as emulsion stabilizers. It employs tromethamine magnesium aluminum silicate as the stabilizer and thickener. Glyceryl stearate SE, a so-called emulsifying wax [208], contains some sodium or potassium stearate and may be somewhat acid-sensitive. Non-soap based components may be more stable. This formulation is prepared by heating the water to 70 to 75°C and then adding the clay while agitating at high shear. Mixing continues until the dispersion is smooth, at which time Part B, at 70 to 75°C, is added with slow agitation. The components of Part C are blended together at 75 to 80°C and then added to the admixture of Parts A and B. Mixing is continued until the product is cool.

Total Sunscreen Cream [209]

PART A	Beeswax (and) PEG-8	15.0 (Gattefossé)
	Mineral oil	22.5
	Apricot kernel oil	7.5
	Mineral oil (and) vegetable oil (and) marigold extract	3.0 (Gattefossé)
	Octyl methoxycinnamate	6.0
PART B	Water	36.3
	Propylene glycol	5.0
	Titanium dioxide	4.0
	Methylchloroisothiazolinone (and) methylisothiazolinone	0.1 (Rohm & Haas)
PART C	Fragrance	0.6

The components of Part A require only simple blending at elevated temperature (75°C). The titanium dioxide in Part B should be blended with the propylene glycol before the remaining ingredients are added and the blend heated to 75°C. Part B is then added to Part A with stirring, which continues during cooling. The product is not to be subjected to homogenization. Part C is added once the product is at room temperature or 25°C. Methylchloroisothiazolinone-/methylisothiazolinone (Kathon® CG) is a broad-spectrum microbicide, a departure from traditional antimicrobial preservatives, such as the parabens, with a more limited spectrum of activity.

Analgesic Balm [210]

Emulsifying wax, NF	15.0
Mineral oil	10.0
Methyl salicylate	10.0
Menthol	5.0
Water	60.0

The emulsifying wax is heated along with half the mineral oil to 55 to 60°C. The methyl salicylate and menthol are mixed to facilitate liquefaction and then blended with the remainder of the mineral oil. Water at 60°C is then added to the oil phase with stirring, and stirring is continued until the product congeals. Two potential problems with this formulation—the volatility of the methyl salicylate and the menthol and their solubility during processing—can be minimized by the addition of a small amount of an oil-soluble surfactant to facilitate their incorporation in the oil phase and reduce their escaping tendency. The emulsifying wax specified, as it combines higher fatty alcohols with a nonionic emulsifer, is relatively unaffected by pH variations in the formulation. The use of such an emulsifier, however, with its fixed hydrophobic/hydrophilic ratio, precludes formulation adjustment insofar as surfactant composition is concerned except that neither the nonionic polysorbate emulsifier nor the cetearyl alcohol is specified in the NF monograph. As a large number of emulsifying waxes can be prepared that meet the monograph requirements but do not have the same physicochemical behavior, product characteristics can vary considerably. Thus, the formulator should be wary of indiscriminate component substitution. The texture or consistency of the product can also be changed by the addition of high melting point waxes or of polyols. An increase in consistency or "self-bodying," caused by gel network formation in the interphase and extending into the continuous phase, may occur as this product ages.

O/W Cream [211]

PART A		
	Mineral oil	40.0
	Stearic acid	3.0
	Glyceryl stearate SE	2.0
	Cetearyl alcohol	1.0
	Sorbitan sesquioleate	2.0
	Triethanolamine	0.5
PART B	Water	50.9
	Sodium lauryl sulfate	0.4
	Carbomer 934	0.2

The oil phase of this cream constitutes 48.5% by weight, but more than 50% by volume of the formulation. Its inclusion among the formulae in this section is based upon the method of preparation devised for it and similar high internal phase volume ratio emulsions by Lin and Shen [211]. The process employed is a modification of the two-stage low energy emulsification process described earlier [197], which involved withholding a portion of the emulsion's intended external phase (α_e) and using it to cool an emulsion concentrate prepared with the remainder of the external phase (β_e) in the conventional manner. The withheld, unheated fractions of the composition are symbolized by α and the heated fractions by β; subscripts e and i refer to the external and internal phases, respectively. Lin and Shen's modification involves a three-stage process in which the internal phase is also divided into a fraction that is withheld (α_i) and a fraction that is to be heated (β_i) in combination with a portion of the external phase (β_e) to form a concentrated emulsion, i.e., $\beta_i + \beta_e$. In the second stage, the unheated remainder of the external phase (α_e) is added to the concentrate. The third stage requires the addition to the emulsion of the unheated remainder of the internal phase (α_i).

The mineral oil and water are each divided into heated and unheated fractions. The waxy substances and oil-soluble surfactants are initially placed in the heated fraction of the internal phase (mineral oil) and the water-soluble surfactant and polymer are dispersed in the heated external phase (water) fraction. For this formulation, there is a linear relationship between the amount of the external phase withheld and the minimum amount of the internal phase that must be withheld if an o/w emulsion is to be formed. Crucial parameters of the Lin and Shen method that should be optimized are the rate of addition of the external phase to the internal phase, and the duration and intensity of agitation.

O/W Hand Lotion [212]

PART A	Dimethicone (200 cs)	0.75
	Cetyl alcohol	1.0
	Petrolatum	3.0
	Stearic acid	4.5
	Mineral oil	6.0
	Propyl paraben	0.05
PART B	Glycerin	5.0
	Triethanolamine	1.25
	Magnesium aluminum silicate	0.50
	Methyl paraben	0.10
	Water	77.85

The solids in Part B may be incorporated with gentle stirring in the aqueous solution of the glycerin and the triethanolamine. Parts A and B are separately heated to 80°C followed by the addition of Part A to Part B with mild agitation. When the product has cooled to 40°C, perfume or fragrance can be added. At 30 to 35°C, it should be suitable for packaging. This emulsion formulation employs a paraben preservative in each phase, although partitioning and redistribution may still occur resulting in ineffectual preservation.

Hydrocortisone Microemulsion [33]

Laureth-23	10.27
Glyceryl oleate (and) propylene glycol	20.54 (ICI Americas)
Isopropanol	14.12
n-Hexadecane	39.69
Water	15.38
Hydrocortisone	8.1 mg/ml

This formulation differs from that reported [33] in that the microemulsion component quantities are cited here on a weight basis. The laureth-23 and glyceryl oleate–propylene glycol are blended together followed by the addition of the hexadecane and the isopropanol. Water is then added slowly with stirring until a clear W/O microemulsion is obtained. Excess hydrocortisone was added to the microemulsion and the dispersion stirred for 3 hours. The dispersion was then quantitatively filtered through a medium-porosity sintered crucible by aspiration. The amount of hydrocortisone incorporated in the microemulsion was estimated gravimetrically from the amount remaining in the crucible and the amount originally dispersed in the microemulsion [33]. This noncommercial method of preparation presents no scale-up problem. Other methods for microemulsion preparation [23] may involve more difficulty as they involve emulsification of the hydrocarbon-water admixture with the surfactant followed by the addition of the cosurfactant (alcohol). The scarcity of pharmaceutically or cosmetically acceptable microemulsion components has limited their development.

Intravenous Taxol Emulsion [14]

Lecithin (soy)	1.5
Poloxamer 188	1.5
Ethyl oleate	2.0
Triacetin	50.0
Taxol	1.0
Water	44.0

Taxol, a plant product with antimitotic activity, is poorly water soluble. Emulsion formulation has been considered as a possible alternative to relatively dilute intravenous solutions that necessitate the administration of large volumes of the drug formulation [14]. A commercial intravenous fat emulsion was unacceptable as a vehicle for taxol because of the drug's poor solubility in the emulsion's soybean oil base. Although taxol has a solubility in soybean oil of only 0.3 mg/ml, its solubility in triacetin is 250 times greater (75 mg/ml). Two drawbacks to the use of triacetin in parenteral emulsions are its water solubility (ca. 1:14) and its potential instability at slightly elevated temperatures (e.g., 40°C) [14]. Unless a monodisperse emulsion can be prepared, some change in the particle size distribution can be anticipated (see discussion below on Ostwald ripening).

W/O/W Emulsion for Multiphasic Solute Incorporation [128]

PART A [primary W/O emulsion]	
Mineral oil	24.0
Hypermer A60	4.0 (ICI)
Distilled water, q.s. ad	100.0
PART B [W/O/W multiple emulsion]	
Primary emulsion [PART A]	80.0
Synperonic PE/F127	0.8 (ICI)
Distilled water, q.s. ad	100.0

Multiple emulsion formation is facilitated by the use of both a hydrophobic surfactant (Hypermer A60, a modified polyester) and a hydrophilic surfactant (Synperonic PE/F127, an ethoxylated propylene oxide copolymer). The preparation of the primary emulsion involves the gradual addition, with stirring at 2000 rpm, of the water, at 80°C, to the oil/hydrophobic surfactant admixture at the same temperature. Stirring is continued until the emulsion temperature reaches about 25°C. Subsequently, the hydrophilic surfactant is dissolved in the water and the multiple emulsion is then prepared by the very slow addition, at ambient temperature, of the primary emulsion to the aqueous solution. Raynal et al. [128] have proposed the above formulation as a means for incorporating different solutes in each of the phases to enhance their stability or prolong their release.

V. EMULSION STABILITY ASSESSMENT

The stability of an emulsion must be considered in terms of the physical stability of the emulsion system per se and the physical and chemical stability of the emulsion components (including pharmacologically active ingredients, if any). The mathematical characterization of pharmaceutical and cosmetic emulsion system instability has been limited, in part, by the inapplicability of the classical theories (i.e., DLVO; von Smol-uchowksi) to polydisperse, nondilute systems—i.e., those with relatively high internal phase volume ratios. The complexity of most emulsion systems of interest is further increased by the physicochemical interactions among the multiple components [213] and by the multibody hydrodynamic interactions [69]. The ultimate definition of emulsion instability requires a rigorous model that incorporates both fluid mechanics and dynamic double layer theory in a general dynamic equation capable of quantitatively describing the number of particles of a given size as a function of time and location. Until these problems can be resolved, one must rely on the approximations provided by relatively simplistic formulations of the phenomena that constitute emulsion instability (e.g., [69,214]).

Physicochemical changes in emulsion components are often accompanied by corresponding changes in emulsion properties; chemical instability generally requires analytical verification. Definitions of product stability based solely upon physicochemical or chemical determinations are arbitrary to the extent that (a) laboratory test conditions may not duplicate the actual storage environment during the course of a product's shelf life; and (b) such tests may not mirror changes in the consumer's perception of product performance. The latter issue, psychophysical aspects of product evaluation, is now the subject of renewed scientific scrutiny [215]. Finally, impaired bioavailability must be a concern in regard to drug-containing formulations. These may require evaluations of the effect of product aging on drug release in vitro as a function of time. A significant change in the rate or extent of drug release may warrant in vivo evaluation to determine the need for reformulation. It should be noted that, by and large, emulsion formulations have not impaired drug bioavailability but have enhanced it. Topical corticosteroid preparations are among those for which bioavailability and efficacy problems have been encountered [216,217].

A. Aggregation, Coalescence, and Ostwald Ripening

Emulsion system instability may involve aggregation of droplets of the internal phase into a single kinetic unit (i.e., floccule), coalescence of droplets to form larger droplets, or phase separation [218]. A more subtle type of instability, referred to as Ostwald ripening, involves the growth of large particles at the expense of small ones because of the greater solubility of the latter particles and the corresponding increase in concentration of the component in the dispersion medium [219]. This increase in droplet size via molecular diffusion can occur even when particles have excellent barriers to coalescence. Stabilization may be achieved by the addition of high boiling point or high molecular weight compounds to the internal phase to reduce the escaping tendency of the diffusible components [220]. It can also be achieved, as noted earlier, by processing the emulsion so that a relatively monodisperse system results.

Multiple emulsions (Fig. 5) pose additional problems for the formulator: instability may be manifested in the coalescence of (a) internal phase droplets of the primary emulsion, (b) droplets of the primary emulsion, and (c) internal phase droplets of the primary emulsion with those of the external continuous phase. To assess the integrity of W/O/W emulsions, Zatz and Cueman [221] have employed water-soluble polymeric dye markers (e.g., polyporphyre, polytartrazine), with negligible solubility and diffusivity in the oil phase. The appearance of these markers in the external continuous (aqueous) phase is indicative of the disruption of the oil film separating the internal and external

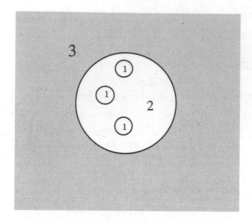

Fig. 5 A multiple emulsion system comprising an external continuous phase, 3, in which droplets of the internal dispersed phase, 2, contain multiple droplets of an inner immiscible phase, 1.

aqueous phases.

The phenomena of aggregation, coalescence, and Ostwald ripening are all reflected in the particle size distribution of the emulsion. As a first approximation, the appearance (i.e., color and opacity) of the emulsion may be indicative of the size of the dispersed phase: if the particle size is greater than 1 µm, the emulsion tends to be milky white; as the size of the dispersed phase decreases, the emulsion becomes less opaque (see Table 7). An emulsion's color and opacity are the result of the absorption, scattering, reflection, and refraction of light. A reduction in the heterogeneity of the particle size distribution of an emulsion—toward a more monodisperse system—and a decrease in the difference between the refractive indices of the phases would tend to reduce the opacity and color of the emulsion. The direct or indirect measurement of particle size or particle size distributions, as a function of time, can help to characterize emulsion stability. Orr [222] has reviewed newer approaches to micromeritic characterization, such as hydrodynamic chromatography and photon correlation spectroscopy, as well as older, well-accepted methods including electrical and optical sensing zone techniques, microscopy, and sedimentation. Klemaszewski and coworkers [223] were among the first to employ a computerized imaging system consisting of a light microscope and a light-sensitive diode array interfaced with a computer to monitor droplet size distribution and the rate of droplet coalescence. Such systems permit the sizing of smaller particles and real-time analyses. Westesen and Wehler [158] evaluated the particle size distribution

Table 7 Emulsion Appearance as a Function of Size of the Dispersed Phase

Particle size, µm	Appearance
> 1	White
0.1–1	Blue-white
0.05–0.1	Opalescent, semitransparent
< 0.5	Transparent

of a model intravenous emulsion by photon correlation spectroscopy (PCS): no droplets with diameters < 140 nm were observed in the unfractionated emulsion. In contrast, transmission electron micrographs yielded a mean particle diameter of about 68 nm, while ^{31}P nuclear magnetic resonance spectroscopy disclosed the presence of approximately 48 mol% of the phospholipid surfactant in particles smaller than approximately 100 nm. PCS measurements, and corresponding chemical analyses, of the *fractionated* emulsion confirmed the impression that the majority of the emulsion droplets were under 100 nm in diameter. The value of PCS in the absence of fractionation of the native emulsion is apparently limited. Finally, particle size analyses of the dispersed phases of a multiple emulsion remain problematical and need to be addressed further given the increasing attention to multiple emulsions as drug delivery systems.

Rheological behavior of an emulsion is also dependent on the emulsion's particle size range and distribution. Sherman [224] demonstrated that the change in emulsion viscosity with time is controlled by the increase in mean particle size. To the extent that emulsions tend to behave in a non-Newtonian manner, viscosity measurements at a single rate of shear, or shearing stress, are of little value. In effect, the complete rheogram should be evaluated; shear stress should be measured as a function of shear rate (or vice versa, depending upon the rheometer) [225]. For emulsion systems displaying time-dependent rheological behavior, sample history (processing, handling) as well as the duration of shear can affect the results. Fong-Spaven and Hollenbeck [226] recommend the non-isothermal evaluation of shear stress at constant shear rate as a means of evaluating emulsion stability.

For emulsions that conform to pseudoplastic (shear-thinning) behavior, Sherman [227] has described a method for predicting viscosity changes during storage based on the time-independent relationship between the viscosity of such emulsions, at a given rate of shear, and mean droplet size, D_m. In general, as D_m decreases, the relative viscosity η_{rel} increases, particularly when D_m falls below 5 μm: small variations in D_m within the range 0 to1 μm for emulsions of a given ϕ cause large changes in η_{rel} [227]. At high rates of shear, viscosity is relatively independent of shear rate and reaches a steady value, η_∞. At low rates of shear, viscosity is shear rate dependent. Sherman's observations provide the basis for calculating rheological changes in emulsions when they are aged, provided the droplet size distribution does not broaden appreciably and that droplet coalescence is the only irreversible structural change in the system. The rate constant governing the increase in D_m can be determined from simple tests extending over a few days. This enables one to predict droplet size at later times and the corresponding viscosity can be derived from the $\eta_\infty - D_m$ relationship established experimentally over a range of ϕ values. Equation (19) is the relationship employed by Sherman [227]:

$$\log \eta_\infty = \left[\frac{0.036\, D_m}{\sqrt[3]{\dfrac{\phi_{max}}{\phi} - 1}} \right] - 0.15 \tag{19}$$

At high shear rates, some droplet distortion may occur leading to values of the maximal volume fraction of the dispersed phase, ϕ_{max}, below the hypothetical 0.74. If the globules are distorted from spheroids to prolate ellipsoids, $\phi_{max} \approx 0.53$. However, droplet distortion is also affected by interfacial tension, the viscosity ratio of the disperse and continuous phases, the rate of shear, D_m, and the physical properties of the interphase. At a shear rate of 1000 s^{-1}, droplets smaller than 10 μm undergo minimal distortion [227]. At low shear rates, some discrepancies may be evident because aged emulsions tend to flocculate and aggregate to a greater extent than freshly prepared emulsions. In spite of its limitations, Sherman's methodology offers an alternative to questionable accelerated aging techniques.

Rheological evaluations of interfacial fluidity of elasticity [228,229] can facilitate the characterization of emulsion stability: high interfacial elasticity is likely to result in stable emulsions [229]. As esoteric as these measurements may be to some formulators, it should be recognized that the rheological properties of the interphase may be quite different from those of the bulk phases comprising the emulsion. Many instruments have been designed to measure interfacial rheological behavior. These include two-dimensional analogs of the Couette rotational viscometer and various interfacial oscillatory devices [228,229]. Chapter 5 in Volume 1 of this treatise includes more detailed information on rheological techniques for the examination of emulsions.

B. Phase Inversion

Phase inversion or emulsion-type reversal (e.g., W/O to O/W) was associated, at one time, with the volume fraction of the internal phase, ϕ [230]: when $\phi \geq 0.74$, uniform, rigid spheres of the internal phase could no longer be accommodated within the continuous phase and the emulsion would invert. The polydispersity and deformability of emulsion droplets, in most systems of practical interest, minimizes the applicability of this rule. Phase inversion, when it does occur, is not usually a function of ϕ but of the nature of the emulsifier and emulsifier concentration [230]. In practice, relatively stable emulsions with $\phi \geq 0.90$ have been prepared [193]; others have been shown to invert at $\phi = 0.25$ [231]. Phase inversion can be a serious problem as emulsion instability or coarsening of texture can be a direct consequence of the inversion. The modified low-energy emulsification technique of Lin and Shen [211] was proposed as a means of reducing the potential for irreversible phase inversion because, for the original process, there appears to be a practical limit to the weight fraction of the unheated phase that can be withheld when ϕ is > 0.30 or the emulsion has a high solids content [232]. The Lin-Shen technique affords less opportunity for phase inversion as the phase ratios are much lower at each stage than in conventional processing.

At the outset, whether the continuous phase is polar or nonpolar can be determined by various simple methods. One can measure the conductivity of the emulsion or, more simply, incorporate the emulsion in an electrical circuit including a lamp. Minimal conductivity or failure of the lamp to glow is indicative of a W/O emulsion, and substantial conductivity or a glowing lamp is associated with an O/W emulsion. A change in conductivity behavior with time is indicative of a multiphase emulsion or of phase inversion. Other more qualitative tests to determine the nature of the continuous phase include the dye solubility test and the dilution test. The former method involves the addition of a water- or oil-soluble dye to the emulsion followed by its microscopic examination. Thus, if a water-soluble dye were added and the droplets of the internal phase are now intensely colored, one has a W/O emulsion. The addition of an oil-soluble dye to the same emulsion would result in the staining of the continuous phase. The dilution test involves observation of the emulsion, following its dilution with oil or water, to see whether separation has been effected. If so, the diluent is not compatible with the continuous phase of the emulsion. When used individually, these simplistic methods can yield incorrect results: the type of emulsion determined by one method should always be confirmed by means of a second method.

Phase inversion can also be detected rheologically or conductometrically. Viscosity increases as ϕ increases because interparticulate and hydrodynamic interactions are accentuated. At some critical ϕ, the emulsion inverts and ϕ becomes much smaller. Consequently, viscosity tends to be considerably lower. One can therefore expect a discontinuity in rheological behavior in the vicinity of the critical ϕ. Similarly, a discontinuity in conductivity behavior as a function of ϕ would be indicative of phase inversion.

C. Component Stability

The physical and chemical instability of emulsion system components is also of concern to the emulsion formulator. Phase solubility and polymorphic changes in components, component migration from one phase to another, and chemical degradation are all of practical consequence. Jass [233] gave examples of marked emulsion deterioration that apparently resulted from temperature- or shear-induced changes in component crystallinity or solubility. Migration of components (partitioning; sorption) from one phase to another can affect the physical, chemical, or microbial stability of the product depending on the nature of the migrating species (e.g., surfactant, antioxidant, or antimicrobial preservative).

Although changes in solubility and crystallinity of emulsion components are often detectable by microscopic examination of the emulsion, identification or analysis of phase components in situ was not possible until recently (see the discussion earlier in this chapter on liquid crystalline phase formation). Louden and coworkers [234] have described the use of nondestructive macro and micro laser Raman spectroscopy to provide detailed qualitative information on the emulsion system and on emulsion components. Quantitative information may also be provided by this approach.

Rheological studies can also provide an indirect means of identifying changes in emulsion components, particularly when the emulsion system is structured or ordered, as with semisolids [225]. The viscoelastic properties of emulsions, in particular, are amenable to rapid, quantitative measurement and can serve as the basis for quality control or stability-indicating methodology [235–239].

In the absence of any demonstrable or significant change in emulsion system properties (e.g., cracking; creaming; phase inversion; altered consistency or color) as a product ages, it is still necessary to establish stability in terms of drug and appropriate nondrug constituents. Selective or specific analyses of each phase, for each component under investigation, can establish whether or not migration or degradation is occurring. It may be necessary to analyze the container or closure to ensure the absence of partitioning or adsorptive interaction with emulsion ingredients. The analyst should be able to account for all of the analyte originally present in the product in terms of a mass balance involving all phases of the emulsion system, the package, and even the processing equipment.

D. Accelerated Stability Testing

Pharmaceutical and cosmetic manufacturers envisage shelf lives for their products of at least 2 to 3 years. Shelf lives of a year or less are impractical insofar as commercial product distribution and sales are concerned. Shelf-life recommendations must be made in accordance with the stability and intended use of the product. The quandary faced by the emulsion technologist is that (a) laboratory stability testing methods are rarely comparable to actual product storage conditions nor absolutely predictive; and (b) product aging protocols specifying actual storage conditions for 2 or 3 years are too protracted to be of immediate practical value to the manufacturer.

The prediction of emulsion product aging and instability is beset with difficulties. Attempts to accelerate the processes that lead to instability, either by thermal or gravitational means, are fraught with error. In many instances, at least for emulsion systems, the results of an accelerated stability test correlate poorly with actual ("real time") product aging.

1. *Thermally Accelerated Stability Testing*

Thermally induced instability is generally assumed to follow the Arrhenius relationship:

$$\ln k = \ln A - \left[\frac{E_a}{R} \right] \frac{1}{T} \tag{20}$$

In Eq. (20), the logarithmic form of the Arrhenius equation, k is the reaction rate constant, A is the Arrhenius constant (associated with reaction entropy and/or collision factors), E_a is the activation energy (a measure of the barrier to the reaction), R is the molar gas constant, and T is absolute temperature ($°K$). Where instability is the result of diffusion or photolytic degradation, E_a is on the order of 2 to 3 kcal/mole and the temperature-dependence of the reaction is negligible. Thus, attempts to thermally accelerate instability would be unproductive at best.

The logarithmic form of the Arrhenius equation indicates that there is a linear relationship between the logarithm of the rate constant and the inverse of absolute temperature. By determining the rate constants for degradation at elevated temperatures, one can estimate k at a lower temperature, by extrapolation, and the corresponding time required for a specific degree of degradation. This approach has been found most useful for predicting a product's shelf life when instability is due to chemical degradation.

Unfortunately, emulsion systems, in contrast to less complex pharmaceutical and cosmetic formulations, seldom obey the Arrhenius relationship. Some reasons for deviations from the equation and the failure of elevated temperature studies to adequately predict stability include the folllowing [240]: (a) emulsifier or stabilizer solubility and phase distribution tend to be temperature-dependent; (b) degradation may occur at higher temperatures but not at lower ones (the mechanism of the reaction or process may change with temperature); (c) temperature-induced phase changes, sometimes drastic, may occur resulting in composition changes and altered rheological behavior; and (d) structural deformation and reformation may vary markedly with time and temperature.

Stratagems and paradigms for accelerated stability testing at elevated temperatures have been described [241]. In the face of an emulsion product's failure to obey the Arrhenius relationship, a formulator may be forced to rely upon room-temperature behavior. Testing protocols that use a heating/cooling cycle, or a freeze-thaw cycle, have been employed for stability testing of emulsions. Even though potential instability problems may be revealed, these methodologies do not provide kinetic data necessary for the estimation of shelf life.

2. *Gravitationally Accelerated Stability Testing*

Centrifugal methods have long been employed by emulsion technologists to induce and accelerate instability by gravitational means. The ultracentrifuge, in particular, has been applied to the evaluation of droplet flocculation kinetics and coalescence [242,243]. These centrifugal test methods have a number of disadvantages that limit their utility with pharmaceutical and cosmetic emulsions. They are neither suitable for very viscous products nor applicable to semisolids. The physical state of the emulsion in the centrifugal field may be quite different from that in a nonstressed environment. For example, the flocculated emulsion region in the ultracentrifuge contains only traces of the continuous phase; the dispersed phase droplets have been deformed considerably so that the droplet content of the emulsion region is markedly increased. Although the centrifugal behavior of emulsions with a low internal phase volume ratio is predictable from droplet size and density data, it does not necessarily correlate with descriptions of "good" or "bad" emulsions [243]. For emulsions with high internal phase volume ratios, correlatability is poorer still, a reflection of the complex hydrodynamics and interparticulate interactions involved. Centrifugal methodology, then, does not eliminate the stability-testing quandary for formulators either.

3. *Miscellaneous Accelerants of Stability Testing*

Stresses other than temperature or gravity—for example, agitation, vibration—may also hasten emulsion product instability. In 1982, Rieger [244] suggested that gentle shaking or vibration could accelerate macroemulsion instability. Rieger's rationale for low shear or vibrational testing of emulsions is based upon the provision of just enough shear to increase the frequency of particle collision and the likelihood of coalescence. If an emulsion behaves rheologically as a shear-thinning system, the tendency to coalesce will be enhanced even more by its exposure to low shear as the result of the decreased viscous resistance to droplet movement. Thus, coalescence may be more likely to occur if the emulsion product is subjected to gentle shear (shaking, rolling, or rocking) or vibration just prior to or during a thermally or gravitationally accelerated stability study [244,245].

Low-shear reciprocating shakers—operating at 10 to 100 cycles/minute and at modestly elevated temperatures (e.g., 40°C)—have been advocated for emulsoin stability testing [245]. Friberg et al. [246] are proponents of "shake testing" of emulsion products in the *final* package (container) because the surface characteristics of the final package may differ from those of laboratory glassware, or other containers, and their closures. An additional benefit of using platform or reciprocating shakers in stability testing of emulsions is that emulsion destabilization is likely to occur during shake testing whenever the continuous phase of an emulsion does not uniformly wet the walls of the container or the lining of the closure because of the formation of a thin film of the dispersed phase on the container or closure surface, thereby increasing the potential for coalescence [245,246]. Shake testing may also provide valuable insight into the vulnerability of an emulsion product to the stresses encountered during shipping and handling [246].

4. *Freeze-Thaw Testing*

Emulsion product stability at freezing temperatures (e.g., −10 to −5°C)—not just at refrigerator conditions (e.g., 4°C)—is a must in the Temperate Zone [245]. Friberg et al.

[246] maintain that cyclical freeze-thaw stability testing is the *only* predictive accelerated testing methodology because the destabilization processes function only during the
freezing and thawing periods and not during storage under frozen conditions. Hence,
repeated freeze-thaw cycling at short intervals should prove informative, even though
shelf-life estimates are generally not provided by these kinds of studies. The utility of
freeze-thaw cycling methodologies is limited further by (a) variable rates of cooling and
heating; (b) temperature nonuniformity in the emulsion system during cycling; and (c)
the thermal lability of emulsion components.

5. *Stability Testing Protocols*

From a thermodynamic point of view, although microemulsion stability is not problematic, the phrase "stable macroemulsion" is an oxymoron. In practice, however, formulators consider a macroemulsion to be stable if there is no evidence of coalescence or
creaming under ambient conditions, or when frozen and thawed repeatedly, or upon
exposure to moderately elevated temperatures (e.g., 40 to 50°C) for various time intervals. Failure under any of these conditions may be allowable in specific instances
(e.g., elevated temperature stability is of no concern with a heat-sensitive drug). For that
matter, creaming or flocculation that can be reversed by simple shaking may not be a
deterrent to product development or marketing.

Stability testing protocols utilized in the evaluation of emulsion products have involved the application of a single stress (or multiple stresses) in a constant, cyclic, step,
progressive, or random manner. The sheer number and variety of accelerated stability
testing protocols proposed in the literature is testimony to the minimal predictivity of
these procedures for macroemulsions. Nonetheless, at present, there is general agreement on at least four aspects of emulsion product stability testing: (a) freshly prepared,
unequilibrated emulsions are not the appropriate subjects of an emulsion product stability
testing protocol: only emulsion products that have had an opportunity to "rest" or equili-
brate (e.g., for 24 or 48 hours) after manufacture should be employed; (b) whenever
possible, comparisons should be made between the "test" emulsion product and a similar
"reference" emulsion product with known stability characteristics and shelf life; (c)
storage and stress conditions should be comparable to those the emulsion product is likely
to encounter during its commercial lifetime, i.e., in the course of shipping, handling,
storage, and use; and (d) each emulsion product necessitates the development of explicit
stability criteria to be employed in conjunction with product-specific stability testing
methods and protocols.

Industrial practice, for most pharmaceutical emulsions, involves storage at 5, 25,
40, and 50°C. Stability at 5 and 40°C for 3 months is considered minimal. Unfortunately, "real-time" ambient temperature testing of emulsion products is not a reasonable
alternative. As Rieger [245] has noted, real-time testing for periods up to or exceeding
2 years has been described as *intolerable* to formulators or manufacturers.

Perhaps the key to the design of the ultimate *accelerated* shelf-life test for emulsion products is to be found within the pages of the definitive monograph by Nelson
[247], which provides an in-depth treatment of "product life" or product performance
testing methodologies and the corresponding statistical and mathematical analyses required. For now, in the absence of a definitive, universally applicable approach to the
stability testing and shelf-life evaluation of emulsions, one is tempted to recall the pro-
posal of Wood and Catacalos [248], who noted the predictive value of the logarithmic
time dependency of emulsion stability or stability-indicating behavior. In effect, if the
logarithm of viscosity, for example, of a stable emulsion were plotted as a function of

the logarithm of time, $d(\log \eta)/d(\log t) \approx 0$. For most emulsions, however, flocculation and/or other phenomena effect changes in system behavior over time so that $d(\log \eta)/d(\log t) \neq 0$. Furthermore, marked deviations from log-log linearity are indicative of even more substantive changes in the emulsion system (e.g., phase separation). The logarithmic compression of the time axis in this and other data transformations (e.g., Weibull plots [249]) or the use of the cumulative sum ("cusum") technique [250] may facilitate the recognition of instability even when room temperature storage must be employed. In this way, the elusive goal of an acceptable stability test protocol for emulsion products may be realized in practice.

ACKNOWLEDGMENT

The author acknowledges with sincere appreciation the contributions of Bernard Idson, Ph.D., which helped make this revision possible.

APPENDIX

Alphabetical Listing of Drugs Incorporated in Macro- and Microemulsions[a]

Drug	Formulation,[b] Administration Route[c]	Reference[d]
amphotericin B	O/W; i.v.	[11, I–1]
anti-inflammatory agents	O/W submicron emulsions; topical	[I–2]
antigens	W/O; i.m.	[I–3, I–4]
antineoplastic agents	O/W; parenteral	[157]
	W/O, W/O/W; intratumor	[I–5]
barbituric acids	O/W; i.v.	[I–6]
benzocaine	O/W; i.v., s.c.	[I–7]
betamethasone esters	O/W submicron emulsion; topical	[I–2]
bleomycin	W/O, O/W; i.m., i.p.	[I–8]
	spray-dried reconstitutible O/W emulsion; i.m., i.p.	[I–8]
	W/O, W/O/W; intratumor	[I–5]
butacaine	O/W; i.v., s.c.	[I–7]
chloroquine	W/O/W; peroral	[I–9; I–10; I–11]
corticosteroids	O/W; i.v.	[I–12]
cyclandelate	O/W; intraarterial	[I–13]
cyclobarbital	O/W; i.v.	[I–6]
cyclosporine	microemulsion; peroral	[145]
	microemulsion; peroral	[35]
cytosine arabinoside	W/O/W; parenteral	[I–14]
dexamethasone palmitate	O/W; i.v.	[I–12]
diazepam	O/W; i.v.	[I–15]
	O/W submicron emulsion; i.v.	[I–16]
diclofenac	O/W submicron emulsion; topical	[I–2]
doxorubicin HCl	W/O	[I–17]
estradiol	microemulsion; topical	[I–18]
5-fluorouracil	O/W; intramural	[I–19]

(*continued*)

Drug	Formulation,[b] Administration Route[c]	Reference[d]
	O/W; rectal	[I-20]
	W/O/W; i.m.	[I-21]
	W/O/W; peroral	[I-22]
griseofulvin[e]	O/W; peroral	[I-23, I-24]
heparin	O/W; intraduodenal	[8]
hexobarbital	O/W; i.v.	[I-6]
hydrocortisone	microemulsion; topical	[33]
indomethacin	O/W/O; peroral	[I-25]
	O/W submicron emulsion; topical	[I-2]
indoxole	O/W; peroral	[7]
insulin	W/O/W; peroral	[146,147]
	microemulsion; rectal	[35]
lidocaine	O/W; i.v., s.c.	[I-7]
	microemulsion; topical	[I-26]
lidocaine-prilocaine[f]	O/W; topical	[I-27]
methotrexate	W/O/W; parenteral	[I-14, I-28, I-29]
miconazole	W/O submicron emulsion; i.v.	[I-30]
mitomycin C	W/O, O/W; i.m., i.p.	[I-31]
naproxen	O/W submicron emulsion; topical	[I-2]
nitgroglycerin	O/W; intraarterial	[I-14]
	O/W; peroral	[I-32]
penclomedine	O/W; i.v.	[157]
pentazocine	O/W/O; peroral	[I-33]
	W/O/W; peroral	[I-34]
perfluorocarbons	P/W; i.v.	[I-35; I-36]
pentobarbital	O/W; i.v.	[I-37]
phenobarbital	O/W; i.v.	[I-6]
physostigmine	O/W; i.m.	[20]
piroxicam	O/W submicron emulsion; topical	[I-2]
prednisolone	O/W/O, W/O/W; ocular	[125]
pregnanolone	O/W; i.v.	[I-38]
propofol	O/W; i.v.	[I-39]
prostaglandin E_1	O/W; pulmonary	[124]
quatacaine	O/W; i.v., s.c.	[I-7]
rhizoxin	O/W; i.v.	[157]
secobarbital	O/W; i.v.	[I-6]
sulfacetamide sodium	W/O/W;	[I-40]
taxol	O/W; parenteral	[14]
terbutaline	W/O/W;	[I-41]
theophylline	O/W; intragastric	[I-42]
thiopental	O/W; i.v.	[I-6, I-37]
vancomycin	O/W; i.v.	[I-43]
vasopressin	microemulsion; peroral	[35]

[a]excluding—in general—formulations prepared extemporaneously by the direct incorporation of drug in an emulsion vehicle

[b]phase composition: O = oil, W = water, P = perfluorocarbon

[c]in some instances, the reference's focus is entirely on formulation: the emulsion system, although intended for a particular route of administration, was not administered to animals or humans

[d]numbers refer to the references in the body of the text; numbers preceded by the letter "I" refer to references that appear only in this appendix

[e]micronized drug suspended in the oil phase

[f]1:1 eutectic mixture emulsified in aqueous system

REFERENCES

1. A. J. Bevacqua, K. M. Lahanas, I. D. Cohen, and G. Cioca, Liquid crystals in multiple emulsions, *Cosmetics Toiletries*, 106(5):53–56 (1991).
2. T. F. Tadros and B. Vincent, Emulsion stability. In: *Encyclopedia of Emulsion Technology*, Vol. 1 (P. Becher, ed.), Marcel Dekker, New York, 1983, pp. 132–133.
3. S. Friberg, M. L. Hilton, and L. B. Goldsmith, Emulsions are not only two liquids, *Cosmetics Toiletries*, 102(2):87–98 (1987).
4. B. A. Mulley and J. S. Marland, Multiple-drop formation in emulsions. *J. Pharm. Pharmacol.*, 22:243–245 (1970).
5. M. M. Rieger, Emulsions. In: *The Theory and Practice of Industrial Pharmacy* (L. Lachman, H. A. Lieberman, and J. L. Kanig, eds.), 3rd ed., Lea & Febiger, Philadelphia, 1986, p. 503.
6. R. J. Gardner, Lipohilicity and the preception of bitterness, *Chemical Senses Flavours*, 4:275–286 (1979).
7. J. G. Wagner, E. S. Gerard, and D. G. Kaiser, The effect of the dosage form on serum levels of indoxole, *Clin. Pharmacol. Ther.*, 7:610–619 (1966).
8. R. H. Engel and S. J. Riggi, Intestinal absorption of heparin: a study of the interactions of components of oil-in-water emulsions, *J. Pharm. Sci.*, 58:1372–1375 (1969).
9. R. Nishigaki, S. Awazu, M. Hanano, and T. Fuwa, The effect of dosage form on absorption of vitamin A into lymph, *Chem. Pharm. Bull.*, 24:3207–3211 (1976).
10. Y. Mizushima, T. Hamano, and K. Yokoyama, Use of a lipid emulsion as a novel carrier for corticosteroids, *J. Pharm. Pharmacol.*, 34:49–50 (1982).
11. S. S. Davis, C. Washington, P. West, L. Illum, G. Liversidge, L. Sternson, and R. Kirsh, Lipid emulsions as drug delivery systems, *Ann. N. Y. Acad. Sci.*, 507:75–88 (1987).
12. T. Takahashi, M. Mizuno, Y. Fujita, S. Ueda, B. Nishioka, and S. Majima, Increased concentration of anticancer agents in regional lymph nodes by fat emulsions, with special reference to chemotherapy of metastasis, *Gann*, 64:345 (1973).
13. T. Kato, Encapsulated drugs in targeted cancer therapy. In: *Controlled Drug Delivery*, vol. 2 (S. D. Bruck, ed.), CRC Press, Boca Raton, 1983, pp. 199–200.
14. B. D. Tarr, T. G. Sambandan, and S. H. Yalkowsky, A new parenteral emulsion for the administration of taxol, *Pharm. Res.*, 4:162–165 (1987).
15. I. D. A. Johnston (ed.), *Advances in Parenteral Nutrition*, MTP Press Limited, Lancaster, England (1978).
16. L. C. Clark, Jr., F. Becattini, and S. Kaplan, Can fluorocarbon emulsions be used as artificial blood, *Triangle*, 11:115–122 (1972).
17. D. L. Parsons, Perfluorochemical blood substitutes, *U.S. Pharmacist*, 10(5):H14–H21 (1985).
18. S. J. Prigal, Emulsion composition, U.S. Patent 3,096,249, 2 July 1963.
19. C. S. L. Chiao and J. R. Robinson, Sustained-release drug delivery systems. In: *Remington: The Science and Practice of Pharmacy* (A. R. Gennaro, ed.), 19th ed., Mack, Easton, 1995, pp. 1669–1671.
20. S. Benita, D. Friedman, and M. Weinstock, Pharmacological evaluation of an injectable prolonged release emulsion of physostigmine in rabbits, *J. Pharm. Pharmacol.*, 38:653–658 (1986).
21. T. P. Hoar and J. H. Schulman, Transparent water-in-oil dispersions: the oleopathic hydromicelle, *Nature*, 152:102–103 (1943).
22. L. M. Prince, ed., *Microemulsions*, Marcel Dekker, New York, 1974.
23. K. Shinoda and S. Friberg, *Emulsions and Solubilization*, John Wiley, New York, 1986.
24. S.-H. Chen and R. Rajagopalan, eds., *Micellar Solutions and Microemulsions*, Springer-Verlag, New York, 1990.
25. P. C. Hiemenz, *Principles of Colloid and Surface Chemistry*, 2nd ed., Marcel Dekker, New York, 1986, pp. 469–470.
26. R. Lostritto, L. Goei, and S. Silvestri, Theoretical considerations of drug release from submicron oil in water emulsions, *J. Parenter. Sci.*, 41:214–219 (1987).

27. E. Ruckenstein and J. Chi, *J. Chem. Soc. Faraday Trans.* 2, 71:1690 (1975); through D. Langevin, Low interfacial tensions in microemulsion systems. In: *Micellar Solutions and Microemulsions*, Springer-Verlag, New York, 1990, p. 216.

28. D. B. Siano, The swollen micelle-microemulsion transition, *J. Colloid Interface Sci.*, 93:1–7 (1983).

29. D. Attwood, Microemulsions. In: *Colloidal Drug Delivery Systems* (J. Kreuter, ed.), Marcel Dekker, New York, 1994, p. 32.

30. F. Lachampt and R. M. Vila, A contribution to the study of emulsions, *Am. Perfum. Cosmet.*, 82(1):29–36 (1967).

31. J. Swarbrick, Phase equilibrium diagrams: an approach to the formulation of solubilized and emulsified systems, *J. Soc. Cosmet. Chem.*, 19:187–209 (1968).

32. F. Lachampt and R. M. Vila, Contribution to the study of emulsions, *Am. Perfum. Cosmet.*, 85(1):27–36 (1970).

33. A. Jayakrishnan, K. Kalaiarash, and D. O. Shah, Microemulsions: evolving technology for cosmetic applications, *J. Soc. Cosmet. Chem.*, 34:335–350 (1983).

34. H. N. Bhargava, A. Narurkar, and L. M. Lieb, Using microemulsions for drug delivery, *Pharm. Technol.*, 11(3):46–54 (1987).

35. W. A. Ritschel, Gastrointestinal absorption of peptides using microemulsions as delivery systems, *Bull. Tech. Gattefossé*, 83:7–22 (1990).

36. S. A. Safran, Theory of structure and phase transitions in globular microemulsions. In: *Micellar Solutions and Microemulsions* (S.-H. Chen and R. Rajagopalan, eds.), Springer-Verlag, New York, 1990, p. 162.

37. J. H. Whittam, W. E. Gerbacia, and H. L. Rosano, Microemulsions: a new technology for the cosmetic industry, *Cosmet. Technol.*, 1(10):35–42 (1979).

38. P. Sherman, Rheological properties of emulsions. In: *Encyclopedia of Emulsion Technology*, Vol. 1 (P. Becher, ed.), Marcel Dekker, New York, 1983, pp. 431–432.

39. S. Bader, F. Brunetta, G. Pantini, and M. Visca, Three-phase emulsions: perfluoropolyether-oil-water, *Cosmet. Toiletries*, 101:45–48 (1986).

40. R. V. Petersen and R. D. Hamill, Studies on nonaqueous emulsions, *J. Soc. Cosmet. Chem.*, 19:627–640 (1968).

41. E. S. R. Gopal, Hydrodynamic aspects of the formation of emulsions. In: *Rheology of Emulsions* (P. Sherman, ed.), Pergamon Press, Oxford, 1963, pp. 15–25.

42. B. Kanner and J. E. Glass, Surface viscosity and elasticity. In: *Chemistry and Physics of Interfaces*, American Chemical Society, Washington, D.C., 1971, pp. 49–61.

43. C. Müller-Goymann, Liquid crystals in emulsions, creams, and gels containing ethoxylated sterols as surfactant, *Pharm. Res.*, 1:154–158 (1984).

44. J. M. Pasternacki-Surian, R. L. Schnaare, and E. T. Sugita, Effect of surfactant phase in perfluorocarbon emulsification efficiency, *Pharm. Res.*, 9:406–409 (1992).

45. D. J. Mitchell, G. J. T. Tiddy, L. Waring, T. Bostock, and M. P. McDonald, Phase behaviour of polyoxyethylene surfactants in water, *J. Chem. Soc. Faraday Trans. I*, 79:975–1000 (1983).

46. D. Attwood and A. T. Florence, *Surfactant Systems: Their Chemistry, Pharmacy and Biology*, Chapman and Hall, New York, 1983, pp. 1–8.

47. R. L. Camp, K. C. Scott, K. F. Schoene, and R. R. Holland, Success of your process may depend on a surfactant, *Res. Develop.*, 27(3):92–97 (1985).

48. C. Fox, Rationale for the selection of emulsifying agents, *Cosmet. Toiletries*, 101(11):25–26, 28, 34, 36, 38–40, 44 (1986).

49. W. C. Griffin, Classification of surface-active agents by "HLB", *J. Soc. Cosmet. Chem.*, 1:311–326 (1949).

50. W. C. Griffin, Calculation of HLB values of nonionic surfactants, *J. Soc. Cosmet. Chem.*, 5:249–256 (1954).

51. Anon., *The Atlas HLB System*, 2nd ed. revised, Atlas Chemical Industries, Wilmington, 1963, p. 19.

52. J. T. Davies and E. K. Rideal, *Interfacial Phenomena*, 2nd ed., Academic Press, New York, 1963, pp. 371–378.
53. K. Shinoda and S. Friberg, *Emulsions and Solubilization*, John Wiley, New York, 1986, pp. 56–68.
54. S. Riegelman and G. Pichon, A critical re-evaluation of factors affecting emulsion stability, I. The hydrophilic-lipophilic balance postulate, *Am. Perfum.*, 77(2):31–33 (1962).
55. P. Becher and R. L. Birkmeier, The determination of hydrophile-lipophile balance by gas-liquid chromatography, *J. Am. Oil Chem. Soc.*, 41:169–172 (1964).
56. K. Shinoda and H. Kunieda, Phase properties of emulsions: PIT and HLB. In: *Encyclopedia of Emulsion Technology*, Vol. 1 (P. Becher, ed.), Marcel Dekker, New York, 1983, pp. 337–367.
57. T. J. Lin, H. Kurihara, and H. Ohta, Prediction of optimum O/W emulsification via solubilization measurements, *J. Soc. Cosmet. Chem.*, 28:457–479 (1977).
58. T. J. Lin, Low-surfactant emulsification, *J. Soc. Cosmet. Chem.*, 30:167–180 (1979).
59. L. I. Osipow, *Surface Chemistry: Theory and Industrial Applications*, Reinhold, New York, 1962, pp. 334–335.
60. T. F. Tadros and B. Vincent, Emulsion stability. In: *Encyclopedia of Emulsion Technology*, Vol. 1 (P. Becher, ed.), Marcel Dekker, New York, 1983, pp. 209–217.
61. J. E. Carless and G. Hallworth, Viscosity of oil-water interfaces and emulsion stability, *Chem. Ind.*, 85:30–31 (1966).
62. B. W. Barry, The self bodying action of the mixed emulsifier sodium dodecyl sulfate/cetyl alcohol, *J. Colloid Interface Sci.*, 28:82–91 (1968).
63. T. Higuchi, Some physical chemical aspects of suspension formulation, *J. Am. Pharm. Assoc.*, *Sci. Ed.*, 47:657–660 (1958).
64. M. Reiner, *Deformation, Strain and Flow*, 2nd ed., H. K. Lewis & Co. Ltd., London, 1960, pp. 243–255.
65. J. R. Van Wazer, J. W. Lyons, K. Y. Kim, and R. E. Colwell, *Viscosity and Flow Measurement*, Interscience Publishers, New York, 1963, pp. 15–17.
66. A. A. Daneshy, Numerical solution of sand transport in hydraulic fracturing, *J. Petr. Technol.*, *January*, 132–140 (1978); through J. Zatz, Physical stability of suspensions, *J. Soc. Cosmet. Chem.*, 36:393–411 (1985).
67. J. Th. G. Overbeek, The interaction between colloidal particles. In: *Colloid Science*, Vol. 1 (H. R. Kruyt, ed.), Elsevier Publishing Co., New York, 1952, pp. 245–277.
68. H. van Olphen, Theories of the stability of lyophobic colloidal systems. In: *Physical Chemistry: Enriching Topics from Colloid and Surface Science* (H. van Olphen and K. J. Mysels, eds.), Theorex, La Jolla, 1975, pp. 5–15.
69. D. H. Melik and H. S. Fogler, Fundamentals of colloidal stability in quiescent media. In: *Encyclopedia of Emulsion Technology* (P. Becher, ed.), Vol. 3, Marcel Dekker, New York, 1988, pp. 3–78.
70. R. I. Feigin and D. H. Napper, Stabilization of colloids by free polymer, *J. Colloid Interface Sci.*, 74:567–571 (1980).
71. M. van den Tempel, Effect of droplet flocculation on emulsion viscosity. In: *Rheology of Emulsions* (P. Sherman, ed.), Pergamon Press, Oxford, 1963, pp. 1–14.
72. R. Darby, Emulsion rheology. In: *Emulsions and Emulsion Technology* (K. J. Lissant, ed.), Part III, Marcel Dekker, New York, 1984, pp. 94–95.
73. P. J. Niebergall, Preparation of buffers at known pH and ionic strength, personal communication, Department of Pharmaceutical Sciences, Medical University of South Carolina, Charleston, SC.
74. J. A. Serrallach and G. Jones, Formation of films at liquid-liquid interfaces, *Ind. Eng. Chem.*, 23:1016–1019 (1931).
75. E. Shotton and R. F. White, Stabilization of emulsions with gum acacia. In: *Rheology of Emulsions* (P. Sherman, ed.), Pergamon Press, Oxford, 1963, pp. 59–71.

76. R. I. Morrison and B. Campbell, Water-soluble cellulose ethers as emulsifying agents, *J. Soc. Chem. Ind.*, 68:333–336 (1949).
77. N. D. Weiner, A. K. Shah, J. L. Kanig, and A. Felmeister, Effect of neutralizing amine on the stability of emulsions prepared with carboxy vinyl polymers. *J. Soc. Cosmet. Chem.*, 20:215–223 (1969).
78. K. P. Oza and S. G. Frank, Drug release from emulsions stabilized by colloidal microcrystalline cellulose, *J. Disp. Sci. Technol.*, 10:187–210 (1989).
79. P. C. Hiemenz, *Principles of Colloid and Surface Chemistry*, 2nd ed., Marcel Dekker, New York, 1986, pp. 4–10.
80. R. Defay, L. Prigogine, A. Bellemans, and D. H. Everett, *Surface Tension and Adsorption*, John Wiley, New York, 1966, pp. 1–4.
81. J. J. Bikerman, The interfacial phase, *Kolloid-Z. Z. Polymere*, 201:46–47 (1965).
82. O. Lutz, M. Vrachopoulou, and M. J. Groves, Use of the Walden Product to evaluate the effect of amino acids on water structure, *J. Pharm. Pharmacol.*, 46:698–703 (1994).
83. O. Lutz and M. J. Groves, The effect of lysine, a water-structure breaker, on the stability of phospholipid-stabilized emulsions, *J. Pharm. Pharmacol.*, 47:566–570 (1995).
84. M. J. Groves, Stability considerations and evaluation methods. In *Multi-Phase Systems for Oral and Parenteral Drug Delivery: Physical and Biopharmaceutical Aspects*, 37th International Industrial Pharmaceutical Research and Development Conference, June 5–9, 1995, Merrimac, WI.
85. A. W. Adamson, *Physical Chemistry of Surfaces*, 5th ed., Wiley, New York, 1990, p. 534.
86. T. R. Briggs, Emulsions with finely divided solids, *J. Ind. Eng. Chem.*, 13:1008–1010 (1921).
87. E. H. Lucassen-Reynders, and M. van den Tempel, Stabilization of water-in-oil emulsions by solid particles, *J. Phys. Chem.*, 67:731–734 (1963).
88. H. van Olphen, *An Introduction to Clay Colloid Chemistry*, Interscience, New York, 1963, pp. 155–187.
89. P. A. Ciullo and D. B. Braun, Clay/carbomer mixtures enhance emulsion stability, *Cosmet. Toiletries*, 106 (5):89–92, 94–95 (1991).
90. H. van Olphen, *An Introduction to Clay Colloid Chemistry*, Interscience, New York, 1963, p. 178.
91. K. J. Lissant, Thermodynamics. In: *Emulsions and Emulsion Technology* (K. J. Lissant, ed.), Part III, Marcel Dekker, New York, 1984, pp. 181–214.
92. J. J. Bikerman, The physical basis of wetting, *Kolloid-Z. Z. Polymere*, 218:52–56 (1967).
93. J. J. Bikerman, *Physical Surfaces*, Academic Press, New York, 1970, p. 295.
94. S. Torza and S. G. Mason, Three-phase interactions in shear and electrical fields, *J. Colloid Interface Sci.*, 33:67–83 (1970).
95. M. E. R. Shanahan, C. Cazeneuve, A. Carre, and J. Schultz, Wetting criteria in three phase solid/liquid/liquid systems, *J. Chim. Phys.*, 79:241–245 (1982).
96. C. F. Lerk, A. J. M. Schoonen, and J. T. Fell, Contact angles and wetting of pharmaceutical powders, *J. Pharm. Sci.*, 65:843–847 (1976).
97. C. F. Lerk, M. Lagas, J. P. Boelstra, and P. Broersma, Contact angles of pharmaceutical powders, *J. Pharm. Sci.*, 66: 1480–1481 (1977).
98. R. Hüttenrauch and S. Fricke, Beziehung zwischen Wasserstruktur und Dispersität der Emulsionen, *Pharmazie*, 41:515–516 (1986).
99. Y. Kumano, S. Nakamura, S. Tahara, and S. Ohta, Studies and practices of water-in-oil emulsions stabilized with amino acids or their salts, 9th International Congress IFSCC, Boston, MA, June 7, 1976; through *Norda Briefs*, No. 477, November 1976.
100. H. Jünginger, A. A. M. D. Akkermans, and W. Heering, The ratio of interlamellarly fixed water to bulk water in O/W creams, *J. Soc. Cosmet. Chem.*, 35:45–57 (1984).
101. R. C. Rowe and J. McMahon, Cryogenic scanning electron microscopy—a novel method for the structural characterisation of semi-solid creams, *Pharm. Int.*, 8:91–93 (1987).
102. G. M. Eccleston, The microstructure of semisolid creams, *Pharm. Int.*, 7:63–70 (1986).

103. H. K. Patel, R. C. Rowe, J. McMahon, and R. F. Stewart, A systematic microscopial examination of gels and emulsions containing cetrimide and cetostearyl alcohol, *Int. J. Pharm.*, 25:13–25 (1985).
104. K. Münzel, Über die Gelstrucktur der Salben, *J. Soc. Cosmet. Chem.*, 19:289–343 (1968).
105. S. Friberg and P. Solyom, The influence of liquid crystalline phases on the rheological behaviour of emulsions, *Kolloid-Z. Z. Polymere*, 236:173–174 (1970).
106. A. T. Florence and D. Whitehill, Stabilization of water/oil/water multiple emulsions by polymerization of the aqueous phases, *J. Pharm. Pharmacol.*, 34:687–691 (1982).
107. D. L. Wedderburn, Preservation of emulsions against microbial attack. In: *Advances in Pharmaceutical Sciences*, vol. 1 (H. S. Bean, A. H. Beckett, and J. E. Carless, eds.), Academic Press, London and New York, 1964, pp. 195–268.
108. M. T. Parker, The clinical significance of the presence of micro-organisms in pharmaceutical and cosmetic preparations, *J. Soc. Cosmet. Chem.*, 23:415–426 (1972).
109. C. R. Woodward Jr. and T. F. McNamara, Microbiological considerations of cosmetic emulsions, *Am. Perfum. Cosmet.* 85:73–76 (1970).
110. J. J. Kabara, ed., *Cosmetic and Drug Preservation: Principles and Practice*, Marcel Dekker, New York, 1984.
111. M. Gay, Testing the efficacy of antimicrobial preservation: pharmacopeial requirements, practical experience, and drug safety, *Pharm. Technol.*, 7 (5):58–61, 64–65, 67, 70 (1983).
112. H. S. Bean, Preservatives for pharmaceuticals, *J. Soc. Cosmet. Chem.*, 23:703–720 (1972).
113. E. R. Garrett and O. R. Woods, The optimum use of acid preservatives in oil-water systems: benzoic acid in peanut oil-water, *J. Am. Pharm. Assoc.*, *Sci. Ed.*, 42:736–739 (1953).
114. N. R. Horn, T. J. McCarthy, and C. H. Price, Interaction between preservatives and suspension systems, *Am. Perfum. Cosmet.*, 86(7):37–40 (1971).
115. R. H. Tilbury, The effect of the hydrophilic-lipophilic balance of nonionic surfactants on the efficiency of preservatives in simple emulsions, *Specialities*, 1(7):3–8 (1965).
116. H. S. Bean, G. H. Konning, and J. Thomas, Significance of the partition coefficient of a preservative in cosmetic emulsions, *Am. Perfum. Cosmet.*, 85(3):61–65 (1970).
117. E. R. Garrett, A basic model for the evaluation and prediction of preservative action, *J. Pharm. Pharmacol.*, 18:589–601 (1966).
118. M. Yamaguchi, Y. Asaka, M. Tanaka, T. Mitsui, and S. Ohta, Antimicrobial activity of butylparaben in relation to its solubilization behavior by nonionic surfactants, *J. Soc. Cosmet. Chem.*, 33:297–307 (1982).
119. M. C. Allwood, Preservative efficacy testing of pharmaceuticals, *Pharm. Int.*, 7:172–175 (1986).
120. G. Sauermann, W. Hofeditz, and W. Engel, Eine Methode zur Bestimmung der Verteilungsgleichgewichte von Konservierungsmitteln in Emulsionen, *J. Soc. Cosmet. Chem.*, 29:767–776 (1978).
121. V. J. Stella, Oxidation and photolysis. In: *Chemical Stability of Pharmaceuticals*, 2nd ed. (K. A. Connors, G. L. Amidon, and V. J. Stella, eds.), John Wiley & Sons, New York, 1986, pp. 82–114.
122. R. Marcuse and P.-O. Fredrikkson, Fat oxidation at low oxygen pressure. II. Kinetic studies on linoleic acid oxidation in emulsions in the presence of antioxidants, *J. Am. Oil Chem. Soc.*, 46:262–268 (1969).
123. K.-H. Foißner, A. Leonhardt, G. Wegner, and K. H. Bauer, Determination of dissolved oxygen in heterogenous systems particularly in emulsions and oily liquids, *Pharm. Res.*, 2:44–46 (1985).
124. Y. Mizushima, K. Hoshi, H. Aihara, and M. Kurachi, Inhibition of bronchostriction by aerosol of a lipid emulsion containing prostaglandin E_1, *J. Pharm. Pharmacol.*, 35:397 (1983).
125. S. M. Safwat, M. A. Kassem, M. A. Attia, and M. El-Mahdy, The formulation-performance relationship of multiple emulsions and ocular activity, *J. Controlled Rel.*, 32:259–268 (1994).

126. L. H. Block, Medicated applications. In: *Remington: The Science and Practice of Pharmacy*, 19th ed. (A. R. Gennaro, ed.), Mack, Easton, 1995, pp. 1577–1597.

127. B. W. Barry, *Dermatological Formulations*, Marcel Dekker, New York, 1983.

128. S. Raynal, J. L. Grossiord, M. Seiller, and D. Clausse, A topical w/o/w multiple emulsion containing several active substances: formulation, characterization and study of release, *J. Controlled Rel.*, 26:129–140 (1993).

129. I. H. Blank, Factors which influence the water content of the skin, *J. Invest. Dermatol.*, 18:433–440 (1952).

130. I. H. Blank, Further observations on factors which influence the water content of the stratum corneum, *J. Invest. Dermatol.*, 21:259–269 (1953).

131. R. R. Warner and N. A. Lilly, Correlation of water content with ultrastructure in the stratum corneum. In: *Bioengineering of the Skin: Water and the Stratum Corneum* (P. Elsner, E. Berardesca, and H. I. Maibach, eds.), CRC Press, Boca Raton, 1994, p. 10.

132. J. Wepierre and M. Adrangui, Factors in the occlusivity of aqueous emulsions, *J. Soc. Cosmet. Chem.*, 33:157–167 (1982).

133. G. L. Flynn, General introduction and conceptual differentiation of topical and transdermal drug delivery systems: differentiation with respect to delivery kinetics. In: *Topical Drug Bioavailability, Bioequivalence, and Penetration* (V. P. Shah and H. I. Maibach, eds.), Plenum Press, New York, 1993, pp. 369–391.

134. A. Rougier, TEWL and transcutaneous absorption. In: *Bioengineering of the Skin: Water and the Stratum Corneum* (P. Elsner, E. Berardesca, and H. I. Maibach, eds.), CRC Press, Boca Raton, 1994, pp. 103–113.

135. M. D. Donovan and D. R. Flanagan, Bioavailability of disperse dosage forms. In: *Pharmaceutical Dosage Forms: Disperse Systems*, 2nd ed., Vol. 1 (H. A. Lieberman, M. M. Rieger, and G. S. Banker, eds.), Marcel Dekker, New York, in press.

136. S.-H. L. Leung, J. R. Robinson, and V. H. L. Lee, Parenteral products. In: *Controlled Drug Delivery: Fundamentals and Applications* (J. R. Robinson and V. H. L. Lee, eds.), 2nd ed., Marcel Dekker, New York, 1987, pp. 455–458.

137. K. Kakemi, H. Sezaki, S. Muranishi, H. Ogata, and S. Isemura, Mechanism of intestinal absorption of drugs from oil in water emulsions. I, *Chem. Pharm. Bull.*, 20:708–714 (1972).

138. K. Kakemi, H. Sezaki, S. Muranishi, H. Ogata, and K. Giga, Mechanism of intestinal absorption of drugs from oil in water emulsions. II, *Chem. Pharm. Bull.*, 20:715–720 (1972).

139. W. I. Higuchi, and T. Higuchi, Theoretical analysis of diffusional movement through heterogeneous barriers, *J. Am. Pharm. Assoc.*, *Sci. Ed.*, 49:589–606 (1960).

140. W. I. Higuchi, Rate of solute transport out of emulsion droplets in micron size range, *J. Pharm. Sci.*, 53:405–408 (1964).

141. A. H. Goldberg, W. I. Higuchi, N. F. H. Ho, and G. Zografi, Mechanisms of interphase transport I: theoretical considerations of diffusion and interfacial barriers in transport of solubilized systems, *J. Pharm. Sci.*, 56:1432–1437 (1967).

142. A. H. Goldberg and W. I. Higuchi, Mechanisms of interphase transport II: theoretical considerations and experimental evaluation of interfacially controlled transport in solubilized systems, *J. Pharm. Sci.*, 58:1341–1352 (1969).

143. A.-H. Ghanem, W. I. Higuchi, and A. P. Simonelli, Interfacial barriers in interphase transport: retardation of the transport of diethylphthalate across the hexadecane-water interface by an adsorbed gelatin film, *J. Pharm. Sci.*, 58:165–174 (1969).

144. S. S. Davis, J. Hadgraft, and K. J. Palin, Medical and pharmaceutical applications of emulsions. In: *Encyclopedia of Emulsion Technology* (P. Becher, ed.), Vol. 2, Marcel Dekker, New York, 1985, pp. 159–238.

145. J. M. Kovarik, E. A. Mueller, J. B. van Bree, W. Tetzloff, and K. Kutz, Reduced inter- and intraindividual variability in cyclosporine pharmacokinetics from a microemulsion formulation, *J. Pharm. Sci.*, 83:444–446 (1994).

146. R. H. Engel, S. J. Riggi, and M. J. Fahrenbach, Insulin: intestinal absorption as water-in-oil-in-water emulsions, *Nature*, 219:856–857 (1968).

147. M. Shichiri, Y. Shimizu, M. Yoshida, R. Kawamori, M. Fukuchi, Y. Shigeta, and H. Abe, Enteral absorption of water-in-oil-in-water insulin emulsions in rabbits, *Diabetologia*, 10: 317–321 (1974).

148. M. Shichiri, Y. Yamasaki, R. Kawamori, M. Kikuchi, N. Hakui, and H. Abe, Increased intestinal absorption of insulin: an insulin suppository, *J. Pharm. Pharmacol.*, 30:806–808 (1978).

149. A. F. Brodin, D. R. Kavaliunas, and S. G. Frank, Prolonged drug release from multiple emulsions, *Acta Pharm. Suec.*, 15:111–118 (1978).

150. M. J. Groves and R. M. A. Mustafa, Measurement of the spontaneity of self-emulsifyable oils, *J. Pharm. Pharmacol.*, 26:671–688 (1974).

151. M. J. Groves and D. A. de Galindez, The self-emulsifying action of mixed surfactants in oil, *Acta Pharm. Suec.*, 13:361–372 (1976).

152. S. A. Charman, W. N. Charman, M. C. Rogge, T. D. Wilson, F. J. Dutko, and C. W. Pouton, Self-emulsifying drug delivery systems: formulation and biopharmaceutic evaluation of an investigational lipophilic compound, *Pharm. Res.*, 9:87–93 (1992).

153. D. Q. M. Craig, The use of self-emulsifying systems as a means of improving drug delivery, *Bull. Tech. Gattefossé*, 86:21–32 (1993).

154. H. C. Meng, Use of fat emulsions in parenteral nutrition, *Drug. Intell. Clin. Pharm.*, 6:321–330 (1972).

155. R. H. Müller, *Colloidal Carriers for Controlled Drug Delivery and Targeting: Modification, Characterization and In Vivo Distribution*, CRC Press, Boca Raton, 1991, pp. 175–176.

156. S. P. Fortmann and D. J. Maron, Disorders of lipid metabolism. In: *Scientific American Medicine*, (D. C. Dale and D. D. Federman, eds.), Scientific American, Inc., New York, 1993, Section 9-II, pp. 1–5.

157. R. J. Prankerd and V. J. Stella, The use of oil-in-water emulsions as a vehicle for parenteral drug administration, *J. Parenter. Sci. Technol.*, 44(3):139–149 (1990).

158. K. Westesen and T. Wehler, Investigation of the particle size distribution of a model intravenous emulsion, *J. Pharm. Sci.*, 82:1237–1244 (1993).

159. R. T. Lyons, Intravenous lipids: an alternate delivery system for drugs and vitamins. In: *Multi-Phase Systems for Oral and Parenteral Drug Delivery: Physical and Biopharmaceutical Aspects*, 37th International Industrial Pharmaceutical Research and Development Conference, June 5–9, 1995, Merrimac, WI.

160. S. Benita and M. Y. Levy, Submicron emulsions as colloidal drug carriers for intravenous administration: comprehensive physicochemical characterization, *J. Pharm. Sci.*, 82:1069–1079 (1993).

161. D. M. Lidgate, T. Trattner, R. M. Shultz, and R. Maskiewicz, Sterile filtration of a parenteral emulsion, *Pharm. Res.*, 9:860–862 (1992).

162. C. J. Herman and M. J. Groves, Hydrolysis kinetics of phospholipids in thermally stressed intravenous lipid emulsion formulations, *J. Pharm. Pharmacol.*, 44:539–542 (1992).

163. M. J. Groves and C. J. Herman, The redistribution of bulk aqueous phase phospholipids during thermal stressing of phospholipid-stabilized emulsions, *J. Pharm. Pharmacol.*, 45:592–596 (1993).

164. H. J. Helbock, P. A. Motchnik, and B. N. Ames, Toxic hydroperoxides in intravenous lipid emulsions used in preterm infants, *Pediatrics*, 91:83–87 (1993).

165. L. Rydhag, The importance of the phase behaviour of phospholipids for emulsion stability, *Fette Seifen Anstrichm.*, 81:168–173 (1979).

166. A. Wade and P. J. Weller, eds., *Handbook of Pharmaceutical Excipients*, 2nd ed., American Pharmaceutical Association/The Pharmaceutical Press, Washington, D.C., 1994.

167. S. Bolton, *Pharmaceutical Statistics: Practical and Clinical Applications*, 2nd ed., Marcel Dekker, New York, 1990, pp. 532–570.

168. N. R. Bohidar, F. A. Restaino, and J. B. Schwartz, Selecting key parameters in pharmaceutical formulations by principal component analysis, *J. Pharm. Sci.*, 64:966–969 (1975).

169. J. B. Schwartz, J. R. Flamholz, and R. H. Press, Computer optimization of pharmaceutical formulations I: General procedure, *J. Pharm. Sci.*, 62:1165–1170 (1973).

170. J. B. Schwartz, J. R. Flamholz, and R. H. Press, Computer optimization of pharmaceutical formulations II: Application in troubleshooting, *J. Pharm. Sci.*, 62:1518–1519 (1973).

171. G. Zografi, An approach to the teaching of factors influencing emulsion formation, *Am. J. Pharm. Ed.*, 31:206–211 (1967).

172. Ternary Plot version 3.0, PAZ Graphics, Toronto, Ontario, Canada.

173. R. Mackay, Use of triangular diagrams in the study of emulsions. In: *Encyclopedia of Emulsion Technology*, vol. 3 (P. Becher, ed.), Marcel Dekker, New York, 1988, pp. 223–237.

174. A. W. Francis and N. O. Smith, Ternary liquid systems, *J. Chem. Ed.*, 46:815–820 (1969).

175. E. Shek, M. Ghani, and R. E. Jones, Simplex search in optimization of capsule formulation, *J. Pharm. Sci.*, 69:1135–1142 (1980).

176. B. S. Everitt, *Graphical Techniques for Multivariate Data*, North-Holland, New York, 1978.

177. K. J. Lissant, Use of glyphs to organize data in multivariant systems. In: *Encyclopedia of Emulsion Technology*, vol. 3 (P. Becher, ed.), Marcel Dekker, New York, 1988, pp. 239–280.

178. S. Ross and I. D. Morrison, *Colloidal Systems and Interfaces*, Wiley, New York, 1988, p. 286.

179. R. R. Scott, A practical guide to equipment selection and operating techniques. In: *Pharmaceutical Dosage Forms: Disperse Systems*, 2nd ed., Vol. 3 (H. A. Lieberman, M. M. Rieger, and G. S. Banker, eds.), Marcel Dekker, New York, in press.

180. S. Ross and I. D. Morrison, *Colloidal Systems and Interfaces*, Wiley, New York, 1988, pp. 56–65.

181. C. Fox, The current state of processing technology of emulsions and suspensions. In: *Cosmetic Science*, vol. 2 (M. M. Breuer, ed.), Academic Press, London and New York, 1980, pp. 1–81.

182. M. M. Breuer, Cosmetic emulsions. In: *Encyclopedia of Emulsion Technology*, vol. 2 (P. Becher, ed.), Marcel Dekker, New York, 1985, pp. 398–403.

183. S. Friberg and R. L. Venable, Microemulsions. In: *Encyclopedia of Emulsion Technology*, vol. 1 (P. Becher, ed.), Marcel Dekker, New York, 1983, pp. 311–312.

184. P. Walstra, Formation of emulsions. In: *Encylcopedia of Emulsion Technology*, vol. 1 (P. Becher, ed.), Marcel Dekker, New York, 1983, pp. 57–127.

185. J. T. Davies and E. K. Rideal, *Interfacial Phenomena*, 2nd ed., Academic Press, New York, 1963, pp. 366–371.

186. H. Lange, Zur Theorie der Stabilität von Emulsionen, *J. Soc. Cosmet. Chem.*, 16:697–714 (1965).

187. C. D. Fox and R. F. Shangraw, Water/oil emulsions prepared by low pressure capillary homogenization II. Stabilizing influence of inorganic electrolytes, secondary emulsifiers, and temperature, *J. Pharm. Sci.*, 55:323–328 (1966).

188. J. T. Davies and E. K. Rideal, *Interfacial Phenomena*, 2nd ed., Academic Press, New York, 1963, pp. 378–382.

189. P. Becher, Effect of preparation parameters on the initial size distribution function in oil-in-water emulsions, *J. Colloid Interface Sci.*, 24:91–96 (1967).

190. M. Reiner, *Deformation, Strain and Flow*, 2nd ed., H. K. Lewis, London, 1960, pp. 212–215.

191. P. Sherman, Rheological properties of emulsions. In: *Encyclopedia of Emulsion Technology*, vol. 1 (P. Becher, ed.), Marcel Dekker, New York, 1983, pp. 405–437.

192. T. Gillespie, The effect of concentration on the viscosity of suspensions and emulsions. In: *Rheology of Emulsions* (P. Sherman, ed.), Pergamon Press, Oxford, 1963, pp. 115–124.

193. K. J. Lissant, The geometry of high-internal-phase-ratio emulsions, *J. Colloid Interface Sci.*, 22:462–468 (1966).

194. M. Primorac, M. Stupar, G. Vuleta, and D. Vasiljevic, Rheological properties of oil/water microemulsions, *Pharmazie*, 47:645–646 (1992).
195. J. M. Church and R. Shinnar, Stabilizing liquid-liquid dispersions by agitation, *Ind. Eng. Chem.*, 53:479–484 (1961).
196. J. Y. Oldshue, *Fluid Mixing Technology*, McGraw-Hill, New York, 1983, pp. 129–130.
197. S. V. Subramanyam and E. S. R. Gopal, Role of interfacial tension and viscosity in the process of emulsification, *Kolloid-Z. Z. Polymere*, 210: 80–81 (1966).
198. T. J. Lin, Low-energy emulsification I. Principles and applications, *J. Soc. Cosmet. Chem.*, 29:117–125 (1978).
199. A. K. Reng, Energy and time-saving production of cosmetic emulsions, *Cosmet. Toiletries*, 101 (11):117–112, 124 (1986).
200. T. J. Lin, Process engineering for cosmetic emulsions. Part I. application of engineering fundamentals, *Am. Perfum. Cosmet.*, 79(11):40,42,44,47–49 (1964).
201. Y. Fujiyama, S. Tahara, and Y. Kumano, Rheological properties of creams upon production scale-up, *J. Soc. Cosmet. Chem.*, 21:625–637 (1970).
202. G. A. Van Buskirk, et al., Workshop III report: scaleup of liquid and semisolid disperse systems, *Pharm. Res.*, 11:1216–1220 (1994).
203. B. Richmond, P. Vescuso, and S. Peterson, *Stella™ for Business*, High Performance Systems, Inc., Lyme, NH, 1987.
204. T. J. Lin, Process engineering for cosmetic emulsions. Part II. model study, scale-up considerations, *Am. Perfum. Cosmet.*, 80 (1):39, 42, 45 (1965).
205. R. Y. Lochhead, W. J. Hemker, J. Y. Castaneda, and D. Garlen, Novel cosmetic emulsions, *Cosmet. Toiletries*, 101(11):125–126, 128, 130, 132, 134, 136, 138 (1986).
206. R. Y. Lochhead, W. J. Hemker, and J. Y. Castaneda, Hydrophobically modified "Carbopol" resins, *Soap Cosmet. Chem. Spec.*, 63 (5):28–29, 32–33, 84–85 (1987).
207. Anon., Formulation ideas, *Soap Cosmet. Chem. Spec.*, 64 (3):83 (1988).
208. A. L. L. Hunting, The history and use of self-emulsifying waxes, *Cosmet. Toiletries*, 101(11): 49–50, 54, 56, 60–62, 64–65, 68 (1986).
209. Anon., *Formulaire Cosmetique*, 3rd ed., Gattefossé, Saint-Priest France, 1987, p. 35.
210. G. E. Schumacher, Emulsifying waxes in bulk compounding formulations, *Am. J. Hosp. Pharm.*, 26:132–133 (1969).
211. T. J. Lin and Y. F. Shen, Low-energy emulsification. Part VI. Applications in high-internal phase emulsions, *J. Soc. Cosmet. Chem.*, 35:357–368 (1984).
212. Anon., Formulation ideas, *Soap Cosmet. Chem. Spec.*, 63 (10):110 (1987).
213. G. M. Eccleston, Application of emulsion stability theories to mobile and semisolid o/w emulsions, *Cosmet. Toiletries*, 101(11): 73–74, 76–81, 84–86, 88, 91–92 (1986).
214. R. A. W. Hill and J. T. Knight, A kinetic theory of droplet coalescence with application to emulsion stability, *Trans. Faraday Soc.*, 61:170–181 (1965).
215. H. R. Moskowitz, *Cosmetic Product Testing, A Modern Psychophysical Approach*, Marcel Dekker, New York, 1984.
216. K. H. Burdick, B. Poulsen, and V. A. Place, Extemporaneous formulation of corticsoteroids for topical usage, *J. Am. Med. Assoc.*, 211: 462–466 (1970).
217. K. H. Burdick, Corticosteroid bioavailability assays, *Acta Dermatovener.*, 67 (Suppl.):19–31 (1972).
218. P. C. Hiemenz, *Principles of Colloid and Surface Chemistry*, 2nd ed., Marcel Dekker, New York, 1986, pp. 384–385.
219. R. Defay, L. Prigogine, A. Bellemans, and D. H. Everett, *Surface Tension and Adsorption*, John Wiley, New York, 1966, pp. 269–273.
220. S. K. Sharma, S. S. Davis, O. L. Johnson, and K. C. Lowe, Physicochemical assessment of novel formulations of emulsified perfluorocarbons, *J. Pharm. Pharmacol.*, 38:5P (1986).
221. J. L. Zatz and G. H. Cueman, Assessment of stability of water-in-oil-in-water multiple emulsions, *J. Soc. Cosmet. Chem.*, 39:211–222 (1988).

222. C. Orr, Determination of particle size. In: *Encyclopedia of Emulsion Technology*, vol. 3 (P. Becher, ed.) Marcel Dekker, New York, 1988, pp. 137–169.

223. J. L. Klemaszewski, Z. Haque, and J. E. Kinsella, An electronic imaging system for determining droplet size and dynamic breakdown of protein stabilized emulsions, *J. Food Sci.*, 54:440–445 (1989).

224. P. Sherman, Changes in the rheological properties of emulsions on aging, and their dependence on the kinetics of globule coagulation, *J. Phys. Chem.*, 67:2531–2537 (1963).

225. L. H. Block and P. P. Lamy, The rheological evaluation of semisolids, *J. Soc. Cosmet. Chem.*, 21:645–660 (1970).

226. F. Fong-Spaven and R. G. Hollenbeck, Thermal rheological analysis of triethanolamine-stearate stabilized mineral oil in water emulsions, *Drug Dev. Ind. Pharm.*, 12: 289–302 (1986).

227. P. Sherman, A method for predicting rheological changes in emulsion products when aged, *J. Soc. Cosmet. Chem.*, 16:591–606 (1965).

228. S. Ross and I. D. Morrison, *Colloidal Systems and Interfaces*, Wiley, New York, 1988, pp. 277–279.

229. D. J. Burgess and N. O. Sahin, Interfacial rheology of β-casein solutions. In: *Structure and Flow in Surfactant Solutions* (C. A. Herb and R. K. Prud'homme, eds.), American Chemical Society, Washington, D.C., 1994, pp. 380–393.

230. S. Ross, Toward emulsion control, *J. Soc. Cosmet. Chem.*, 6:184–192 (1955).

231. T. F. Tadros and B. Vincent, Emulsion stability. In: *Encyclopedia of Emulsion Technology*, Vol. 1 (P. Becher, ed.), Marcel Dekker, New York, 1983, pp. 228–229.

232. T. J. Lin, T. Akabori, S. Tanaka, and K. Shimura, Low-energy emulsification. III. Emulsification in high α range, *Cosmet. Toiletries*, 95 (12):33–39 (1980).

233. H. E. Jass, Effect of process variables on the stability of some specific emulsions, *J. Soc. Cosmet. Chem.*, 18:591–598 (1967).

234. J. D. Louden, H. K. Patel, and R. C. Rowe, A preliminary examination of the structure of gels and emulsions containing cetostearyl alcohol and cetrimide using laser Raman spectroscopy, *Int. J. Pharm.*, 25:179–190 (1985).

235. B. W. Barry and B. Warburton, Some rheological aspects of cosmetics, *J. Soc. Cosmet. Chem.*, 19:725–744 (1968).

236. S. S. Davis, Viscoelastic properties of pharmaceutical semisolids I. Ointment bases, *J. Pharm. Sci.*, 58:412–418 (1969).

237. S. S. Davis, Viscoelastic properties of pharmaceutical semisolids II. Creams, *J. Pharm. Sci.*, 58:418–421 (1969).

238. G. B. Thurston and S. S. Davis, The viscoelastic properties of a soap-stabilized oil-in-water emulsion, *J. Colloid Interface Sci.*, 69:199–208 (1979).

239. M. M. Breuer and H.-C. Tsai, Measuring the viscoelastic properties of aerosol shaving foams, *J. Soc. Cosmet. Chem.*, 35:59–71 (1984).

240. D. G. Pope, Accelerated stability testing for prediction of drug product stability. 2., *Drug Cosmet. Ind.*, 127 (6): 48, 52, 56, 58, 60, 62 (1980).

241. K. A. Connors, G. L. Amidon, and V. J. Stella, eds., *Chemical Stability of Pharmaceuticals*, 2nd ed., John Wiley, New York, 1986, pp. 135–159.

242. R. D. Vold and R. C. Groot, Parameters of emulsion stability *J. Soc. Cosmet. Chem.*, 14:233–244 (1963).

243. E. R. Garrett, Prediction and evaluation of emulsion stability with ultracentrifugal stress, *J. Soc. Cosmet. Chem.*, 21:393–415 (1970).

244. M. M. Rieger, The predictive determination of emulsion stability, *Cosmet. Toiletries*, 97(8):27–31 (1982).

245. M. M. Rieger, Stability testing of macroemulsions, *Cosmet. Toiletries*, 106 (5):59–60, 62–66, 69 (1991).

246. S. E. Friberg, L. B. Goldsmith, and M. L. Hilton, Theory of Emulsions. In: *Pharmaceutical Dosage Forms: Disperse Systems*, 2nd ed., (H. A. Lieberman, M. M. Rieger, and G. S. Banker, eds.), Chapter 3, Vol. 1, Marcel Dekker, New York, pp. 53–90.

247. W. Nelson, *Accelerated Testing: Statistical Models, Test Plans, and Data Analyses*, John Wiley, New York, 1990.

248. J. H. Wood and G. Catacalos, Prediction of the rheologic aging of cosmetic lotions, *J. Soc. Cosmet. Chem.*, 14:147–156 (1963).

249. J. E. Ogden, A Weibull shelf-life model for pharmaceuticals, *Pharm. Technol.*, 2 (10):45–49, 58 (1978).

250. S. H. C. du Toit, A. G. W. Steyn, and R. H. Stumpf, *Graphical Exploratory Data Analysis*, Springer-Verlag, New York, 1986, pp. 252–259.

References for Appendix I

I-1. D. Forster, C. Washington, and S. S. Davis, Toxicity of solubilized and colloidal amphotericin B formulations to human erythrocytes, *J. Pharm. Pharmacol.*, 40:325–328 (1988).

I-2. D. I. Friedman, J. S. Schwarz, and M. Weisspapir, Submicron emulsion vehicle for enhanced transdermal delivery of steroidal and nonsteroidal antiinflammatory drugs, *J. Pharm. Sci.*, 84:324–329 (1995).

I-3. J. Freund, and M. V. Bonanto, The effect of paraffin oil, lanolin-like substances and killed tubercle bacilli on immunization with diphtheric toxoid and bact. typhosum, *J. Immunol.*, 48:325–334 (1944).

I-4. B. A. Mulley, Medicinal emulsions. In: Emulsions and Emulsion Technology (K. J. Lissant, ed.), Marcel Dekker, New York, 1974, pp. 291–349.

I-5. T. Takahashi, S. Ueda, K. Kono, and S. Majima, Attempt at local administration of anticancer agents in the form of fat emulsion, *Cancer*, 38:1507–1514 (1976).

I-6. R. Jeppsson, Effects of barbituric acids using an emulsion form intravenously, *Acta Pharm. Suec.*, 9:81–90 (1972).

I-7. R. Jeppsson, Comparison of pharmacological effects of some local anesthetics when using water and lipid emulsion as injection vehicles, *Acta Pharm. Toxicol.*, 36:299–311 (1975).

I-8. Y. Nakamoto, M. Hashida, S. Muranishi, and H. Sezaki, Studies on pharmaceutical modification of anticancer agents. II. Enhanced delivery of bleomycin into lymph by emulsions and drying emulsions, *Chem. Pharm. Bull.*, 23:3125–3131 (1975).

I-9. J. A. Omotosho, The effect of acacia, gelatin and polyvinylpyrrolidone on chloroquine transport from multiple w/o/w emulsions, *Int. J. Pharm.*, 62:81–84 (1990).

I-10. R. S. Okor, Retard release from a flocculated emulsion system, *Int. J. Pharm.*, 65:133–136 (1990).

I-11. A. Vaziri and B. Warburton, Slow release of chloroquine phosphate from multiple taste-masked w/o/w multiple emulsions, *J. Microencaps.*, 11:641–648 (1994).

I-12. Y. Mizushima, T. Hamano, and K. Yokoyama, Use of a lipid emulsion as a novel carrier for corticosteroids, *J. Pharm. Pharmacol.*, 34:49–50 (1982).

I-13. R. Jeppsson and S. Ljungberg, Intraarterial administration of emulsion formulations containing cyclandelate and nitroglycerin, *Acta Pharm. Suec.*, 10:129–140 (1973).

I-14. C. J. Benoy, R. Schneider, L. A. Elson, and M. Jones, Enhancement of the cancer chemotherapeutic effect of the cell cycle phase specific agents methotrexate and cytosine arabinoside when given as a water-oil-water emulsion, *Eur. J. Cancer*, 10:27–33 (1974).

I-15. J. P. Fee, P. S. Collier, and J. W. Dundee, Bioavailability of three formulations of intravenous diazepam, *Acta Anaesthesiol. Scand.*, 30:337–340 (1986).

I-16. M. Y. Levy and S. Benita, Short- and long-term stability assessment of a new injectable diazepam submicron emulsion, *J. Parenter. Sci. Technol.*, 45:101–107 (1991).

I-17. S. Lin, S. Wu, and W. Lui, In vitro release, pharmacokinetic and tissue distribution studies of doxorubicin hydrochloride (Adriamycin HCl®) encapsulated in lipiodolized w/o and w/o/w multiple emulsions, *Pharmazie*, 47:439–443 (1992).

I-18. F. Fevrier, Microemulsions for topical application, *Bull. Tech. Gattefossé*, 83:23–31 (1990).

I–19. H. Ohta, K. Takagi, Y. Noguchi, I. Ohashi, T. Takahashi, S. Watanabe, T. Takekoshi, K. Ohashi, and Y. Kato, Endoscopic intramural injection of anti-neoplastic emulsion, *Gann*, 75:641–649 (1984).

I–20. S. Watanabe, B. Nishioka, Y. Fujita, T. Ueda, O. Kojima, K. Morisawa, E. Yamane, M. Umehara, and S. Majima, Comparative studies on absorption patterns of the drug after intrarectal administration of 5-FU emulsion and 5-FU solution, *Jpn. J. Surg.*, 10:105–109 (1980).

I–21. J. A. Omotosho, T. L. Whateley, and A. T. Florence, Release of 5-fluorouracil from intramuscular w/o/w multiple emulsions, *Biopharm. Drug Dispos.*, 10:257–268 (1989).

I–22. J. A. Omotosho, A. T. Florence, and T. L. Whateley, Absorption and lymphatic uptake of 5-fluorouracil in the rat following oral administration of w/o/w multiple emulsions, *Int. J. Pharm.*, 61:51–56 (1990).

I–23. T. R. Bates and J. A. Sequeira, Bioavailability of micronized griseofulvin from corn oil-in-water emulsion, aqueous suspension, and commercial tablet dosage forms in humans, *J. Pharm. Sci.*, 64:793–797 (1975).

I–24. T. R. Bates and P. J. Carrigan, Apparent absorption kinetics of micronized griseofulvin after its oral administration on single- and multiple-dose regimens to rats as a corn oil-in-water emulsion and aqueous suspension, *J. Pharm. Sci.*, 64:1475–1481 (1975).

I–25. J. K. Pandit, B. Mishra, D. N. Mishra, P. K. Choudhary, In vitro release of indomethacin from multiple o/w/o emulsions, *Indian Drugs*, 25:408–412 (1988).

I–26. J. Carlfors, I. Blute, and V. Schmidt, Lidocaine in microemulsion—a dermal delivery system, *J. Disp. Sci. Technol.*, 12:467–482 (1991).

I–27. A. A. Nyqvist-Mayer, A. F. Brodin, and S. G. Frank, Phase distribution studies on an oil-water emulsion based on a eutectic mixture of lidocaine and prilocaine as the dispersed phase, *J. Pharm. Sci.*, 74:1192–1195 (1985).

I–28. L. A. Elson, B. C. V. Mitchlev, A. J. Collings, and R. Schneider, Chemotherapeutic effect of a water-oil-water emulsion of methotrexate on the mouse L1210 leukaemia, *Rev. Eur. Etudes Clin. Bio.*, 15:87–90 (1970).

I–29. J. A. Omotosho, T. L. Whateley, and A. T. Florence, Methotrexate transport from the internal phase of multiple w/o/w emulsions, *J. Microencaps.*, 6:183–192 (1989).

I–30. M. Y. Levy, I. Polacheck, Y. Barenholz, and S. Benita, Efficacy evaluation of a novel submicron miconazole emulsion in a murine cryptococcosis model, *Pharm. Res.*, 12:223–230 (1995).

I–31. Y. Nakamoto, M. Fujiwara, T. Noguchi, T. Kimura, S. Muranishi, and H. Sezaki, Studies on pharmaceutical modification of anticancer agents. I. Enhancement of lymphatic transport of mitomycin C by parenteral emulsions, *Chem. Pharm. Bull.*, 23:2232–2238 (1975).

I–32. H. Ogata and H.-L. Fung, Effect of sesame oil emulsion on nitroglycerin pharmacokinetics, *Int. J. Pharm.*, 5:335–344 (1980).

I–33. B. Mishra and J. K. Pandit, Prolonged release of pentazocine from multiple o/w/o emulsions, *Drug Dev. Ind. Pharm.*, 15:1217–1230 (1989).

I–34. B. Mishra and J. K. Pandit, Multiple water-oil-water emulsions as prolonged release formulations of pentazocine, *J. Controlled Rel.*, 14:53–60 (1990).

I–35. N. Jing and B. A. Cooper, Stable perfluorocarbon emulsions using XMO-10 as surfactant: potential oxygen-carrying plasma expanders, *Biomaterials, Artif. Cells, Artif. Organs*, 18:107–117 (1990).

I–36. G. K. Hanna, M. C. Ojeda, and T. A. Sklenar, Application of computer-based experimental design to optimization of processing conditions for perfluorocarbon emulsions, *Biomaterials, Artif. Cells, Immobiliz. Biotechnol.*, 20:849–852 (1992).

I–37. S. Ljungberg and R. Jeppsson, Intravenous injection of lipid soluble drugs: a preliminary report, *Acta Pharm. Suec.*, 7:435–440 (1970).

I–38. S. Høgskilde, J. W. Nielsen, P. Carl, and M. B. Sørensen, Pregnanolone emulsion—a new steroid preparation for intravenous anaesthesia: an experimental study in mice, *Anaesthesia*, 42:586–590 (1987).

I-39. G. C. Cummings, J. Dixon, N. H. Kay, J. P. Windsor, E. Major, M. Morgan, J. W. Sear, A. A. Spence, and D. K. Stephenson, Dose requirements of ICI 35,868 (propofol, 'Diprivan') in a new formulation for induction of anaesthesia, *Anaesthesia*, 39:1168–1171 (1984).

I-40. E. Fredro-Kumbaradzi, M. Sturpar, G. Vuleta, and A. Simov, Release of sulfacetamide sodium from multiple w/o/w emulsions, *Pharmazie*, 46:607–608 (1991).

I-41. M. Mathew and C. S. Thampi, Evaluation of multiple w/o/w emulsions containing terbutaline sulfate, *Eastern Pharm.*, 33:181–182 (1990).

I-42. L. Diamond, A comparison of the gastrointestinal absorption profiles of theophylline from various vehicles, *Arch. Int. Pharmacodyn*, 185:246–253 (1970).

I-43. A. J. Repta, Formulation of investigational anticancer drugs. In: Topics in Pharmaceutical Sciences (D. D. Breimer and P. Speiser, eds.), Elsevier, New York, 1981.

3

Antacids and Clay Products

Richard J. Harwood

Private Formulations, Inc., Edison, New Jersey

Joseph R. Luber

Johnson & Johnson Merck Consumer Products Co., Fort Washington, Pennsylvania

Edward W. Sunbery

Merck & Co., Inc., West Point, Pennsylvania

I. INTRODUCTION

As the reader of Volume 2 of *Pharmaceutical Dosage Forms: Disperse Systems* learns, there are a number of factors that can affect the performance, stability and physical properties of a suspension formulation. The purpose of this chapter is to give the formulator of liquid antacid products and/or clay products an insight into how the physical/chemical properties of these formulations and the practical aspects of drug efficacy can be intertwined.

II. DEVELOPMENT OBJECTIVES

A. Antacids

The formulation of antacid suspension preparations requires trade-offs between efficacy and stability. For example, a very stable suspension containing aluminum hydroxycarbonate and magnesium hydroxide can be prepared if the pH is carefully adjusted and the particle size is carefully controlled. However, use of a phosphate buffer may result in a less efficacious product, even though, technically and scientifically speaking, addition of such a buffer would stabilize the product. The process of trading off one desire for another could be called optimization. Optimization in the product development laboratory sometimes results in selecting a balance between the desires of the formulator and those of the marketing organization. In the example above, the formulator would have to select a less efficacious buffer to prevent the insoluble aluminum phosphate from forming so that marketing's desire of having the highest acid neutralizing capacity (ANC) per unit volume (dose) could be obtained.

Antacids are substances that react with acid in the stomach and, ideally, raise the pH of the stomach contents to between 4 and 5. Antacids neutralize only existing acid; they do not affect the amount or rate of gastric acid secreted. Antacids do not neutralize all stomach acid. With usual therapeutic doses they do not raise and cannot maintain gastric pH higher than 4 to 5. When the pH is increased from 1.3 to 2.3, 90% of the acid is neutralized, and at pH of 3.3, 99% is neutralized. Antacids also inhibit the conversion of pepsinogen to pepsin, which depends on the degree of acid neutralization. Pepsin is most active between pH 1.5 and 2.5. At pH 4 (or greater) pepsin activity is completely inhibited [1]. For an in-depth discussion of the in vitro interaction between aluminum hydroxycarbonate and pepsin, the reader is referred to the papers by Sepelyak et al. [2,3]. All antacid products contain at least one of the four primary neutralizing ingredients: sodium bicarbonate, calcium carbonate, aluminum salts, and magnesium salts [4]. Pinson and Weart [4] and Garnett [5] describe the ideal antacid product attributes. These attributes include:

Potent/Efficient. Small amounts of the product should neutralize large amounts of gastric acid.

Effective/Long-Acting. The antacid should neutralize gastric acid for a prolonged period of time without causing either rebound acid secretion or release of carbon dioxide after reacting with gastric acid.

Safe. The product should not affect electrolyte balance or blood glucose or cause diarrhea or constipation. The product should neither interfere with other drugs the patient is taking nor contain large amounts of the other ingredients that might exacerbate concomitant disease(s).

Inexpensive. The patient may be taking the product for a long time.

Palatable. A prerequisite for successful antacid therapy. Palatability of antacids is an important issue because the products must be dosed at a high frequency to provide consistent suppression of gastric acidity. Therapeutic failure can result when patients do not comply with dosing regimen [6].

No commercially available product fulfills all of these criteria. Aluminum hydroxycarbonate is known to cause constipation. Magnesium hydroxide causes laxation. Sodium carbonate can cause systemic alkalosis, does cause acid rebound, and releases carbon dioxide. Calcium carbonate may induce gastric hypersecretion [7–10] and also releases carbon dioxide. In high potency antacids, hexitols (such as mannitol and/or sorbitol) are added to reduce the tendency of the product to gel. However, sorbitol can cause laxation if large amounts are ingested. The taste of an antacid can be affected by the additives. Potassium citrate, which can be used as a buffer, tastes unpleasant. Parabens, which are used as preservatives, impart a numbing sensation and aftertaste, which is accentuated by peppermint [11].

B. Clays

The clays (kaolin, bentonite, hectorite, attapulgite, and magnesium aluminum silicate) are chemically inert and are frequently used in nonprescription antidiarrheal preparations. Clays are usually administered in large doses and are, therefore, formulated as flavored suspensions to improve palatability. Generally, clays used as hydrocolloids and adsorbents are silicates, which differ only in their metallic composition.

White and Hem [12] summarized the structure and properties of clays as follows:

> The basic structure of clays consists of octahedra of aluminum and magnesium in combination with silica tetrahedra which are uniquely arranged to produce the surface charge, morphology, and surface area characteristic of each type of clay. A surface charge may arise from either isomorphous substitution, i.e., aluminum in place of silicon, magnesium in place of aluminum, etc., or broken bonds at the edges of the clay. The surface charge arising from isomorphous substitution is negative and is characterized by the cation-exchange capacity.

> Clays can be classified morphologically as platy or fibrous. A platy morphology is seen in the clays which have a layer-like structure. The kaolin group consists of sheets of silica tetrahedra and aluminum octahedra shared in a 1:1 ratio. These minerals have little or no isomorphous substitution and normally are nonswelling in aqueous solutions. Smectites belong to the 2:1 (ratio of silica tetrahedra to aluminum and/or magnesium octahedra) structural group of clays and include montmorillonite, hectorite, and saponite. In these clays an aluminum or magnesium octahedral sheet is sandwiched between two silica tetrahedral sheets. Isomorphous substitution occurs in both the tetrahedral and octahedral sheets of the 2:1 minerals and gives rise to moderate to high cation-exchange capacities. The viscosity-enhancing properties of the 2:1 platy clays is related to the ability of the clay to swell and immobilize large quantities of water between the layers.

> The fibrous clays such as sepiolite and attapulgite are 2:1-type minerals but the laths are elongated along the x-axis, resulting in ribbons of the 2:1 layer attached at their longitudinal edges. A cross section of the fiber reveals a checkerboard arrangement of 2:1 ribbons and channels with no possibility of expansion. The fibrous clays are effective viscosity-enhancing agents because the fibers become entangled in brush heap-like arrangements.

> The morphology of the clay also influences the adsorptive properties of the clays. The 2:1 platy clays, which can swell, are able to accommodate solute molecules in the extensive interlayer space. The channels of the fibrous clays have a fixed geometry which is too small to accept molecules larger than water, ammonia, or perhaps primary alcohols.

III. PRODUCT DEFINITION

In the development of any pharmaceutical dosage form, the first step is to have the marketing group and product development group agree on what the product is expected to do clinically and what the form of the product should be. In the case of a liquid antacid suspension or clay suspension the flavor, colors, and viscosity requirements are criteria that need to be established by marketing within the constraints of what the formulator is able to accomplish in the laboratory and, eventually, what can be done in large-scale production. The product development group and the marketing group have to agree on dose requirements and the physical/chemical/biological properties of the antacid and/or clay product.

IV. DEVELOPMENT PROCESS (THE FORMULATOR'S CONCERNS)

The objective of this chapter is to present to the reader a practical approach for the development of a typical antacid and/or clay product. This section deals with what the formulator should think about before even beginning to mix the ingredients.

All of the antacid and clay materials to be discussed exhibit surface charges. In the case of materials such as magaldrate and bentonite, there is a permanent surface charge due to isomorphous substitution. For other materials such as aluminum hydroxide and magnesium hydroxide, a pH-dependent surface charge exists as the result of ionization of surface hydroxyls and carbonates.

The formulator must be cognizant of how surface charge of each component in the suspension can influence the physical and chemical attributes of the final formulation. The physical properties of suspensions are affected by particle interactions. Therefore, the control of particle interactions is particularly important in the formulation and production of antacid and clay suspensions [13].

The interfacial properties of particles play a major role in determining the type of network that will develop in a suspension. There are three basic types of interparticle relationships: dispersed, flocculated, and coagulated. In the dispersed system, the overall repulsive forces are greater than the attractive forces, and, therefore, the particles remain separate. However, dispersed systems eventually settle. The settling occurs slowly and the sedimentation volume is fairly low. Once settled, the cake is difficult to redisperse. In the flocculated system, the attractive forces are slightly stronger than the repulsive forces. The particles are initially attracted to one another, but the repulsive forces prevent them from moving too close to each other. A loose network results. The particles settle out as a loosely aggregated floc. Settling time is moderate, and the sedimentation volume is high. This network can easily be disrupted by the mild shear of shaking. In the coagulated system, the attractive forces are stronger than the repulsive forces, and the resulting network is strongly held together. The aggregates settle into a cake that is difficult to redisperse by shaking. Sedimentation volume is low.

As mentioned above, one of the key factors affecting the interactions of particles in suspension is surface charge. The source of a surface charge can be classified as either a permanent charge or a pH-dependent charge. In the latter case, the magnitude of the charge is dependent on the pH of the suspension. The pH also determines whether the surface charge is positive or negative. For particles with pH-dependent-surface charges, a concept known as the point of zero charge can be useful in understanding the interactions of the suspended particles. The *point of zero charge* (PZC) is defined as the pH of a suspension at which the net surface charge is zero [14]. For example, Feldkamp et al. [14] reported that the apparent viscosity of amorphous carbonate-containing aluminum hydroxide suspension was found to be maximum when the pH of the suspension was adjusted to the PZC. Therefore, the formulation of antacid and clay product suspensions that consist of charged solids must be approached cautiously. The following illustrates the complexity of developing a stable/efficacious formula.

Pure aluminum hydroxide has a PZC equal to 9.65. However, the aluminum hydroxide used in the formulation of antacids typically contains a substantial amount of carbonate. The substitution of the dibasic carbonate ion for the hydroxyl ion causes a decrease in the PZC of the aluminum hydroxycarbonate. The extent of charge depends on the amount of carbonate. Typical commercial aluminum hydroxycarbonates used as antacids have a mole ratio of carbonate to aluminum of 0.2 to 0.4. The PZC is decreased to 8 with the former and to 6 with the latter. The incorporation of tribasic ions, such as phosphate or citrate, into the aluminum hydroxide has even a greater effect on the PZC [15]. Knowledge of the PZC-pH relationship enables the formulator to better understand the physical properties of a suspension.

Figure 1 shows the effect of the pH on the viscosity of a suspension of aluminum hydroxycarbonate. The figure demonstrates that when the pH of the suspension is above or below the PZC, the particles have a net surface charge and repel each other. The suspension would be characterized as dispersed, and because the particles have little interaction, the viscosity is low. However, as the pH of the suspension nears the PZC, the particles exhibit a very low surface charge. The suspension would be characterized as flocculated, and because there is a great deal of interparticle interaction, the viscosity is high.

The PZC is determined via a titration. At several ionic strengths, the raw material is titrated with either acid or base. A plot is made: amount of acid or base versus pH. The ionic strength is varied by the addition of potassium chloride to the test medium. The PZC is found at the intersection of the curves for the different ionic strengths. Figure 2 shows a typical plot.

Another example that shows the magnitude of the effect that surface charge has on the rheological properties of a suspension is demonstrated in the case of bentonite. This platelike material has a permanent negative charge on its faces. However, the edges of these plates have a pH-dependent charge. Therefore, when the pH of the suspension is lower than the point of zero charge, the plate edge will be positively charged. This results in an edge-to-face attraction of particles. This produces a three-dimensional "house of cards" network that causes the suspension to be quite thixotropic and viscous. However, when the pH of the suspension is above the point of zero charge, the edge

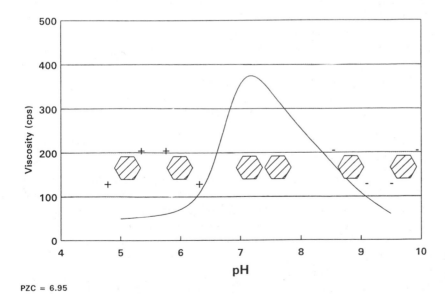

PZC = 6.95

Fig. 1 Effect of pH on the viscosity of aluminum hydroxycarbonate suspension. Adapted from Feldkamp et al. [14].

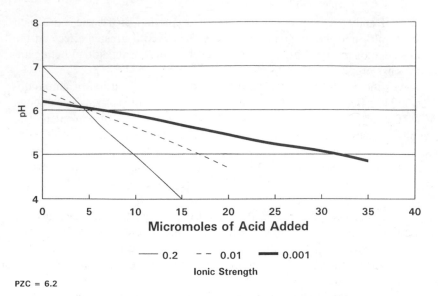

PZC = 6.2

Fig. 2 Point of zero charge titration of aluminum hydroxycarbonate.

of the particle exhibits a negative charge. In this system, the particles repel each other and do not form a three-dimensional network, the suspension is not thixotropic and the viscosity is reduced.

An example of the effect that surface charge has on the acid reactivity of an antacid suspension is found in the manufacture of a product with aluminum hydroxycarbonate and magnesium hydroxide. When aluminum hydroxycarbonate and magnesium hydroxide are both present in a suspension, the two interact. The PZC of magnesium hydroxide is pH 10; the PZC of a typical aluminum hydroxycarbonate is usually between pH 6 and 7. The pH of the overall suspension is 8 and therefore the aluminum hydroxycarbonate will have a negative surface charge and the magnesium hydroxide a positive surface charge. Consequently, the smaller aluminum hydroxycarbonate particle will coat the larger magnesium hydroxide particle. Because aluminum hydroxycarbonate reacts with acid at a slower rate than magnesium hydroxide, the result of the coating is a decrease in the rate of acid neutralization of the product.

It has been determined that the inclusion of polyols into such a formulation will reduce the magnitude of the above interaction. Figure 3 demonstrates the effect of pH on the amount of mannitol bound to a sample of aluminum hydroxycarbonate, which has a PZC of 6.3 [16]. The figure shows that the maximum binding of the mannitol occurs above the PZC. Shah et al. [16] found that the adsorption occurs through hydrogen bonding: the mannitol serves as a proton donor, and the aluminum hydroxycarbonate surface as the proton acceptor. This can occur only when the suspension pH is above the PZC: the pH at which the aluminum hydroxycarbonate is negatively charged, and therefore a proton receptor.

The pH stat titragram (see Section VIII.D for a description), at pH 3.0, of magnesium hydroxide exhibits a rapid rate of acid neutralization (see Fig. 4). Conversely, the titragram for aluminum hydroxycarbonate displays a relatively slower reaction rate (see

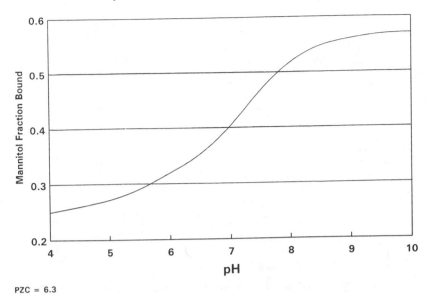

PZC = 6.3

Fig. 3 Effect of pH on the adsorption of mannitol by aluminum hydroxycarbonate suspension. Adapted from Shah et al [16].

Fig. 5). A titragram of a mixture of the two materials would be expected to have a fast initial rate of reaction caused by the neutralization of the magnesium hydroxycarbonate (see Fig. 6), followed by a slower rate of neutralization as the aluminum hydroxide reacts. However, titragrams of these mixtures exhibit a reverse profile, with the initial neutralization rate being a slow one, which is then followed by a fast rate of reaction.

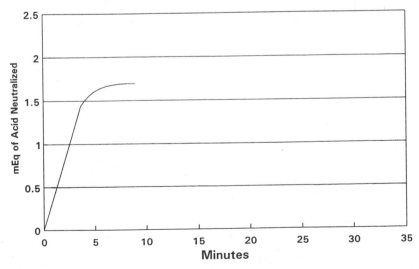

Fig. 4 pH stat titragram at pH 3.0 of magnesium hydroxide. Adapted from Vanderlaan et al. [17].

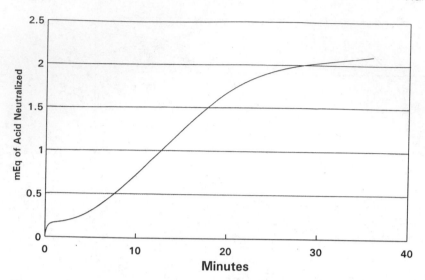

Fig. 5 pH stat titragram at pH 3.0 of aluminum hydroxycarbonate. Adapted from Vanderlaan et al. [17].

The cause of this phenomenon was described above: the relatively small particle size of the aluminum hydroxide allows it to electrostatically adsorb onto the surface of the larger magnesium hydroxide particle, resulting in the latter's surface being completely coated with the aluminum hydroxide.

V. COMPONENTS OF ANTACID OR CLAY SUSPENSIONS

A typical antacid or clay suspension formulation contains, in addition to the active ingredients, a number of excipients that, in combination, are designed to deliver to the patient a pleasant tasting, microbial-free, acid-reactive antacid or absorbent clay.

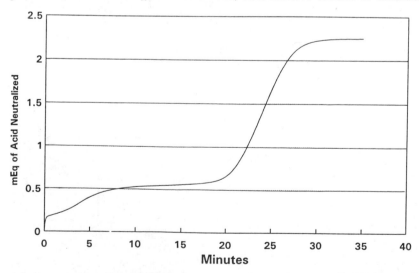

Fig. 6 pH stat titragram at pH 3.0 of a 5:1 mixture of magnesium hydroxide and aluminum hydroxycarbonate. Adapted from Vanderlaan et al. [17].

The ingredients of an antacid or clay suspension typically belong to one of the following categories:

Active ingredients (antacids, antiflatulents, and clays)
Suspending agents
Sweetening system
Preservative system
Anticaking/antigelling agent
Flavor and mouthfeel system
Coloring agents

In an effort to determine a list of the ingredients likely to compose each of the above seven categories, a survey was made of currently marketed products. Below are typical ingredients found in each category.

A. Active Ingredients

1. *Antacids*

The code of Federal Regulations includes in its monograph entitled "Antacid Products For Over-the-Counter (OTC) Human Use" [18] a rather extensive list of antacid raw materials. Most current antacid suspensions are composed of one or more of the following materials: aluminum hydroxide, magnesium hydroxide, calcium carbonate, magnesium carbonate, magaldrate, and magnesium trisilicate. The characteristics of each of the antacid raw materials are listed as follows.

a. *Aluminum Hydroxide.* This raw material is often found either alone or in combination with magnesium hydroxide in many antacid suspensions. The theoretical stoichiometry of its reaction with hydrochloric acid is

$$Al(OH)_3 + 3\ HCl \rightarrow AlCl_3 + 3\ H_2O$$

In order for the above reaction to occur within the relatively short gastric residence time, the aluminum hydroxide must be in an amorphous form. However, aluminum hydroxide undergoes rapid polymerization, which leads to more crystalline forms. Such crystalline forms of aluminum hydroxide, such as Gibbsite, show little reaction with hydrochloric acid in gastric juice.

In actuality, the aluminum hydroxide that is found in most antacid suspensions is an aluminum hydroxycarbonate. It has been shown [19] that the presence of carbonate anion during the precipitation of aluminum hydroxide has a stabilizing effect on its acid reactivity by minimizing polymerization.

Unlike many other antacids, aluminum hydroxide has the ability to buffer the gastric pH between 3 and 4. This is demonstrated *in vitro* in the Rossett-Rice Test [20] (see Section VIII.D for a description). An ideal antacid is capable of buffering the gastric pH between 3 and 5. By raising the pH above 3, pepsin is largely inactivated [21]; if the pH is raised above 5, however, acid rebound may occur [20].

Aluminum hydroxide is classified as a nonsytemic antacid because it exerts its action in the stomach and is not absorbed. Theoretically, it is capable of neutralizing 29.4 mEq of hydrochloric acid per gram of dried material. Its sodium content is relatively low. It has the ability of adsorbing pepsin, phosphates, and bile salts [22]. It causes constipation in high doses. Finally, it has the ability of delaying gastric emptying.

For use in antacid suspensions, aluminum hydroxide typically is in the form of a gel or pourable liquid. In some cases, it may be used in powder form. Though use of the gel form generally results in the most reactive suspensions with the best mouthfeel, the gel's high viscosity prohibits its use in high potency suspensions. In addition, the gels require more vigorous agitation during processing to properly disperse the active homogeneously. The powder form of aluminum hydroxide, because of its large particle size, results in poor mouthfeel and low acid reactivity.

b. *Magnesium Hydroxide.* This raw material is rarely used alone in antacid suspensions. It is commonly found in combination with aluminum hydroxide. The stoichiometry of its reaction with hydrochloric acid is

$$Mg(OH)_2 + 2\ HCl \rightarrow MgCl_2 + 2\ H_2O$$

Magnesium hydroxide is a crystalline material known as the mineral brucite. Crystalline magnesium hydroxide reacts rapidly with hydrochloric acid. It quickly raises the gastric pH above 3. However, unlike aluminum hydroxide, it is unable to buffer the gastric contents between pH 3 and 5. Rossett-Rice testing indicates that the pH rises to between 8 and 9. Such a high pH can trigger acid rebound.

Magnesium hydroxide is classified as a nonsystemic antacid. It has a pH-dependent surface charge. It is capable of neutralizing 34.3 mEq of hydrochloric acid per gram on a dried basis. It is very low in sodium. It produces a laxating effect. It binds some bile salt but does so to a lesser extent than aluminum hydroxide.

For use in antacid suspensions, magnesium hydroxide is typically in the form of a gel. However, it occasionally may be used as a pumpable liquid or a powder. Various viscosity grades of the gel are manufactured. Typically, low viscosity gels are used in high potency suspensions.

Magnesium hydroxide, when used in combination with aluminum hydroxide, results in a suspension that reacts with hydrochloric acid quickly. Such a suspension buffers the gastric contents between pH 3 and 5. The suspension will exhibit an improved laxation–constipation balance. However, due to the electrostatic attraction of the two antacids, antigelling agents are needed to prevent excessively high viscosity of the suspension.

c. *Calcium Carbonate.* This raw material is used both alone or in combination with aluminum and magnesium hydroxide. The stoichiometry of its reaction with hydrochloric acid is

$$CaCO_3 + 2\ HCl \rightarrow CaCl_2 + CO_2 + H_2O$$

Calcium carbonate is a crystalline mineral known as calcite. Crystalline calcium carbonate reacts rapidly with hydrochloric acid. It quickly raises the gastric pH above pH 3. Rossett-Rice testing indicates the pH is maintained at 7, which may trigger acid rebound.

Calcium carbonate is classified as a nonsystemic antacid because it does not tend to cause a systemic alkalosis. However, chronic use of large doses of calcium carbonate may cause renal pathology or some systemic alkalosis [23]. Calcium carbonate has a constipating effect when used in large doses. It may cause flatulence because of the release of carbon dioxide when reacted with hydrochloric acid.

It is available in several grades, differing in particle size. In general, the particle size is varied by adjusting the concentration of the reactants used in its manufacture. In suspensions the light grade, exhibiting a mean particle size in the range of 1 to 4 μm, is typically used.

d. *Magnesium Trisilicate.* This material, having the general formula $2\ MgO \cdot 3SiO_2 \cdot xH_2O$, has a long history of use as an antacid and as an adsorbent. The stoichiometry of its reaction with hydrochloric acid is

$$2\ MgO \cdot 3\ SiO_2 \cdot xH_2O + 4\ HCl \rightarrow 2\ MgCl_2 + 3\ SiO_2 + (x + 2)\ H_2O$$

Magnesium trisilicate is a weak antacid. Because of its slow onset of action, it is not able to meet the current pH requirements for nonprescription antacids [24]. Therefore, it is typically used in conjunction with other antacid raw materials. The hydrated silicon dioxide is a by-product of the above reaction. Traces of silicon dioxide may be absorbed and excreted in the urine [25].

In the stomach, unreacted magnesium trisilicate may adhere to the ulcer crater and provide some cytoprotective action [26]. Magnesium trisilicate is classified as a nonsystemic antacid. The acid-consuming capacity over a 4-hour period at 37°C for magnesium trisilicate is approximately 15 mEq of hydrochloric acid per gram of dried material [27].

Magnesium trisilicate does not inactivate pepsin in solutions below pH 6 [28]. It does bind some bile acids, but it does so to a lesser extent than aluminum hydroxide [22]. It has a laxative effect in large doses. It is supplied as a fine white odorless powder.

e. *Magnesium Carbonate.* Depending on the method of manufacture, this material varies in composition from basic hydrated magnesium carbonate of the formula $(MgCo_3)_4 \cdot Mg(OH)_2 \cdot 5H_2O$ to a hydrated magnesium carbonate of the formula $MgCO_3 \cdot nH_2O$. The stoichiometry of its reaction with hydrochloric acid is

$$(MgCO_3)_4 \cdot Mg(OH)_2 \cdot 5\ H_2O + 10\ HCl \rightarrow 5\ MgCl_2 + 4\ CO_2 + 11\ H_2O$$

Basic hydrated magnesium carbonate is a fast-acting antacid, with an acid-neutralizing capacity equal to 20.6 mEq of hydrochloric acid per gram. During in vitro testing, it raises the pH beyond 5 and thus may cause acid rebound. It also can cause laxation in moderately high doses. It may cause flatulence because of the release of carbon dioxide when reacted with hydrochloric acid.

It is available as a white bulky powder in either light or heavy grades. The density of the powder is dependent on concentration of reactants, temperature during precipitation and extent of aging during manufacture. Typically, the light grade is used in the manufacture of antacid suspensions.

f. *Magaldrate.* Malgaldrate, a member of the hydrotalcite family, has a magnesium hydroxide–like structure in which aluminum ions displace one of every three magnesium ions in the brucite lattice. Because this leaves the lattice with a net positive charge, anions are sandwiched between alternate magnesium–aluminum layers. In the case of magaldrate, this anion is largely sulfate. The structure of magaldrate is

$$Mg_4 \cdot Al_2\ (OH)_{12}SO_4 \cdot H_2O$$

The stoichiometry for magaldrate's reaction with hydrochloric acid is

$$Mg_4 \cdot Al_2\ (OH)_{12}\ SO_4 \cdot H_2O + 12\ HCl \rightarrow MgSO_4 + 3\ MgCl_2 + 2\ AlCl_3 + 13\ H_2O$$

This material has a rapid onset of action and has shown its ability to buffer between pH 3 and 5 in in vitro testing. It has an acid-neutralizing capacity of approximately 25.6 mEq of hydrochloric acid per gram. It disturbs neither electrolyte balance nor bowel function [29], and its sodium content is very low. It is supplied both in powder form and as a paste for use in suspensions.

2. Clays

a.   *Kaolin.*   Kaolin is a native hydrated aluminum silicate of the general formula $Al_2O_3 \cdot 2SiO_2 \cdot 2H_2O$. It is a natural product. Most kaolin deposits are contaminated with ferric oxide (hence the red color of ordinary clay) and some other impurities such as calcium carbonate and magnesium carbonate [30]. Therefore, to purify kaolin it is treated with hydrochloric acid or sulfuric acid and then washed. Kaolin particles are platelike. It has little charge on its faces, but is negatively charged on the edges. Kaolin does not swell appreciably in water. It adsorbs toxic substances and increases the bulk of feces. Its particle size is about 0.5 to 1 μm. The pH of a 20% slurry is about 6. It may be microbiologically contaminated and is usually sterilized after mining. Kaolin contains approximately 0.2% sodium. Kaolin has a low surface area (7–30 m^2/gm). Kaolin's cation exchange capacity is low (3–15 mEq/100 gm). Because of its absorptive properties, kaolin may absorb some other drugs [31].

b.   *Bentonite.*   Bentonite, a native hydrated aluminum silicate, has the general formula $Al_2O_3 \cdot 4SiO_2 \cdot H_2O$. Hectorite is structurally identical to bentonite. However, the molecular lattice of hectorite contains small amounts of lithium and fluorine. Bentonite and hectorite are in the montmorillonite family of clays. Bentonite contains some iron oxide, calcium carbonate, and magnesium carbonate as impurities.

It contains about 1.5 % sodium. It is insoluble in water but swells to about 12 times its volume in water. It forms thixotropic suspensions. It is hygroscopic and therefore should be stored in sealed containers. Bentonite is precipitated by acid, but acid-washed material does not have any suspending ability. Bentonite is used as a suspending agent, emulsion stabilizer, and absorbent. The pH of its suspensions is about 10. It has a high surface area (600–800 m^2/gm). Its particles are platelike and have a negative charge. It has a high cation-exchange capacity (80–100 mEq/100 gm). It should be sterilized after mining. It is incompatible with strong electrolytes and positively charged particles. Its gelling properties are reduced by acids but increased by alkalies such as magnesium oxide.

c.   *Attapulgite.*   Attapulgite is a hydrous magnesium aluminum silicate. It can be "activated" by thermal treatment and is used in finely divided form. Its general formula is $MgO \cdot Al_2O_3 \cdot SiO_2 \cdot H_2O$. It is a fibrous mineral with little or no cation-exchange capacity. It has a moderately high surface area (125–160 m^2/gm), which has a higher adsorptive capacity than kaolin. Its suspensions are thixotropic and have a pH of about 8.5. The maximum viscosity is achieved at pH's between 6 and 8.5 It is available in two grades: a regular activated form (particle size—2.9 μm) that has good adsorptive properties but little colloidal properties, and a colloidal activated form (particle size—0.14 μm) that has good colloidal and adsorptive properties.

d.   *Magnesium Aluminum Silicate.*   Magnesium aluminum silicate is a magnesium bentonite in which magnesium replaces some of the aluminum in the bentonite structure. It has a three-layer lattice of octahedral aluminum and two tetrahedral silica sheets. The aluminum is substituted to varying degrees by magnesium. Sodium and potassium are substituted for the total balance of electrical charge at the surface. It has platelike particles and is supplied either in flake or micronized powder forms. It swells in water to many times its volume, and its swelling capacity is greater than bentonite. It forms thixotropic pseudoplastic suspensions and can be repeatedly wetted and dried without losing its swelling capacity. The pH of its suspensions is about 9 and it is stable from pH 3.5 through 11. It has a moderately high cation-exchange capacity. The viscosity of its suspensions increases with heat, age, and the addition of electrolytes. It prevents caking of other solids in suspension with it. Magnesium aluminum silicate contains about 1.5% sodium. It has been known to alter the bioavailability of some drugs.

3. *Antiflatulents*

a. *Simethicone.* This material is a mixture of the dimethylpolysiloxane polymer and silicon dioxide. Because of its ability to reduce the surface tension of gas bubbles, simethicone has antifoaming properties. It is often used in combination with antacids to provide antiflatulent properties to the suspension. It is available as a 30% aqueous emulsion for use in suspensions. Various emulsifiers have been used in the manufacture of the emulsion.

The concentration of simethicone normally used in antacid suspensions ranges from 20 to 40 mg per 5 mL.

B. Suspending Agents

Suspending agents are used to prevent rapid settling and caking of some antacid raw materials. They are often capable of improving the mouthfeel of antacids, which, as a rule, are gritty and chalky. Only suspending agents that are stable at relatively high pH's (7.5–9.5) should be considered.

Because many antacid raw materials have some limited solubility, suspending agents that may undergo cross-linking in the presence of polyvalent cations should be avoided. Of course, sequestrants may be used to improve the stability of anionic suspending agents.

Suspensions develop large aggregates during repeated freeze–thaw cycles; these settle rapidly and cause a grainy texture. Some polymeric suspending agents are effective in improving the freeze–thaw stability of a suspension. Hydroxypropyl methylcellulose, methylcellulose, sodium carboxymethylcellulose, sodium alginate, and povidone (PVP) have all been shown to offer protection against this phenomenon.

1. *Antacid Suspensions*

The following includes suspending agents commonly found in antacid suspensions.

a. *Avicel RC 591 (FMC Corporation).* Avicel RC 591 consists of 89% microcrystalline cellulose and 11% sodium carboxymethylcellulose. It is stable over a broad pH range. Avicel RC 591 forms thixotropic gels at low concentrations that show shear-thinning with mild agitation. It is flocculated by cationic polymers and surfactants.

b. *Alginates.* Alginates are high molecular weight anionic hydrophilic polysaccharides. Alginates are natural products derived from brown seaweed. The viscosity of their solutions decreases with increasing temperature, but this is partially reversible. Alginate solutions are typically pseudoplastic and stable between pH 4 and 10. Alginates form precipitates with polyvalent cations (except magnesium) and are incompatible with quaternary nitrogen compounds.

c. *Methylcellulose–Hydroxypropyl Methylcellulose.* The methyl ether of cellulose and its hydroxypropyl derivative form water-soluble nonionic polysaccharide polymers. They are soluble in cold water and insoluble in hot water. Their solutions are typically pseudoplastic and nonthixotropic. The viscosity of these solutions decreases as temperature is increased until the gel point is reached. They have some surface-active properties, can function as emulsifiers, and may cause foaming. They are stable in the pH range from 3 to 11.

d. *Guar Gum.* Guar gum is a high molecular weight nonionic polysaccharide polymer. It is a natural product and is a cold water–swelling polymer. Its solutions are pseudoplastic and nonthixotropic. The viscosity of its solutions decreases reversibly as temperature increases. Prolonged heating causes irreversible loss of viscosity. It is susceptible to biological attack. Guar gum has good pH stability.

e. *Hydroxypropylcellulose.* This is the hydroxypropyl derivative of cellulose. It is a nonionic polysaccharide polymer with optimal stability between pH 6 and 8. It is soluble in water below 40°C and precipitates above 45°C. Its solutions are pseudoplastic and nonthixotropic. It possesses some surface-active properties and, therefore, may cause foaming. It is incompatible with the parabens [32].

f. *Xanthan Gum.* Xanthum gum is a high molecular weight natural anionic polysaccharide polymer. Its solutions are pseudoplastic. When shear is discontinued the original viscosity is regained almost immediately. The viscosity of its solutions show little change as the temperature is increased. Xanthan gum exhibits good pH stability, but its solutions may gel at high pH in the presence of divalent cations and may gel in the presence of trivalent cations at neutral pH. Sequestrants are effective in preventing gelation.

g. *Carboxymethylcellulose.* This is a carboxymethyl derivative of cellulose. It is an anionic high molecular weight polysaccharide polymer. Its solutions are precipitated by trivalent cations. However, sequestrants are effective in preventing this. Carboxymethylcellulose solutions show a loss in viscosity as temperature increases. Its solutions are pseudoplastic and typically thixotropic; they are stable between pH 5 and 9.

h. *Magnesium Aluminum Silicate.* Magnesium aluminum silicate is a clay that is sometimes used in antacid suspensions to impart thixotropy and to improve dispersion of settled materials and thus prevent caking. The formulator should be aware of potential interaction between the magnesium aluminum silicate and active antacid ingredients caused by the surface charge of each ingredient.

C. Sweetening System

The major function of the ingredients found in this category of excipients is to improve the palatability of the actives. Besides the obvious sweetness that these ingredients impart to the formulation, some members of the category are effective in improving the mouthfeel of the suspension. Also, some sweeteners, because of their absorption onto the surface of aluminum hydroxide, are able to reduce its polymerization and, therefore, stabilize its acid-neutralizing reactivity [33]. In a similar manner, some sweeteners are capable of preventing adverse interactions between aluminum–magnesium mixtures [34]. These interactions take the form of excessive viscosity increases or even gelation and reduction of acid-neutralizing capacity.

Selection of the proper sweetening system often requires a series of compromises. One must balance such properties as palatability, cost, caloric content, dental concerns, laxation effects, and ability to mask objectionable-tasting substances.

1. *Typical Sweeteners for Antacid Suspensions*

a. *Sucrose.* Sucrose is a good-tasting sweetener capable of adding to the consistency of a suspension and improving mouthfeel. It has a caloric content of 4 calories per gram. It may cause an increase in the incidence of dental caries and must be used with care in patients with diabetes. It may cause cap-locking because of crystallization of the sucrose in the threads of the bottle neck.

b. *Sorbitol.*   Sorbitol is approximately half as sweet as sucrose. It is good-tasting and improves mouthfeel. It has a caloric content of 4 calories per gram. However, it is only partially absorbed and, therefore, it is often considered to be noncaloric. It is an osmotic diuretic and can cause diarrhea. It retards the likelihood of cap-locking. It stabilizes aluminum hydroxide reactivity by preventing the polymerization during the aging process and protects aluminum hydroxide–magnesium hydroxide mixtures by slowing their interaction [34].

c. *Mannitol.*   Mannitol is a good-tasting sweetener that has a cooling effect in the mouth. It has a caloric content of 4 calories per gram. However, it is only partially absorbed and, therefore, it is often considered noncaloric. It is fairly expensive. It is an osmotic diuretic and can cause diarrhea. It stabilizes the reactivity of aluminum hydroxide by preventing the polymerization aging process [33].

d. *Saccharin.*   Saccharin is a synthetic sweetener approximately 500 times as sweet as sucrose. However, it has a bitter and unpleasant aftertaste. It has a low water solubility, but the sodium and calcium salts, which are readily soluble, are often used. It has no caloric value. It is inexpensive because the amount required per dose is low.

e. *Glycerin.*   Glycerin is a pleasant-tasting sweetener with a warm aftertaste, and it improves mouthfeel. It has a caloric content of 4.3 calories per gram and should be administered with caution to diabetic patients. It is an osmotic diuretic that can cause diarrhea. It is able to reduce the likelihood of cap-locking. It is fairly expensive. It is capable of stabilizing the reactivity of aluminum hydroxide by preventing the polymerization aging process.

f. *Glycyrrhizinates.*   Ammonium glycyrrhizinate and monoammonium glycyrrhizinate are natural sweeteners approximately 50 times sweeter than sucrose. They are potent flavor enhancers. They are useful in masking the taste of bitter substances. They are foaming agents. They are moderately expensive.

D. Preservative System

The preservative systems of liquid pharmaceutical products are undergoing increasing scrutiny by regulatory agencies, both in the United States and abroad. Suspensions containing clays and/or antacids are no exceptions. The goal of an ideal preservative system is to provide effective microbiological control of bacteria, yeast, fungi and molds without adverse effects on the palatibility or physical properties of the product. The microbiological control should, ideally, be effective during the shelf life of the product.

Because of the high pH of antacid suspensions, the formulator has relatively few preservatives from which to choose. At pH 8, the pH of a typical antacid suspension, preservatives such as the benzoates and sorbates are ineffective due to ionization. Some clay suspensions can be formulated at somewhat lower pH's. This allows the use of benzoates and sorbates. Those few preservatives that are effective at pH 9 typically have limited chemical stability.

In combination with the preservative system used in the formulation, several processing steps may be employed during the manufacture of suspensions to ensure that the products are packaged with little or no microbiological contamination. However, these processing treatments can provide only short-term microbiological protection. Use of a combination of preservatives occasionally results in some synergistic effects.

1. *Preservatives*

Following are preservative ingredients and processes often used in the manufacture of antacid suspensions. The major attributes of each are outlined as well.

a. *Chlorine.* Sodium hypochlorite (common bleach) is an effective agent that kills most bacteria and some yeast, fungi, and protozoa. It is most stable in alkaline pH, though it is more effective in acidic pH. Overall, it is only effective in the short term. Sodium hypochlorite is used in treatment of water at a concentration of approximately 5 ppm available chlorine. It is often used in combination with other preservatives. It may affect the product's flavor.

b. *Hydrogen Peroxide.* Peroxide is an effective agent against most organisms. It has no long-term effects and must be used in combination with other preservatives. It may affect the product's flavor.

c. *Parabens.* Methyl, ethyl, propyl, and butyl esters are the most often used parabens. They are effective against molds, yeasts, and fungi. They are not as active against gram-positive bacteria and are less effective against gram-negative bacteria. The parabens show an additive effect when used in combination with each other. They generally exhibit effective short to medium range preservative action. They have an adverse effect on the flavor. They impart a bitter, numbing taste sensation. They are relatively inexpensive and exhibit low toxicity.

d. *Pasteurization.* Pasteurization is effective against most organisms. The process kills by coagulating proteins of the microorganisms. The temperature criteria and holding times must be determined experimentally for each product. The process has no long-term effects and must be used in combination with other preservatives in any multidose product.

e. *Ozonation.* Ozonation is effective against most organisms. There is no long-term effect. Therefore, it must be used in combination with other preservatives. Ozone may affect the flavor of the product.

E. Anticaking–Antigelling Agents

These materials are used to provide for the redispersal of settled solids. They are also supposed to prevent gelation of antacid suspensions. Listed below are ingredients typically used to prevent caking and/or gelling.

EDTA. This excipient is used to sequester polyvalent cations that may cause the cross-linking of some suspending agents, thus leading to increased viscosity or gelation.

Citric acid or potassium citrate. These sequesterants are used in suspensions containing aluminum hydroxide to lower the product's viscosity and to prevent interaction of aluminum hydroxide with magnesium compounds.

Potassium Phosphate. Potassium phosphate is used both as a buffering and a sequestering agent.

Silica. Cab-O-Sil, Aerosil, and Quso are commercial forms of silica. They are very effective anticaking agents, although they may affect both the product viscosity and mouthfeel in high concentrations. They also can reduce the degree of sedimentation of a suspension.

F. Flavor–Mouthfeel System

The flavor and mouthfeel systems are an important part of any antacid suspension. Because many consumers of antacids use the products for extended periods of time, the palatability of a suspension is of utmost importance.

The selection of a flavor involves the evaluation of the following criteria: (a) stability at high pH, (b) stability in glass or plastic bottle, (c) ability to mask the taste of undesirable flavor components, (d) appeal to most segments of the patient population, and (e) availability in dry form, if comparable chewable tablet is planned.

When evaluating various flavor systems for an antacid suspension, one should monitor the initial taste, mouthfeel, chalkiness, grittiness, and aftertaste.

The following flavors are typically found in currently marketed antacid suspensions: (a) mints (peppermint, spearmint, and wintergreen), (b) citrus (lemon, lime, and orange), (c) cream (vanilla), and (d) anise.

Nonflavor ingredients are often used to improve the mouthfeel of an antacid. They include: (a) mineral oil, (b) milk solids, (c) glycine, and (d) natural and artificial gums.

G. Coloring Agents

All water-soluble coloring agents have a charge and can interact with oppositely charged compounds such as antacids and clays. The resulting compound is water insoluble. This can make the suspension color appear very heterogeneous.

The best way to prevent such an interaction is to use a colored lake.

H. Water

A final ingredient in all antacid and clay suspensions, one having a profound effect on the palatability and stability of the product, is water. Water is the major ingredient in antacid and clay suspensions. It acts both as the vehicle and as the solvent for various components in the suspension.

It should not be overlooked that the quality of water is not necessarily a constant. The water's method of preparation, its handling and its storage are crucial to the development of a suitable antacid and/or clay suspension product. Water requires careful consideration and monitoring.

Various grades of water are available. They include tap water, distilled water, deionized water, filtered water, and chlorinated water. The major impurities in water are calcium, magnesium, iron, silica, and sodium. These cations are usually combined with carbonate, bicarbonate, sulfate, and chloride anions.

Deionization can be accomplished by distillation, ion exchange, or reverse osmosis. The prevention of growth of microorganisms in the water must also be addressed. Such processes are chlorination, ozonation, ultraviolet light, heating, and filtration are effective in limiting this growth.

A final word of caution: All experiments and scaleup testing should be conducted with the same grade of water as that used in the production facility.

VI. ANTACID SUSPENSION FORMULATION

A formulated antacid suspension must meet many specific requirements. The proper blending of various factors is needed in order to accomplish the objectives. Following is a list of typical objectives for an antacid suspension to meet:

> O.T.C. monograph
> Contribution of at least 25% of labeled ANC by each active ingredient
> Desired potency requirement (milliequivalents of HCl neutralized per mL)
> Listing of acceptable antacid actives
> Antiflatulents included?
> Permitted sweetener content (artificial versus natural)
> Laxation/constipation balance
> Permitted sodium content
> Viscosity range
> Flavor preferences
> Color preferences

In general, the role of an antacid is to raise the pH of the gastric contents and, subsequently, to reduce the amount of acid emptied into the duodenum.

It should be pointed out that over 95% of the hydrogen ion concentration is neutralized at pH 3.5 A further consequence of the raising of the gastric pH is the reduction in the activity of the enzyme pepsin and the conversion of pepsinogen to pepsin. Finally, antacids can also have bile acid–binding properties.

A. Type of Antacid Suspension

There are currently over 200 marketed antacid suspensions. Although these products vary widely in composition, they can be divided into the four types of suspension listed below.

1. *Single-strength suspensions.*   These products have the capacities to neutralize 10 to 15 milliequivalents of hydrochloric acid per 5 mL dose.
2. *Double-strength suspensions.*   Typically, these products have the capacity to neutralize 20 to 30 milliequivalents of hydrochloric acid per 5 mL dose.
3. *Antacids containing antiflatulents.*   These products may be either single or double strength. However, they generally contain between 20 and 40 mg of simethicone per 5 mL dose.
4. *Floating antacid suspensions.*   These products usually have a low acid neutralization capacity. They also contain both soluble alginate and a carbonate-containing antacid, which, upon ingestion and contact with the gastric acid, form a low-density barrier that floats on the surface of the gastric contents. These products are specifically used for the treatment of reflux esophagitis.

B. Examples of Antacid Suspension Formulations

1. *Antacid Formula*

This antacid formulation does not require gums or thickening agents but relies on the viscosity characteristics of the antacids to maintain the desired body and mouthfeel characteristics. A teaspoonful of the following formula should contain about 225 mg of aluminum hydroxide (equivalent to dried aluminum hydroxide gel, USP calculated as 50% Al_2O_3), and about 200 mg of magnesium hydroxide.

	% w/w
Aluminum hydroxide gel [8.9% Al_2O_3]	24.0
Magnesium hydroxide paste [29.5% $Mg(OH)_2$]	12.9
Sorbitol, USP	2.0
Mannitol, USP	0.25
Methylparaben, USP	0.10
Flavors	0.10
Citric acid, anhydrous, USP	0.06
Propylparaben, USP	0.05
Sodium saccharin, USP	0.03
Purified water	60.5

GENERAL PROCEDURE

1. Charge a large mixing tank with purified water at about 40% of the total water required.
2. Add the sorbitol to a smaller mixing tank, and dilute with an equal amount of purified water. This mixing tank should have a dynamic mixing system. Next, add the citric acid and sodium saccharin followed by the parabens, which have to be dispersed well under dynamic conditions.
3. Add magnesium hydroxide paste to the large mixing tank with continuous agitation.
4. Pump the contents of the smaller tank into the large vessel. Rinse the small tank with purified water into the larger one.
5. Next, add the aluminum hydroxide gel followed by the flavors.
6. Add the remainder of the purified water to the desired end volume or weight.
7. Mix until uniform.

If marketing wants a product with an antiflatulent, simethicone can be added to the product.

2. *Antacid/Antiflatulent Formula*

The following example should yield a product providing a dose of about 200 mg of magnesium hydroxide and about 200 mg of aluminum hydroxide with about 20 mg of simethicone per teaspoonful.

	% w/w
Aluminum hydroxide gel [8.9% Al_2O_3]	21.0
Magnesium hydroxide paste [29.5% $Mg(OH)_2$]	12.9
Sorbitol, USP	6.0
Simethicone, USP [90.5% simethicone]	0.37
Hydroxypropyl cellulose	0.33
Methylparaben, USP	0.16
Flavors	0.12
AVICEL, RC-591	0.11
Citric acid, anhydrous, USP	0.06
Methylcellulose	0.03
Propylparaben, USP	0.03
Sodium saccharin, USP	0.02
Purified water	58.87

GENERAL PROCEDURE

1. Charge the mixing tank with the purified water at about 40% of the total water required.
2. In another smaller mixing tank, disperse the methylcellulose with a high-shear mixture in 1.5% of the above purified water. Once the methylcellulose is completely dispersed, add the simethicone. When the mixture is uniform pump into the large tank while mixing. Wash out with 1.0% of the purified water.
3. Mix the methyl and propyl parabens into a slurry with about 2% of the purified water. Add the paraben slurry to the large mixing tank with agitation. Wash out the small tank with 1/2% of the purified water.
4. Mix the AVICEL and hydroxypropyl cellulose with about 13% of the purified water with vigorous agitation in a smaller vessel. Keep agitating while making the remainder of the formulation.
5. Add the magnesium hydroxide paste to the large manufacturing tank with continuous agitation. Pump in the gums from Item No. 4 and rinse with 1% of the purified water. Next add the aluminum hydroxide gel.
6. Add the citric acid, sodium saccharin, and sorbitol solution.
7. Next add the flavorings and the remainder of the purified water to the desired end volume or weight.
8. Mix until uniform.

If an extra-strength product is desired by marketing, the formulator will have to use a lower viscosity grade of antacid raw materials. In order to provide a low-viscosity grade of aluminum hydroxide and/or magnesium hydroxide, manufacturers increase the particle size of the suspended actives. The reason is straightforward if the reader considers the following explanation by Hem [35].

> Reducing the particle size while maintaining a constant volume fraction causes a colloidal system to have more particles dispersed in the same volume of vehicle. Thus, the particles are closer to each other and therefore are more likely to interact. The effect of particle size on the distance between particles is illustrated by sequentially reducing individual particle volume by half while maintaining the same total volume of solids. Although the surface area does not increase substantially upon two divisions, the average interparticulate distance decreases significantly. Since the magnitude of interparticle forces depends inversely upon separation distance, the force exerted on a given particle by all other particles during a small displacement from its equilibrium position will be greater if the average interparticle distance is small. Conversely, at low particle density, the particles will be less influenced by each other.

The formulator may choose to add one or more suspending agents to decrease sedimentation and to improve consumer acceptance.

3. *Extra-Strength Antacid Formula*

The formula listed on the next page is designed to deliver about 400 mg of magnesium hydroxide, about 400 mg of aluminum hydroxide, and about 30 mg of simethicone per teaspoonful.

	% w/w
Aluminum hydroxide gel [8.9% Al_2O_3]	42.0
Magnesium hydroxide paste [29.5% $Mg(OH)_2$]	25.8
Sorbitol solution, USP	18.0
Simethicone, USP [90.5% simethicone]	0.55
Citric acid, anhydrous, USP	0.10
Methylparaben, USP	0.09
Guar gum	0.07
Methylcellulose	0.04
Propylparaben, USP	0.04
Flavors	0.02
Purified water	12.99

GENERAL PROCEDURE

1. Add aluminum hydroxide gel to a large mixing tank and agitate.
2. In another smaller mixing tank, disperse the methylcellulose with a high-shear mixer in 1.5% of the above purified water. Once the methylcellulose is completely dispersed, add the simethicone and pump into the large tank while mixing until the mixture is uniform. Wash out with 1% of the purified water.
3. In another mixing tank with high-speed agitation, add gum, citric acid, parabens, and one third of the sorbitol. Disperse thoroughly and completely for a period of time and add to large mixing tank and wash out with about 1% of purified water. Add remainder of sorbitol solution to large mixing tank.
4. Add magnesium hydroxide paste.
5. Bring up to volume with purified water.
6. Add flavoring.
7. Mix until uniform.

4. *Aluminum Hydroxide Formula*

The following formula can be prescribed for patients requiring aluminum hydroxide therapy. Such patients are typically receiving dialysis treatment and require elimination of phosphate. Aluminum phosphate is very insoluble and is eliminated via the feces.

Aluminum hydroxide	362.8 g[a]
Sorbitol solution, USP	282.0 mL
Syrup, USP	93.0 mL
Glycerin, USP	25.0 mL
Methylparaben, USP	0.9 g
Propylparaben, USP	0.3 g
Flavor	q.s.
Purified water, a sufficient quantity to make	1000 mL

[a]Equivalent to approximately 300 mg aluminum hydroxide/5 mL.

GENERAL PROCEDURE

1. Dissolve the methyl- and propylparaben in the sorbitol solution, syrup, glycerin, and 50 mL water previously mixed in a suitable container, by heating to 60°C with rapid stirring.

2. Cool to room temperature and add the antacid product, stirring thoroughly to disperse antacid.
3. Add the flavor and sufficient water to make 1000 mL.
4. Homogenize. Hand homogenizers, homomixers, and colloid mills are all satisfactory and yield products with comparable viscosities.

5. *Magaldrate Formula*

The following formula shows that magaldrate does not need any special buffering to stabilize the system.

	% w/w
Magaldrate gel [25% magaldrate, assay]	43.2
Hydroxypropyl methylcellulose, USP	0.15
Sodium saccharin, USP	0.03
Flavors	0.1
Methyl- and propylparaben	0.13
Purified water, a sufficient quantity to make	100

GENERAL PROCEDURE

1. Charge mixing tank with about one-half of required purified water.
2. Add magaldrate gel to tank with agitation.
3. In smaller tank disperse hydroxypropyl methylcellulose with one-fourth of the required purified water with dynamic agitation. Next add sodium saccharin and parabens.
4. Pump contents of small vessel into larger mixing tank and rinse with purified water.
5. Add flavors, plus the remaining purified water.
6. Mix until uniform.

Table 1 is presented in order for the reader to troubleshoot formulations and to help the formulator resolve common problems that are usually associated with antacid products. Most of the time it is necessary to balance the pH/PZC ratio and to check particle size of the homogenized suspension at the same time. These two formulation variables usually need to be optimized in order to balance these sometimes opposing factors. The effect of pH on the apparent viscosity of two suspensions that have two different particle sizes was shown by Hem [35]. Hem pointed out that a suspension containing smaller particle size particles exhibited a tenfold increase in apparent viscosity at the PZC whereas a suspension consisting of larger particle sizes shows only a fourfold increase in apparent viscosity at the PZC.

VII. CLAY SUSPENSION FORMULATION

The factors listed below must be addressed by the formulator in order to prepare an efficacious product:

Desired potency (adsorptive capacity)
List of acceptable clay actives
Permitted sweeteners (artificial versus natural)

Table 1 Trouble Shooting

Observation	Potential problem	What to look for
Premature settling (dispersible cake)	—Particle size too large —Insufficient suspending agent —pH/PZC not in balance	—Additional homogenization may be needed —Add more, or change agent —Check PZC of raw material(s) and pH of suspension
Premature settling (nondispersible cake)	—pH/PZC not in balance —Electrolyte balance —Particle size too small	—Check PZC of raw material(s) and pH of suspension —Either add or eliminate salt —Reduce processing energy input
Viscosity too high	—pH/PZC not in balance —Particle size too small	—Check PZC of raw material(s) and pH of suspension —Reduce processing energy input
Viscosity too low	—Particle size too large —Material not fully hydrated —Suspending agent not fully hydrated (fish eyes in test sample) —pH << PZC >> pH	—Need additional homgenization —Let stand for more time —Let stand for more time —Check PZC of raw material(s) C and pH of suspension
Gritty mouthfeel	—Particle size too large —Particles agglomerate —Viscosity too low	—Need additional homogenization —Either add or eliminate salt —See above
Chalky mouthfeel	—Particle size too small —Viscosity too high —pH/PZC balance	—Reduce processing energy input —See above —Check PZC of raw material(s) and pH of suspension

Viscosity range
Flavor preference
Color preference

In general, the role of a clay product is its adsorbent action in the gastrointestinal tract. Adsorbents are generally used to treat mild diarrhea. An FDA panel has determined that clay adsorbents are safe, and effective in treating diarrhea [36]. Attapulgite has been classified as safe and effective for the treatment of diarrhea [37].

A. Examples of Clay Suspension Formulations

Kaolin is often mixed with pectin. Such a mixture is used to control diarrhea. A typical formula is as follows:

	% w/w
Kaolin	17.5
Pectin	0.47
Glycerin	1.75
Magnesium aluminum silicate	0.88
Sodium carboxymethylcellulose	0.22
Saccharin	0.09
Flavor	q.s
Preservative	q.s
Purified water	q.s

GENERAL PROCEDURE

1. Dry-blend magnesium aluminum silicate and sodium carboxymethylcellulose.
2. Add the blend to water slowly and agitate continually until smooth.
3. Add kaolin and continue stirring.
4. Blend pectin, saccharin, glycerin, flavor, and preservative.
5. Add mixture in (4) to other components.
6. Mix until smooth.

Although it could be considered "old fashioned," bentonite magma can be made quite easily and can provide bulk to the bowel contents.

	% w/v
Bentonite	5.0
Flavors	q.s
Saccharin	0.09
Preservative	q.s
Purified water	q.s

GENERAL PROCEDURE

1. Place about half of the purified water in a tank equipped with a high-shear blender.
2. Add bentonite to the water with the blender in operation.

3. Add flavors, saccharin, and preservative and mix until uniform.
4. Add purified water to volume and mix until uniform.

Colloidal attapulgite, as mentioned previously, has been approved as a safe and effective antidiarrheal agent. A formula is listed below.

	% w/v
Colloidal attapulgite	14
Flavors	q.s
Saccharin	0.09
Methylparaben	0.2
Propylparaben	0.05
Purified water	q.s

GENERAL PROCEDURE

1. Heat 20% of the purified water to 60°C.
2. Add and dissolve the parabens.
3. Place about half of the purified water in a tank equipped with a high-shear blender.
4. Add colloidal attapulgite to the water with the blender in operation.
5. Add the paraben solution, saccharin, and flavors and mix until uniform.
6. Add purified water to volume and mix until uniform.

The following is a formula for a topical pharmaceutical product that contains bentonite.

	% w/w
Calcium hydroxide solution	55.80
Bentonite (Albagel® 4444 or 4446)[a]	3.44
Carboxymethylcellulose, sodium	0.06
Calamine	7.83
Zinc oxide	7.83
Glycerin	1.96
Water	23.08

[a]Whittaker, Clark and Daniels, Inc.

GENERAL PROCEDURE

1. Prepare a calcium hydroxide solution by adding 3 grams of calcium hydroxide to 1 liter of purified water. Mix vigorously for 1 hour. Allow undissolved calcium hydroxide to settle to the bottom of the container. Use only the clear, supernatant liquid in the formula. Add sufficient water to make 1 liter.
2. Prepare a bentonite magma by adding the bentonite and the sodium carboxymethylcellulose to the calcium hydroxide solution with rapid mixing until the bentonite is completely hydrated and the sodium carboxymethylcellulose is dispersed.
3. In a separate vessel, blend the calamine and zinc oxide.
4. Add the glycerin into the powders. Mix until uniform.
5. Begin adding the bentonite-containing suspension with mixing until all of the suspension is blended into the mixture.

VIII.   EVALUATION OF THE STABILITY OF CLAY AND ANTACID SUSPENSIONS

Careful evaluation of any suspension is necessary in order to ensure the product is stable and effective during its shelf life. A proper evaluation of the product can only be performed when the methods for its analysis have been validated.

Stability studies should be performed in all packages and sizes in which the product will be marketed. Stability of the product should be evaluated at room temperature and several elevated temperatures. The product should also be examined after several freeze–thaw cycles.

The product should be evaluated using at least three different lots of actives and suspending agents. Laboratory scale batches can provide useful data. However, several full-scale batches, manufactured at each production site, should be evaluated. Because of the many physical changes that occur during the first few days following the manufacture of a suspension, the product should be monitored especially carefully during this time period.

Four main areas of testing are necessary to ensure proper stability evaluation of a suspension. They include the chemical, physical, and microbiological testing of the product, and the physical evaluation of the container. Below are some of the various individual tests.

A.   Container Evaluation

The following should be monitored: (a) torque on closure, (b) swelling of the container, (c) discoloration of the container, and (d) stability of cap-liner.

B.   Microbiological Testing of the Product

Microbial testing of the initial product should determine the number of microbiological organisms in the suspension and the absence of pathogenic organisms. Preservative effectiveness testing at various stability points (for example, samples stored at room temperature for 6, 12, 18, and 24 months) should be completed to determine the ability of the preservative system to combat the introduction of various organisms. The chemical stability of the preservative system should be monitored at various time periods (for example, samples stored at room temperature for 6, 12, 18, and 24 months) to show that the preservative system is stable for the shelf life of the product.

C.   Physical Testing of the Product

The following is a list of physical properties that need to be monitored:

    Color—change in hue or intensity
    Odor—decrease in characteristic odor, occurrence of abnormal odor
    Taste—change in mouthfeel, chalkiness, grittiness, etc., occurrence of abnormal
        tastes
    Appearance—changes in the texture
    Sedimentation rate and volume
    Redispersability
    Zeta potential—monitor changes that correspond to the state of flocculation of the
        particle

Particle size
Viscosity—if possible, perform at several shear rates
Specific gravity

D. Chemical Testing of the Product

The following is a list of chemical tests that may be needed to show that an antacid product is stable:

Actives content—aluminum, magnesium, calcium, clay
Carbonate content
Acid Neutralization Capacity [38]

> This test measures the number of milliequivalents (mEq) of hydrochloric acid that one dose of product can neutralize in 15 minutes. The procedure is as follows:
>
> A sample, equivalent to the minimum recommended dose of the product is added to a container containing 70 mL of water. The container's temperature is maintained at 37°C.
>
> After mixing for 1 minute, 30.0 mL of 1.0 N hydrochloric acid is added.
>
> Mix for 15 minutes. Then, titrate with 0.5 N sodium hydroxide to a stable pH of 3.5.
>
> The number of mEq of hydrochloric acid neutralized by the product is then calculated.

Preliminary Antacid Test [39]

> This test determines the ability of a dose of product to raise the pH of 5 mEq of hydrochloric acid to above pH 3.5 in 10 minutes.

pH stat test [40]

> This test has immense value in evaluating antacid formulations. As previously mentioned, when aluminum hydroxycarbonate and magnesium hydroxide are combined in a suspension, an interaction occurs resulting in the slower acting aluminum hydroxycarbonate coating the faster acting magnesium hydroxide. The pH stat test is the ideal tool for observing this interaction. Refer again to Figs. 4, 5, and 6.

Rossett-Rice test [41]

> This is an in vitro test used to simulate the production of hydrochloric acid in the stomach. The sample of product is added to a known volume of acid, and the pH of the mixture is monitored versus time. Additional acid is continually added to the test mixture at a specified rate. The procedure is as follows:
>
> The sample is added to a container containing 70 mL of 0.1 N hydrochloric acid and 30 mL water. The mixture is maintained at 37°C.
>
> While monitoring the pH versus time, 0.1 N hydrochloric acid is added at a rate of 4 mL per minute. The addition of acid is continued until the pH drops below 3.0.
>
> Measurements are made of the time to onset of action (time from when the product is added to the acid until the pH rises above 3.0); the maximum pH attained (the pH should not go above 5); and the duration of activity (the time the pH remains above 3.0).
>
> Modifications to the methodology are often performed. These modifications include: removal of test medium at the same rate as the addition of the acid, incorporation of pepsin to the acid solution, and adjustment of the initial acid

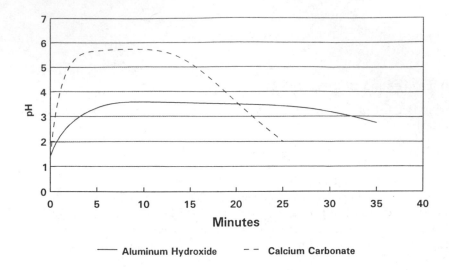

Fig. 7   Rossett-Rice titragram of aluminum hydroxide and calcium carbonate (500 mg sample).

concentration. Figure 7 shows the typical pH versus time plots for aluminum hydroxide and for calcium carbonate using the standard test procedure.

E. Special Tests

Pepsin inactivation—measures the ability of the product to bind and inactivate the enzyme pepsin

Bile acid binding—measures the capacity of the product to bind bile acids

Defoaming test

IX. PROCESSING EQUIPMENT

A. Manufacturing

The processes for manufacturing and packaging antacids or clay suspensions require the use of a wide variety of processing equipment. The equipment requirements are divided into the following basic categories:

1. Holding and mixing equipment
    a.   manufacturing tanks
    b.   bulk holding tanks
2. Transfer equipment
    a.   pumps
3. Specialty equipment
    a.   particle reduction equipment
    b.   deaerators
    c.   pasteurizers

It is not the intent of this chapter to cover a detailed description of each of these categories. However, the following basic rules of thumb may be helpful when selecting appropriate equipment for a specific product.

B. Holding Equipment

Manufacturing and/or holding tanks should be manufactured of Type 304-or 316-grade stainless steel, with a design meeting 3A sanitary standards [42, 43]. This will ensure ease of cleaning and reduce the chance of microbial contamination. Such a system can easily be expanded for multiproduct use or for future increased capacity employing other equipment meeting 3A sanitary standards.

Load cells on tanks facilitate production of a consistent quality product. Load cells reduce processing time and help to calculate product yield quickly. Errors associated with liquid volume variation caused by temperature and air entrapment are eliminated. The only problem with load cells is that they have limited use on jacketed tanks used to heat and/or cool product during processing. Because of variations in the mass of liquid in the tank jacket, it is often impossible to accurately determine the mass inside the tank.

The tanks should be fitted with agitators capable of efficiently wetting large quantities of powders and dispersing gel or magma-type raw materials. This usually requires multiple high-speed mixers. Ideally, a sweep mixer should be used in combination with the high-speed mixer to reduce the likelihood of large quantities of gels or powders settling at dead spots in the tank.

Agitator selection and the related topic of tank baffles will not be covered in this chapter. Ideally the selected agitator should have the capability of efficiently wetting and/ or dispersing large quantities of powders or liquids in a solvent. The various agitator manufacturers can supply specific technical performance data on their products.

Many of the raw materials used in the manufacture of antacid suspensions are suitable for bulk storage systems. Some forms of the antacids are in pumpable liquid form. The storage system for these materials must be designed to properly maintain the uniformity of the material and also prevent microbial contamination. Similarly, excipients such as sorbitol, glycerin, and liquid glucose must be stored in a suitable fashion.

C. Transfer Equipment

Transfer of liquids from one container to another is accomplished with a transfer pump. Pump selection is generally a function of product viscosity and application. The less viscous products generally use centrifugal-type pumps. They are generally less expensive, easier to clean, and have more pumping capacity. However, centrifugal pumps do not develop the back pressure required for applications such as filtration. The pumping rate of a centrifugal pump is also difficult to control. The more viscous liquids generally require rotary gear or positive displacement pumps. These pumps have easily controlled pumping rates, operate under great back pressure, and add minimal air to the product.

Bulk powder storage systems are often used for dry antacid or clay raw materials. Air conveyor systems transfer the materials from the storage area to the manufacturing area.

D. Specialty Equipment

The manufacture of the liquid products under discussion usually requires special equipment to create a finished product with high quality.

1.   The *hydration*, *wetting*, *or dispersion* of hydrophobic excipients may be accomplished through the use of slurry tanks and/or specialized mixing equipment. The selection of the type of equipment used is determined by the nature of the material to be processed. The use of jacketed slurry tanks is advised in order to have the capability of heating or cooling. A mixer (either high-shear or low-shear type) should be attached to the tank to assure content uniformity during the processing.

Tri-Clover Inc. (Kenosha, Wisconsin) developed the Tri-Blender. The Tri-Blender enables the addition of large volumes of powders to the manufacturing tank. The Tri-Blender (see Fig. 8) is a modified centrifugal pump equipped with a diffuser tube located in the eye of the pump impeller. Its basis of operation is simple. Liquid is pumped into the liquid inlet through the impellers. The liquid flow through the equipment produces a partial vacuum in the diffuser tube. A valve between the diffuser tube and a hopper holding the dry powder prevents air from being introduced into the blending chamber. When the powder is ready for addition via the hopper, the valve is opened and the powder is pulled into the blending chamber. The use of such equipment reduces tank requirements and manufacturing time.

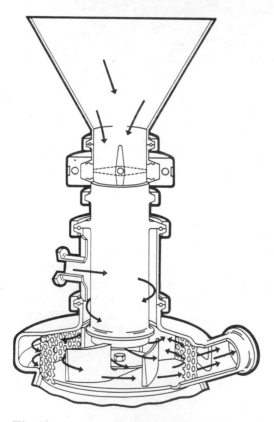

Fig. 8   Cut-away schematic of the Tri-Blender®. Courtesy of Tri-Clover Inc. (Kenosha, WI).

2. *Wet milling equipment* is used to ensure the dispersal of powder or gel aggregates. Colloid mills or homogenizers are typically used for this purpose. Particle size reduction may be accomplished by mills that work on one or more of the following principles:

     a. A suspension may be pumped through rotating flat or toothed plates. The particle size is controlled by adjusting the speed of rotation and/or the distance between the plates. Fig. 9 shows a dual slotted in-line mixer emulsifier.

     b. A suspension may be pumped under pressure through an orifice. The particle size can be controlled by adjusting the size or type of the orifice and the pressure of the liquid before entering the orifice. Figure 10 shows a cross section of a valve used to provide control of the orifice size of the APV Gaulin Rannie Homogenizer (Wilmington, Massachusetts).

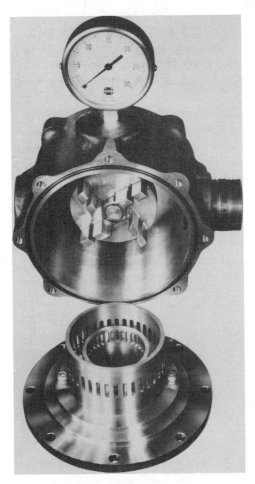

Fig. 9 Dual slotted head for an in-line mixer emulsifier. Figure courtesy of Charles Ross and Sons Company (Hauppauge, NY).

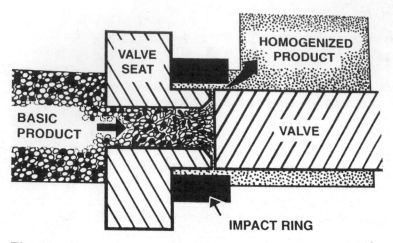

Fig. 10 Cross section of a homogenzing valve used to provide control of the orifice size on a homogenizer. Figure courtesy of APV Homogenizers Gaulin Rannie (Wilmington, MA).

      c. A centrifugal-type pump may be equipped with an obstructive screen to help break up the particles. Such a system is typified by the Ross Mixer Emulsifier (Hauppauge, New York). The typical flow pattern of such a mixer is shown in Fig. 11.

    3.   The mixing and milling may entrap air in a liquid formulation. *Deaerators* are used to remove the entrapped air. Deaerators are built to act on the principle that entrapped air near the atmosphere/liquid interface will expand and burst in the presence of a particle vacuum. Deaerators are partial vacuum chambers in which liquid is cascaded as a thin stream so that the entrapped air is easily brought to the atmosphere/liq-

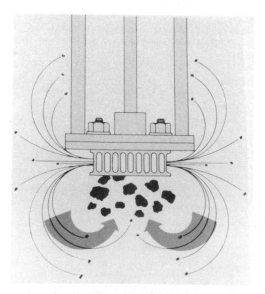

Fig. 11 Typical flow pattern of a centrifugal-type pump equipped with a screen. Figure courtesy of Charles Ross and Sons Company (Hauppauge, NY).

uid interface. Koruma (represented in the United States by Romaco, Inc., Morris Plains, NJ) makes deaerators to augment its line of dispersing and homogenizing equipment. Krieger A. G. (represented in the United States by GEI Processing, Towaco, NJ) manufactures vacuum/mixing/homogenizing equipment as well. Figure 12 shows a cut-away drawing of the vessel of such equipment. It should be pointed out that the Krieger unit can be equipped with a Clean-In-Place system. Figure 13 shows the process flow pattern in a Krieger processing vessel and Fig. 14 shows the Clean-In-Place (CIP) flow pattern utilizing the Krieger homogenizer and agitator tools without spray balls.

4.   A *pasteurizer* is a system of devices that act in unison to sterilize a product by heating a relatively heat labile product to a moderate temperature for the specific time needed to kill pathogenic bacteria and to delay the growth of other bacteria.

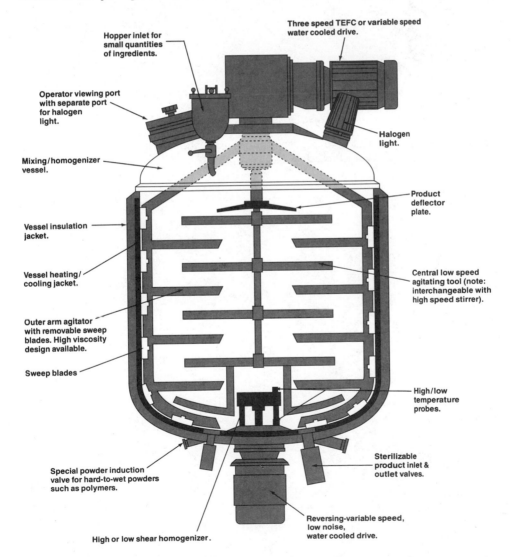

Fig. 12   Schematic of a Krieger vacuum mixer/homogenizer. Figure courtesy of GEI Processing, Inc. (Towaco, NJ).

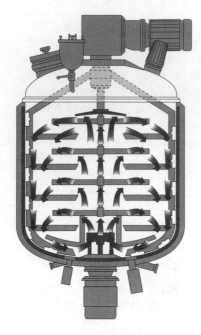

Fig. 13 Process flow pattern showing the expected material flow within a Krieger processing vessel. Figure courtesy of GEI Processing Inc. (Towaco, NJ).

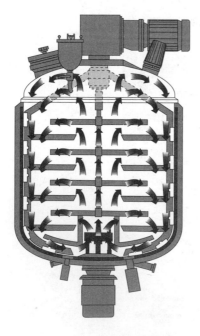

Fig. 14 Clean-In-Place (CIP) flow pattern utilizing the Krieger homogenizer and agitator tools without spray balls. Figure courtesy of GEI Processing, Inc. (Towaco, NJ).

E. Packaging

There are three categories of liquid filling equipment: (a) gravity fill, (b) vacuum fill, and (c) pressure fill. There are two types of fill control: (a) volume control or (b) weight control.

As discussed with transfer pumps, the type of filling equipment operation is largely determined by product viscosity. The more viscous liquids are filled with pressure and pressure/vacuum assisted equipment. The less viscous liquids are filled by gravity-type fillers.

Fill control is determined by product viscosity and container design. The more viscous liquids and liquids in opaque bottles are fill-checked by weight. The less viscous liquids in translucent or transparent containers are filled to volume. Filling to volume presents a more uniform quality appearance when bottles are displayed together on a store shelf.

ACKNOWLEDGMENTS

Sincere appreciation is extended to Barcroft Company for providing antacid formulations/procedures that have been used as models in this chapter and to Whittaker, Clark, and Daniels for providing clay formulations/procedures that were used as models in this chapter.

REFERENCES

1. J. B. Pinson and C. W. Weart, Antacid products. In: *Handbook of Non-Prescription Drugs*, *Tenth Edition*, American Pharmaceutical Association, Washington, D. C., 1993, pp. 150–151.
2. R. J. Sepelyak, J. R. Feldkamp, T. E. Moody, J. L. White and S. L. Hem, Adsorption of pepsin by aluminum hydroxide I: adsorption mechanism, *J. Pharm. Sci.*, 73(11), 1514–1517 (1984).
3. R. J. Sepelyak, J. R. Feldkamp, T. E. Moody, J. L. White, and S. L. Hem, Adsorption of pepsin by aluminum hydroxide II: Pepsin Inactivation, *J. Pharm. Sci.*, 73(11), 1517–1522 (1984).
4. J. B. Pinson and C. W. Weart, Antacid products. In: *Handbook of Non-Prescription Drugs*, *Tenth Edition*, American Pharmaceutical Association, Washington, D. C., 1993, pp. 175–176.
5. W. R. Garnett, In: *Handbook of Non-Prescription Drugs*, *Ninth Edition*, American Pharmaceutical Association, Washington, D.C., 1990, p. 256.
6. N. Bahal-O'Mara, R. W. Force, and M. C. Nahata, Palatability of 14 over-the-counter antacids, *Am. Pharmacy* NS34(1): 31–35 (1994).
7. J. S. Fordtran, Acid rebound, *N. Engl. J. Med.*, 279:900 (1968).
8. R. F. Barreras, Calcium and gastric secretions, *Gastroenterology*, 64:1168 (1973).
9. R. M. Case, Calcium and gastrointestinal secretions, *Digestion*, 8:269 (1973).
10. J. E. Hade and H. M. Spiro, Calcium and acid rebound: A Reappraisal, *J. Clin. Gastroenterol.*, 15(1):37–44 (1992).
11. N. K. Patel, L. Kennon, and R. S. Levinson, Pharmaceutical suspensions. In: *The Theory and Practice on Industrial Pharmacy*. Third Edition (L. Lachman, H. A. Lieberman, J. L. Kanig, eds.), Lea & Febiger, Philadelphia, 1986, p. 498.
12. J. L. White and S. L. Hem, Pharmaceutical aspects of clay–organic interactions, *I and EC Prod. Res. Dev.*, 22:665–671 (1983).

13. P. P. Wu, J. R. Feldkamp, J. L. White, and S. L. Hem, Effect of surface charge of carbonate-containing aluminum hydroxide on particle interactions in aqueous suspensions, *J. Colloid Interface Sci.*, 10(2):601–603 (1986).

14. J. R. Feldkamp, D. N. Shah, S. L. Meyer, J. L. White, and S. L. Hem, Effect of adsorbed carbonate on surface charge characteristics and physical properties of aluminum hydroxide gel, *J. Pharm. Sci.*, 70:638 (1981).

15. E. Scholtz, J. Feldkamp, J. White, and S. Hem, Point of zero charge of amorphous aluminum hydroxide as a function of adsorbed carbonate, *J. Pharm. Sci.*, 74(4):478 (1985).

16. D. Shah, J. Feldkamp, J. White, and S. Hem, Effect of the pH-zero point of charge relationship on the interaction of ionic compounds and polyols with aluminum hydroxide gel, *J. Pharm. Sci.*, 71(2):266 (1982).

17. R. Vanderlaan, J. White, and S. Hem, Effect of interaction of aluminum hydroxycarbonate gel and magnesium hydroxide gel on acid neutralization, *J. Pharm. Sci.*, 68(12): 1498 (1979).

18. *Code of Federal Regulations, Title 21*, Part 331, U.S. Government Printing Office, Washington, D.C., 1992.

19. N. Kerkhof, J. White, and S. Hem, Role of carbonate in acid neutralization of aluminum hydroxide gel, *J. Pharm. Sci.*, 66(11): 1533 (1977).

20. S. Hem, Physicochemical properties of antacids, *J. Chem. Ed.*, 52:383 (1975).

21. D. Piper and B. Fenton, pH Stability and activity curves of pepsin with special reference to their clinical importance, *Gut*, 6:506 (1965).

22. K. H. Holtermuller and P. Herzog, Antacids: Pharmacology and clinical efficacy—A critical evaluation. In: *Therapeutic Agents for Peptic Ulcer Disease, Drugs and Peptic Ulcer*. Vol. I (C. J. Pfeiffer, ed.), CRC Press, Boca Raton, FL, 1982, pp. 105–122.

23. E. A. Swinyard, Gastrointestinal drugs. In: *Remington's Pharmaceutical Sciences*, 18th ed. (A. R. Gennaro, ed.), Mack Publishing, Easton, PA, 1990, p. 776.

24. E. A. Swinyard, Gastrointestinal drugs. In: *Remington's Pharmaceutical Sciences*, 18th ed. (A. R. Gennaro, ed.), Mack Publishing, Easton, PA, 1990, p. 778.

25. J. E. F. Reynolds, ed., *Martindale The Extra Pharmacopoeia*, 30th ed., The Pharmaceutical Press, London, 1993, p. 890.

26. A. Osol, G. Farrar, and R. Pratt, eds., *The Dispensatory of the United States of America*, 25th ed, J. B. Lippincott Co., Philadelphia, 1960, p. 780.

27. *The United States Pharmacopeia XXII*, United States Pharmacopeial Convention, Inc., Rockville, MD, 1990, p. 798.

28. A. Osol, G. Farrar, and R. Pratt, eds., *The Dispensatory of the United States of America*, 25th Ed. J. B. Lippincott Co., Philadelphia, 1960, p. 781.

29. E. A. Swinyard, Gastrointestinal drugs. In: *Remington's Pharmaceutical Sciences*, 18th ed. (A. R. Gennaro, ed.), Mack Publishing, Easton, PA, 1990, p. 776.

30. E. A. Swinyard, Gastrointestinal drugs. In: *Remington's Pharmaceutical Sciences*, 18th ed. (A. R. Gennaro, ed.), Mack Publishing, Easton, PA, 1990, p. 796.

31. R. L. Longe, Antidiarrheal products. In: *Handbook of Nonprescription Drugs*, 10th ed. American Pharmaceutical Association, Washington, D.C., 1993, p. 210.

32. *KLUCEL, Hydroxypropyl Cellulose, Physical and Chemical Properties*, by Aqualon Company, Bulletin 250–2D (1991).

33. S. Nail, J. White, and S. Hem, Structure of aluminum hydroxide gel I: Initial precipitate, *J. Pharm. Sci.*, 65(8):1195 (1976).

34. R. Vanderlaan, J. White, and S. Hem, Formation of hydrotalcite in mixtures of aluminum hydroxycarbonate and magnesium hydroxide gels, *J. Pharm. Sci.*, 71(7):780 (1982).

35. S. L. Hem, in Program Notes from *Twenty Second Annual Educational Conference on Industrial Pharmacy*, Arden House-Harriman, NY, February 8–13, 1987.

36. *Federal Register*, 40, 12924 (1975).

37. *Federal Register*, 51, 16146, (1986).

38. *The United States Pharmacopeia XXII*, United States Pharmacopeial Convention, Inc., Rockville, MD, 1990, p. 1625.

39. *The United States Pharmacopeia XXII*, United States Pharmacopeial Convention, Inc., Rockville, MD, 1990, p. 1624.

40. M. Brody and W. Bacharach, Antacids. I. Comparative biochemical and economic considerations, *Am. J. Dig. Dis.*, 4:435 (1959).

41. N. E. Rossett and M. L. Rice, Jr., An in-vitro evaluation of the efficacy of the more frequently used antacids with particular attention to tablets, *Gastroenterology*, 26:490 (1954).

42. International Association of Milk, Food and Environmental Sanitarians, United States Public Health Service and The Dairy Industry Committee, 3-A Sanitary standards for polished metal tubing for dairy products, *Journal of Milk and Food Technology*, 39(10):(1976).

43. International Association of Milk, Food and Environmental Sanitarians, United States Public Health Service and The Dairy Industry Committee, 3-A Sanitary standards for sanitary fittings for milk and milk products Number 63–00 (08–17 as Amended), *Dairy, Food and Environmental Sanitation*, 13(12):738–750 (1993).

4

Oral Aqueous Suspensions

Clyde M. Ofner III, Roger L. Schnaare, and Joseph B. Schwartz

Philadelphia College of Pharmacy and Science, Philadelphia, Pennsylvania

I. INTRODUCTION

Oral aqueous suspensions constitute the largest percentage of pharmaceutical suspensions and are used primarily to overcome undesirable properties of the drug. The formulation of a pharmaceutical suspension is often a challenge and in most cases unique because the physical and chemical properties of drugs are different. In addition, a concern exists in all disperse systems, including suspensions, which is to develop a formulation that provides consistent doses throughout the prescribed shelf life of the product. This chapter is a summary of pertinent information to assist the formulator in the preparation of marketable oral aqueous suspension products with an emphasis on the essential principles involved in the process.

Oral aqueous suspensions can be described as two-phase systems composed of water-insoluble drug substances that are dispersed in a continuous aqueous medium. One of the most common reasons to formulate a drug as a suspension is poor aqueous solubility. Another reason for these formulations is that suspensions minimize drug degradation. Drug molecules susceptible to aqueous degradation are protected from reacting with water in the interior of the suspended drug particles. Only the very small soluble fraction of the drug is exposed to water in the solution. Suspensions are also used to mask the unpleasant taste from dissolved drug in solution, which is particularly useful for products intended for pediatric or geriatric patients.

II. CHARACTERISTICS OF ORAL AQUEOUS SUSPENSIONS

A. Efficacy

Drug suspensions are often pharmacologically very effective and they may be less complicated to manufacture than other dosage forms. Their effectiveness may be attributed to a number of factors. For example, drugs formulated as suspensions may be more bioavailable than comparable tablets or capsules [1,2]. Suspensions are often more effective than tablets or capsules in the pediatric and geriatric patient population, because these patients generally find suspensions easier to swallow. Also, dose flexibility, such as one-half or one-third of a dose, is more convenient with suspensions than with solids, and as a result, patients are more inclined to comply with their dosage instructions.

The bioavailability of oral aqueous suspensions has been studied by comparison with other oral dosage forms, by comparison with different suspending agents, and by comparison with different routes of administration. Bioavailability of some oral aqueous suspensions can be as high as that from I.V. solutions. For example, the estimated bioavailability of a methocarbamol suspension given to rates depended on the dose concentration and ranged from 7% to 112% of the drug formulated in an I.V. polyethylene glycol aqueous solution [3].

Several studies have shown bioequivalence between oral aqueous suspensions and other comparable oral formulations. For example, a suspension of the antibiotic cefuroxime axetil was slightly less bioavailable but statistically bioequivalent to the tablet formulation when tested in 12 healthy volunteers [4]. A similar comparison of propyphenazon in rabbits showed biological equivalence between suspension and tablet formulations [5]. A comparison of three oral formulations of cisapride, a gastrointestinal stimulant, demonstrated no significant differences between the bioequivalence of a suspension, tablet, and solid formulation in healthy men even though the solution produced the shortest time to attain peak plasma drug concentrations [6]. In a study involving 17 cancer patients, peak plasma drug concentrations (C_{max}) were lower from an aqueous medroxyprogesterone acetate suspension than those from a syrup formulation, but the wide intersubject spread in the plasma levels in both groups did not allow any statistical significance to be assigned to this difference [7]. Particle size reduction has produced some suspension formulations that are more bioavailable than comparable tablets or capsules [8]. Particle size reduction to submicron dimensions has been used to increase bioavailability of poorly water-soluble drugs [9].

Other oral suspension formulations have been shown to be bioequivalent to tablets and oral drug solutions. The extent of absorption of a sustained-release formulation of carbinoxamine and phenylpropanolamine was slightly less than that of an aqueous solution of the same drugs in 20 healthy subjects, but the two preparations were statistically bioequivalent [10]. The slightly greater area under the curve (AUC) value and C_{max} of a cefotaxime reconstitutable suspension compared to the values of a tablet formulation in 12 healthy volunteers were not statistically significant and indicated that the two preparations were bioequivalent [11].

The viscosity of the external or continuous phase can influence drug absorption from suspensions. The effects of several suspending agents on drug absorption from a nitrofurantoin suspension was studied in 11 subjects. A viscosity increase slowed absorption and lengthened the duration of action by 2 hours without decreasing bioavailability [12]. Viscosity enhancers, however, decreased the extent of intestinal absorption of sulfafurazole from an aqueous solution in rats; AUC decreased inversely with viscosity [13].

In some cases of poor bioavailability from oral aqueous suspensions, reformulation for alternate routes of administration may be desired. An oral aqueous suspension of artemisinin to treat plasmodium infections was rapidly but incompletely absorbed in 10 male volunteers. Its bioavailability was only 32% that of an I.M. injectable suspension of the same drug in oil. In addition, I.M. injection and rectal administration of the aqueous suspension produced very low and variable drug concentrations in serum indicating poor and erratic absorption [14]. In this case the I.M. suspension formulated with an oil medium produced the highest bioavailability compared with three other routes of administration formulated with an aqueous medium.

Drug suspensions are subject to formulation factors that if not recognized can result in a deleterious effect on the final product and the patient. Nonuniform mixing of the product results in variations of drug concentration. Difficult redispersion of the drug from a sediment, or in the worst case, from caking, will result in over- or underdosing. An undetected polymorphism of the drug can alter its solubility and cause crystal growth. Other, less direct, parameters to be considered once the suspension leaves the manufacturer include the consequences of exposure to extreme heat or cold temperatures, risks of microbial growth, extraction of harmful container components, and change in drug concentration caused by the loss of aqueous vehicle as the result of evaporation or leaking.

B. Desired Attributes

Specific desired attributes of a suspension drug product may depend on the physical/chemical nature of the drug. Required characteristics of suspensions in general are listed in Table 1. In addition to the drug, a typical suspension may contain several other ingredients, including:

Wetting agent
Suspending agent
Protective colloid
Flocculating agent
Sweetener
Preservatives
Buffer system
Flavor
Color
Sequestering agent
Antifoaming agent

The appropriate selection and combination of these ingredients are the goal of the formulator.

III. PRINCIPLES OF FORMULATION

Because the specific properties of various suspended drugs differ, no single procedure will always produce a successful suspension product. Different methods have been de-

Table 1 Requirements of Oral Suspension Formulations

1. The dispersed particles should be small and uniform; they should not settle fast.
2. If the particles settle, they should be easily redispersed.
3. There should be no excess viscosity to interfere with pouring and redispersal.
4. The redispersal should produce a uniform dose for administration.
5. The suspension should be chemically and physically stable for the shelf life of the product.
6. The final formulation should be pleasing to the patient; it should have an agreeable odor, color, and taste.

veloped with varying degrees of success. However, certain principles have been recognized that are fundamental for all successful formulations. This section contains a general discussion of these principles. Specific examples are discussed with sample formulas. Ingredients are discussed in more detail in the next section. For additional information on suspension formulation, see the excellent reviews by Haines and Martin [15–17], Nash [18,19], and Idson and Scheer [20]. For more information on the colloidal and surface-chemical aspects of suspensions, see the review by Schott and Martin [21].

A. Particle Size

One of the most important considerations in the formulation of a suspension is the particle size of the drug. As the insoluble drug settles, a nonuniform distribution results. A major goal of the formulator is to slow or even prevent sedimentation of the drug particle. Particle sedimentation can lead to caking, which is dense packing of the sediment. Redispersal of a caked suspension is difficult if not impossible. Redispersal of a caked sediment presents a potential danger to the patient. The patient will receive an overdose of the drug if the administered dose from the suspension contains many particles of the broken but previously caked drug sediment. It should be pointed out that as long as the sediment is easily redispersed to produce a uniform drug concentration, sedimentation is not a risk to the patient and is frequently not considered a formulation problem. The relationship of factors that describes the rate of particle settling, or sedimentation, is Stokes' law:

$$v = \frac{d^2(\rho_2 - \rho_1)g}{18\eta} \tag{1}$$

where v = sedimentation rate of an average particle
    d = mean particle diameter
    ρ_2 = particle density
    ρ_1 = density of the dispersion medium
    g = acceleration due to gravity
    η = viscosity of the dispersion medium.

Equation (1) illustrates that the largest factor to influence sedimentation rate is particle diameter because the rate is directly proportional to the square of particle diameter; consequently, smaller particles settle slower than larger particles. If the particles are less than approximately 3 μm, and their density does not differ by more than 20% from that of the vehicle, then the particles could remain suspended due to Brownian motion.

In practice, there is a limit to particle size reduction. After reducing particles to a certain size, further reduction can be costly because of the time and equipment involved. Furthermore, suspensions of particles in the colloidal size range have additional problems caused by the enhanced consequences of interactions between very small particles that have an extremely large total particle surface area. One example of such problems is the change in driving force of particle motion from gravity for larger particles to the driving force of Brownian motion for colloidal-sized particles. Such particle motion can produce particle aggregation followed by settling of the aggregates and finally caking.

Equation 1 was derived under conditions not entirely applicable to pharmaceutical suspensions. More theoretical expressions have been reported [22] but Stokes' law is accurate for illustrating the factors that affect sedimentation of suspended particles.

B. Viscosity

Equation (1) illustrates the inverse relationship between viscosity of the dispersion medium and rate of particle settling. An increase in viscosity produces a reduced sedimentation rate and increases physical stability. Viscosity is also increased by the volume fraction of the particles [23]. The formulator must be aware that the presence of the drug itself increases viscosity. The most common method of increasing viscosity is by adding a suspending agent. Too high a viscosity, however, is undesirable if it interferes with pouring and redispersal of the settled particles.

According to Eq. (1), sedimentation rate is also lowered by reducing the density difference between particles and the dispersion medium. Increasing the vehicle density has not been a particularly successful way to control the sedimentation rate because water is the most common vehicle and the additional ingredients do not greatly increase its density. Traditionally, particle size and viscosity have been the properties of suspension products that have received the most attention by formulators.

Also illustrated in Eq. (1) is that suspending agent viscosity will slow but not prevent sedimentation. As early as 1959 Meyer and Cohen [24] suggested that yield value, or the point of an effective infinite viscosity in which there is no flow, was an important mechanism of permanent suspensions in order to prevent sedimentation. The mechanism has been examined [25]. The theoretical yield value (YV) for a suspension must balance or exceed the force of gravity on the settling particles. The equation for spherical particles is:

$$YV = \frac{V(\rho_2 - \rho_1)g}{A} \qquad (2)$$

where V = particle volume
ρ_2 = density of particle
ρ_1 = density of dispersion medium
g = acceleration due to gravity
A = cross-sectional area of the particle = πR^2 for radius, R

Using Carbomer 934P as the suspending agent, Meyer and Cohen produced a sand suspension that lasted for several years. These investigators calculated a theoretical yield value for sand (density = 2.60 g/cm^3 radius = 0.030 cm) and for marbles (density = 2.55 g/cm^3 radius = 0.800 cm) of 63 and 1622 dynes/cm^2, respectively. The concentrations of the agent required to suspend the "particles" were 0.18% and 0.4%, for sand and marbles, respectively.

The yield value of a dispersion medium can be experimentally determined using a rotational viscometer by plotting shear stress (dyne/cm^2) as a function of shear rate (sec^{-1}). The resulting curve, shown in Fig. 1, does not pass through the origin but intersects the axis of shear stress as in curve A, or by extrapolation of the linear portion of the curve as in curve B. The intersection, at C or D, is the yield value. The apparent viscosity of the material is the slope of the curve and for most pharmaceutical systems varies with shear rate, as in curve A. The entire curve, therefore, is usually required to describe the viscosity of these systems.

A dispersion medium in which the suspending agents has a molecular structure that entraps drug particles, thereby severely retarding or preventing sedimentation, is called a structured vehicle [26]. If sedimentation is prevented, then the material has a yield value. This structure must not be so rigid as to prevent flow during pouring from the

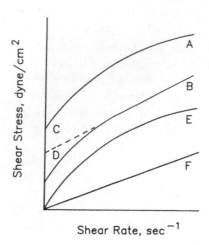

Fig. 1 Rheologic flow behavior. Key: Plastic flow, A and B, with yield values C and D; pseudoplastic flow, E; Newtonian flow, F.

container. These vehicles should be shear-thinning—that is, have high viscosities at negligible shear rates during shelf storage and low viscosities at high shear rates during shaking.

If the molecular structure of the suspending agent producing the increased viscosity is broken down by agitation during shaking but then re-forms upon aging, the suspending agent is thixotropic. The apparent viscosity of thixotropic suspensions is therefore dependent on their previous shear history, including the duration of shearing. This property is useful for pharmaceutical suspensions because the structure formed on standing produces high viscosity or even a yield value and retards or prevents sedimentation. Redispersion by shaking with shear stress greater than the yield value prior to administration temporarily breaks down the structure, reduces the yield value to practically zero, and lowers the apparent viscosity. The suspension then pours easily from the container. After administration and on standing, the structure re-forms to impede sedimentation. Colloidal clays such as bentonite are an example of suspending agents that are thixotropic.

One type of rheologic flow illustrated in Fig. 1 is plastic flow (curves A and B). If the curve passes through the origin (i.e., has no yield value), the material exhibits pseudoplastic flow (curve E). Pseudoplastic materials are shear-thinning; the viscosity varies with shear rate. If the viscosity of a material is unaffected by shear rate, then the plot is linear, the plot passes through the origin, and the material exhibits Newtonian flow (curve F). The yield value of plastic materials is an advantage in a suspending medium. The shear-thinning ability, or the lowered viscosity during shaking, is an advantage of pseudoplastic materials, but the absence of a yield value is a disadvantage. Suspending agents exhibiting Newtonian flow are used infrequently because they lack both yield value and shear-thinning properties. Additional background on the rheology of pharmaceutical materials is available in volume one of this series and in standard pharmacy texts [27,28].

C. Wetting

Most drugs are hydrophobic and, when suspended, frequently float on the vehicle surface as the result of poor wetting. A wetting agent enhances the ability of the dispersion medium, or suspension vehicle, to spread on the surface of the drug particle. Wettability of the drug particle can sometimes be evaluated by measuring the contact angle [29]. If poor wetting can be differentiated from moderate wetting, the number of wetting agents to be tested can be reduced. Low concentrations of surfactants are commonly used as wetting agents to aid dispersion of the particles in the suspension vehicle.

Excess wetting agent may lead to foaming or unpleasant taste. An additional caution with wetting agents is the increased possibility of caking because the coated particles resist aggregate formation, settle individually, and may form a dense or caked sediment.

D. Mixing

Although not usually considered an aspect of suspension formulation, mixing is the major operation of suspension particles and is very important because inadequate mixing results in nonhomogeneity of the drug dispersed in the vehicle. A few pertinent points directly related to formulation are discussed. Good reviews on the principles and equipment are available in other chapters of this volume and other sources [30–32].

The initial dispersion of the drug in the vehicle medium is a mixing operation. If the drug is hydrophobic, a wetting agent should be included. Sometimes shearing forces from equipment, such as a ball mill or colloid mill, are used to break up particle aggregates for enhanced wetting and dispersion of the drug.

In some cases, mixing has an unusual purpose. Restoration of the structure associated with thixotropic suspensions is slow if the suspension is viscous. Gentle agitation from low shear rates may accelerate structure restoration, producing high apparent viscosity or thixotropic gels with a yield value [26].

The addition of suspending agents, such as sodium carboxymethylcellulose, to build viscosity increases the difficulty of mixing. The equipment must have the capacity to mix viscous material, but excessive shearing and its concomitant heat production can degrade polymeric suspending agents and should be avoided. Often the completed suspension is passed through a colloid mill to break up excessive particle aggregates and to ensure adequate mixing of the final product.

E. Flocculation

Early formulation efforts were concerned with reduction of the sedimentation rate and ease of redispersing the settled particles. One approach still used is to employ a protective colloid [21]. These agents, such as proteins or gums, adsorb and coat the drug particles and impede aggregation. The result is usually an unsightly appearance of sediment and clear supernatant because the particles eventually settle. If the particles are easily redispersed, however, the appearance does not preclude use of the product. Many antacid suspensions are formulated in this manner but placed in an opaque container to hide the appearance of separated sediment.

Maintaining the drug in suspension with little or no separation results in a more elegant, permanent suspension and is more consistent with modern suspension technology. One such approach is flocculation, which is the formation of loose, low density, particle aggregates [26,33,34]. The flocs settle and produce a loose, inefficiently packed sediment that is less dense and easier to redisperse than a sediment produced by deflocculated, or individual, particles. If the flocculated particles have a sufficient concentration prior to settling, a continuous structure is produced that results in a yield value and little sedimentation. The yield value can therefore be used as an indicator for the extent of flocculation [28]. With the use of flocculating agents, adequate control of floc-

Table 2 Comparison of Properties of Flocculated and Deflocculated Suspension Particles

Deflocculated
1.   Particles exist in suspension as separate entities.
2.   Sedimentation rate is slow because each particle settles separately and particle size is minimal.
3.   The sediment is formed slowly.
4.   The sediment eventually becomes closely packed due to weight of upper layers of sediment. Repulsive forces between particles are overcome, caking results and the sediment is difficult, if not impossible, to redisperse.
5.   The suspension has a pleasing appearance because the suspended material remains suspended for a relatively long time. The supernatant also remains cloudy, even when settling is apparent.

Flocculated
1.   Particles form loose aggregates.
2.   Sedimentation rate is high because particles settle as a floc, which is a collection of particles.
3.   The sediment is formed rapidly.
4.   The sediment is loosely packed and possesses a scaffold-like structure. Particles do not bond tightly to each other and a hard, dense cake does not form. The sediment is easy to redisperse in order to re-form the original suspension.
5.   The suspension is somewhat unsightly because of rapid sedimentation and the presence of an obvious, clear supernatant region. This can be minimized if the volume of sediment is made large. Ideally, volume of sediment should equal volume of the product.

Source: Ref. 35.

culation ideally results in a suspension that does not noticeably separate [35]. Table 2 is a comparison of the properties of flocculated and deflocculated suspension particles.

The use of electrolytes to control the extent of flocculation, known as controlled flocculation, has been used successfully in a number of systems [15–17, 33–35]. Electrolytes reduce the electrical barrier, or zeta potential, between particles and allow them to approach each other and to form flocs. The most efficient electrolytes are those with a charge opposite to that of the particle. The efficiency increases as the valence of the electrolyte increases. For example, a negatively charged particle, such as kaolin, would be very efficiently flocculated with aluminum chloride. This approach requires determinations of zeta potential of the drug particle as a function of electrolyte concentration. The concentration producing zero or a low absolute value of zeta potential should produce optimum flocculation.

Flocculation may occur unintentionally. Other ingredients such as protective colloids, wetting agents, suspending agents, and electrolytes can act as flocculating agents. Colloidally dispersed solids are also an effective method of inducing flocculation [36].

F. Chemical Incompatibilities

Formulators must be aware of the potential chemical incompatibilities between suspension ingredients. These problems may not be immediately apparent. The suspending agents, which are often large anionic molecules such as sodium carboxymethylcellulose, will usually precipitate or gel with cationic molecules. Possible cationic ingredients are the drug, wetting agents, electrolytes, and flocculating agents. Anionic surfactants are usually incompatible with cationic surfactants. Surfactants are used as wetting or flocculating agents. Incompatibilities also exist between di- and trivalent electrolytes and surfactants of opposite charge. Buffers may occasionally react with the drug or suspending agent. Colorants may react with surfactants.

G. Principles of Particle Interactions in Liquid

A discussion of some theory of particle interactions is included to increase conceptual understanding of the principles in the prior sections. The topics of surface free energy, forces of attraction, surface potential, and forces of repulsion are briefly discussed. Several sources are available for more detailed information [37–40].

When a solid material is decreased in size, the total surface area of the subdivided material increases. As the surface area increases, so does the surface free energy, or the positive free energy. Basically, this means that the molecules at the surface have a higher energy state than the molecules below the surface (i.e., within the particle). In order to attain a more energetically stable state, the particles tend to aggregate, which reduces the surface area and lowers the positive free energy toward zero. The clumping of particles, particularly hydrophobic particles such as steroids or sulfur, illustrates this "natural" mechanism of a reduction in free energy.

An alternate mechanism of reducing surface free energy is the adsorption of surface-active materials such as surfactants. After this wetting step, the reduced free energy results in less tendency to reduce surface area and less, if any, clumping is observed. In practice however, the dispersed particles usually settle and caking often results.

The terminology used to describe particle aggregation varies. Some investigators differentiate between coagulation and flocculation to describe the result of specific interactions. The term flocculation is used for all "loose" particle aggregation in this brief discussion.

The forces of attraction between these hydrophobic particles originate at the molecular level and are predominately van der Waals forces of attraction. The rate of particle flocculation caused by these forces can be measured under controlled conditions. Comparison of measured rates constants with theoretical rates constants reveals many examples in which flocculation occurs much slower than expected [40]. These cases indicate a component of repulsion that opposes and reduces attraction.

The forces of repulsion are the result of the presence of an electrical charge on the surface of the particles. Charges of the same sign produce forces of electrostatic repulsion. The charge may originate from different sources. The material may have an ionic composition, such as insoluble salts; or electrolytes from the continuous liquid phase may adsorb to the particles; or surfactant ions may adsorb to the particles.

The charge on the particle results in a surface potential, ψ_0, at the particle surface. Counterions, or ions of a charge opposite to that on the particle, must be present for electro-neutrality and consequently can counteract the potential. The distance at which the potential drops to zero depends on the concentration of counterions. This region of decreasing potential ends gradually at a distance where its ionic composition approaches that of the bulk liquid and is called the electrical double layer. It ranges in thickness from 10 to 1000 Å and decreases as the concentration of electrolyte increases. It is illustrated by the dashed circle and line D in Fig. 2 (a). The Stern layer is within the double layer and represents a first layer of charge. It is composed of counterions adsorbed directly to the surface of the particle and is represented by line S. Line P represents the sur-

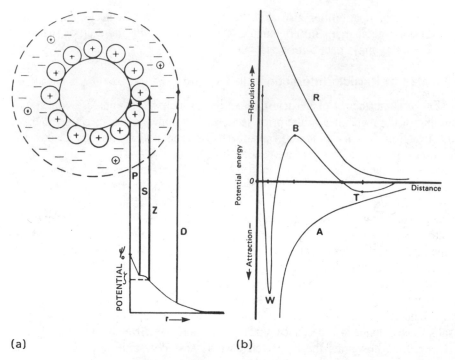

(a)   (b)

Fig. 2 Components of particle interactions. (a) Decreasing potential at various points: particle surface, P; Stern layer, S; plane of shear, Z; electrical double layer, D. (b) Potential energies between two identically charged particles: curve of electrostatic energy of repulsion, R; van der Waals energy of attraction, A; and net interaction energy, WBT. (From Refs. 37 and 38.)

face of the particle. The potentials at the corresponding distances from the particle surface are also shown in Fig. 2(a).

The electrokinetic or ζ (zeta) potential has practical importance because it can be experimentally measured. A charged particle suspended in water will migrate toward an electrode of the opposite charge in an electrical field. Ions in the Stern layer and bound water of hydration are carried along with the particle. The plane of shear that separates the bound water from the free bulk water is represented by line Z in Fig. 2 (a). This plane is a small distance from the particle surface and therefore has a lower potential than the surface. The zeta potential is frequently used to describe energies of interactions between particles because it can be measured directly.

The energies of attraction and repulsion were used to develop a quantitative theory of particle interactions known as the DLVO theory. The forces of electrostatic repulsion and van der Waals attraction are compared. While the theory does not explain all of the experimental data, it provides a very useful basis for understanding particle interactions in suspensions (and in emulsions).

Figure 2 (b) illustrates the DLVO theory in which the potential energy of interaction between two identically charged particles is plotted as a function of the interparticle distance. If the y-axis is viewed as the plane of a particle surface, then the x-axis measures the distance of an approaching particle and the curves describe the forces encountered. The upper curve, labeled R, represents the electrostatic energy of repulsion and curve A represents the van der Waals energy of attraction. Both forces, and their resultant energies, decrease as interparticle distance increases but they do not decrease in an identical manner. The algebraic sum of these curves is the middle curve labeled with the points, W, B, T; it gives the total or net energy of interaction between two like charged particles. If the particles are of opposite charge then electrostatic attraction is added to van der Waals attraction to easily overcome repulsion and rapidly aggregate the particle.

The chemical nature and particle size of the material primarily determines the extent of interparticle attraction. Electrostatic repulsion, however, is subject to more variables. It is largely influenced by surface potential and thickness of the double layer. Zeta potential is also governed by these factors and its magnitude is therefore an indicator of interparticle repulsion. As a consequence of these factors, and probably because it can be measured directly, this parameter has been correlated to the stability of dispersion [39]. Electrolytes and ionic surfactants are among the additives that influence zeta potential.

Curve WBT of net interaction energy illustrates aspects of an energy barrier and an energy well regarding particle aggregation. A shallow well, or secondary minimum, exists at the distance corresponding to point T on the curve. At a closer interparticle distance corresponding to point B, an energy barrier repels any approaching particle with less kinetic energy than the potential energy at B. If the approaching particle has sufficient energy to overcome the barrier, then van der Waals attraction dominates up to point W in the primary minimum where the particles touch. Energetically, this point represents a very stable situation.

Although the DLVO theory enjoys almost universal acceptance, disagreement exists on some details. Some investigators believe that flocculation exists in the secondary minimum, others believe it to exist in the primary minimum. The variables of major influence, however, are well described and their effects can be used to advantage by the formulator.

If a hydrophobic particle is wetted with an anionic surfactant to aid dispersion, then the adsorbed charges give the particle a sufficient zeta potential such that interparticle repulsion dominates to prevent flocculation. As an electrolyte is added in increasing concentrations, the thickness of the repulsive double layer is reduced and consequently, the zeta potential is reduced which allows closer approach of particles to each other. Flocculation occurs as the absolute value of the zeta potential shifts to a certain range closer to zero. Generally, this occurs at zeta potentials less than 25 mV. Most of the zeta potential and electrostatic repulsion from the anionic surfactant is countered because of electrolyte cation adsorption and van der Waals attraction then dominates. The flocs, as voluminous particle aggregates, have a high sedimentation volume and are easily redispersed. An example of this system is described in a study that uses the DLVO theory to interpret suspension stability [41]. The investigators used griseofulvin as the drug particle, ammonium dodecyl polyoxyethylene sulfate as the anionic surfactant, and aluminum chloride as the electrolyte.

In some situations, the continued addition of the electroylte after the zeta potential was shifted to near zero leads to further adsorption of the counterion in which a charge gradually builds. The magnitude of the zeta potential then increases, which promotes repulsion and deflocculation. An example of this is the addition of phosphate anions to suspensions of positively charged particles of bismuth subnitrate. The zeta potential of the particle starts as positive, is reduced to zero, and builds a negative charge from the continued addition of the phosphate anion. When the zeta potential is near zero the sediment of such a suspension is voluminous, with no caking. When the magnitude of the zeta potential is high, the sediment is small, and a high tendency for caking exists.

IV. COMMONLY USED INGREDIENTS

This section contains material on the ingredients used in suspension formulation, including the primary ingredient—the drug. Many ingredients are presented in tabular form for ease of comparison. Suspending, flocculating, and wetting agents are discussed separately and the remaining ingredients are discussed collectively.

A. Drug Particles

Some drugs are known to pose specific problems to the formulator. Particle size reduction and characteristics of the drug, such as polymorphism and crystal growth, are discussed.

In most pharmaceutical suspensions the range of particle diameters is between 1 and 50 μm. Common methods of particle size reduction include dry-milling, spray-drying, micropulverization, and fluid-energy grinding, of which the last two are considered industry standards [18,42]. Recent reviews of particle size reduction are available [43,44].

Particles are micropulverized by a high-speed attrition impact mill. Because the particles are seldom less than 10 μm, a buildup of electrostatic charge on the powder surface is not routinely a problem. The distribution of particle sizes obtained usually ranges from 10 to 50 μm. This broad range is the primary disadvantage of micropulverization, but the particles are suitable for most oral suspensions.

Micronizing with a fluid-energy mill readily reduces particle size below 5 μm. The primary disadvantage of this method is the electrostatic charge built up on the powder surface; powder collection is, therefore, very difficult. The cost of a fluid-energy source and dust collection equipment in addition to that of the mill might be considered a second disadvantage.

Colloidal particles can be prepared by precipitation. Three methods used are organic solvent precipitation, precipitation by pH changes of the medium, and chemical reaction. A precipitation reaction is illustrated in an example formula in a subsequent section. The interested reader is referred to a review for additional information on precipitation methods [45].

The unrecognized existence of different polymorphic forms of the drug can present several problems. Polymorph conversion is usually from a less stable and more soluble form to a more stable form. The more stable polymorph is less soluble and may produce crystal growth, unanticipated sedimentation, and possibly caking. A slow conversion rate may result in adverse consequences after manufacture. The different solubilities of the polymorphs can produce changes in concentration of the administered dose. Changes in bioavailability can occur because solubility changes alter absorption [1]. Cortisone, prednisolone, riboflavin, sulfathiazole, many barbiturate derivatives, and chloramphenicol palmitate [46] are examples of drugs that exhibit polymorphism. The temperature, solvent for crystallization, and cooling rate are important factors in obtaining both the desired polymorph and in controlling its rate of formation. A change in the particle shape is also important and can influence the rate of sedimentation [47]. Melting point and x-ray diffraction patterns are other physical properties that differ between polymorphs.

Crystal growth often occurs in the absence of polymorphism [48]. Drugs frequently formulated as suspensions in which crystal growth was investigated include sulfathiazole and methylprednisolone [49]. Protective colloids that inhibit crystal growth provide one means of preventing caking. Polymers employed to inhibit crystal growth include polyvinylpyrrolidone [50] and methylcellulose [51]. The effect of several surfactants on carbamazepine crystal growth and aqueous solubility has also been examined. The authors of these studies concluded that benzalkonium chloride [52] and polysorbate 80 [53] stopped crystal growth at a certain level, but sodium lauryl sulfate [53] and poloxamer 184 [54] accelerated growth and could produce very large crystals.

B. Suspending Agents

Several classes of suspending agents are discussed in this section. Suspending agents are used to impart increased viscosity and retard sedimentation. The formulator must select the most appropriate agent, alone or in combination, and at the appropriate concentration. Factors to consider during selection include suspending ability in the system; chemical compatibility with all ingredients, especially the drug; effect of pH range on the drug; length of time for hydration; appearance; source; reproducibility of these considerations from batch to batch; and cost. Even if chemically compatible, the suspending agent and drug may interact. For example, reduced dissolution behavior of nitrofurantoin was reported in the presence of methylcellulose [55].

Table 3 is a compilation of some pertinent characteristics of most suspending agents currently used. The agents are divided into classes of cellulose derivatives, clays, natural gums, synthetic gums, and miscellaneous agents. Although a few little-used agents are included in the table, a suspending agent such as calcium carboxymethylcellulose is not, because it is very similar to an agent that is included. Not all agents listed are suitable for individual use; some must be used in combinations. For each agent the rheologic flow behavior, maximum viscosity, pH range, ionic charge, range of useful concentration, and references are listed. The types of rheologic behavior listed are plastic, pseudoplastic, Newtonian, and thixotropic. An agent may exhibit more than one type of rheology; changes are listed in the order of concentration exhibiting that behavior. The viscosity range is designated by the maximum value reported from pertinent concentrations and grades at room temperatures. These values are dependent on the conditions of measurement such as shear rate, concentration, spindle size, and the instrument. They are intended only for general comparison. Stable pH ranges of the agents and common concentrations are listed. One value is listed if no range was reported. The concentration units of percent vary but they are usually weight per volume (w/v) or weight per weight (w/w). Additional details of the values in this table are available in the listed references. For incompatibilities and proprietary preparations of many suspending agents consult the monographs in Martindale [56].

1. *Cellulose Derivatives*

Cellulose derivatives are semisynthetic and have good batch-to-batch reproducibility of their characteristics. Excluding sodium carboxymethylcellulose, these agents are nonionic and, therefore, are chemically compatible with most ingredients. Most are available in grades of different viscosities. These agents usually exhibit pseudoplastic flow and have

Table 3 Summary of Suspending Agents[a]

	Agent	Class	Rheologic behavior
1	Microcrystalline cellulose	Cellulose	Plastic/thixotropic
2	Microcrystalline cellulose with carboxymethylcellulose sodium	Derivative	Plastic/thix
3	Powdered cellulose		Plastic/thix[b]
4	Ethylmethylcellulose		Pseudoplastic
5	Carboxymethylcellulose sodium		Pseudoplastic
6	Hydroxypropyl methylcellulose		Pseudoplastic
7	Methylcellulose		Pseudo/plastic
8	Ethylcellulose		Pseudoplastic[b]
9	Ethylhydroxyethylcellulose		Pseudoplastic
10	Hydroxyethylcellulose		Plastic
11	Hydroxypropyl cellulose		Pseudoplastic
12	Attapulgite	Clay	Plastic/thix[b]
13	Bentonite		Plastic/thix
14	Hectorite		Plastic/thix
15	Montmorillonite		Plastic/thix
16	Magnesium aluminum silicate		Plastic/thix
17	Silica gel	Colloidal	Pseudo/plastic[b]
18	Silicon dioxide, colloidal		Plastic/thix[b]
19	Acacia	Natural	Newtonian
20	Agar	Gum	Plastic
21	Carrageenan		Newt/pseudo
22	Guar gum		Newt/pseudo
23	Locust bean gum		Pseudoplastic
24	Pectin		Newt/pseudo
25	Na alginate		Pseudoplastic
26	Propylene glycol alginate		Pseudoplastic
27	Tamarind gum		Pseudoplastic
28	Tragacanth		Newt/pseudo
29	Xanthan gum		Plastic
30	Carbomer 934	Synthetic	Plastic
31	Povidone	Gum	Newt/pseudo
32	Gelatin	Miscellaneous	Plastic
33	Glycyrrhizin		Pseudoplastic
34	Pregelatinized starch		Plastic
35	Sodium starch glycolate		Pseudoplastic[b]

	Viscosity range (cps)	pH range	Ionic charge	Concentration range (%)	References
1	<25	5–7	0	1–5	[59],[60]
2	<200	3.5–11	–	0.5–2	[59],[61],[62]
3	—	5–7.5	0	10	[56],[63],[64]
4	<60	7	0	2.5	[56]
5	<6000	3–11.5	–	1–2	[18],[24],[65], [66],[67]
6	<5250	6–8	0	0.3–2	[21],[56],[66]
7	<8000	2–12	0	1–5	[18],[65],[66]
8	<100	7	0	5	[56]

Table 3 Continued

	Viscosity range (cps)	pH range	Ionic charge	Concentration range (%)	References
9	—	—	0	0.1–2	[56]
10	<4000	6.5–8.5	0	0.5–2	[59],[66],[67],[68]
11	<6500	5–8.5	0	1–10	[69],[70]
12	—	6–8.5	–	10	[71],[72]
13	<800	3–10	–	1–6	[60],[73]
14	<120	—	–	3–5.5	[74]
15	—	3–10	–	1–5	[72]
16	<2200	3–11	–	0.5–5	[18],[59],[61]
17	—	4–8	0	5	[56]
18	low	3.5–4.4	0	0.25–1.0	[60],[75],[76]
19	<10	4–10	–	2.0	[77],[78]
20	—	4.5–9	–	0.1–2	[79]
21	<1000	4–10	–	1–2	[18],[56],[64],[73]
22	<12000	1–10.5	0	0.6–1.5	[12],[75],[80]
23	<6000	3–11	0	0.4–2.5	[24],[81]
24	<1000	2–9	–	1–3	[18],[71],[73]
25	<10000	4–11.5	–	0.5–2.5	[12],[18],[24],[65]
26	<10000	2.5–7	–	1.5–3	[59],[73]
27	—	2.5–9.5	0	0.5–2	[82]
28	<9700	2.5–9	–	0.2–4	[24],[59],[66]
29	<8000	2–13	–	0.3–3	[83]
30	<40000	5–11	–	0.1–0.4	[24],[60],[84],[85]
31	<95	5.5–11.5	0	5–10	[86],[87]
32	—	3–8	+/–	<1	[88]
33	<370	3.5–5.5	–	0.5–2	[89]
34	—	—	0	1	[59],[90]
35	<6	3–7.5	–	1–2	[59],[90]

aSee text for explanation of column headings.
bView of authors based on behavior of similar agents.

no yield value. However, microcrystalline and powdered cellulose are not water soluble and produce dispersions that exhibit plastic flow and have yield values. A good review of the pharmaceutical uses of these cellulose derivatives is available [57].

Combinations are used to increase suspending ability. Microcrystalline cellulose has been used in combination with hydroxypropyl methylcellulose, sodium carboxymethyl-cellulose, and methylcellulose. The combination of microcrystalline cellulose and sodium carboxymethylcellulose is used extensively. It disperses quickly in cold water and needs little hydration time. The presence of sodium carboxymethylcellulose adds sufficient structuring to retard sedimentation of the cellulose, and, at total concentrations of the combination above 1%, its presence results in thixotropic gels. The presence of the anionic derivative also extends the usefulness over a larger pH range.

Methylcellulose also produces gels and is available in several viscosity grades. This agent is soluble in cold and insoluble in hot water. It is dispersed in hot water and a subsequent temperature reduction dissolves the agent. Agents with properties and uses similar to those of methylcellulose include ethylmethylcellulose, and ethylhydroxy-ethylcellulose.

Table 3 includes other suspending agents with uses similar to those of methylcellulose. Hydroxypropyl methylcellulose is often used in ophthalmic preparations because of its clarity; a high viscosity grade is available for use in suspensions. Ethylcellulose is insoluble in water and rarely used as a suspending agent. Less insoluble grades with a lower degree of substitution are available. Hydroxyethylcellulose is soluble in cold or hot water but is reported to have poor suspending ability [58,59].

Sodium carboxymethylcellulose is extensively employed as a suspending agent. Because it is anionic it is usually incompatible with cationic drugs. Solutions are usually pseudoplastic but certain grades exhibit thixotropy. Hydroxypropyl cellulose is soluble in both water and alcohol. This agent is pseudoplastic at high shear and has been used as a protective colloid. Water-soluble cellulose derivatives are all subject to microbial degradation and require preservatives.

2. Clays

The second class of suspending agents in Table 3 is the clays. They are hydrated aluminum and/or magnesium silicates, which in water hydrate further to from viscous colloidal dispersions. They exhibit thixotropy and are very useful for stabilizing suspensions. These agents should be dispersed in water with high shear for optimum dispersion and hydration. Clays are most stable between pH 9 and 11 but can be used within a broader pH range. Ethanol and electrolytes may reduce the viscosity of these agents.

Magnesium aluminum silicate is used extensively. Its innocuous taste often produces a more acceptable suspension than other suspending agents. Bentonite is recognized for its swelling ability. Equal concentrations of bentonite and sodium carboxymethylcellulose for a total of 5% produce a good structure vehicle with both pseudoplastic and thixotropic behavior [27]. Hectorite possesses greater swelling ability than bentonite, but its disadvantage is cost and supply. Attapulgite, bentonite, and magnesium aluminum silicate in concentrations of 0.1% to 1% have been used as flocculating agents to aid the suspension of many drugs in a sorbitol or syrup base [18].

Silicon dioxide and its hydrate, silica gel, are considered in this section because their colloidal nature is similar to that of clays. Like the clays, these agents are water insoluble. At sufficient concentrations their dispersions gel and exhibit thixotropy. These agents are usually employed in combination with other suspending agents. For example, colloidal silicon dioxide, used alone at a concentration of 1%, was reported to be an unsatisfactory suspending agent for chalk and sulfamethazine [59].

3. Natural Gums

The natural gums are common suspending agents. This group, listed in Table 3, includes those of tree exudate, seed or root, and seaweed origin. These agents are nontoxic, readily available, and inexpensive. They are water soluble and produce solutions of high viscosity. Most are anionic and therefore are incompatible with cationic ingredients. These agents, however, are susceptible to bacterial and mold growth. In the past, many imported tree gums and seed pods were so heavily contaminated that they overwhelmed any added preservative [69]; this problem does not usually occur today. Another disadvantage is batch variation in color, viscosity, gel strength, and hydration rate. Because of these disadvantages and the anionic charge of natural gums, other agents such as the cellulose derivatives are often preferred.

Acacia, tragacanth, and pectin have been employed as suspending agents for many years. Tragacanth solutions are very viscous and have been employed to suspend dense particles. Several different viscosity grades are available. Pectin solutions have low viscosity; use of this agent is decreasing. Guar gum and locust bean (or carob) gum are nonionic. Guar gum is recognized as producing solutions of very high viscosity; locust bean gum is infrequently used because of its limited water-thickening and swelling properties at room temperatures. Tamarind gum, or specifically tamarind seed polysaccharide, is seldom used in the pharmaceutical industry although it is nonionic, disperses readily in cold water, and forms viscous solutions at concentrations less than 2%. This agent is relatively unaffected by the pH of the solution.

Agar, the alginates, and carrageenan are seaweed extracts. Agar is resistant to microbial growth and produces strong gels. It has been used to suspend barium sulfate. The alginates form solutions of high viscosity. They exhibit Newtonian flow at concentrations below those listed in Table 3. The propylene glycol form is used at low pH values and is available in a grade for dispersal by vigorous hand shaking. Carrageenans are water soluble and anionic. The commercially available types are kappa, iota, and lambda. The kappa and iota types form gels; gels from the latter type are thixotropic. Lambda carrageenan does not gel.

Use of xanthan gum is increasing for several reasons. It is a high molecular weight natural polysaccharide produced from microbial fermentation by an organism originally isolated from the rutabaga plant [83]. It has good batch-to-batch uniformity, few microbial contamination problems because it is unusually resistant to enzymes, and it is soluble in both hot and cold water. Xanthan gum is particularly useful as a suspending agent because of its shear-thinning or pseudoplastic behavior and because it has a yield value (the combination being plastic behavior). The apparent yield value of a 1% solution was reported as 20 to 50 dyne/cm^2 [83]. At low rates of shear, but high enough to exceed the yield value, the solution has a high viscosity. At high shear rates, such as mixing or pumping, the solution has a low viscosity. Another very useful property of xantham gum is that its solution viscosity is almost independent of temperature and pH. In addition, it is usually more resistant to degradation or fracture from prolonged shearing than other polymeric suspending agents. For example, a 1% solution was sheared at 46,000 sec^{-1}, which is comparable to that encountered in a colloid mill, and no viscosity loss was reported after 1 hour [83].

4. *Synthetic Gums*

The synthetic agents have the advantage of good batch-to-batch uniformity and no microbial contamination. Carbomer is widely used because its solutions have a very high viscosity and a yield value. At concentrations above 0.4% it forms gels. Povidone, which is polyvinylpyrrolidone, should be used with other suspending agents because it has a low solution viscosity. It is used more often as a protective colloid.

5. *Miscellaneous*

The starches are not widely used but were evaluated as comparable or better than several other suspending agents, including alginates, tragacanth, and magnesium aluminum silicate [59]. Glycyrrhizin is reported to have good suspending characteristics [89]. Its solution is pseudoplastic and exhibits thixotropy. Gelatin may be anionic or cationic, depending on the pH of the medium and the type of gelatin. Interactions between this agent and drugs have been investigated [91]. Under appropriate conditions, this agent is compatible with most ingredients. It has a disadvantage in that it lacks good batch-to-batch uniformity.

C. Flocculating Agents

Flocculating agents enable particles to link together in loose aggregates or flocs. As described previously, these flocs settle rapidly but are easily redispersed. These agents can be divided into four classes: surfactants, hydrophilic polymers, clays, and electrolytes. Typical agents are listed in Table 4.

Both ionic and nonionic surfactants have been used as flocculating agents. Concentrations employed range from 0.001% to as high as 1.0% (w/v). Nonionic surfactants are preferred because they are chemically compatible with more ingredients. The flocculating agent may be the same material as the wetting agent. Excess concentrations may produce a bad taste, foaming, or caking.

Hydrophilic polymers have wide use as flocculating agents. These substances have a high molecular weight with long carbon chains and include many materials that at higher concentrations (> 0.1%) are employed as suspending agents. Xanthum gum has been used to flocculate sulfaguanidine, bismuth subcarbonate, and other drugs [92,93]. Hydrophilic polymers may act both as protective colloids to prevent caking and as flocculating agents to form loose flocs. The use of surfactants alone or in combination with a protective colloid in conjunction with a structured suspending vehicle is reported as a common and successful method of flocculation [61]. Bentonite, at 1.7%, produces very good flocculation of bismuth subnitrate suspensions [36]. Clays at concentration equal to or above 0.1% are reported to successfully flocculate most drugs suspended in a sorbitol or syrup base [18].

The presence of electrolytes can enhance flocculation and lower the necessary surfactant concentration. For example, sulfamerazine suspensions were flocculated with sodium dodecyl polyoxyethylene sulfate. Addition of the appropriate amount of sodium

Table 4 Typical Flocculating Agents

Agent	Class	Ionic charge
Sodium lauryl sulfate	Surfactant	Anionic
Docusate sodium		Anionic
Benzalkonium chloride		Cationic
Cetylpyridinium chloride		Cationic
Polysorbate 80		Nonionic
Sorbitan monolaurate		Nonionic
Carboxymethylcellulose sodium	Hydrophilic polymer	Anionic
Xanthan gum		Anionic
Tragacanth		Anionic
Methylcellulose		Nonionic
Polyethylene glycol		Nonionic
Magnesium aluminum silicate	Clay	Anionic
Attapulgite		Anionic
Bentonite		Anionic
Potassium dihydrogen phosphate	Electrolyte	Anionic
Aluminum chloride		Cationic
Sodium chloride		Anionic/cationic

chloride increased flocculation and reduced the required surfactant concentration [94]. An electrolyte may be the sole flocculating agent. Sulfaguanidine, wetted by a suitable surfactant, was flocculated by aluminum chloride [95]. Electrolytes as flocculating agents are apparently not routinely utilized in the industry, yet offer a means of attaining optimum flocculation.

D. Wetting Agents

Surfactants, hydrophilic polymers, and certain clays are used as wetting agents to aid in the dispersion of hydrophobic drugs. The USP 23 [96] includes 24 surfactants as official wetting and/or solubilizing agents. Sodium carboxymethylcellulose, bentonite, aluminum magnesium silicate, and colloidal silicon dioxide are also reported to aid dispersion of hydrophobic drugs. Glycerin, propylene glycol, and alcohol are widely employed. Concentrations of alcohol used as a wetting agent include 0.008%, 0.1%, and 0.26%.

The formulator selects the wetting agent for optimum dispersion of the drug at the lowest effective concentration. The agent selected will vary depending on its ability to wet the surface of the drug. The Hiestand [34] method of selecting a wetting agent provides a comparison of their wetting ability. A narrow hydrophobic trough holds the powder at one end while a solution of the wetting agent is placed at the other end. The better agents will have a faster rate of penetration through the powder. Another test evaluates the wetting ability by dripping a solution of the wetting agent onto the drug powder spread over a piece of gauze. The better wetting agents carry more powder through the gauze than the poorer agents.

E. Sweeteners

Frequently sweeteners are included in suspensions to produce a more palatable medication. Drugs may have a bitter taste, and suspending agents, particularly clays, may have a bland taste. A viscous sweetener, such as sorbitol solution, or syrup (sucrose) also can be used to impart viscosity to retard sedimentation. High-fructose corn syrup has also been used for this dual purpose. Other common sweetening agents include mannitol, sodium saccharin, and aspartame. Aspartame is used extensively at low concentrations because of its high potency.

F. Additional Ingredients

Table 5 contains some typical buffers, flavoring agents, colorants, and preservatives. Buffers are used to control the pH of the formulation. Suspension pH is often adjusted to ensure that the drug remains insoluble. If too much drug is in solution the drug may recrystallize and alter the particle size, shape, and distribution. The tendency of particles to fuse together is also increased. In addition, the poor taste of a drug in solution may be amplified.

The optimum pH for each ingredient may not coincide. The pH may be selected on the basis of solubility or stability of the drug. The polymeric suspending agents, however, have the greatest viscosity at the pH of their maximum solubility. The suspending agent should be stable at the pH of the system for the shelf life of the product. Certain preservatives, such as sodium benzoate, are effective only at low pH values in which the molecule is predominately un-ionized.

Table 5 Typical Buffering Agents, Flavors, Colorants, and Preservatives Used in Suspensions

Agent	Class
Ammonia solution, strong	Buffering
Citric acid	
Fumaric acid	
Sodium citrate	
Cherry	Flavor
Grape	
Methyl salicylate	
Orange	
Peppermint	
D&C Red No. 33	Colorant
FD&C Red No. 3	
FD&C Red No. 40	
D&C Yellow No. 10	
FD&C Yellow No. 6	
Butylparaben	Preservative
Methylparaben	
Propylparaben	
Sodium benzoate	

Flavoring agents also enhance patient acceptance of the product; they are a necessity in suspensions intended for pediatric patients. Some prevalent flavors used in formulations intended for children include raspberry, pineapple, and bubble gum. To maintain full effectiveness of the flavoring agent in some commercial suspensions, the manufacturer recommends that the product be stored at refrigerator temperatures. In such cases, the formulator must consider both the positive and adverse consequences of the increased viscosity caused by the temperature reduction. Flavoring agents are usually oils and require solvents.

Colorants are intended to provide a more aesthetic appearance to the final suspension. As relatively large cations or anions, these agents may be chemically incompatible with other ingredients. For example, anionic D&C Yellow No. 10 interacts with quaternary ammonium compounds such as surfactants. Some colorants have been implicated as a potential source of cancer, and the formulator must realize that a selected agent, in the future, may be banned by the Food and Drug Administration. FD & C Yellow No. 5 is a noted allergen, and its presence must be listed on the label.

Preservatives are required in most suspensions because the suspending agents and sweeteners are often good growth media for microorganisms. Some natural gums are sources of contamination, and the preservative must be effective against these contaminating organisms. Clays are susceptible to mold growth. In some suspensions the drug imparts a pH at which no preservative is stable. An example is magnesium hydroxide suspension. Antimicrobial surfactants, such as cetylpyridinium chloride, must be used with caution because of their potential incompatibilities.

The parabens are frequently employed as preservatives. These agents may require small concentrations of a solvent to remain in solution. Alcohol, glycerin, or propylene glycol are often used as these solvents at concentrations $\leq 10\%$. These solvents can also be used for other water-insoluble ingredients such as flavors. Other, less common, excipients include a sequestering, or chelating, agent, such as edetate disodium, an antifoaming agent such as simethicone, or bitterness modifiers such as sodium chloride.

V. PREPARATION OF SUSPENSIONS

A. General Guidelines

There are three general approaches to the formulation of suspensions, as illustrated in Fig. 3. All three have the common preliminary step of dispersing the wetted particles in the medium to achieve a uniform dispersion of deflocculated particles. The approach labeled A in Fig. 3 is to suspend the deflocculated particles in a viscosity-enhancing agent or a structured vehicle. This approach produces individual particles that settle slowly but are seldom completely suspended.

The second approach, labeled B in Fig. 3, incorporates a flocculating agent to produce a flocculated suspension as the final product. In practice, this approach is not commonly used because the flocs settle rapidly leaving a clear supernatant. Usually a suspending agent, with properties of a structured vehicle, is added to the flocculated suspension. The flocculated particles are suspended better than deflocculated particles in a structured vehicle, often yielding no noticeable separation. Upon shaking, the high shear thins the vehicle, and the suspension is easily poured from the container. After use, the vehicle regains its structure, producing a high viscosity to retard, if not prevent, sedimentation of the flocculated particle. The approach of combining flocculated particles and structured vehicle is labeled C in Fig. 3.

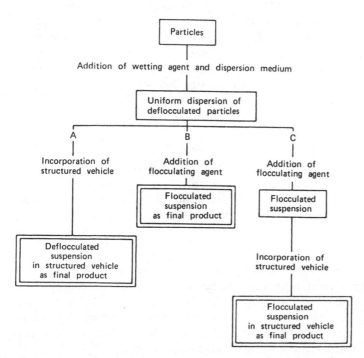

Fig. 3 General guidelines to suspension formulation. (From Ref. 35.)

B. Specific Guidelines

Each procedure requires some trial and error. The following guidelines have been recommended [20].

1. Disperse the drug by slow addition to a water, water-glycol, or glycol system containing the wetting agent. Addition of wetting system to the powder requires prolonged levigation and is more difficult on a large scale.

2. Add all other excipients that require solution in as dilute a system as possible. Concentrated solutions can cause reactions or precipitation on the liquid surface of the bulk phase.

3. Ensure that the solvent system maintains ingredients in solution. Precipitation can occur if the bulk vehicle cannot dissolve the solute.

4. Provide sufficient water for ease of dispersion and hydration of suspending agent(s) and protective colloids.

5. If the suspension is to contain more than one drug, ascertain mutual compatibility.

6. Use sufficient drug excess to compensate for loss during manufacture and to maintain the labeled amount during the shelf life of the product.

7. Flavors (as oils) can be added to most suspension vehicles if the final batch is processed through a colloid mill.

8. Process the batch through a colloid mill to ensure dispersion of the drug. The mill will break up large soft agglomerates.

9. Process the batch through deaerating equipment. Suspensions may contain large quantities of air from the surface of the drug particles or from incorporation during milling and mixing. These suspensions are unsatisfactory.

10. Avoid excessive water loss, particularly if prolonged heating is required. Use an excess of water to compensate for a significant loss.

11. Avoid excessive shearing and high temperatures, which can degrade colloids.

12. Consider the percentages of un-ionized preservatives at various pH values.

13. Follow Good Manufacturing Practices as published by the FDA and described in Chapter 12, "Drug Regulatory Affairs," in Volume 3 of *Disperse Systems*.

VI. STABILITY

Determining the stability of a suspension entails evaluation of the complete product. The batch should be evaluated in the final package. More than one batch should be evaluated to compare different lots of drug and other ingredients to the criteria established with the first batch. The product should be evaluated after manufacture, after storage at all test temperatures, and after all conditions of stress testing.

A. Chemical Stability

The drug within suspended particles is not likely to undergo chemical degradation; only the small but finite fraction of drug in solution is susceptible to degradation. A method of determining the stability of drugs in suspension has been reported [97]. The method is based on three assumptions which are: (a) degradation takes place only in solution and is first order, (b) the effect of temperature on drug solubility conforms to classical theory, and (c) dissolution is not rate limiting on degradation.

Suspending agents are also subject to degradation with age. The functional parameter, viscosity, can be examined at elevated temperatures to determine aging characteristics [98]. The viscosity change for sodium alginate followed first-order degradation. Concentration of the agent had a negligible influence on the stability. An increase in concentration of sodium carboxymethylcellulose, however, produced a decrease in the rate of viscosity change.

The antimicrobial activity can be reduced by chemical degradation or incompatibility of the preservative. If an unexpected pH change occurs, the effectiveness of the preservative may be reduced substantially. A loss of activity may also occur from adsorption of the preservative onto the drug particle [99].

B. Physical Stability

Several physical tests are employed to evaluate physical ability of suspensions. Tables 6 and 7 list these tests, which are divided into passive and active types [20]. The most common tests are evaluations of sedimentation by sedimentation volume and degree of flocculation [100]. Flocculation and deflocculation of suspension particles can be evaluated by rate of filtration [101], rate of settling, and the filtration of suspension and refiltration of filtrate through the formed filter bed [102].

Not all tests listed in Tables 6 and 7 are required to evaluate suspension stability. Fewer tests than these, as well as additional tests, have been used. The stability of suspensions containing primidone and prednisone was well characterized by the following common tests: turbidity measurements, viscosity measurements, sedimentation volumes, and redispersibility of sediments [103].

Stability testing of suspensions is a difficult problem faced by formulators. There are no standardized tests available to determine stability and shelf life. Evaluation of suspension physical stability is an area of ongoing research. For example, the effects of surface charge on dye adsorption and suspension stability were examined in a titanium dioxide aqueous suspension. Both suspension stability and dye adsorption were dependent on the pH of the suspension and the point of zero charge (PZC) of the suspended titanium dioxide [104]. Another example is the evaluation of a spreading coefficient parameter as a method of predicting the aggregation of powders dispersed in

Table 6 Passive Tests for Evaluation of Physical Stability of Suspensions

1. Aesthetic appeal (appearance, color, odor, taste)
2. pH
3. Specific gravity
4. Sedimentation rate
5. Sedimentation volume
6. Zeta potential measurement
7. Compatibility with container
8. Compatibility with cap-liner
9. Microscopic examination (photomicrographs)
10. Determine crystal size
11. Determine uniform drug distribution

Source: Adapted from Ref. 20.

Table 7 Active Tests for Evaluation of Physical
Stability of Suspensions

1. Redispersibility
2. Centrifuge
3. Rheological measurements
4. Stress tests (vibration to simulate transportation)
5. Accelerated shock cycles
6. Freeze–thaw cycles
7. Use tests

Source: Adapted from Ref. 20.

aqueous suspensions [105]. The remainder of this section on stability concerns strategies for the evaluation of suspensions. For additional information see the excellent review by Weiner [106].

It should be clear what type of stability is under investigation because not all formulations use the same system of stabilization. The factors affecting rate of settling, flocculation, and caking are different. Different types of instabilities require different testing procedures and will result in different degrees of reliability for determining a shelf life.

Protocols for stability testing should consider special properties of the product that may be troublesome as well as special conditions the product may encounter. If controlled flocculation is the strategy used to stabilize a suspension, it must be made certain that the energy barrier (which stabilizes the product) will protect the product from destabilizing factors such as vibration caused by shipping. Therefore, a reciprocating shaker is useful to test this type of product.

Accelerated stability testing is difficult and risky. Testing at elevated temperatures ($>25°C$) is often used but the higher temperatures cause large changes in physical properties of the so-called inactive ingredients. Irreversible changes may occur from the precipitation or breakdown of polymers in the dispersion that can substantially alter viscosity. Higher temperatures will dramatically change the solubility of the suspended drug. During cycling from hot to cold temperatures, the saturated layer around the suspended particles will change, resulting in a greater tendency for aggregation of particles, particularly in suspensions that do not have a uniform particle size [106]. Higher temperatures will also affect the hydration of polymer additives, which affects the ability of the polymer to stabilize the suspension.

VII. TYPICAL FORMULAS

Examples of formulations that illustrate systems of suspensions are described in this section. The systems range from those with no suspending agents to those with combinations of agents. The objective of the suspending agents may vary. Ease of redispersal and good flow properties are the goals of some formulations such as the antacid-demulcent suspension in part F. The absence of sedimentation is the goal of other formulations such as the sulfamethazine suspension in part D.

A. Drug Particles from Precipitation Reaction

1. *Milk of Magnesia, USP*

This simple formulation illustrates a precipitation reaction to produce the drug in a colloidal size range and the subsequent preparation of the suspension. The reaction between a magnesium salt and sodium hydroxide yields magnesium hydroxide as a colloidal precipitate. The ingredients for this reaction and the preparation of the suspension [107] follow.

Magnesium sulfate	300 g
Sodium hydroxide	100 g
Distilled water, qs	1000 mL

The magnesium salt is dissolved in about 650 mL of distilled water in a large container and heated to boiling. The sodium hydroxide is dissolved in 1000 mL of distilled water and added slowly to the boiling solution of magnesium sulfate; continue the boiling for 30 minutes. Transfer the mixture to a cylindrical container of not less than 5000 mL and fill with hot distilled water. Allow the mixture to stand until a separation occurs and remove the supernatant liquid. Wash repeatedly with hot distilled water until sulfates have practically been eliminated, as indicated by testing the supernatant liquid with barium chloride T.S. Concentrate the mixture by evaporation until it contains not less than 7% magnesium hydroxide [107].

Current preparations usually employ a suspending agent because caking has been known to occur. A nonionic suspending agent, such as methylcellulose, could be used. A flavoring oil or blend of oils is often used but the amount is limited to 0.5 mL for each 1000 mL of product. The addition of 0.1% of citric acid reduces the interaction between the magnesium hydroxide and the glass. If a plastic container is used, then citric acid is not required. An opaque container is preferred so that the sediment is not visible. A preservative should be used.

B. Viscous Sweetener as Suspending Agent

1. *Antacid Aluminum Hydroxide*

A viscous solution of the sweetener such as syrup or sorbitol solution may supply sufficient viscosity to suspend the drug. The following formula employs syrup and sorbitol solution for both sweetness and viscosity [108]. The preservatives are methylparaben and propylparaben.

Aluminum hydroxide compressed gel	362.8 g
Sorbitol solution, USP	282.0 mL
Syrup, NF	93.0 mL
Glycerin, USP	25.0 mL
Methylparaben, NF	0.9 g
Propylparaben, NF	0.3 g
Flavor	qs
Purified water, USP to	1000.0 mL

The parabens are dissolved in a heated mixture of the sorbitol solution, glycerin, syrup and a part of the water. The mixture is cooled and the aluminum hydroxide is added with stirring. The flavor is added followed by sufficient purified water to volume. A hand homogenizer, homomixer, or colloid mill is then used to homogenize the suspension.

The preparation of aluminum hydroxide compressed gel can be divided into two parts. The first part is the preparation of the aluminum hydroxide gel. The gel is then dried, or compressed, at a low temperature until it has the required amount of Al_2O_3. One process for the preparation of aluminum hydroxide gel follows. Dissolve 1000 g of $Na_2CO_3 \cdot 10H_2O$ in 400 mL of hot water and filter. Dissolve 800 g of ammonium alum in 2000 mL of hot water and filter into the carbonate solution with constant stirring. Then add 4000 mL of hot water and remove all gas. Dilute to 80,000 mL with cold water. Collect and wash the precipitate and suspend it in 2000 mL of purified water flavored with 0.01% peppermint oil and preserve with 0.1% of sodium benzoate. Homogenize the resulting gel [109].

C. Viscosity from Active Ingredients

1. *Kaolin Mixture with Pectin*

Kaolin and pectin, the active ingredients, provide some viscosity of the system. Glycerin is the wetting agent. Sodium saccharin is the sweetener, peppermint oil is for flavor. The preservative is benzoic acid. The formula follows.

Kaolin	200 g
Pectin	10 g
Tragacanth	5 g
Sodium saccharin	1 g
Glycerin	20 mL
Benzoic acid	2 g
Peppermint oil	0.75 mL
Purified water, qs	1000 mL

Mix kaolin with 500 mL of the purified water. Triturate pectin, powdered tragacanth, and sodium saccharin with glycerin. Add to this mixture, with constant stirring, benzoic acid dissolved in 300 mL of boiling purified water. Continue mixing until all the pectin is dissolved and allow the mixture to stand until it cools to room temperature. Add peppermint oil and the kaolin-water mixture, thoroughly mix, and finally add sufficient purified water to make 1000 mL. The quantity of tragacanth and pectin may be altered in order to obtain a product with suitable consistency in the preparation of larger amounts. If, however, the proportion of pectin in the formula is altered by more than 10%, then the pectin content of the preparation must be clearly stated on the label [109].

D. Plastic Suspending Agent

1. *Sulfamethazine suspension*

Carbomer 934 is used in this formula as the suspending agent to produce good suspensions with practically no sedimentation [84]. The wetting agent is sodium lauryl sulfate. The sweeteners are sodium saccharin and sugar (sucrose). Citric acid and sodium hydroxide are used to control pH. The preservatives are the sodium salts of methyl and propylparaben, which are not listed in the USP. Substitution with methyl and propylparaben at the same concentrations may be acceptable.

Sulfamethazine	10.00 g
Carbomer 934	0.50 g
Sodium lauryl sulfate	0.02 g
Sodium saccharin	0.08 g
Sugar (sucrose, granular)	40.00 g
Methyl sodium hydroxy benzoate	0.20 g
Propyl sodium hydroxy benzoate	0.02 g
Flavor mixture	1.00 g
Citric acid	0.20 g
1.0 N sodium hydroxide solution to pH 5.5	(approx. 10 mL)
Purified water, qs	100.00 mL

The flavor mixture consists of vanilla 1.00 mL, caramel 3.00 mL, and glycerin 100.00 g. Carbomer 934 is hydrated for 24 hours in a solution of the sodium lauryl sulfate in 30 mL of water. The sulfamethazine powder is suspended in the vehicle and the aid of a mixer. The preservatives and sugar are dissolved in the remaining 40 mL of water by heating. After the solution has cooled to room temperature, the sodium saccharin and citric acid are added to the cooled solution. The solution is then added to the suspension, the flavor mixture added, the pH adjusted to 5.5, and the final suspension mixed in a homogenizer.

E. Pseudoplastic Suspending Agents

Two formulas in this section illustrate the use of different pseudoplastic suspending agent. Methylcellulose is used in the first formula and sodium carboxymethylcellulose is used in the second formula.

1. *Kaolin-Pectin Suspension*

This formula has a slightly lower solids concentration than the similar formula in part C, and uses methylcellulose 4000 cps as the suspending agent [110].

Kaolin	20.00%
Pectin	0.50%
Methylcellulose 4000 cps	0.75%
Methylparaben	0.20%
Propylparaben	0.04%
Butterscotch imitation flavor	0.01%
Vanillin	0.01%
Sorbitol solution USP	20.00%
Distilled water, qs	100.00%

Minor modifications in procedure were tested without the butterscotch imitation flavor in three preparations of 100 g [111]. The differences between these preparations are not large but the suspension prepared by the third procedure was considered the most elegant.

Mix the kaolin with half the water. In another container, disperse the pectin in the remaining half of the water and heat to near boiling. To this hot solution of pectin, add the parabens and disperse the methylcellulose while mixing. Allow the methylcellulose mixture to hydrate and cool for 4 hours followed by 5 minute's exposure to ice bath temperatures. To this solution, add the kaolin-water mixture, sorbitol solution, and flavors using an electrical mixer to complete the preparation. After 7 days standing, the suspension was a thixotropic gel with a yield value but no supernatant.

The second procedure eliminates the exposure of the methylcellulose to cold temperature but extends the hydration time to overnight. An additional minor change is to mix the pectin in water for 1 hour with a magnetic stirrer prior to heating. After 7 days, the sediment of this suspension appeared clumpy, represented approximately 93% of total suspension volume, and did not flow upon inversion (indicating a yield value).

The third procedure eliminated both the cold temperatures and overnight hydration. The methylcellulose mixture was hydrated for only 4 hours. After 7 days, the sediment flowed smoothly and represented approximately 93% of total volume.

Ease of redispersal of the three suspensions after seven days decreased from procedure 3 > procedure 2 > procedure 1. After 30 days, the suspension prepared by the third procedure exhibited a sediment volume of 99% and could be poured, although slowly. The order of redispersability did not change and the remaining two preparations did not flow upon inversion. Because viscosity was somewhat high the formulator may wish to reduce the concentration of methylcellulose.

2. *Antacid Suspension*

The suspending agent used in this formula [110] is low-viscosity, pharmaceutical grade, sodium carboxymethylcellulose.

Aluminum hydroxide	4.00%
Magnesium hydroxide	4.00%
Sodium carboxymethylcellulose, 7LP	1.00%
Methylparaben	0.20%
Propylparaben	0.04%
Saccharin calcium	0.02%
Peppermint oil	0.01%
Distilled water, qs	100.00%

Hydrate the suspending agent in some hot water and allow it to stand overnight. The hydroxides are mixed in some water to which the saccharin and the parabens, as a propylene glycol solution, are added. The slurry is added to the solution of NaCMC with mixing. Add the flavor and the remaining water. Homogenize the suspension by passing it through a colloid mill.

F. Combination of Pseudoplastic and Thixotropic Agents

In many cases, these combinations produce suspensions with more stability, better flow properties, and equal redispersion capacity to suspensions using either agent alone.

1. *Sulfamethazine Suspension*

The formula in part D is modified to use the combination of sodium carboxymethylcellulose and magnesium aluminum silicate as the suspending agents [84]. The viscosity of a 2% solution of the cellulose derivative was reported as 72 cp. The suspension is prepared in the same manner as described in part D except that the pH is not adjusted; the final pH of the suspension is 7.4. In addition, the preservatives, as described in part D, may be replaced with methyl- and propylparaben.

Sulfamethazine	10.00 g
Magnesium aluminum silicate	0.60 g
Sodium carboxymethylcellulose	1.30 g
Sodium lauryl sulfate	0.02 g
Sodium saccharin	0.08 g
Sugar (sucrose, granular)	40.00 g
Sodium methyl hydroxy benzoate	0.20 g
Sodium propyl hydroxy benzoate	0.02 g
Flavor mixture	1.00 g
Purified water, qs	100.00 g

2. *Antacid-Demulcent Suspension*

Caking is a major problem in suspensions containing a high concentration of solids. Suitable redispersion and flow properties are attained with different concentrations of the suspending agents illustrated above [110]. A medium-viscosity type of the cellulose derivative is used.

Aluminum hydroxide	4.00%
Magnesium trisilicate	12.00%
Magnesium aluminum silicate	0.80%
Sodium carboxymethylcellulose, 7MP	0.60%
Methylparaben	0.20%
Propylparaben	0.04%
Peppermint oil	0.01%
Sorbitol solution, USP	20.00%
Distilled water, qs	100.00%

Hydrate the magnesium aluminum silicate and the sodium carboxymethylcellulose in some hot water and allow them to stand overnight. The hydroxide is mixed in some water; the sorbitol and parabens are added. The slurry is pumped into the gelled suspending agents and mixed. The trisilicate is added slowly with vigorous agitation and mixed until it is well dispersed. The flavor is added with agitation and the suspension brought to full volume. Pass the suspension through a colloid mill into a tank fitted with a strainer.

Combinations of similar agents are used in other successful formulations. Examples include magnesium aluminum silicate and sodium alginate in a griseofulvin suspension [112] and bentonite and carboxymethylcellulose in a sulfamethoxazole/trimethoprim suspension [113]. The exact ratio of suspending agents will vary with processing conditions and selection of other ingredients.

REFERENCES

1. M. Gibaldi, *Introduction to Biopharmaceutics*, Lea & Febiger, Philadelphia, 1971, p. 37.
2. L. N. Sansom, W. J. O'Reilly, C. W. Wiseman, L. Stern, and J. Derham, *Med. J. Aust.*, 2:593–595 (1975).
3. R. Obach, J. Prunonosa, A. Menargues, M. Nomen, and J. Valles, *Biopharm. Drug Dispos.*, 9:501–511 (1988).
4. F. Kees, U. Lukassek, K. G. Naber, and H. Grobecker, *Arzneim. Forsch.*, 41:843–846 (1991).

5. R. Shekerdjiiski, V. Paskov, N. Lambov, P. Gencheva, D. Rachev, S. Titeva, and E. Minkov, *Pharmazie* 42:184–186 (1987).

6. J. A. Barone, Y. C. Huang, R. H. Bierman, J. L. Colaizzi, J. F. Long, D. A. Ker, A. Van Peer, R. Woestenborghs, and J. Heykants, *Clin. Pharm.* 6:640–645 (1987).

7. F. Pannuti, E. Strocchi, A. Longhi, R. Comparsi, and C. M. Camaggi, *Chemioterapia*, 5:237–239 (1987).

8. J. D. Strum, J. L. Colaizzi, T. S. Goehl, J. M. Jaffe, and R. I. Poust, *J. Pharm. Sci.*, 67:1399–1402 (1978).

9. N. Kondo, T. Iwao, H. Masuda, K. Yamanouchi, Y. Ishihara, N. Yamada, T. Haga, Y. Ogawa, and K. Yokoyama, *Chem. Pharm. Bull.*, 41:737–740 (1993).

10. A. Stockis, E. Lebacq, S. Deroubaix, A. M. Allemon, and H. Laufen, *Arzneim Forsch.*, 42:1478–1481 (1992).

11. F. Kees, K. G. Naber, G. Sigl, W. Ungethum, and H. Grobecker, *Arzneim. Forsch.*, 40:293–297 (1990).

12. M. M. Soci and E. L. Parrott, *J. Pharm. Sci.*, 69:403–406 (1980).

13. M. Marvola, J. Pirjola, and A. Huikari, *Int. J. Pharm.*, 3:13–22 (1979).

14. H. A. Titulaer, J. Zuidema, P. A. Kager, J. C. Wetsteyn, C. B. Lugt, and F. W. Merkus, *J. Pharm. Pharmacol.*, 42:810–813 (1990).

15. B. A. Haines and A. N. Martin, *J. Pharm. Sci.*, 50:228–232 (1961).

16. B. A. Haines and A. N. Martin, *J. Pharm. Sci.*, 50:753–756 (1961).

17. B. A. Haines and A. N. Martin, *J. Pharm. Sci.*, 50:756–759 (1961).

18. R. A. Nash, *Drug Cosmet. Ind.*, 97:843–951 (1965).

19. R. A. Nash, Drug and Cosmetic Ind., 98:39–43, 128–133 (1966).

20. B. I. Idson and A. J. Scheer, Suspensions. In: *Problem Solver* (J. Wallace, ed.), FMC Corporation, 1984, pp. 1–31.

21. H. Schott and A. N. Martin, Colloidal and surface-chemical aspects of dosage forms. In: *American Pharmacy* (L. W. Dittert, ed.), Lippincott, Philadelphia, 1974, pp. 103–174.

22. J. T. Carstenson and K. S. E. Su, *J. Pharm. Sci.*, 59:666–670 (1970).

23. P. C. Hiemenz, *Principles of Colloid and Surface Chemistry*, Marcel Dekker, New York, 1986, pp. 193–200.

24. R. J. Meyer and L. Cohen, *J. Soc. Cosmet. Chem.* 10:143–154 (1959).

25. S. L. Hem, J. R. Feldkamp, and J. L. White, Basic chemical principles related to emulsion and suspension dosage forms. In: *Theory and Practice of Industrial Pharmacy* (L. Lachman, H. A. Lieberman, J. L. Kanig, eds.), Lea & Febiger, Philadelphia, 1986, pp. 140–143.

26. E. N. Hiestand, *J. Pharm. Sci.*, 53:1–18 (1964).

27. H. Schott, Rheology. In: *Remington: The Science and Practice of Pharmacy* (A. R. Gennaro, ed.), Mack, Easton, PA, 1995, pp. 292–311.

28. A. Martin, *Physical Pharmacy*, Lea & Febiger, Philadelphia, 1993, pp. 453–476.

29. A. Martin, *Physical Pharmacy*, Lea & Febiger, Philadelphia, 1993, p. 384.

30. J. Y. Oldshue, *Pharm. Sci.*, 50:523–530 (1961).

31. R. J. Lantz and J. B. Schwartz, Mixing. In: *Pharmaceutical Dosage Forms: Tablets*, Vol. 2 (H. A. Lieberman, L. Lachman, J. B. Schwartz, eds.), Marcel Dekker, New York, 1990, pp. 1–70.

32. E. G. Rippie, Mixing. In: *The Theory and Practice of Industrial Pharmacy* (L. Lachman, H. A. Lieberman, J. L. Kanig, eds.), Lea & Febiger, Philadelphia, 1986, pp. 3–20.

33. A. Martin, *J. Pharm. Sci.*, 50:513–517 (1961).

34. E. N. Hiestand, *J. Pharm. Sci.*, 61:268–272 (1972).

35. W. Higuchi, J. Swarbrick, N. Ho, A. Simonelli, A. Martin, Particle phenomena and coarse dispersions. In: *Remington's Pharmaceutical Sciences* (A. R. Gennaro, ed.), Mack, Easton, PA, 1985, pp. 311–317.

36. H. Schott, *J. Pharm. Sci.*, 65:855–861 (1976).
37. H. Schott, Colloidal dispersions. In: *Remington: The Science and Practice of Pharmacy* (A. R. Gennaro, ed.), Mack, Easton, PA, 1995, pp. 261–269.
38. W. Higuchi, J. Swarbrick, N. Ho, A. Simonelli, A. Martin, Particle phenomena and coarse dispersions. In: *Remington's Pharmaceutical Sciences* (A. R. Gennaro, ed.), Mack, Easton, PA, 1985, pp 308–311.
39. K. J. Mysels, *Introduction to Colloid Chemistry*, Wiley-Interscience, New York, 1959.
40. P. C. Hiemenz, *Principles of Colloid and Surface Chemistry*, Marcel Dekker, New York, 1986, pp. 611–731.
41. B. A. Mathews and C. T. Rhodes, *J. Pharm. Sci.*, 59:521–525 (1970).
42. A. J. Scheer, *Drug Cosmet. Ind.*, 128:40–44 (1981).
43. R. J. Lantz, Size reduction. In: *Pharmaceutical Dosage Forms: Tablets,* Vol. 2 (H. A. Lieberman, L. Lachman, J. B. Schwartz, ed.), Marcel Dekker, New York, 1990, pp. 107–200.
44. E. L. Parrott, Milling. In: *The Theory and Practice of Industrial Pharmacy* (L. Lachman, H. A. Lieberman, J. L. Kanig, eds.), Lea & Febiger, Philadelphia, 1986, pp. 21–46.
45. K. N. Patel, L. Kennon, and S. R. Levinson, Pharmaceutical suspensions. In: *The Theory and Practice of Industrial Pharmacy* (L. Lachman, H. A. Lieberman, J. L. Kanig, eds.), Lea & Febiger, Philadelphia, 1986, p. 487.
46. S. Banerjee, A. Bandyopadyay, R. C. Bhatttacharjee, A. K. Mukherjee, and A. K. Halder, *J. Pharm. Sci.*, 60:153–155 (1971).
47. A. Heyd and D. Dhabhar, *Drug Cosmet. Ind.*, 125:42–45, 146 (1979).
48. C. M. G. Macie and A. J. W. Grant, *Pharm. Int.*, 7:233–237 (1986).
49. S. C. Mehta, P. D. Bernardo, W. I. Higuchi, and A. P. Simonelli, *J. Pharm. Sci.*, 59:638–644 (1970).
50. A. P. Simonelli, S. C. Mehta, and W. I. Higuchi, *J. Pharm. Sci.*, 59:633–637 (1970).
51. J. D. Mullins and T. J. Macek, *J. Am. Pharm. Assoc. (Sci. Ed.)*, 49:245–248 (1960).
52. S. Luhtala, P. Kahela, and E. Kristoffersson, *Acta. Pharm. Fenn.*, 99:59–67 (1990).
53. S. Luhtala, *Acta Pharm. Nordica*, 4:85–90 (1992).
54. S. Luhtala, *Acta Pharm. Nordica*, 4:271–276 (1992).
55. N. B. Shah and B. B. Sheth, *J. Pharm. Sci.*, 65:1618–1623 (1976).
56. *Martindale, The Extra Pharmacopoeia*, 30th ed., The Pharmaceutical Press, London, 1993, pp. 1217–1221.
57. V. Kumar and G. S. Banker, *Drug Dev. Ind. Pharm.*, 19:1–33 (1993).
58. J. H. Chapman and E. L. Neustadter, *J. Pharm. Pharmacol.*, 17:S138 (1965).
59. C. A. Farley, *Pharm. J.*, 216:562–566 (1976).
60. H. Schott, *J. Pharm. Sci.*, 59:1492–1496 (1970).
61. A. Scheer, *Drug Cosmet. Ind.*, 128:53–55, 102–105 (1981).
62. B. A. Miller, *Pharm. J.*, 231:384 (1983).
63. National Formulary, 18th ed., United States Pharmacopoeial Convention, Rockville, MD, 1995, p. 2232.
64. L. G. Galt and R. V. Josephson, *Am. J. Hosp. Pharm.*, 39:1009–1012 (1982).
65. S. Kabre, H. DeKay, G. Banker, *J. Pharm. Sci.*, 53:495–499 (1964).
66. D. Johnston, M. R. Gray, C. S. Reed, F. W. Bonner, and N. H. Anderson, *Drug Dev. Ind. Pharm.*, 16:1893–1909 (1990).
67. H. Asche, *Pharm. Acta Helv.*, 49:277–284 (1974).
68. C. Chauveau, H. Maillols, H. Delonca, *Pharm. Acta Helv.*, 61:292–297 (1978).
69. B. Idson and M. O. Bachynsky, *Drug Cosmet. Ind.*, 122:38–46, 153–155 (1986).
70. R. W. Butler and E. D. Klug, Hydroxypropylcellulose. In: *Handbook of Water-Soluble Gums and Resins* (R. L. Davidson, ed.), McGraw-Hill, New York, 1980, pp. 13-3.
71. B. Joynt and D. Zuck, *Can. J. Pharm. Sci.*, 3:93–96 (1968).

72. J. A. Polon, *J. Soc. Cosmet. Chem.*, 21:347–363 (1970).
73. P. W. Gerding and G. J. Spierandio, *J. Am. Pharm. Assoc. Pract. Ed.*, 15:356–359 (1954).
74. J. E. Carless and J. Ocran, *J. Pharm. Pharmacol.*, 24:637–644 (1972).
75. G. Catacalos and J. Wood, *J. Pharm. Sci.*, 53:1089–1093 (1964).
76. G. Dondi and A. Zanotti Gerosa, *Boll. Chim. Farm.*, 120:606–617 (1981).
77. V. Das Gupta, *Am. J. Hosp. Pharm.*, 38:363–264 (1981).
78. B. Meer, Gum arabic. In: *Handbook of Water-Soluble Gums and Resins* (R. L. Davidson, ed.), McGraw-Hill, New York, 1980, pp. 8-1-8-24.
79. W. Meer, Gum agar. In: *Handbook of Water-Soluble Gums* (R. L. Davidson, ed.), McGraw-Hill, New York, 1980, p. 7-5.
80. A. M. Goldstein, E. N. Alter, and J. K. Seaman, Guar gum. In: *Industrial Gums,* (R. L. Whistler, ed.), Academic Press, New York, 1973, pp. 303–321.
81. F. Rof, Locust bean gum. In: *Industrial Gums* (R. L. Whistler, ed.), Academic Press, New York, 1973, pp. 323–337.
82. P. S. Rao and H. C. Srivastava, Tamarind. In: *Industrial Gums* (R. L. Whistler, ed.), Academic Press, New York, 1973, pp. 394–411.
83. I. W. Cottrell, K. S. Kang, and P. Kovacs, Xanthan gum. In: *Handbook of Water-Soluble Gums and Resins* (R. L. Davidson, ed.), McGraw-Hill, New York, 1980, pp. 24-1-24-30.
84. M. C. B. Van Oudtshoorn and F. J. Potgieter, *Pharm. Weekblad*, 106:909–915 (1971).
85. A. Delgado, V. Gallardo, A. Perera, and F. Gonzalez Caballero, *J. Pharm. Sci.*, 79:709–715 (1990).
86. M. Barzegar-Jalali and J. R. Richards, *Int. J. Pharm.*, 2:195–201 (1979).
87. M. A. Kassem and A. G. Mattha, *Pharm. Acta Helv.*, 45:18–27 (1970).
88. N. Patel, L. Kennon, R. Levinson, Pharmaceutical suspensions. In: *The Theory and Practice of Industrial Pharmacy* (L. Lachman, H. A. Lieberman, J. L. Kanig, eds., Lea & Febiger, Philadelphia, 1986, p. 490.
89. E. Azaz and R. Segal, *Pharm. Acta Helv.*, 55:183–188 (1980).
90. K. Sabra and D. B. Deasy, *J. Pharm. Pharmacol.*, 35:275–278 (1983).
91. C. M. Ofner III and H. Schott, *J. Pharm. Sci.*, 76:715–723 (1987).
92. A. Felmeister, S. Kuchtyak, S. Kozioi, C. J. Felmeister, *J. Pharm. Sci.*, 62:2026–2027 (1973).
93. J. S. Tempio and J. L. Zatz, *J. Pharm. Sci.*, 70:554–558 (1981).
94. J. V. Bondi, R. L. Schnaare, P. J. Niebergall, and E. T. Sugita, *J. Pharm. Sci.*, 62:1731–1733 (1973).
95. R. D. C. Jones, R. A. Matthews, and C. T. Rhodes, *J. Pharm. Sci.*, 59:518–520 (1970).
96. *United States Pharmacopeia/National Formulary*, 23rd ed., United States Pharmacopeial Convention, Inc., Rockville, MD, 1995, p. 2207.
97. J. Tingstad, J. Dudzinski, L. Lachman, E. Shami, *J. Pharm. Sci.*, 62:1361–1363 (1973).
98. G. Levy, *J. Pharm. Sci.*, 50:429–435 (1961).
99. A. A. H. Khalil and R. N. Nasipuri, *J. Pharm. Pharmacol.*, 25:138–142 (1973).
100. J. Swarbrick, Coarse dispersions: Suspensions, emulsions, and lotions. In: *American Pharmacy* (L. W. Dittert, ed.), Lippincott, Philadelphia, 1974, pp. 196–197.
101. V. K. La Mer, R. H. Smellie, and P. Lee, *J. Colloid Sci.*, 12:230–239 (1957).
102. A. Dakkuri and B. Ecanow, *J. Pharm. Sci.*, 65:420–423 (1976).
103. H. Schott and A. E. Royce, *Colloids Surfaces*, 19:399–418 (1986).
104. T. T. Ortyl and G. E. Peck, *Drug Dev. Ind. Pharm.*, 17:2245–2268 (1991).
105. S. A. Young and G. Buckton, *Int. J. Pharm.*, 60:235–241 (1990).
106. N. Weiner, *Drug Dev. Ind. Pharm.*, 12:933–951 (1986).
107. A. Osol and G. Farrar, eds., *United States Dispensatory*, Lippincott, Philadelphia, 1955, p. 771.
108. H. C. Ansel, *Introduction to Pharmaceutical Dosage Forms*, Lea & Febiger, Philadelphia, 1985, p. 213.

109. K. G. Tolman, Gastrointestinal and liver drugs. In: *Remington: The Science and Practice of Pharmacy* (A. R. Gennaro, ed.), Mack, Easton, PA, 1995, p. 887.
110. G. E. Schmacher, *Am. J. Hosp. Pharm.* 26:85 (1969).
111. C. M. Ofner III and R. L. Schnaare, Unpublished data.
112. *Grifulvin V, Package Insert*, Ortho Pharmaceutical Corporation, Raritan, NJ, 1985.
113. H. J. Von Dechow, D. Dolcher, G. Hubner, S. Kim, K. Lammerhirt, C. H. Pich, and E. Schmidt-Bothelt, *Arzneim. Forsch.*, 26:596–613 (1976).

5

Topical Suspensions

Hridaya N. Bhargava

Massachusetts College of Pharmacy and Allied Health Sciences, Boston, Massachusetts

Daniel W. Nicolai

Stiefel Research Institute, Inc., Oak Hill, New York

Bharat J. Oza

Oza Enterprises, Summit, New Jersey

I. INTRODUCTION

Pharmaceutical suspensions constitute a drug delivery system in which insoluble solid particles are dispersed as discrete units or as a network of particles in a continuous liquid medium. Pharmaceutical suspensions are used for oral, injectable, or topical applications. Nearly all pharmaceutical suspensions have particles greater than $0.1\mu m$, though the size and shape of individual particles may vary.

Suspensions form an important class of pharmaceutical dosage form and offer distinct advantages. Many of the more recently developed drugs are generally hydrophobic with limited aqueous solubilities. A suspension is an ideal delivery system for insoluble and bitter-tasting drugs. Suspensions allow masking of taste and thus improve patient compliance. They are a suitable form of drug delivery for the topical application of dermatologic materials to the skin and sometimes to the mucous membrane. Compared to the solubilized system, suspensions offer better chemical stability of drugs. Drugs from suspensions are more readily bioavailable than from a tablet or a capsule [1,2]. Lately, suspensions are becoming increasingly popular as intramuscular injections for depot therapy.

Formulation of a safe, effective, stable, and pharmaceutically elegant suspension is more difficult and challenging than formulation of tablets or capsules. Some of the difficulties that a formulator should overcome during the development of a suspension are nonhomogeneity of dosage, sedimentation, compaction of sediment, aggregation of suspended particles, difficulty with redispersion, and masking of taste and of undesirable odor.

For the most part, this discussion will focus on aqueous topical suspensions and theoretical considerations such as wetting, crystal growth, surface tension, zeta potential, preformulation, preparation, testing, and stability of suspensions. However, many of the areas that are covered are applicable to nonaqueous suspension or emulsion suspensions.

II. DESIRABLE ATTRIBUTES OF A SUSPENSION

An acceptable and therapeutically effective suspension should possess the following attributes:

1. Ideally, the suspended material should not settle readily at the bottom of the container. However, suspensions, being thermodynamically unstable, do tend to settle and should therefore be readily redispersible into a uniform mixture upon shaking and must not cake.
2. Physical characteristics such as particle size and viscosity should remain fairly constant throughout the shelf life of the product.
3. Its viscosity must promote free and even flow from the container. For external application, the product should be fluid enough to spread freely over the affected area and yet must not be so mobile as to run off the intended area of application.
4. The topical suspension should dry quickly and provide a protective elastic film that will not rub off readily.
5. It should be safe, effective, stable, and pharmaceutically elegant during its shelf life.
6. Resuspension should produce a homogeneous mix of drug particles such that same amount of drug can be removed repeatedly.

III. A SYSTEMATIC APPROACH TO SUSPENSION FORMULATION

A systematic approach to a pharmaceutical suspension, whether intended for systemic or topical usage, involves several steps. It requires:

1. Identification and knowledge of the site of drug release and its therapeutic effect
2. Preformulation studies on pure drug
3. Selection of compatible excipients and validation of their specifications
4. Identification and selection of the method of manufacturing
5. Preparation of trial formulations for in vitro and in vivo testing and evaluations
6. Pilot plane scale-up of the formula
7. Development and evaluation of in-process test methods
8. Performance of stability studies
9. In vivo safety and efficacy data
10. Validation of manufacturing process, stability data, method of analysis, and other data required for submission with an Investigational New Drug application (IND), New Drug Application (NDA), and Abbreviated New Drug Application (ANDA).

IV. THEORETICAL CONSIDERATIONS

The difficulties in the development of a reasonably stable suspension, and problems associated with the evaluation of such products are, for the most part, related to their nonequilibrium state. A conceptual understanding of the thermodynamics of these dispersions, particularly concerning their surfaces or interfacial free energy, will facilitate a successful formulation of such systems. A strategy that fails to utilize surface behavior to stabilize unstable formulations thermodynamically is unlikely to be productive, whereas a strategy based on an appreciation of the surface properties of the system is much more likely to succeed [3].

An understanding of interfacial properties, wetting, particle interaction, electrokinetics, aggregation, sedimentation, and rheological concepts will be of immense help to the formulator. Many of the concepts and equations presented may not be used directly for the purpose of formulation; rather, they provide an understanding of the interactions involved in the formulation of a suspension.

A. Interfaces

Interface is defined as the boundary between two phases [3]. Usually an interior molecule has "equal" forces pulling at it equally in all directions. However, at the interface, molecules are subjected to a highly unbalanced force field, because they are in contact with other molecules exhibiting different forces of attraction. As a result of this, molecules situated at the phase boundary contain potential forces of interaction that are not satisfied relative to the situation in the bulk phase [4]. Interfaces possess positive free energy, meaning molecules at the interface have a higher energy state than if they were located in the bulk. The greater the preference of the molecule for the bulk phase as compared to interface, the greater the interfacial free energy. The formulator attempts to reduce this positive free energy value to zero by reducing the amount of interface or varying the composition of the interface.

Although interfacial free energy is not directly measurable, interfacial tension values are obtainable. Surface or interfacial tension, however, should be looked upon as a mathematical approximations of surface or interfacial free energy.

B. Wetting

The introduction of solid particles into a vehicle is the critical step in the preparation of a pharmaceutical suspension and requires adequate wetting of the solid particles for a stable dispersion.

Wetting of solid materials in the most general sense implies replacement of air on a solid surface by liquid. The process of wetting involves surfaces and interfaces. Usually, slightly lyophobic powders present no major problem and can be wetted easily. Strongly lyophobic powders, however, may float in an aqueous medium because of high interfacial energy between the vehicle and the powder.

Three types of wetting have been distinguished: (a) spreading wetting, (b) adhesional wetting, and (c) immersion wetting. All types of wetting depend on the balance of surface forces [5].

In spreading wetting, a liquid in contact with substrate spreads over the substrate and displaces air from the surface. If a liquid displaces air from the surface completely, the liquid is said to wet the surface completely [5].

If the liquid L in Fig. 1 spreads from C to B, covering an area A, then the decrease in surface-free energy of the system occurs due to a decrease in area of the substrate/air interface. This decrease in surface free energy is $A \times \gamma_{SA}$, where γ_{SA} is the inter-

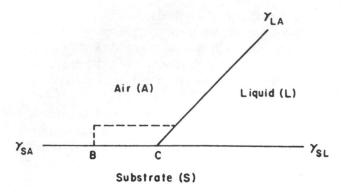

Fig. 1 Spreading wetting.

facial free energy per unit area of the substrate in equilibrium with liquid-saturated air above it.

At the same time, the free energy of the system increases because of the increase in liquid/substrate and liquid/air interfaces. The increase in surface free energy of the system due to the increase in the liquid/substrate interface is $A \times \gamma_{SL}$, where γ_{SL} is the interfacial free energy per unit area at the liquid/substrate interface. The increase in surface free energy of the system due to the increase in the liquid/air interface is $A \times \gamma_{LA}$, where γ_{LA} is the surface tension of liquid L.

The quantity, which is a measure of the driving force behind the spreading process, is usually called the spreading coefficient $S_{L/S}$ and is defined by the equation:

$$S_{L/S} = \gamma_{SA} - (\gamma_{SL} + \gamma_{LA}) \qquad (1)$$

In general, a liquid will spread spontaneously if the spreading coefficient $S_{L/S}$ is positive, and it will not spread spontaneously if $S_{L/S}$ is negative.

1. *Critical Surface Tension*

Critical surface tension provides a way to characterize solid surfaces. The concept of critical surface tension (γ_C) for spreading on a low energy surface was developed by Zisman and coworkers [6,7]. Generally, a liquid whose surface tension is equal to or less than the critical surface tension of a solid spreads readily. Table 1 gives the critical surface tension values of some powders [8].

Knowledge of the critical surface tension helps in determining the necessity for and the selection of a wetting agent. Usually, compounds that have a critical surface tension below 30 dynes/cm^2 require a wetting agent.

2. *Contact Angle and Its Measurement*

The contact angle is an angle that a liquid makes when it is at equilibrium with other phases. A drop of liquid at rest upon a solid assumes a shape that is controlled by three forces: surface tension of the liquid, surface tension of the solid, and interfacial tension between the solid and the liquid. The contact angle (Θ) is a measure of the relative strength of the combined forces [8]. In many applications the contact angle is the only value required for evaluating wetting properties. For applications that require determi-

Table 1 Critical Surface Tension Values for
Some Powders

Substance	Critical surface tension (dyne/cm)
Sulfadiazine	33
Aspirin	32
Salicylic acid	31
Sulfur	30
Magnesium stearate	22

Source: Ref. 8. Reprinted with permission from the publisher,
the Society of Cosmetic Chemists, New York, NY.

nation of surface or interfacial energies, Θ is analyzed in terms of vector forces using Young's equation [8], as described below:

$$\gamma_S = \gamma_{L/S} + \gamma_L \cos \Theta \tag{2}$$

where γ_S, $\gamma_{L/S}$, and γ_L are surface tension of solid, interfacial tension of liquid/solid, and surface tension of the liquid, respectively.
Rearranging Eq. (2) gives

$$\cos \Theta = \frac{\gamma_S - \gamma_{L/S}}{\gamma_L} \tag{3}$$

Complete wetting occurs if $\cos \Theta = 1$. For all wetting processes, reduction of the surface tension of liquid (γ_L) is always beneficial and reduction of the interfacial tension between liquid and solid ($\gamma_{L/S}$) may also be beneficial.

To date, numerous papers on measurements of contact angle have been published [8–10]. Contact angles have been measured on macroscopic smooth planar substrates by placing a droplet of a liquid or a solution on a substrate and determining the contact angle by any of the number of techniques reviewed by Adamson [10]. The contact angle can be measured directly by the use of a microscope fitted with a goniometer or indirectly by measuring height h and diameter d of a droplet and using the Bartell relationship [11] and as given by Eq. (4).

$$\tan \frac{\Theta}{2} = 2 \frac{h}{d} \tag{4}$$

3. *Modification of Wetting by Surfactant*

Water has a rather high surface tension and generally does not spread spontaneously over substrates that have low surface free energy. For any liquid to wet the substrate, the spreading coefficient must be positive. The addition of a surfactant to water reduces its surface tension and in some instances may reduce the interfacial tension between water and the substrates well, resulting in a positive spreading coefficient. However, addition of a surfactant to water does not always increase the spreading coefficient. In cases where the substrate is porous or when adsorption of the surfactant occurs at the liquid/solid interface, the use of a surfactant may decrease wetting [5].

To save time in surfactant selection, a systematic scheme of identifying the relatively few surfactants, suitable for any given application was introduced in the late 1940s. This is called the HLB system (the letters HLB stand for "hydrophile–lipophile balance"). In the HLB system, each surfactant is assigned a numerical value, which is called its HLB value. A surfactant with a low HLB value tends to be oil soluble; one that has a high HLB value will tend to be water soluble. Any surfactant that lowers the surface tension of water below 30 dynes/cm^2 will cause spontaneous wetting [8].

C. Zeta Potential

Electrical charges may be developed on suspended particles as the result of ionization of chemical groups on a solid surface, adsorption of the surfactant molecule on a solid surface, or adsorption of electrolytes from the solution on a solid surface. The particle charge gives rise to surface potential ψ_z. The potential will drop to zero at some distance away from the surface depending on the concentration of counterions in the external phase. The region in which the influence of the surface charge is appreciable is called the electrical double layer [12,4]. In the double layer, the first layer is tightly bound and moves with the particle; the second layer is more diffuse, as illustrated in Fig. 2.

The magnitude of charge is defined as the difference in electrical potential between the charged solid surface and the bulk of the solution. There are several potentials that can be defined but the important one for formulation of a suspension is zeta potential, ζ. Zeta potential is defined as the difference in potential between the surface of the tightly bound layer of ions on the particle surface and the electroneutral region of the solution. The application of zeta potential measurements to the formulation of suspensions has been investigated by Haines and Martin [13].

When the zeta potential is relatively high, 25 mV or more (which depends on the particular system being used), the repulsive forces exceed the attractive London forces and particles are dispersed and the system is deflocculated. On the other hand, when the zeta potential is lowered (less than 25mV), the attractive forces exceed the repulsive forces, and the particles come together leading to flocculation.

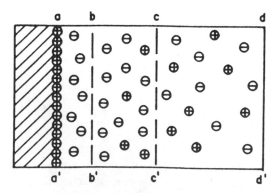

Fig. 2   The electrical double layer at the surface of separation between two phases showing distribution of ions. (From A. Martin, J. Swarbrick and A. Cammarata, Interfacial phenomena. In: *Physical Pharmacy* 4th ed., p. 387. Reprinted with permission from the publisher, Lea & Febiger, Philadelphia, PA.)

D. Crystal Growth, Aggregation, and Caking

The basic concern in almost all suspension systems is to decrease the rate of settling and permit easy resuspendability of any settled particulate matter. Physical instability of the suspension results from crystal growth, aggregation, or caking.

1. *Crystal Growth*

The following factors affect the potential for crystal growth in a pharmaceutical suspension:

1. Particle size distribution
2. Dissolution and recrystallization
3. Changes in pH and temperature
4. Polymorphism and solvate formulation [14].

Small particles are more soluble than larger particles because of a higher surface energy per unit mass. The Ostwald-Freundlich equation:

$$\ln \frac{C_1}{C_2} = \left(\frac{2\,M\gamma}{\rho\,RT} \frac{1}{R_1} - \frac{1}{R_2} \right) \tag{5}$$

where
C = solubility of particles of radii R_1 and R_2
M = molecular weight
γ — surface energy of solid
ρ = density of solid
R = gas constant
T = absolute temperature

The Ostwald-Freundlich equation shows that the solubility (C_1) is higher for smaller particles (R_1) than the solubility (C_2) is for larger particles (R_2). Variable particle size can also result from various factors including: (a) preparation of suspension, (b) changes in pH, and (c) temperature changes. Causes of this recrystallization phenomena include polymorphism, solvate formation, and temperature fluctuation [14].

To retard or eliminate crystal growth, the formulator must consider many factors, including the theory behind crystal growth and particle size distribution of the drug, the use of the right polymorph and solvate forms, the conducting of temperature cycling, and the selection of the appropriate viscosity of the product.

2. *Aggregation and Caking*

Suspensions are thermodynamically unstable systems and, when left undisturbed for a long period of time, lead to aggregation of particles, sedimentation, and eventually caking. Particles held together strongly are called aggregates, and the compaction of strongly adhering aggregates that settle at the bottom of the container forms a cake. Caking is one of the most difficult problems encountered in the formulation of a suspension. Caking cannot be eliminated by reducing particle size or increasing the viscosity of the medium. Once the cake is formed it cannot be remedied. However, cake formation can be anticipated and prevented.

When particles are held together in a loose open structure, the system is said to be in the state of flocculation. The flocculated particles settle rapidly in the suspension to form sediment with large volume but are readily redispersed.

To resolve the problem of caking, one must consider forces of attraction and repulsion between particles in the suspension. Flocculation and aggregation are brought about by the forces that reside at the surface of the particles. These forces depend on the nature of the species, distance of separation, orientation of the molecule, and the nature of the medium.

Much of the present day theory regarding charge on suspended particles results from the work of four scientists, Derjaguin, Landau, Verwey, and Overbeek, and is often called the DLVO theory [15]. The theory quantitatively describes the stability of lyophobic colloids and is universally accepted. It involves the comparison of two types of forces: London and van der Waals attractive forces and forces of repulsion caused by interaction of electrical double layers surrounding each particle. The DLVO theory details the factors [16,17] involved in controlling the rate at which the particles in suspension come together or aggregate [15]. The process of aggregation of particles will accelerate the rate of sedimentation and thus affect redispersibility. The following total energy of interaction between the two particles is defined by equation:

$$V_T = V_R + V_A \tag{6}$$

where
V_T = total energy of interaction
V_R = total repulsive forces
V_A = total attractive forces

Figure 3 shows the total energy of interaction curves between suspended particles of three general types [15,18].

Curve A applies when V_R is greater than V_A; that is, the term V_T is always positive because of high potential at the double layer. In such cases the suspension would exhibit good resistance to aggregation and indefinite stability, provided particles are not sufficiently large to sediment under gravity.

Curve B shows a high potential energy barrier V_M, which must be surmounted if particles are to approach one another sufficiently close to enter the deep primary en-

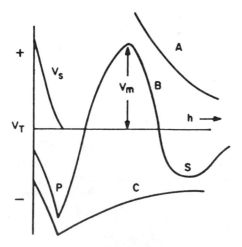

Fig. 3 The total energy of interaction between two particles, as a function of interparticulate distance h. (From Ref. 18. Reproduced with permission of the copyright owner, the American Pharmaceutical Association.)

ergy minimum at P. The value V_M required to just prevent this is probably equivalent to a zeta potential of about 50 mV. Aggregates that do form at P are likely to be very tightly bound together because h, the interparticulate distance, is small. Thus, to redisperse the product, virogous shaking is required. Curve B also has a secondary minimum S. Aggregations formed by particles in this region can break up readily with shaking [18].

Curve C prevails when attractive forces completely overwhelm the electrostatic repulsion (i.e., $V_A > V_R$) and rapid coagulation occurs [18].

Curve V_S exhibits the stabilizing effect of the surfactants absorbed on the substrate. It shows a sharp cutoff point at a distance equal to 2d, where d is the thickness of the adsorbed surfactant layer. The strongly hydrated nature of the surfactant head group impedes particle-particle contact, which would result in aggregation and thus stabilize the suspension [15]. In such suspensions, which are stabilized by adsorbed surfactant molecules, the total energy of interaction, V_T, existing between two particles is obtained by adding the contribution from repulsion V_S, V_A, and V_R. The total energy of interaction, V_T, is then given by Eq. (7).

$$V_T = V_A + V_R + V_S \tag{7}$$

Schneider et al. [19] have prepared a computer program to calculate the repulsion and attraction energies in pharmaceutical suspensions.

Several differences between flocculated and deflocculated suspensions are evident and summarized in Table 2. Overflocculation is undesirable as it leads to the growth of excessively large particles that interfere with uniformity in the viscosity and appearance of the suspension. The concept of "controlled flocculation" applies to a pharmaceuti-

Table 2 Relative Properties of Flocculated and Deflocculated Particles in Suspension

Deflocculated	Flocculated
1. Particles exist in suspension as separate entities	Particles form loose aggregates
2. Rate of sedimentation is slow because each particle settles separately and particle size is minimal.	Rate of sedimentation is high because particles settle as a floc, which is a collection of particles.
3. A sediment is formed slowly.	A sediment is formed rapidly.
4. The sediment eventually becomes very closely packed as the result of weight of upper layers of sedimenting material. Repulsive forces between particles are overcome and a hard cake is formed that is difficult, if not impossible, to redisperse.	The sediment is loosely packed and possesses a scaffold-like structure. Particles do not bond tightly to each other and a hard, dense cake does not form. The sediment is easy to redisperse, so as to reform the original suspension.
5. The suspension has a pleasing appearance, because the suspended material remains suspended for a relatively long time. The supernatant also remains cloudy, even when settling is apparent.	The suspension is somewhat unsightly because of rapid sedimentation and the presence of an obvious, clear supernatant region. This can be minimized if the volume of sediment is made large. Ideally, volume of sediment should encompass the volume of the suspension.

Source: Ref. 4. Reprinted with permission from the publisher, Mack Publishing Co., Easton, PA.

cal suspension. The theory and technique of controlled flocculation was first introduced by Haines and Martin [13]. Scientists have tested and advanced the concept, finding it to be helpful in the formulation of suspensions. Mathews and Rhodes, in a series of papers [20–25] dealing with physicochemical factors involved in suspension formulation, evaluated the use of "controlled flocculation" for suspension stability. Various therapeutic agents such as hydrocortisone and norgestrel were formulated using a controlled flocculation technique to stabilize the suspension [24]. The theory of controlled flocculation is still the subject for further investigation, and certain aspects of the theory have been criticized [26].

E. Flocculents

Particle flocculation affects sedimentation rate, as well as the degree of compaction that takes place within the sediment. Flocculents function either by reducing the electrostatic repulsive forces or by providing additional interparticle attraction. Electrolytes function as flocculating agents in a suspension containing charged particles by reducing interparticulate repulsion; thus, the balance shifts in favor of the attractive van der Waals forces bringing particles together [8]. Formula adjuvants such as surface-active agents and polymers, chosen for their effect on wetting and rheological behavior, respectively, may also influence flocculation.

1. *Electrolytes*

The electrolytes needed to effect optimum flocculation depend on the valence and type of interacting ion; the Schulze-Hardy rule [27] summarizes this, stating that the valence of the ions having a charge opposite to that of the lyophobic particle determines the effectiveness of a electrolyte in aggregating the particle. The aggregating efficiency increases with the valence of the ion. Trivalent ions are more efficient than divalent ions, which in turn are more efficient than monovalent ions.

Mathews and Rhodes [21] studied the influence of several salts and anionic wetting agents on the flocculation characteristics of suspensions. In the absence of a salt the suspension was deflocculated, but the addition of a salt flocculated the system. Their studies found aluminum chloride to be a much more efficient flocculentn than calcium chloride, which was found to be more efficient than sodium chloride. They further extended their work on the flocculation of sulfamerazine hydrocortisone and griseofulvin suspensions and found the efficiency of the electrolytes to be of the same order in all three suspensions and in agreement with the Schulze-Hardy rule.

2. *Surface-Active Agents*

Ionic and nonionic surface-active agents have been reported to produce flocculation [28–32]. The flocculation produced by a surfactant depends on its physicochemical properties and its concentration. The surface-active agent is adsorbed on the electrical double layer, causing neutralization or reversal of the charges, thus lowering the zeta potential. Otsuka et al. [30] studied adsorption of nonionic polyethoxylated octyl and nonylphenols on sulfathiazole and naphthalene and observed that the surfactant with a large hydrophilic chain length significantly influenced flocculation of sulfathiazole, but there was little influence of the hydrophobic chain length on the flocculation behavior of naphthalene. Liao and Zatz [29,30] investigated the effect of nonionic surfactants on the flocculation behavior of a suspension containing benzocaine and butamben. Assessing the apparent viscosity, sedimentation volume and refiltration as a flocculation probe they reported that the flocculation of benzocaine was a function of the surfactant concentration, polyoxyethylene chain length, and particle size.

3. *Polymers*

Polymers are considered to differ from surfactants because polymers have a very high molecular weight with many active centers spaced along the chain. On the other hand, a surfactant has low molecular weight with few active centers on a single molecule [28]. The polymers act as flocculating agents by adsorption as well as by liquid bridging of particles. In the case of polymers, a part of the polymer chain is adsorbed at the solid-liquid interface with the remaining part projecting out into the dispersion medium. The adsorption phenomenon of polymers is independent of changes in temperature, solvent, and even the adsorbent surface [28].

Zatz et al. [34] studied flocculation of negatively charged sulfamerazine by a cationic polymer and reported that at low concentration of the polymer, the sedimentation volume was not affected, but at a critical value a significant rise in sedimentation volume was observed, indicating the suspension had flocculated. Their findings suggest that at a small concentration or in the absence of a polymer, particles were separated by their negative charge. Flocculation occurred at a critical polymer concentration and was caused by the bridging of particles by the polymer [33]. Felmeister, Reiss, and Healy separately [34–36] studied the influence of xanthan gum, an anionic polysaccharide, on the flocculation characteristics of suspensions of sulfaguanidine and bismuth subcarbonate. Addition of xanthan gum resulted in a flocculated suspension. Tiempo and Zatz [37,38] studied the effect of xanthan gum on the flocculation properties of aluminum hydroxide and magnesium carbonate suspensions. Addition of xanthan gum increased the extent of the flocculation. They studied flocculation mechanism and concluded that a number of factors influence the adsorption of a polymer at the solid-liquid interface.

Zatz [39] reported that a magnesium carbonate suspension became highly flocculated in the presence of xanthan gum but deflocculated on addition of docusate sodium, an anionic surfactant. The nonionic surfactant polysorbate 40 had no effect on the flocculation state of a suspension. If xanthan gum and docusate sodium both were present, the flocculation state depended on the relative concentration of the two substances, as both are anionic and compete for the same surface site on the magnesium carbonate particle.

F. Sedimentation

The majority of factors that govern the physical stability of a suspension are the result of unequal gravitational pull on the suspended particles and the medium, and are depicted by Stokes' equation:

$$V = \frac{d^2 (\rho - \rho_0) g}{18 \eta} \qquad (8)$$

Where
V = sedimentation velocity
d = particle diameter
ρ = particle density
ρ_0 = medium density

g = gravitational constant
η = viscosity of continuous external phase.

Thus, physical stability of a suspension can be improved by increasing the viscosity of the external phase as the rate of sedimentation is an inverse function of viscosity. However, too high a viscosity is undesirable, especially if the suspending medium is Newtonian, because in such a system it is difficult to redisperse the material that has settled. Also, the rate of sedimentation is proportional to the particle diameter and a reduction in particle size will reduce the rate of sedimentation significantly.

According to Stokes' law the rate of sedimentation is reduced if the difference in densities $(\rho - \rho_o)$ of the dispersed phase and the continuous phase can be reduced significantly. It is possible to increase the density of the liquid by using polyols like glycerin or sorbitol and thus bringing it closer to the dispersed solid, but this technique is rarely used to stabilize pharmaceutical suspensions.

G. Rheology

The rheological behavior of a pharmaceutical suspension furnishes the formulator with a means of exercising the greatest control over sedimentation and optimization of the physical stability of the system. The choice of the type of rheology depends to a large extent on the type of bodying agent and its intended application. If the medium is viscous enough, like castor oil or glycerin, a bodying agent may not be necessary to enhance the viscosity. However, if the medium is nonviscous, like alcohol or water, a bodying agent may be necessary to impart the desired viscosity to the medium. For example, a suspension for topical application should be fluid enough to permit proper shaking and pourability yet should not flow readily from the skin. It should also provide sufficient resistance against the gravitational settling while in the container.

A fluid may exhibit Newtonian or non-Newtonian flow. The non-Newtonian type of behavior includes pseudoplastic, plastic thixotropic, or dilatant flow characteristics, as shown in Fig. 4. The combination of desired attributes requires careful selection of an additive that will impart non-Newtonian flow characteristics to the suspension.

1. *Pseudoplasticity*

The viscosity of a system exhibiting pseudoplastic flow is inversely proportional to the shear rate. As shear stress is increased, the resistance to flow decreases (Fig. 4a), and the system becomes more fluid. This shear-thinning behavior is called pseudoplasticity. The apparent viscosity of such a system therefore cannot be defined in terms of one value. Many colloidal systems, especially polymer solutions, exhibit pseudoplastic flow.

2. *Plasticity*

Plastic behavior is characterized by the presence of a yield value (Fig. 4b). Some materials such as semisolids do not flow at low shear stress. A Bingham body does not flow until shearing stress equals or exceeds the yield value. Once the shear stress equals or exceeds the yield value, the composition begins to flow. This system exhibits solid-like behavior under quiescent conditions. This property of plastic flow may effectively inhibit sedimentation altogether in a suspension. Agitation temporarily disrupts the rigid network of solids, making it possible to pour or apply the suspensions to the skin.

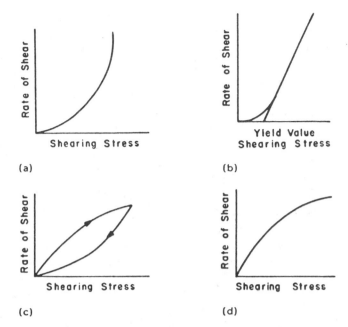

Fig. 4 Plots of rate of shear as a function of shearing stress for: (a) simple pseudoplastic; (b) plastic; (c) thixotropic; and (d) dilatant flow. (Reprinted from Ref. 15, p. 333, by courtesy of Marcel Dekker, Inc., New York, New York.)

3. *Thixotropy*

Thixotropy, which may be seen in both plastic and pseudoplastic systems, is characterized by the fact that the rate of shear at any given shearing stress can vary depending on whether the rate of shear is increasing or decreasing. Thixotropy is a measure of the breakdown and then rebuilding of the structure of the system. Thixotropic systems contain a structural network of colloidal particles. At rest, this structure confers some degree of rigidity on the system, but when disrupted by shear, the system begins to flow. Upon removal of shear stress, the structure begins to re-form. The reformation of structure is time dependent and can take from several minutes to hours or days. During this time, the product can be poured from the container. The apparent viscosity of a thixotropic system depends not only on the shear rate and shear stress, but also on duration under shear.

The most apparent characteristic of a thixotropic system is the presence of a hysteresis loop, which is formed by the up and down curve of the rheogram (Fig. 4c). The area of a hysteresis loop has been proposed as a measure of thixotropic breakdown and rebuilding of the structure and can be easily obtained [40].

4. *Dilatancy*

A dilatant system exhibits an increase in the resistance to flow when stress is exerted; thus, the system returns to its original state of fluidity when the stress is removed (Fig. 4d). A dilatant system is the reverse of a pseudoplastic system and is a shear-thickening system.

Pharmaceutical suspensions that exhibit plastic or thixotropic rheological behavior generally exhibit good physical stability. Such a suspension may prevent sedimentation, aggregation, and caking by virtue of its high yield value at rest, yet reduce viscosity significantly to permit its application. On the other hand, pseudoplastic or dilatant flow characteristics are undesirable in a suspension as they impart physical instability to the product.

V. PREFORMULATION

The first step in the systematic development of any pharmaceutical dosage form is the careful examination of preformulation test results. The compilation of physicochemical properties is known as preformulation. In today's environment of drug development, it is imperative that the formulator have a complete profile of the physicochemical properties of the drug substance available before initiating formulation development. The use of preformulation parameters maximizes the chances of success in formulating an acceptable, safe, efficacious, and stable product and at the same time provides the basis for optimization of the drug product quality.

A typical preformulation program should begin with the description of the organoleptic qualities of the drug substance. The color, odor, and taste are of immense value in developing an aesthetically acceptable suspension. Appropriate flavor, dyes, and adjuvants can be used to alleviate problems of unpalatable taste, unsightly appearance, or unpleasant odor, but only if they do not compromise efficacy or stability of the drug in the suspension. Some descriptive terms for organoleptic attributes of a drug product are listed in Table 3.

Other significant preformulation parameters include purity of the drug, particle size, shape and surface area, static charge, solubility, dissolution, partition coefficient, ionization constant, crystal properties and polymorphism, chemical and physical stability, solid state and aqueous stability, absolute and bulk density, hygroscopicity, flowability, and excipient compatibility [41]. Of these, crystal properties, particle size and surface area, dissolution, flow characteristics, and drug excipient compatibility are of prime importance in the formulation of suspensions.

A. Crystal Properties

Most organic drug substances exist in more than one crystalline form or lattice configuration, a feature called polymorphism. Polymorphs may exhibit differing physical properties; for example, x-ray diffraction patterns, solubility, dissolution, density, vapor pressure, melting point, crystal form, compaction behavior, flow properties, solid state

Table 3 Suggested Terminology to Describe Organoleptic Properties of Pharmaceutical Powders

Color	Odor	Taste
Off white	Pungent	Acidic
Cream yellow	Sulfurous	Bitter
Tan	Fruity	Bland
Shiny	Aromatic: odorless	Intense; sweet; tasteless

Source: Ref. 41

stability, and absorption rate [42]. Though a drug can exist in more than one polymorphic form, only one of these forms is thermodynamically stable, and the other unstable (metastable) forms will revert to the stable form in time [43]. Many solids can be prepared in the desirable polymorphic form by selecting an appropriate solvent for recrystallization and the appropriate rate of cooling.

Polymorphs of several drugs have been extensively investigated. Cortisone acetate exists in four polymorphic forms but only one is stable in aqueous medium. Amorphous penicillin exhibits less chemical stability than the crystalline salt [43]; metastable sulfathiazole dissolves more rapidly than the more stable sulfathiazole [42].

The use of a metastable polymorph may result in the following: (a) crystal growth; (b) caking; (c) reduced bioavailability; (d) crystal transition, which produces changes in physical and biological characteristics; and (e) reduced chemical stability.

The transition from one structural arrangement to another can be achieved by temperature fluctuations. One polymorphic form of the drug can be reversibly changed to another one. The crystal habit (external shape of crystal), although not as important as polymorphism, also plays a role in product properties, especially if the particle size is small. An increase in temperature during shipment and storage of a suspension may lead to increased solubility, with subsequent dissolution of small crystals. When the temperature decreases, however, the dissolved drug tends to recrystallize to larger crystals. Thus, fluctuations in temperature may change the particle size distribution and crystal habit and may lead to caking. The crystal growth of some drugs has been significantly retarded by the use of a surface-active agent or a polymer. They seem to act by adsorbing at the surface of the crystal [4].

Various techniques are available to study crystal properties. These include microscopy, infrared spectrophotometry, x-ray powder diffraction, and thermal analysis [42].

B. Particle Size and Surface Area

Several chemical, physical, and biological properties of drug substances are influenced by particle size and surface area. The rate of sedimentation, content uniformity, taste, texture, and chemical stability are dependent on the particle size. Control of particle size is directly related to flow properties, segregation, and demixing. The relationship between particle size and particle surface area is an inverse one; that is, reduction in particle size leads to an increase in the surface area. Although a decrease in particle size favors suspendability, the high surface energy of a micronized powder caused by the large surface area may result in poor wettability and agglomeration in suspension.

In most pharmaceutical suspensions, the particle diameter is between 1 and 50 μm; a topical suspension should have a particle size less than 35 μm to be impalpable to the touch—otherwise, grittiness results.

The most efficient method of producing particles of optimum size is by dry milling prior to incorporation into the dispersion medium. However, this method is not appropriate when processing potentially explosive ingredients such as benzoyl peroxide for which wet milling or homogenization of the finished product may be more desirable. Among the several methods of producing small uniform drug particles are micropulverization, fluid energy grinding, spray drying, and controlled precipitation [44]. Micropulverizers, using high speed attrition, or impact mills are capable of reducing the particle size to an acceptable range for most oral or topical suspensions. Fluid energy grinding is quite effective in producing particles less than 10 μm in size. Particles of extremely small dimensions and desired shape can also be produced by the spray-drying technique. It produces free-flowing monodispersible powder. Particles of less than 5 µm can be prepared by controlled precipitation with the aid of ultrasound. This involves shock cooling of a hot, saturated solution of the drug in conjunction with ultrasonic insonation of its solvent environment [45].

Several techniques and tools are used to monitor particle size. The most widely used technique is microscopy, which is capable of measuring particles of 0.3 µm or larger. Sieving is another technique for particles in the 40 µm or higher range. Screen analysis data serves as a qualitative guideline in evaluating raw materials. A variety of instruments is available (see listing in Appendix, p. 199). These instruments are based on light scattering[a] (see Appendix), light blockage,[b] or blockage of electrical conductivity[c] [41]. Most of these instruments measure the numbers and sizes of particles and readily convert them to weight and size distribution. The most widely used technique to measure surface area utilizes the Brunauer, Emmet, Teller (BET) theory of adsorption using an inert gas as an adsorbate at a specific partial pressure [41].

C. Dissolution

Several in vivo/in vitro correlation studies have shown that the absorption of many poorly soluble drugs, administered in suspension form, is dissolution rate limited, thus confirming the necessity for dissolution rate determination of suspensions [46].

Therefore, knowledge of the intrinsic dissolution rate of the drug aids in determining whether a drug is absorbed easily. The intrinsic dissolution rate of a drug is its own dissolution rate in a given solvent and is expressed as mg dissolved per minute per square centimeter [41]. Usually, drugs with intrinsic dissolution rate in water of less than 0.1 mg per minute per square centimeter exhibit absorption rates [47] and would require modification in their dissolution rate for adequate bioavailability. The dissolution rate of a drug can be improved by reducing particle size, coprecipitation, or by the addition of small quantities of an appropriate surface-active agent.

D. Flow Properties

The flow properties of a drug in powder form are an important parameter for the manufacturing of a suspension and should be studied at an early stage of development. Good flow of powder is essential for mixing and for homogeneous drug content. Powders with low density and static charge exhibit poor flow and may be modified to achieve proper flow.

Flow characteristics of a powder are commonly expressed by the "static angle of repose." Most pharmaceutical powders have angle of repose values between 25 and 45° [41]. A low angle of repose is indicative of superior flow properties. There are a number of methods available to measure angle of repose. The method of Pilpel [48] uses a container with a platform. First, the container is filled with the powder. Then the powder is drained out from the bottom, leaving a cone. The angle of repose is then measured using a cathetometer [41].

E. Drug-Excipient Compatibility

Drug-excipient studies are designed to select the basic list of excipients that may be used to develop a final suspension formulation. Some commonly used excipients in a suspension include a dispersing agent, wetting agent, suspending agent, flocculent, preservative, sequestrant, antioxidant, color, and fragrance, and these should be tested for their compatibility with the drug.

An aqueous suspension containing drug, dispersion medium, and an excipient should be stored at elevated temperature of 50°C or 60°C and at 6000 foot-candle lights, with constant agitation for 2 to 12 weeks. The ratio of drug to the excipient concentration is at the discretion of the preformulation scientist and should be consistent with the ratio most likely to be encountered in the final formulation.

The samples are drawn at predetermined time intervals and examined for physical and chemical integrity of the drug and the excipient. Parameters such as color change, crystal shape, caking, pH, and quantitative assay for the drug should be examined by commonly used techniques; for example, thin layer chromatography, differential thermal analysis, and diffuse reflectance spectroscopy [41]. The excipients that show minimal or no degradation of the drug after 8 to 12 weeks at elevated temperatures are chosen, as they are compatible with the drug and the product probably would exhibit satisfactory stability for about 2 years at ambient temperatures. A change in physical attributes (pH, color, crystal shape, etc.) of the drug-excipient mixture, on the other hand, is indicative of physicochemical change and suggests incompatibility. This, too, will aid in the selection of an appropriate colorant, buffer, and other excipients of the formulation.

VI. SUSPENSION EXCIPIENTS

A pharmaceutical suspension seldom contains a drug and a vehicle alone. Usually, it contains several formula adjuvants. These excipients may enhance its physical and chemical stability, microbiological integrity, and aesthetic attributes. Today, formulators have a large number of raw materials to choose from to develop a safe, effective, and stable suspension.

The main considerations for excipient selection are compatibility with the drug, stability at a specific pH and temperature, compatibility with other adjuvants of the formula, ease of processing, and cost. All excipients preferably should be selected from the Generally Recognized As Safe (GRAS) list.

A. Dispersing Agents

There are four general classes of dispersing agents that can be used to prepare an optimum dispersion. Their use depends on the type of dispersion, their required concentration, and the physicochemical properties of the solid to be dispersed. They are classified as (a) wetting agents, (b) deflocculant or true dispersing agents, (c) protective colloids, and (d) inorganic electrolytes.

1. Wetting Agents

Wetting agents are surfactants that lower the contact angle between the solid surface and the wetting liquid. Surfactants that adsorb significantly to the vapor-liquid and solid-liquid interface facilitate wetting. Sometimes alcohol, glycerin, or other polyols such as polyethylene glycol or propylene glycol are used in the initial stages to disperse the solid particles, thereby allowing the vehicle to penetrate.

Ionic as well as nonionic surfactants have been used as wetting agents. Anionic surfactants are most effective for drugs with negative zeta potential, and cationic surfactants are most effective for drugs with positive zeta potential. Good examples of anionic wetting agents are dioctyl sodium sulfosuccinate (docusate sodium) and sodium lauryl sulfate (SLS). Table 4 indicates the effect of increasing concentration of a surfactant, dioctyl sodium sulfosuccinate, on the surface tension and the contact angle of water with magnesium stearate, a hydrophobic tablet lubricant [4].

Two groups of nonionic surfactants used as wetting agents are ethoxylates and poloxamers. A large variety of ethoxylated surfactants exist. In principle, any compound with a reactive hydroxyl group can serve as a starting material for the preparation of an ethoxylated surfactant by reacting it with ethylene oxide.

$$R\!-\!OH + \left(\underset{O}{CH_2\!-\!CH_2}\right)_n \longrightarrow R\!-\!O\ (CH_2\!-\!CH_2\!-\!O)_n\ H$$

Most frequently used starting materials are fatty acids, fatty alcohols, phenols, sterols, sucrose, fatty esters, and fatty amides. Ethoxylation allows control of the physicochemical properties of nonionic surfactants resulting in a diverse range of HLB values; for example, sorbitan mono-oleate has a HLB value of 4.3 and polyoxyethylene sorbitan mono-oleate (polysorbate 80) with 20 moles of ethylene oxide has a HLB value of 15.0.

Nonionics are favorite wetting agents because of their insensitivity to pH, presence of electrolytes, and low toxicity potential.

Although using an ethoxylated surfactant offers many advantages, it has disadvantages as well. Some of the disadvantages include complexation with phenolic/ester preservatives such as parabens and their inactivation and degradation as the result of oxidation.

Poloxamers are synthetic block copolymers of ethylene oxide and propylene oxide. Their molecular weight ranges from 1,000 to 150,000. In a molecule the hydrophilic

Table 4   Effect of Dioctyl Sodium Sulfosuccinate Concentration on the Surface Tension of Water and the Contact Angle of Water with Magnesium Stearate

Concentration, $m \times 10^6$	Surface tension	Contact angle
1.0	6.01	120°
3.0	49.8	113°
5.0	45.1	104°
8.0	40.6	89°
10.0	38.6	80°
12.0	37.9	71°
15.0	35.0	63°
20.0	32.4	54°
25.0	29.5	50°

Source: Ref. 4. Reprinted with permission from the publisher, Mack Publishing Co., Easton, PA.

poly(oxyethylene) sandwiches the hydrophobic poly(oxypropylene). The poly(oxyethylene) on the ends of the molecule constitutes 10% to 80% of the final molecule. The general structure of poloxamer is:

$$HO-(CH_2-CH_2O)_A - \left(\begin{array}{c} CH-CH_2-O \\ | \\ CH_3 \end{array}\right)_B - (CH_2-CH_2-O)_C H$$

where A and C are statistically equal.

High molecular weight poloxamers are ideal for viscosity control and have excellent dispersing power. The hydrophobic group here is polypropylene oxide polymer, whose multiple ether linkage promotes adsorption on to the particle surface [3].

Table 5 lists some selected wetting and solubilizing agents [49].

Irrespective of the type of wetting agent selected, it should be compatible and should be used in the minimum amount necessary to produce adequate dispersion. Excessive amounts may lead to foaming, solubilization, and unpleasant taste or odor.

2. Deflocculants or True Dispersing Agents

Invariably, as a result of wetting, the particles are deflocculated. True dispersing agents or deflocculants are polymerized organic salts of sulfonic acid of both the aryl-alkyl as well as the alkyl-aryl type that alter the charges through physical adsorption [45]. However, most of these polyelectrolytes are not generally considered safe for internal use. One deflocculating agent, lecithin, has been widely used.

Table 5 Wetting and
Solubilizing Agents

Benzalkonium chloride
Benzethonium chloride
Cetylpyridinium chloride
Docusate sodium
Nonoxynol 10
Octoxynol 9
Poloxamer
Polyoxyl 50 stearate
Polyoxyl 10 oleyl ether
Polyoxyl 20 cetostearyl ether
Polyoxyl 40 stearate
Polysorbate 20
Polysorbate 40
Polysorbate 60
Polysorbate 80
Sodium lauryl sulfate
Sorbitan monolaurate
Sorbitan mono-oleate
Sorbitan monopalmitate
Sorbitan monostearate

Source: Ref. 49.

3. *Protective Colloids*

Protective colloids that are adsorbed by solid particles increase the strength of the double layer through hydrogen bonding and thus reduce the molecular interaction and aid in dispersion. These agents do not reduce the interfacial or surface tension. These are discussed in detail under suspending agents.

4. *Inorganic Electrolytes*

Inorganic electrolytes can be used to disperse drug particles. Though they are relatively inexpensive, they are not very efficient. Their efficiency as dispersing agents varies with the size and valence of the electrolyte. Some commonly used inorganic electrolytes are trisodium phosphate, alum (aluminum potassium sulfate), aluminum chloride, and sodium chloride.

B. Suspending Agents

Suspending agents are used to prevent sedimentation by affecting the rheological behavior of a suspension. There are many factors that determine the selection of pseudoplastic and plastic suspending agents for a particular preparation.

An ideal suspending agent should have the following attributes:

1. It should produce a structured vehicle.
2. It should have high viscosity at low shear.
3. Its viscosity should not be altered by temperature or on aging.
4. It should be able to tolerate electrolytes and should be applicable over a wide pH range.
5. It should exhibit "yield stress."
6. It should be compatible with other formula excipients.
7. It should be nontoxic.

Modern technology has provided the pharmaceutical scientist with a variety of suspending materials for formulating and developing superior suspensions. Among the suspending agents, hydrocolloids have played an important role. All hydrocolloids increase the viscosity of water. They do so by binding the water molecule or by trapping the water molecule between their intertwined macromolecular chain, thus limiting the mobility of water. This increase in viscosity has a significant effect on the rate of sedimentation at low shear and is responsible for the improved physical stability of the suspension.

There are numerous hydrocolloids approved for pharmaceutical use and they may be used as suspending agents either alone or in combination. They can be broadly classified into four categories:

1. *Cellulose derivatives*: microcrystalline cellulose (MCC), carboxymethyl cellulose, hydroxypropyl methylcellulose, etc.
2. *Polysaccharides and gums*: alginates, carrageenan, xanthan gum, acacia, tragacanth, avicel, etc.
3. *Synthetic polymers*: carbomer, polyvinylpyrrolidone, poloxamer, etc.
4. *Clays*: magnesium aluminum silicate (veegum), bentonite, etc.

Lately, synthetic suspending agents are preferred because of their batch-to-batch consistency and superior microbial integrity.

1. *Cellulose*

a. *Sodium Carboxymethylcellulose.* Carboxymethylcellulose (CMC), an anionic polymer, is a long-chain cellulose ether prepared by reacting alkali and cellulose with sodium monochloroacetate (Fig. 5). It is available in low, medium, or high viscosity grades.

It dissolves rapidly in hot or cold water, giving a clear solution, but forms aggregates when first wet with water. Its solution characteristics depend on the average chain length and degree of substitution [50]. As the molecular weight of CMC increases, the viscosity of its solutions increases. The high or medium viscosity type of CMC in solution exhibits pseudoplastic flow characteristics. However, solutions of low molecular weight CMC are less pseudoplastic than those of high molecular weight CMC.

The viscosity of CMC solution is influenced by the temperature and pH. On prolonged exposure to heat, the polymer degrades with a permanent reduction in viscosity. CMC solutions exhibit maximum viscosity and stability at pH 7 through 9. At a pH above 10, there is an increase in viscosity and at a pH below 4.0, the viscosity decreases significantly due to hydrolysis of the polymer [50].

Carboxymethylcellulose solutions have poor tolerance for electrolytes especially di- and trivalent cations, as they precipitate the polymer. CMC is compatible with other nonionic cellulose derivatives, clays, and commonly used preservatives but is incompatible with cationic drugs [50].

b. *Microcrystalline Cellulose.* Some forms of microcrystalline cellulose (MCC), such as Avicels (FMC Corp.), provide for a smoother, more uniform suspension vehicle. MCC is a linear, long-chain cellulose polmer. The Avicel MCC grades used in aqueous dispersions are Avicel RC/CL. These products are made by adding sodium carboxymethyl cellulose of medium viscosity (89%) to MCC.

Avicel RC 591 is not water soluble, but disperses quickly in water. Avicel RC 591 gels are highly thixotropic with finite yield values at low concentrations. Its use in a formulation results in a well-structured suspension vehicle that will retard phase separation.

Avicel RC 591 dispersions are stable over a wide pH range (4 to 11), and show little change in their viscosity after exposure to increased temperatures, or after being subjected to freeze and thaw cycles. Avicel RC 591 is compatible with other hydrocolloid clays, and most preservatives and colorants, but is incompatible with cationic drugs and electrolytes [51].

c. *Hydroxypropyl Methylcellulose.* Hydroxypropyl methylcellulose (HPMCs) are linear polymers consisting of polymeric anhydro-glucose (cellulose) units to which a methyl and hydroxypropyl substitution have been attached (Fig. 6). Commercial designations of HPMC products are based on their viscosity values at room temperature [52].

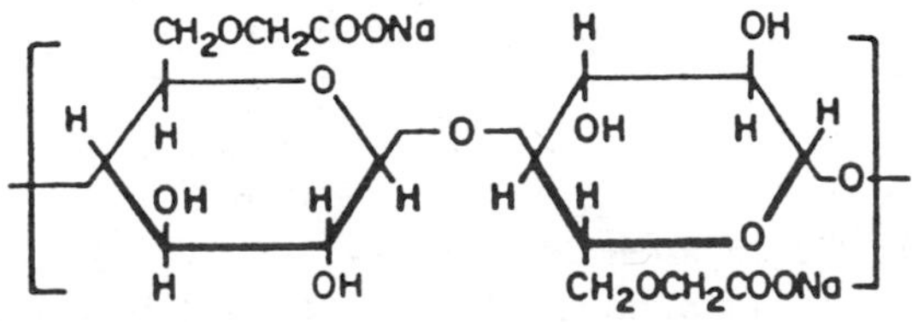

Fig. 5 Structure of sodium carboxymethylcellulose.

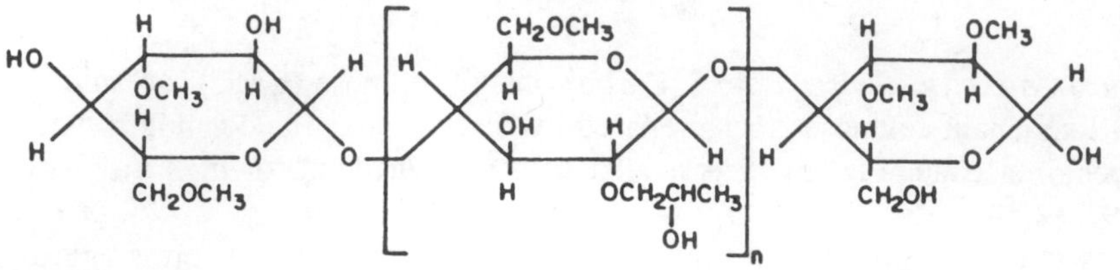

Fig. 6 Structure of hydroxypropyl methylcellulose.

Hydroxypropyl methylcellulose swells in water with successive hydration and its solutions are prepared by dispersion in hot water (about 80°C) with agitation to assure better wetting, followed by the addition of cold water or even ice to obtain proper temperature (0 to 5°C) for optimal hydration. [52]. HPMC forms a clear solution and the apparent viscosity is proportional to the molecular weight or chain length of the polymer. In general, the solution of a high molecular weight HPMC exhibits pseudoplastic flow.

The rheology of an aqueous solution of HPMC is affected by temperature, pH, and the presence of other solutes. Because HPMC is nonionic, the viscosity of its solution is generally stable over a wide pH range. On prolonged exposure to a pH above 10 or below 3, HPMC solutions exhibit a permanent reduction of viscosity caused by hydrolysis of the polymer. It also degrades at high temperatures as well, a factor that should be considered for the shelf life of the product.

HPMC solutions have better tolerance for electrolytes than CMC solutions do, but electrolytes in large concentration precipitate HPMC from solution [52]. HPMC is compatible with preservatives, other celluloses, and clay-type suspending agents as well as other excipients used in pharmaceutical suspensions.

2. *Xanthan Gum*

Xanthan gum is a high molecular weight, specially designed anionic polysaccharide that functions as a hydrocolloid and suspending agent. Xanthan gum contains three different monosaccharides: mannose, glucose, and glucuronic acid (as salt). Each repeating block of polymer chain has five sugar units (two glucose, two mannose, one glucuronic acid). The main chain is made of β-D-glucose units linked through the 1 and 4 positions. The two mannose units and glucuronic acid units make up the side chain. The terminal β-D-mannose unit is glycosidically linked to the 4 position of β-D-glucuronic acid, which in turn is linked to the 2 position of α-D-mannose. This side chain is linked to the 3 position of every other glucose residue on average in the polymer main chain. Roughly half of the terminal D-mannose residue carries a pyruvic acid residue linked ketolically to the 4 and 6 positions,. The non-terminal D-mannose unit on the side chain has an acetyl group at the 6 position (Fig. 7).

Xanthan gum is soluble in hot and cold water and imparts high viscosity at low concentration with pseudoplastic flow characteristics [53]. Aqueous xanthan gum systems exhibit gel behavior at a very low pH. Gel persistence under shear, viscosity, and pseudoplasticity all increase with xanthan gum concentration [54]. Compared to other cellulosic agents and or polysaccharides, xanthan gum solutions are unusually resistant

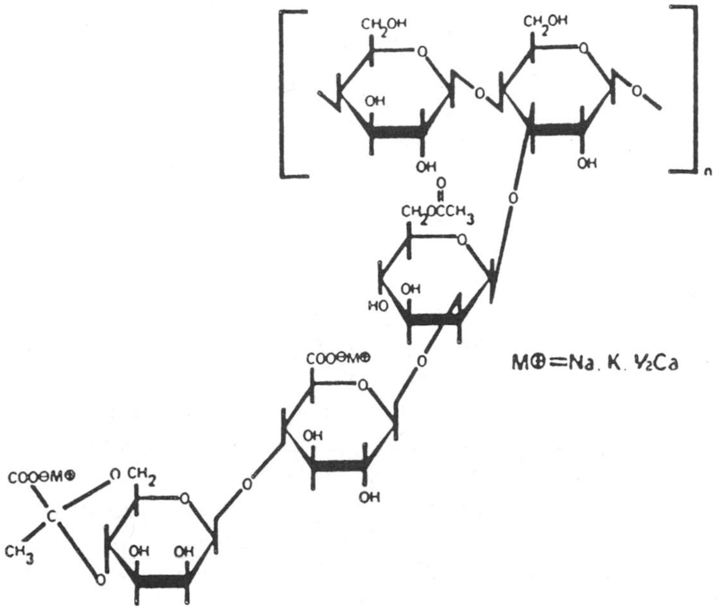

Fig. 7 Structure of xanthan gum. (Reproduced from the *Kelco Xanthan Gum Booklet*, 5th ed., with permission of proprietor Merck & Co., Inc., Kelco Division, San Diego.)

to prolonged shear. A 1% xanthan gum solution sheared at 46,000 reciprocal seconds for 1 hour exhibited no significant loss of viscosity [53].

Temperature has very little effect on the viscosity of xanthan gum solutions. The small change in viscosity that does occur with temperature is reversible [53]. This temperature independence of viscosity is unique to xanthan gum and is a very desirable attribute for product shelf life. Products containing xanthan gum stored at elevated temperatures are stable and exhibit minimal loss of viscosity. There is no significant change in the viscosity of a solution over a wide pH range of 1 to 10.

Solutions of xanthan gum are compatible with virtually all mono- and divalent cations like sodium, calcium, and magnesium over a wide pH range and with many pharmaceutical adjuvants such as polyols, alcohol, acidulants, chelating agents, and preservatives. Because of its anionic nature, xanthan gum is incompatible with cationic drugs and preservatives. It is not influenced by a freeze–thaw cycle and is resistant to enzymatic degradation. However, xanthan gum solutions are susceptible to microbiological degradation on prolonged storage and do require a preservative to maintain the microbial integrity of the product.

3. Carbomer

Carbomer resins are high molecular weight polymers of acrylic acid (Fig. 8). They are available in several grades. The choice of the proper carbomer resin may require evaluation of all grades because formulations must often meet several requirements.

Carbomers represent a family of polymers that impart plastic behavior to aqueous systems at a relatively low concentration. Nearly any required level of viscosity can be achieved by simply adjusting the concentration of polymer. Initial viscosity development

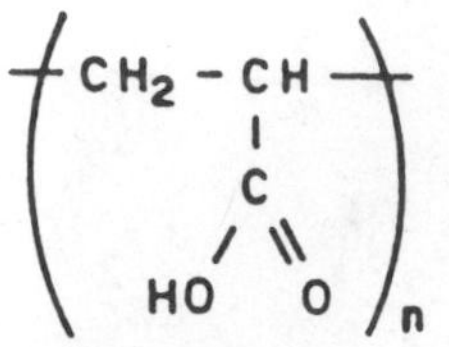

$$\left(\!\begin{array}{c} CH_2 - CH \\ | \\ C \\ \diagup \ \diagdown\diagdown \\ HO \quad O \end{array}\!\right)_n$$

Fig. 8 Structure of polyacrylic acid.

occurs as a result of partial swelling of the polymer by water molecules. Final swelling along with the development of viscosity and yield value occurs when the acid polymer is neutralized with an organic or inorganic base [55]. Irrespective of the type of carbomer resin, neutralization is essential to develop the unique rheological properties of these resins. Much of the work on carbomer rheology has been summarized by Barry [56]. At low concentration, carbomer solutions are pseudoplastic, becoming plastic at higher concentrations. The combination of yield value and high consistency accounts for their good suspending properties. Meyer and Cohen [57] made permanent suspensions of silica and using 0.25% carbomer. For the same stability of suspension, 3% polysaccharide gum concentration was required. Their work showed that the formation of a permanent suspension is dependent on the critical yield value and not the viscosity. Berney and Deasy [58] indicated the suitability of carbomer[e] to prepare a pharmaceutically stable, nonsedimenting, readily pourable suspension of 10% sulfadimidine [58]. Swafford and Nobles [59] successfully developed a topical suspension of calamine and neocalamine using carbomer.

The viscosity of carbomer resin is influenced by temperature and pH. Carbomer resins are not subject to hydrolysis or oxidation under normal conditions and resist thinning at elevated temperatures when exposed for a short period of time but there is a loss of viscosity after prolonged exposure. Carbomer resin solutions offer maximum viscosity control at pH 5.5, but loss of viscosity and precipitation of acrylic acid polymer occur at a lower pH.

Even a small amount of soluble electrolyte decreases the viscosity and the efficiency of carbomer solutions. Salts cause deswelling, and divalent salts cause more drastic loss of viscosity than monovalent salts. Carbomer resins are compatible with commonly used formula excipients and hydrocolloids.

The stability of carbomer resin solutions is sensitive to ultraviolet (UV) light, which causes a significant reduction in the viscosity. The combination of a chelating agent such as the sodium salt of ethylenediaminetetraacetic acid and a water-soluble UV absorber is an effective stabilizer for carbomer resin against UV light [55]. Carbomer resin solutions are not attacked by bacteria and fungi; however, they do not prevent their growth in aqueous system [55].

New entries into the market are the new water-swellable, high molecular weight cross-linked polymers and copolymers of acrylic acid marketed by BF Goodrich under the trade names Pemulen® and Noveon®. By modifying cross-link types and levels as well as hydrophilic comonomer characteristics in cross-linked polymers, a wide range of performance characteristics can be achieved [60]. Pemulen are high molecular weight polymers with larger hydrophilic and smaller oleophilic portions. Pemulen are compatible with a broad spectrum of raw materials used in topical formulations. Pemulen require neutralization to desired pH with water-soluble base to impart swelling properties. Pemulen have limited tolerance for electrolytes and are incompatible with cationics.

4. *Magnesium Aluminum Silicate*

Various inorganic clays have the property of swelling in water. Important representatives of this group are colloidal aluminum silicates, bentonite, and magnesium aluminum silicate (MAS), which are differentiated by their crystal structure.

Magnesium aluminum silicate is derived from natural smectite clays characterized by an expanding lattice structure [61]. It is preferable to other clays because of its whiter color and greater uniformity. Several grades of MAS are available that differ in viscosity, particle size, acid demand, and salt stability.

Water dispersions of 1% to 2% MAS are thin but increase in viscosity with an increased concentration of MAS. These dispersions exhibit pseudoplastic rheological behavior with yield value and impart thixotropy to the suspension. Hence, MAS functions well as a suspending agent. It is a superior suspending agent because it prevents caking without affecting pourability or spreadability of the suspension.

Magnesium aluminum silicate dispersions are influenced by heat, and the viscosity of the dispersion increases on prolonged exposure to elevated temperatures. Magnesium aluminum silicate is stable over a wide pH range of 6 to 11.

Electrolytes also thicken MAS dispersions because MAS is partially flocculated by electrolytes [61]. This increases both the viscosity and the yield value.

Magnesium aluminum silicate is compatible with many commonly used formula adjuvants, especially anionic and nonionic hydrocolloids. Syman observed that blends of MAS and CMC provide synergistic viscosity and excellent electrolyte tolerance, combining the high yield value of MAS and the smooth flow properties of CMC [62]. Schumacher [63] uses blends of MAS with CMC and other gums in an antacid suspension and observed that MAS in the flocculated state enhanced the stability of the antacid suspensions. For a synergistic effect, MAS/CMC ratios of 9:1 to 2:1 are most commonly used. Ciullo [64] investigated rheological properties of MAS and xanthan gum combinations (Fig. 9). A minor inclusion of xanthan gum in MAS dispersions provided synergism in both the viscosity and the yield value. The combination showed a modification of the thixotropy of MAS in the presence of xanthan gum. The excellent yield value obtained suggest superior stabilization of the suspension [64].

Magnesium aluminum silicate dispersions allow the growth of bacteria, and need a bacteriostat to maintain their microbiological integrity. Magnesium aluminum silicate possesses cation exchange capacity and drug adsorption properties for various cationic and nonionic drugs. Anionic drugs are found to be weakly bound [65].

C. Buffers

A large number of modern therapeutic agents are either weak acids or weak bases. Their physicochemical properties, therapeutic efficacy, and stability can be influenced by a change in the pH of their environment. The same is true of organic excipients, such as preservatives, suspending agents, and chelating agents, used in the formulation of a suspension. Furthermore, buffer salts may also act as flocculating agents. Thus, the selection of a proper buffer to maintain optimum pH is critical. The selection of a buffer should meet the following criteria [66]:

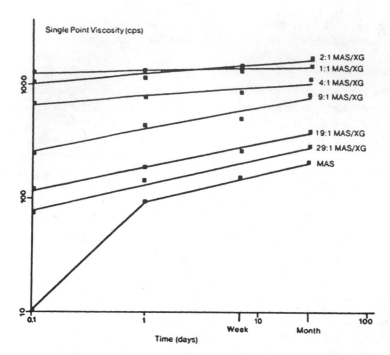

Fig. 9 Three percent magnesium aluminum silicate/xanthan gum dispersions showing progressive flattening of the MAS aging curve with increasing levels of XG. (From Ref. 64. Reprinted with permission from the publisher, the Society of Cosmetic Chemists, New York.)

1. A buffer must have adequate buffer capacity in the desired pH range.
2. A buffer must be compatible with the flocculating agent.
3. A buffer must be biologically safe for the intended use.
4. A buffer should have little or no deleterious effect on the stability or efficacy of the product.
5. A buffer should permit incorporation of an acceptable flavor, fragrance, and color in the product.

Windheuser [67] has reported commonly used buffers and their effective buffer ranges (Fig. 10).

D. Humectants and Cosolvents

Humectants and cosolvents are used as formula adjuvants in oral as well as in topical suspensions. Humectants such as glycerin, sorbitol, and polyethylene glycol retard the crystallization of solubilized solids in an aqueous suspension. They impart desired consistency and good taste and help prevent "cap locking." Cosolvents increase the solubility of weak electrolytes or nonpolar molecules in water. These nonpolar molecules may include the preservatives, antioxidants, flavors, or fragrances. Generally, the drugs in suspension should exhibit practically no solubility in the cosolvent or humectant chosen. Commonly used cosolvents are alcohol, polyethylene glycol, propylene glycol and 1,3-butylene glycol. These are acceptable for use in oral as well as in topical preparations.

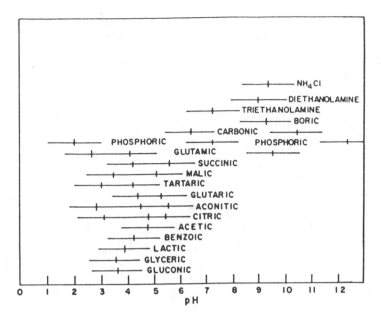

Fig. 10 Commonly used pharmaceutical buffers and their effective buffer ranges. (From Ref. 67. Reprinted with permission from the publisher, Parenteral Drug Association, Philadelphia.)

E. Preservatives

Stringent regulatory and compendial limits coupled with numerous product recalls have increased the importance of formulating a well-preserved suspension. Injectable and ophthalmic suspensions must be sterile, but oral and topical suspensions that come into prolonged contact with tissues and organs of the human body must meet very high standards of microbial integrity. Microbial growth is a potential health hazard and a source of infection. All oral and topical suspensions must be free of pathogens such as *Escherichia coli, Pseudomonas aeruginosa, Staphylococcus aureus, Candida albicans, Aspergillus niger,* and *Salmonella* species [49].

The presence of microorganisms is not only hazardous to the health of patients but can also bring about undesirable physicochemical changes in the suspension. The physical changes may include discoloration, loss of viscosity and modification of rheological behavior, and gas and odor formation. The chemical changes may include hydrolysis of drug or formula excipients such as hydrocolloid and preservative, inactivation of the preservative system, change in pH, and so forth.

Preservation of a suspension poses several problems to a formulator. Suspensions may contain carbohydrates, clay, polysaccharides, electrolytes, gum, cellulose derivatives, surfactant, polar solvent, and other excipients, many of which are excellent nutrients for the growth of microorganisms. Processing containers, equipment, packaging components, and operators may also contribute to the microbial contamination of the product.

Therefore, pharmaceutical suspensions should contain an antimicrobial preservative that will eliminate infecting microorganisms (bacteria, yeast, and fungi) and should be manufactured and packaged in accordance with current Good Manufacturing Practices.

Factors affecting the efficacy of a preservative include solubility in aqueous phase, partitioning between polar and nonpolar phases, dissociation due to change in pH, and interaction with the other ingredients in the formula. Though none exists, an ideal preservative should have a broad spectrum of activity; be capable of sustained action; have few chemical or physical incompatibilities; be effective over a wide pH range and not influence the pH of product; be nontoxic, nonirritant, and nonsensitizing; be colorless and odorless (or nearly so); be economical; and be easily formulated [68].

From a large number of available preservatives, a formulator chooses a preservative system for a particular product. The formulator is aided by the knowledge of a few basic guidelines during each stage of development such as the history of similar raw materials and formulas, routes of administration, package design, frequency of use, manufacturing process and product life.

A preservative system usually consists of a combination of preservatives to ensure microbial integrity of the product in case one of the preservatives is inactivated either by a contaminant in the product or by one of the challenge organisms.

In a broad chemical sense, a preservative may be an alcohol, acid, ester, quaternary ammonium compound, phenol and its derivatives including halogenated phenols, or aldehyde and formaldehyde donors. The formaldehyde donors in combination with parabens are the most frequently used preservatives in topical suspensions. However, many of the aldehyde and formaldehyde donors are not approved for internal use. Table 6 gives a classification of some commonly used preservatives [68].

F. Sequestrants

The presence of metal ions causes oxidative degradation of many drugs and excipients used in suspensions. Metal ions in such cases act as catalysts in the degradation processes. Removal of these free metal ions from the formulation improves its integrity, acceptability, and stability. For the most part, sequestrants react with metal to form metal-sequestrant complexes and thereby block the reaction site of metal ions. In order to form a sequestrant-metal complex, two general conditions must be satisfied [69].

1. A sequestrant must have proper stearic and electronic configuration in relation to the metal being complexed.
2. The surrounding environment—such as pH, ionic strength, and solubility—must be conducive to complex formation.

The rate at which the metal-sequestrant complex is formed depends on the rate of rupture of the proceeding complex. In a well-defined system, relative inefficiency of different sequestrants for a given metal can be compared by inspecting the stability constant of each metal complex. Generally, the higher the stability constant (log K), the more stable is the metal-sequestrant complex. The stability constants of some metal-sequestrant complexes have been reported [69].

Some commonly used sequestrants in pharmaceuticals are ethylenediaminetetraacetic acid (EDTA) and its salts, citric acid, glutamic acid, 8-hydroxyquinoline, etc. The theoretical quantity of sequestrant required can be calculated but actual usage levels in the particular formula should be established in the laboratory by the formulator.

G. Antioxidants

Many polydisperse preparations deteriorate on storage because the therapeutic agent or the adjuvant is subject to oxidative degradation. The degradation can result in reduced potency of the drug or a change in the color, odor, taste, viscosity, or other characteristic of the product.

Table 6 Limited Chemical Classification of Some Contemporary Preservatives

Acids and their salts	Esters	Quaternary compounds	Phenols	Formaldehyde and formalde-hyde donors	Miscellaneous
Benzoic acid and its salt	Methylparaben	Benzalkonium chloride	Ottasept		Ethyl alcohol
Formaldehyde	Benzyl alcohol				Myacide SP
	Propylparaben	Cetylpyridinium chloride	Irgasan DP 300	Bronopol	Kathon CG
Sorbic acid and its salts	Butylparaben			Ucarcide	Oxadine A
		Benzethonium chloride		MDMH	Omadine
				Dowicil 200	Phenoxetox
				Germall II	
				Germall 115	
				Glydant	

Source: Ref. 68.

Many pharmaceuticals are prone to autoxidation, a free radical reaction initiated by UV radiation in the presence of a trace amount of oxygen. The autoxidation may be catalyzed by metal ions. The addition of a small amount of an antioxidant inhibits the formation of highly reactive free radicals and the chain reaction by providing a hydrogen atom or an electron to the free radical.

Antioxidants are classified into two major groups. True antioxidants such as butylated hydroxyanisole (BHA), tocopherols, and alkyl gallates perform by blocking and breaking the free radical chain reaction. These antioxidants are generally oil soluble. A second group of antioxidants is composed of reducing agents such as sodium bisulfate and ascorbic acid, which have a lower redox potential than the chemical they protect. They are preferentially oxidized and also react with free radicals. They are generally water soluble.

An ideal antioxidant should be nontoxic, nonirritant, and nonsensitizing as well as effective in low concentration. It should be odorless, tasteless, colorless, stable over a wide pH range, and compatible with formula excipients. Its decomposition products should be nontoxic and nonirritant.

The selection of an antioxidant can be made on sound theoretical grounds based on the difference of redox potential between the drug and the antioxidant. In practice, however, a combination of two antioxidants and a chelating agent or a weak acid has been found to be more effective [56]. The comparative value of an antioxidant's efficiency is measured by subjecting the pharmaceutical system to standard oxidative conditions and periodically analyzing for the drug and the antioxidants [70].

H. Colors

Colors are incorporated into pharmaceutical oral or topical suspensions for several reasons. First, colors give aesthetic appeal and impart pleasing appearance to the product, thereby providing it with a marketing advantage. Second, colors may be used to identify products or similar appearance or to mask the discolored degraded excipient or drug, thereby maintaining the appearance of the formulation for its entire shelf life. Finally, colors help minimize the possibility of a mix-up during manufacture.

Dyes and other organic colorants may degrade via oxidation, hydrolysis, photolysis, or other routes, and their solubility and stability may be pH dependent. Before selecting a dye for a particular formulation, its physicochemical properties should be examined.

Dyes are incorporated into a suspension as aqueous solutions. At times it may be necessary to utilize a combination of a water-soluble dye and an inorganic pigment to obtain homogeneity of color and the desired shade.

A formulator should use only FD&C colors or D&C colors in oral suspensions. Additionally, one can use D&C external colors for topical suspensions. However, not all colorants are universally approved and each country has its own list of approved colorants. For example, FD&C Red No. 40 is an approved colorant for food, drugs, and cosmetics in the United States, but its use is not approved in Canada. On the other hand, FD&C Red No. 2 (amaranth) is approved in Canada but its use is prohibited in the United States. The list of approved colors and dyes is revised on a continuing basis.

Hence, before formulating a product that may be marketed in several countries, it would be wise to check the current status of each dye in each country. Dye suppliers are excellent sources of information on this subject. Such information may also be obtained from the Division of Colors & Cosmetics of the Food and Drug Administration. Colorants currently in use are listed in CTFA International Color Handbook [71].

I. Fragrances

Even a well-designed topical pharmaceutical suspension with optimum efficacy, safety, and stability requires the aesthetic appeal necessary to ensure patient acceptability. An unpleasantly scented product may result in patient noncompliance and in the possibility of the patient switching to a competitive product. Odor of the product can be a determining factor between commercial success or failure for an OTC product. Although consumers may not apply as stringent criteria of acceptability to a pharmaceutical suspension as to a cosmetic suspension, one would still prefer a product that has a pleasant odor—or at least no unpleasant odor. Fragrances are used to mask an unpleasant odor and impart aesthetic appeal to the product.

VII. PREPARATION OF A SUSPENSION

A suspension can be prepared by the precipitation method or by the dispersion method. The precipitation method is tedious, complex, and time consuming. The precipitation of a drug can be accomplished by controlling the pH or by the use of appropriate solvents. This method is not widely used for the preparation of oral or topical suspensions. The dispersion method utilizes dispersion of fine particles in an appropriate vehicle.

The development of a suspension formula involves some degree of trial and error. Several trial formulations are produced to include the optimum level of excipients needed to impart the desired physical attributes. Suspensions can be formulated by any of the following three methods [4] as illustrated in Fig. 11.

1. Deflocculated suspension in a structured vehicle as the final product
2. Flocculated suspension as the final product
3. Flocculated suspension in a structured vehicle as the final product

All three methods of preparation require uniform dispersion of the deflocculated particles and preparation of an appropriate vehicle. The decision of whether to develop a deflocculated or flocculated suspension will be determined by the physicochemical properties of the drug and its application. Generally, suspensions developed with controlled flocculation in a structured vehicle are preferred. As a rule, the steps involved in the preparation of such formulations on laboratory batch or small pilot batch scale are:

1. Preparation of a dispersion of the drug
2. Preparation of a structured vehicle, followed by addition of the drug dispersion
3. Addition of other formula adjuncts
4. Deaeration, followed by making up to final volume
5. Homogenization

A. Drug Dispersion

In the preparation of a suspension, particle-particle attractive forces among powder particles may be overcome by high shear action of a colloid mill or by the use of a wetting agent. Normally, an anionic surfactant is preferred but nonionics may also be

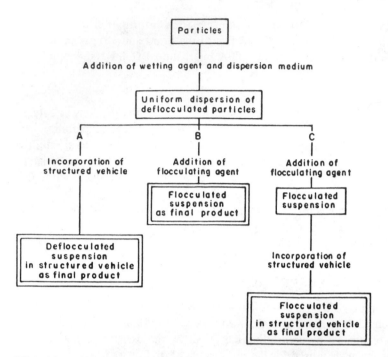

Fig. 11 Alternative approaches to the formulation of suspensions. (From Ref. 4, p. 296, Reprinted with permission from the publisher, Mack Publishing Co., Easton, PA.)

used. The minimum amount of wetting agent should be used. A concentrated solution of the wetting agent in the vehicle may be used to prepare the slurry. The drug-dispersion slurry may be prepared through a colloid mill[f] (Gaulin type) to provide optimum wetting. Alcohol or glycerin may be used in the initial stages to disperse the particles and facilitate the penetration of the vehicle into the powder mass. Alternately, the drug can be dispersed by slow addition to the water or to a water-glycerol system containing a wetting agent.

B. Preparation of Structured Vehicle and Addition of Drug Dispersion

Structured vehicles are aqueous solutions of suspending agents: hydrocolloids, polysaccharides, clays, or a combination of these. The vehicle suspension may be water, glycerin alone, or a combination of several solvents. Usually a structured vehicle is preferred.

The uniform dispersion of hydrocolloids or clays in water is the key to rapid preparation of the vehicle. Generally speaking, a warm medium hydrates hydrocolloids/clays more readily and is preferred over a cold medium, though not all hydrocolloids require a warm medium. A solution of hydrocolloid or drug can be made in short time if the dry hydrocolloid is dispersed properly. Clays however, take more time to hydrate. Subsequent to the preparation of a structured vehicle, the drug dispersion may be added to it. Any one of the following methods can be employed to obtain good dispersions of hydrocolloids or clays: high shear mixer, use of an eductor, or dry mixing.

1. *High-Shear Mixing*

Good dispersion can be achieved with a high-shear mixture that develops a good vortex. Alternatively, a rotor-stator processing system can be utilized. The powdered hydrocolloid should be sifted slowly into the upper wall of the vortex so that individual granules are wetted. The addition should be completed before thickening destroys the vortex and starts to incorporate air into the system.

2. *Use of an Eductor*

Possibly the best dispersion of a hydrocolloid can be obtained by using a funnel and mixing eductor (Fig. 12). Sufficient water is added to the tank fitted with a high-shear mixer. The mixer is turned on, and the hydrocolloid is poured into a funnel that is attached to the top of an aspirator while the water is running. In this process, individual particles are coated with water before reaching the bulk of water in the tank and subsequent lumping of the hydrocolloid is prevented.

3. *Dry Mix Dispersion*

Often a formulation contains other water-soluble ingredients like citric acid that can be preblended with a hydrocolloid to facilitate dispersion. A blend of hydrocolloid and other dry ingredients is added slowly to water with high-shear mixing, and dispersion of the hydrocolloid is attained in a short time.

4. *Addition of Other Formula Adjuncts*

Formula adjuncts such as a chelating agent, antioxidant, humectant, preservative, color, and fragrance are added to the vehicle directly or are presolubilized in an appropriate

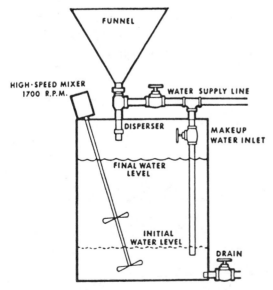

Fig. 12 Typical installation of Kelco funnel and mixing eductor. (Reproduced from the *Kelco Xanthan Gum Booklet*, 5th ed., with permission of proprietor Merck & Co., Inc., Kelco Division, San Diego.)

cosolvent. Generally, preservatives such as propylparaben, fragrances, and antioxidants require presolubilization in a cosolvent such as propylene glycol or alcohol before their addition to the aqueous medium. The time of addition and the temperature at the time of addition of some excipients will depend on their physicochemical properties. Usually, temperature-sensitive materials such as fragrances are added at a relatively low temperature and generally toward the end of the manufacturing process.

C. Deaeration and Making Up to Final Volume

The batch is processed through deaerating equipment just prior to making up to final volume. A suspension with a large amount of entrapped air will not be pharmaceutically acceptable because excess air will affect the rheological properties, drug dosage, color, density, and fill volume.

D. Homogenization

Finally, the suspension is passed through a homogenizer to efficiently reduce the particles dispersed phase.

VIII. PILOT PLANT SCALE-UP

Scientists expend large amounts of time developing topical suspension formulations that not only meet the criteria of safety, efficacy, and stability, but also conform to exacting specifications. In addition, the laboratory formulas should be reproducible on large-scale production equipment at a reasonable cost. To be acceptable, a formula must be capable of being manufactured and packaged in commercial quantities, often with equipment that only remotely resembles the laboratory equipment.

Often it is necessary and advisable to scale up laboratory formulas in a pilot plant. The goal, then, of a pilot plant is to facilitate the transfer of the product from laboratory into mass production. The ease with which a new product and its manufacturing processes are brought into routine production reflect the effectiveness of the pilot plant [72].

Suspensions require more attention during scale-up than do simple solutions because of additional processing. Variability in the quality of a product may result from:

1. Raw materials
2. Equipment
3. Processing

Early intelligent decisions to define and control these variables can yield significant economic benefits, as well as prevent unnecessary headaches and delays. If necessary, it is not unusual to make slight modifications in product formulas and processes in order to meet the demands of production equipment.

A. Raw Materials

One of the responsibilities of pilot plant function is approval and validation of active and inactive raw materials in a given formula. Even a slight change in morphology, particle size and particle size distribution, or rate of solubility may result in different bulk density, density ratio charge, flow properties and handling properties, or raw materials and ultimately may alter the quality and integrity of the product [72]. Reliance on a single source of a raw material may leave a company vulnerable with respect to supplies and price. Evaluation of alternate suppliers, approval of raw material, or any change in the specifications of raw material require that several batches of the product be prepared with each raw material and their performance in the formulation and stability of finished product be compared to standard product [72].

B. Processing Equipment

Formulation development work on a topical suspension is usually carried out with relatively simple equipment. For example, addition and dispersion of suspending agents—which on a laboratory scale—may merely involve sprinkling the material into a liquid vortex may require the use of a vibrating feeder or other novel approaches of dispersion in the pilot plant and manufacturing procedure [73].

Additionally, the manufacturing of topical suspensions requires several pieces of equipment. Many types and variations of mixing, dispersion, particle size reduction, and filling equipment can be used to manufacture a suspension. By selecting a given type of equipment, not only are certain operating techniques made possible as a result of the individual capabilities of the equipment, [72] but also there is the opportunity to produce a product with desirable physical and chemical attributes while maintaining economical production.

It is essential that the equipment used during scale-up be the same as that which would be used in the final manufacturing process of the product. Pilot plant design and equipment are available from manufacturers of full-sized production equipment. Ideally, the pilot plant laboratory will have the equipment to prepare batches in volumes in the 10 to 100 liter range.

Based on known characteristics of processing, types of mixers, homogenizers, filters, and filling equipment, each with its own advantages and limitations, should be critically examined. The selection of each piece of equipment will depend on the state of matter of the dispersed phase. Tabibi [74] has listed various mixers and mills generally used in the preparation of disperse systems.

C. Processing

Once the manufacturing process has been proposed and accepted, and various pieces of equipment needed to mix, mill, homogenize, filter, and fill have been evaluated and selected, the next step in the scale-up and transfer of laboratory formula to production is to analyze "process parameters flexibility."

Process parameters flexibility analyzes a number of operating parameters such as [75]:

1. Rate and order of addition of components
2. Mixing rate and intensity
3. Mixing time
4. Rate of heating and overall time
5. Rate of cooling and overall time

6. Homogenization (particle size reduction, condition and effectiveness)
7. Filter screen size

All these process parameters can be critical to the production of a stable product. Experience has shown that a vast number of process parameters will ultimately affect the physicochemical or microbiological attributes of topical suspensions. Knowledge of the effects of these critical process parameters on "in-process" and finished product quality is the basis for process optimization and validation. For example, mixing at too high a speed may result in an incorporation of excessive air into the product—which if not removed can influence the stability of the product. The temperature, rate of addition, and time required to hydrate suspending agents are often critical; unless this hydration process is complete, the suspension may not conform to its specifications. Topical suspensions should be constantly agitated or recirculate these during transfer, otherwise solids may "settle out," resulting in loss of homogeneity of drug in the product.

During the scale-up process, critical process parameters, (mixing rate, mixing time, rate of cooling, rate of heating, homogenization, etc.) should be altered intentionally to ascertain the resultant effects on product quality and yield. Such process data should be accumulated from a series of batches. For example, if a colloid mill is used for homogenization in the scale-up process, several variations in experimental variables should be considered to determine the aperture setting, RPM, length of process time required, and so on. If the data show that the homogenization process parameters repeatedly produced a similar product that conforms to specifications, then the process has been validated.

Current Good Manufacturing Practice regulations require that manufacturing processes be validated so as to demonstrate quantitatively that a manufacturing process does what it purports to do.

To initiate the validation process, a set of specification ranges of desired characteristics should be established. For a topical suspension, for example, a specification range should be established for important characteristics including appearance, pH, density, viscosity, particle size, sedimentation volume, zeta potential, total drug content, and drug content uniformity.

It is necessary that all the information from each of these validation runs be documented in order to know what was done and to provide a record of the conditions under which the experiment was conducted. Validation runs should include a condition that puts the most stress on the process (worst case), thereby making it most likely that the product characteristic will fall outside specifications. Process specifications can then be established to ensure that this "worst case" condition will not occur.

A checklist of GMP items that should be part of scale-up includes the following:

1. Equipment qualification
2. Process validation
3. Regularly scheduled preventive maintenance of equipment
4. Regular process review and revalidation
5. Relevant Standard Operating Procedure
6. Use of competent technically qualified personnel
7. Adequate provision for training of personnel
8. A well-developed technology transfer system
9. Validated cleaning procedures
10. Orderly arrangement of equipment so as to ease material flow and prevent cross-contamination

Table 7 details some problems and suggested remedies in preparation, scale-up, and production of topical suspensions [51].

IX. EVALUATION OF A SUSPENSION

There are many dimensions of a suspension dosage form that are indicative of its quality, stability, acceptance, and performance. Appearance, color, odor, pH, density, viscosity, sedimentation parameters, ease of redispersibility, particle size, zeta potential, dissolution, labeled potency, microbial integrity, and human safety are all important parameters to consider in evaluating suspensions.

A. Sedimentation Parameters

The study of sedimentation includes two different parameters: sedimentation volume and degree of flocculation.

1. *Sedimentation Volume*

In an acceptable suspension the sediment formed should be easily redispersed to yield a homogeneous (uniform) product. The sedimentation volume F is defined as the ratio of the final, equilibrium volume of the sediment, V_u to the total volume, V_o, before settling, as expressed in Eq. 9 [40].

$$F = \frac{V_u}{V_o} \times 100 \tag{9}$$

where
 F = sedimentation volume
V_u = volume of sediment and
V_o = volume of suspension before settling

For example, if 200 ml (V_o) of a well-shaken formulation is placed in a graduated cylinder and it is found that the equilibrium volume of sediment V_u is 40 ml then

$$F = \frac{40}{200} = 0.2$$

Calculated as percentage sedimentation,

$$F = \frac{40}{200} \times 100 = 20\%$$

Usually, the higher the value of F, the more acceptable the product.

2. *Degree of Flocculation*

A more useful parameter to measure sedimentation is the degree of flocculation (β). Sedimentation volume F gives only a qualitative account of flocculation. The degree of flocculation is calculated by using Eq. (10)

$$\beta = \frac{\text{Ultimate sediment volume of flocculated suspension}}{\text{Ultimate sediment volumne of deflocculated suspension}} \tag{10}$$

Table 7 Some Problems, Causes, and Suggested Remedies in Production of Suspensions

Problem	Cause	Remedy
Caking	Crystal growth, fusing of crystals, to form aggregates	Modify particle size characteristic Increase density and viscosity of vehicle Check zeta potential Formulate a flocculated system
	Deflocculated systems	Apply controlled flocculation concept (See details in chapter)
Crystal growth	Polymorphism: combination of crystalline and amorphous entities	Lower interfacial tension to reduce free surface energy of particles Modify drug precipitation procedure
	Too much surfactant, causing drug to be solubilized and precipitated	Check surfactant concentration and HLB Change content of suspension vehicle
	Extreme differences in crystal size	Modify particle size reduction procedure to yield narrow particle size range
	Temperature changes resulting in cooling of an already saturated solution	Create protective coating around particles with protective colloids (barriers to free energy)
Deflocculation	Excessive electrolyte concentration	Check drug properties, surfactant, polymer content, electrolyte level Check ionic charge of drug, flocculating and suspending agents Try controlled flocculation
Drug potency (decrease)	Crystal growth	Check ionic charge of drug and suspending agent
	Suspension is not homogeneous	Check particle size and distribution
	Variations in particle size	Check ionic charge of flocculating and suspending agents
	Too large particle size Suspension is air-filled	Check mixing technique methods, filling methods

Observation	Action
pH change — Insufficient buffer system	Maximize buffer system, avoiding overuse of salts and buffers
Altered surface charge of particles	Check ionic character of drug, surfactant and polymers
Drug decomposition	Check drug stability, route of degradation, and decomposition products
Redispersibility (poor) — Bacteriological	Check preservative system
Deflocculation	Formulate a flocculated system; Apply controlled flocculation system
Settling — Particle size uniformity questionable	Modify particle size characteristics
Insufficient quantity of suspending agent—low yield value	Increase concentration of suspending agent in small increments to increase yield value
Flotation agent — Electrolyte effect	Check electrolyte quantities and ionic charges
Hydrophobic drug is not adequately wetted by suspension vehicle due to air adhering to the wetted or insufficiently unwetted particle	Use appropriate hydrophobic wetting—a nonionic surfactant to reduce contact angle at particle interface
Physical breakdown of suspension system (sudden, severe) — Severe flocculation of suspending agent	Check electrolyte content
Color change — Change in suspending agent; characteristics not detected by quality control check of specifications; Change in raw material manufacturing method	Check with raw material supplier to confirm lot conformity and method of manufacture
Dye reaction with drug or any excipient or formula; Poor color retention of colorant	Check reactivity properties of dye (colorant); Dye may decompose in light or air or at pH of vehicle
Suspension extremely air-filled	Deaerate product
Suspending agent is flocculating	Check electrolyte content
Fragrance change — Reactive fragrance constituents (Aldehydes oxidize, react easily with amines; esters hydrolyze at high pH, phenol aromatic amine, etc.)	Reexamine fragrance components relative to their organic chemical class

Source: Ref. 51.

that is,

$$\beta = \frac{F}{F_\infty}$$

where F_∞ is sedimentation volume of the deflocculated suspension.

The degree of flocculation is therefore an expression of increased sediment volume resulting from flocculation. If, for example, β has a value of 5.0 (Fig. 13), this means that the volume of sediment in a flocculated system is five times that in the deflocculated state. If a second flocculated formulation results in a value of β of, say, 6.5, this latter suspension obviously is preferred if the aim is to produce as flocculated a product as possible [4].

B. Ease of Dispersibility

Stanko and Dekay [76] first proposed the use of redispersibility to evaluate a pharmaceutical suspension. Various modifications of their basic principle have been described. Stanko and Dekay [76] placed a sedimented suspension in a 100 mL graduated cylinder and rotated it through 360° at 20 rpm. The end point was taken when the base of the graduated cylinder was free of sediment. The number of revolutions necessary to achieve the end point was recorded [76]. Matthews evaluated the above method to measure redispersibility of suspensions [77]. Dekay and Lesschaft [78] measured redispersibility by shaking in a 90° arc and not a complete revolution. The ultimate test of redispersibility is the uniformity of the suspended drug delivered from the product.

C. Rheological Measurements and Viscosity

The viscosity of suspensions can be of particular importance, especially for a topical suspension. It is important to measure viscosity at a low shear rate to evaluate the structure achieved on storage.

Viscometers are used to measure the viscosity of high shear rate systems as well as low shear rate systems. They are divided into two types:

1. Those that operate at a single rate of shear
2. Those that allow more than one shear rate to be examined

The first type is a useful quality-control tool. However, to measure the rheological behavior of plastic, pseudoplastic, or thixotropic materials, it has limited value as it only

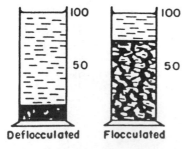

Fig. 13 Sedimentation parameters of suspensions. Deflocculated suspension: F = 0.15. Flocculated suspension: F = 0.75; B = 5.0. (From Ref. 4, p. 296. Reprinted with permission from the publisher, Mack Publishing Co., Easton, PA.)

provides a single point measurement on the rheogram. The second type of viscometer[j] is capable of operating at several shear rates and is therefore preferred because it develops the entire rheogram.

D. Zeta Potential Measurement

Zeta potential measurements are of significant importance to the physical stability of suspensions. Zeta potential can be measured in a microelectrophoresis cell. A sample of the disperse system is mounted on a special microscope slide across which a known potential is applied. The speed of movement of the particles across the field is a function of the zeta potential and is determined visually. The zetameter is a commercial micro-electrophoresis apparatus for easy, fast, and reproducible operations. This apparatus should be standardized using particles of known zeta potential [79].

E. Particle Size Measurement

Particle size measurements permit evaluation of aggregation or crystal growth. Any change in particle size affects the sedimentation rate, ease of redispersibility, caking, and efficacy properties of a disperse system. Commonly used techniques to estimate and detect changes in particle size are microscopy and use of the Coulter counter.[l] Particle size measurement can be rapid and simple or detailed and complex, depending upon the exact nature of the product.

F. Centrifugation

Centrifugation has been explored as a possible method of evaluating suspensions because sedimentation rate is influenced by the gravitational force. However, to date, no reliable correlation has been established to justify its application in establishing the performance or the stability of the suspension over its shelf life. However, it serves as an excellent tool to monitor batch to batch variation.

G. pH Measurement

pH is an important physical parameter as some drugs exhibit maximum stability at a specific pH value, and fluctuation in pH is not desirable. The measurement of the pH value provides good control over the manufacturing process and shelf life of the product.

H. Density Measurement

The density measurement provides qualitative information on the amount of air entrapped in a suspension during manufacture, floating of sedimentation, and lumping of dispersed particles. These measurements provide for better product control during production. There are several methods to measure density but the most widely used employ the precision hygrometer or a pycnometer.

I. Dissolution

In general, most dissolution apparatuses that are used for tablets or capsules can be employed to determine the dissolution rate of drug in suspension. The USP apparatus II (paddle) has been used frequently at a rotation speed of 25 to 50 rpm [47]. However, a rotating filter apparatus by Shah [80], as shown in Fig. 14, has gained wide accep-

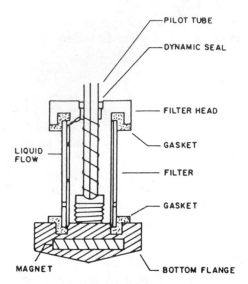

Fig. 14 Rotating filter assembly. (From Ref. 80. Reproduced with permission of the copyright owner, the American Pharmaceutical Association.)

tance for suspension testing because it provides mild laminar liquid agitation and functions as an in situ nonclogging filter [46].

J. Preservative Efficacy Test

A suspension is adequately preserved if it withstands a laboratory challenge test and resists microbial insults during manufacturing and use. Preservative efficacy testing enables the formulator to ensure microbial integrity of the product. In recognition of the importance of preservative efficacy testing, several officials and nonofficial guidelines have been developed such as the guidelines of the United States Pharmacopeia [49] and the guidelines of the Cosmetics, Toiletries and Fragrance Association [81].

K. Safety Tests

According to federal regulations administered by the Food & Drug Administration, pharmaceutical manufacturers must substantiate the safety of the pharmaceutical products they market and each ingredient contained in the product. The first stage of safety substantiation is preclinical toxicity testing, which includes acute oral toxicity; acute, subacute, and chronic dermal toxicity; skin irritation; eye irritation; and skin sensitization tests. These tests are performed using various species of animals, followed by human testing [81]. Each product must be individually tested for dermal toxicity, eye or skin irritation, photoallergic reaction, or other toxic side effects. To obtain information on toxicity, the test should be performed in a well-planned manner on the final product [81].

X. STABILITY

Drug stability is a critical element in the accurate and appropriate delivery of drug therapy. Both the therapeutic adequacy of treatment and safety of therapy can be adversely affected by drug instability. The necessity and importance of stability testing during the development of pharmaceutical testing is well recognized, not only by regulatory agencies, but also by the pharmaceutical industry. From regulatory considerations, there are several sections of the Federal Food and Drug & Cosmetics Act that relate to the stability of drug products [83].

A New Drug Application (NDA) requires a complete description of stability studies indicating the methods of analysis for the drug substance. If the drug does not meet criteria of stability and purity, it is considered adulterated [83].

It is required that all prescription drug products for human use have an "expiration date" with storage conditions on the labels. It is also required that the company producing the drug include a written description of the testing program to cover stability characteristics of the drug substance and drug product, and that this program be followed [84].

The purpose of stability testing is to provide evidence of the quality of the drug substance or drug product, and how it varies with time under the influence of a variety of environmental conditions (heat, humidity, light, air, etc.). Information gathered from stability testing enables the establishment of recommended storage conditions, retest periods, and shelf life [85]. A good stability program exposes the weaknesses of a product, demonstrates that weaknesses can be protected by a "barrier," and demonstrates that this barrier has no effect on the safety of efficacy of the dosage form.

The diversity of topical suspensions and the complexity of stability parameters precludes the existence of simple, rigid, and universally accepted stability guidelines. No single stability protocol could reasonably be expected to ensure the quality and integrity of every topical suspension from every manufacturer.

An important document relating to the stability testing of pharmaceuticals was first developed in 1984 and later updated in 1987 [86]. The FDA guidelines for submitting documentation for the stability of human drugs and biologicals are designed to give one an understanding of the stability performance of a given product. The process begins in the early development phases and continues through registration and monitoring of a marketed product. The guidelines give common definitions, such as the following:

Bulk drug substance: The pharmacologically active component of drug product before formulation [87].

Batch: A defined quantity of product processed in a single process or series of processes, so that the resultant product could be expected to be homogeneous [87].

Expiration date: The date placed on the immediate container label of drug product that designates the date through which the product is expected to remain within specifications, if stored correctly [88].

Accelerated stability testing: Studies designed to increase the rate of chemical and physical change of a drug by using exaggerated storage conditions (elevated and below normal temperatures, heat, high humidity, and light) as part of a formal stability-testing program [88].

Shelf life: The period during which a pharmaceutical product, if stored correctly, is expected to comply with specifications, as determined by stability studies on a number of batches of product. The shelf life is used to establish the expiration date of each batch [89].

Real-time stability studies: Evaluation of experiments to determine physical, chemical, biological and microbiological characteristics of a drug product during and beyond the expected time of shelf life and storage of samples at expected storage conditions in the intended market. The results are used to establish shelf life, as well as to confirm projected shelf life and recommended storage conditions [89].

Stability-indicating methodology: Quantitative analytical methods that are based on the characteristic structural, chemical, and biological properties of each active ingredient of the drug product, and that will distinguish each active ingredient from its degradation products, so that active ingredient content can be accurately measured [88]. The method should be specific, accurate, precise, reproducible, and rugged.

The guidelines include various phases of stability testing, reflecting the development of a suspension. Table 8 shows the phases and their activities.

Mounting concerns over duplication of data and continued debate over what constitutes sufficient data for registration of a pharmaceutical in different countries prompted the formation of an International Conference on Harmonization (ICH). It consists of a working group of experts from the European Community (EC), Japan, and the United States. ICH developed "The Guidelines on Stability of New Drug Substances and Products" in October 1993 [85]. Recognizing the potential of harmonization, the ICH has recommended adoption of the Guidelines by the regulatory agencies of all three Conference groups. The document has already been accepted in the EC, and is under review by the FDA and its counterpart in Japan.

Some advantages of harmonizing protocol design are:

1. Inherent simplicity for worldwide filing
2. Decreased stability testing for global products
3. Bracketing and matrix design permitted
4. Detailed photosensitivity testing

FDA guidelines, as well as the ICH Tripartite Guidelines, primarily address the information required in the registration applications for new molecular entities and associated drug products. Generally, these are prescription drug products that progress from IND status through NDA status. However, there are different storage conditions (such as the addition of RH to established temperatures) and minimum time requirements, as well as defined parameters for long-term accelerated testing for the generation of stability data required in the preparation of dossiers for registration in ICH guidelines.

Once the ICH Guidelines are adopted by the United States and Japan, the stability data generated in one country will be mutually acceptable to the EC, Japan, and the United States.

The stability testing protocols of generic and OTC products differ from studies of a product containing a New Chemical Entity (NCE). Manufacturers of generic products are not required to perform stability tests on the individual drug substances, only on the finished products. Such companies have access to (once) privileged information concerning drug substances and their stability. In reviewing an ANDA, the regulatory authorities may be able to establish a tentative shelf life for a potential product on the basis of minimal core data. The World Health Organization (WHO) has developed guidelines for stability testing of generic and OTC products for global distribution [88]. The guidelines primarily address the information required in the registration applications.

Table 8 Phase of Stability Testing

Protocol elements	Activities or results
Preformulation [87]	
Objectives	Determine any reactivities of the new drug substance
	Establish storage conditions and packaging requirements for the new drug substance
Study design	Short-term studies under accelerated conditions, looking for gross changes
Tests	Potency, appearance, physical properties, degradation products, etc.
	Storage conditions geared to possible degradative conditions of heat, light, moisture, oxidants, catalysts, pH, etc.
Schedules	As appropriate to allow estimates of stability parameters
Samples	Representative of the batch
Evaluation	Review of data to estimate relevant stability parameters
Excipient Compatibility [90]	
Objective	Delineate any interaction between probable formulation excipient and the drug substance
Study design	Short-term; accelerated studies designed to elucidate gross changes
Tests	Assay for potency and appearance; other tests
Storage conditions	Environment geared to probable degradative sensitivities—exaggerated heat, light, humidity, etc.
Schedules	Established on rate of degradation
Samples	Representative batch of the drug and selected excipients
Evaluation	Flexible and comparative
Study design	Short-term; accelerated studies designed to elucidate gross changes
Tests	Assay for potency and appearance; other tests
Storage conditions	Environment geared to probable degradative sensitivities—exaggerated heat, light, humidity, etc.
Schedules	Established on rate of degradation
Samples	Representative batch of the drug and selected excipients
Evaluation	Flexible and comparative

(continued)

Table 8 Continued

Protocol elements	Activities or results
Toxicology [90]	
Objectives	Ensure that potency and level of significant degradation products are documented throughout the life of the supplies
	Develop supporting data for subsequent stability studies of the formulated drug
Study design	Generally short to medium term
Tests	Assay for potency, significant degradation products and significant physical characteristics
Storage conditions	Under the same conditions as storage of clinical supplies
Schedule	More frequent testing for unstable drug
Samples	Representative of each formulation of toxicology supplies
Evaluation	Regular evaluation of data to ascertain continued suitability of the supplies, usually involving direct comparison with established criteria
Formulation Comparison [89]	
Objectives	Determine any physical formulation changes and significant drug substance degradation products
	Collect preliminary information on possible stability-limiting factors
Study design	Short-term studies under accelerated conditions, looking for gross changes
Tests	Potency, significant degradation products, physical properties, plus individual tests relevant to specific dosage forms
Storage conditions	Geared to possible degradative conditions of heat, light, moisture, etc.
Schedules	As appropriate to allow estimation of stability parameters
Samples	Representative of the batch
Evaluation	Direct comparison of raw data, comparison of rates, etc., to estimate relative stability parameters
Clinical Supplies [89]	
Objectives	Determine the values of the critical quality parameters of formulations utilized to establish safety and efficacy
	Ensure that only satisfactory material is used
Study design	Medium-term studies looking for changes in critical quality parameters
Tests	Basic attributes such as potency, significant degradation products, physical properties plus individual tests relevant to specific dosage form
Storage conditions	Conforming to label storage conditions
Schedules	More frequent for less stable formulations
Samples	Representative of each formulation and container-closure system
Evaluation	Periodic evaluation to ensure continued suitability of supplies by direct comparison to established specifications or statistical evaluation

Proposed Product [89]

Objectives
- Assess stability performance to define stability-limiting parameter factors and storage conditions
- Confirm degradation pathways in the market formulation
- Establish initial expiration-dating period

Study design
- Both short-term studies at accelerated conditions and long-term studies at proposed label storage conditions

Tests
- Potency, significant degradation products, physical properties, plus individual tests relevant to specific dosage form

Storage conditions
- Accelerated: geared to known reactivities

Schedules
- More frequent testing for less stable formulations

Samples
- Representatives of the formulation and container-closure systems; the least protective container-closure should be included

Evaluation
- Direct comparison of raw data with proposed standards or statistical analysis with a determined confidence level

Established Product [89]

Objectives
- Confirmation of stability performance determined in preceding stages

Study design
- Long-term studies

Tests
- Significant quality attributes as determined in preceding stages

Storage conditions
- Consistent with the label storage conditions

Schedules
- Based on relative stability of the product and the relative sensitivities of the various stability parameters

Samples
- Representatives of the product
- Lot selection rotated among the various marketed container-closure systems
- Periodic evaluations to allow timely decision making

Evaluation
- Evaluation by comparison of results with the established statistical profile

A. Stability Protocol

Design of stability testing protocols varies from product to product. A good protocol should allow a degree of flexibility that encompasses a variety of different practical situations and the various characteristics of the topical suspension being evaluated.

A stability protocol should be a written document that will demonstrate trends and provide predictive power in settling the choice of storage conditions. The program should include specifications and reliable and specific test methods, sample size, test intervals, storage conditions, and number of batches. For a topical suspension, physical, chemical, and microbiological characteristics should be examined: appearance, odor, density, total drug content, uniformity of drug content, redispersibility, dissolution, sedimentation volume, crystal size, pH, rheological behavior, and preservative efficacy.

The above specifications should cover features that are susceptible to change during storage conditions and that may influence quality, safety, and efficacy of the product.

Test Samples

For registration purposes of the product, samples from three production batches, or two production and one pilot lot, should be tested. Batches should be representative of the manufacturing process of pilot or production scale. Where possible, batches should be manufactured using different lots of drug substance as well as excipients.

B. Storage Test Conditions and Testing Frequency

The time length of studies and the storage conditions should be sufficient to reveal any possible instabilities caused by storage, shipment, and subsequent use. Current FDA guidelines and ICH Tripartite guidelines include different storage conditions. The details of storage conditions and testing frequency specifications are listed in Tables 9 and 10.

1. Accelerated (Stress) Stability Studies

Because most pharmaceutical suspensions contain organic drugs or excipients that may degrade via oxidation, photolysis, hydrolysis, racemization, or decarboxylation, their rate

Table 9 Current FDA Guidelines

Conditions	Storage time (months)											
	0	1	2	3	6	9	12	18	24	36	48	60
50°C		x	x	x								
40°C		x	x	x	x							
30°C	x	x	x	x	x	x	x	x	x	x	x	x
40°C & 75% RH		x	x	x								
30°C/Light		x	xx or as necessary									
Cold (2 and 8°C)			x	x		x	x		x	x	x	

Cyclic Testing: Three freeze-and-thaw cycles
1. Long-term testing at 30°C with ambient RH.
2. Accelerated testing at 40°C and 75% RH with 3 months' data required for submission.

Source: Ref. 84.

Table 10 ICH Guidelines

Conditions	Storage time (months)										
	0	1	2	3	6	9	12	24	36	48	60
50°C		x	x	x							
40°C & 75% RH		x	x	x	x						
30°C & 60% RH			x	x	x	x					
25°C & 60% RH		x	x	x	x	x	x	x	x	x	x
Light				To be determined							
Temperature ± 2°C											
RH ± 5°C											

Cyclical Testing: Three freeze-and-thaw cycles
1. Long-term testing at 25°C and 60% RH.
2. Accelerated testing at 40°C and 75% RH with 6 months' data required for submission.
3. 30°C and 60% RH with 12 months' data required for submission if significant changes at 40°C and 75% RH.
4. 12-month data at 25°C and 60% RH required for submission.

Source: Ref. 85.

of degradation can be influenced by heat, moisture, light, or air. Accelerated stability studies are designed to increase the rate of chemical or physical degradation of drugs or excipients by using exaggerated storage conditions with the purpose of determining kinetic parameters of degradation reactions and to predict the shelf life of a product at normal storage conditions. Results from accelerated stability studies help to establish inherent stability conditions [88] and support the suitability of the analytical method [85].

For suspensions, centrifugation as well as freeze-and-thaw cycles should be integral parts of stress in monitoring of crystal growth, caking, and redispersibility phenomena. Generally, for accelerated stability testing, suspensions are stored inverted and straight at 45°C or 50°C, 35°C or 40°C, room temperature or 30°C, 40°C & 75%, light and at 4°C. Additionally, they are subjected to three freeze-and-thaw cycles, and centrifuged for 30 minutes at 3000 rpm.

2. *Microbial Stability*

Topical suspensions generally contain a preservative or preservative system to control microbial contamination of the product. Preservative content should be monitored, at least at the beginning and end of the projected expiration dating period [86]. This may be accomplished by performing a chemical assay for preservatives or by performing the Antimicrobial Preservative Effectiveness Test of the USP. This includes subjecting the product to the microbial limit test, USP, which is designed to confirm the absence of pathogenic organisms in the product [86].

3. *Analytical Methods*

All analytical methods should be validated for precision, accuracy, reproducibility, and specificity and should be stability indicating. Where applicable, the standard deviation should be recorded [91].

4. *Stability Report*

A stability profile is established for internal use, registration purposes, and so forth, detailing the design and concept of the study as well as results and conclusions. The results should be presented as tables and graphs for each batch. Testing results should be given both at the time of manufacture and at different times during storage of the product [92].

C. Predicting Shelf Life

The use of kinetic and predictive studies for establishing tentative expiration dates is well accepted by regulatory agencies worldwide. Techniques for estimating shelf life of a suspension from accumulated data at elevated temperatures utilizes Arrhenius' equation to extrapolate shelf life of the product at lower temperatures. Application of Arrhenius' equation only applies when the stability-limiting factor is of a chemical nature. It is not applicable for physical parameters such as caking, viscosity, or redispersibility. Usually, a product exhibiting satisfactory stability for 3 months at 50°C or 6 months at 40°C has a potential of 2 years of shelf life.

Tingstad and his coworkers [93] have developed a simplified method for determining the stability of a drug substance in a suspension. The approach is based on the assumption that degradation takes place only in solution and is of a first order rate process. Also, the effect of temperature on drug solubility and reaction rate conforms with classical theory, and dissolution is not rate-limiting for degradation [94].

A simple means of estimating shelf life using a set of computer-prepared tables is described by Lintner [95]. The method has proved to be quite reliable in predicting the shelf life of active ingredients in the product.

To make a shelf-life prediction from elevated temperatures, three or more storage temperatures are necessary. One could measure intact drug by a highly selective method, measure total drug content nonselectively and estimate the decomposition products, or selectively measure both drug and decomposition products [96]. As a general rule, the FDA accepts the data from accelerated stability testing on three pilots for a tentative expiration date of up to 2 years. Currently a product with adequate stability for 3 months at 40°C and 75% relative humidity (RH) is generally granted an expiration date of 2 years. However, if the FDA agrees with ICH guidelines, minimum stability for 6 months at 40°C and 75% RH would be required. Final determination of an expiration date is based on real-time data from several batches that have been stored at storage conditions and assayed at regular intervals per recommendation of the Food and Drug Administration. If results of a real-time study do not conform to the predictive studies, an appropriate adjustment in expiration date must be made.

XI. ILLUSTRATIVE EXAMPLES

This section includes a number of formulas that illustrate the use of some of the excipients discussed in this chapter.

A patent by Young includes the following examples of suspending benzoyl peroxide in a hydro-alcoholic vehicle [97]

Formula No. 1	% by weight
Benzoyl peroxide (on an anhydrous basis)	5.00
Water	57.95
Ethyl alcohol	30.00
Polyoxyethylene (9) lauryl ether	3.00
Colloidal magnesium aluminum silicate	2.50
Hydroxypropyl methylcellulose	1.50
Citric acid	0.05

PROCEDURE: Water is heated to approximately 70°C. While stirring, add the colloidal magnesium silicate to the water and continue to stir for approximately 1 1/2 hours. While continuing to stir, add the hydroxypropyl methylcellulose. Continue to stir for an additional 15 minutes. Then cool to 50°C and add the polyoxethylene [9] lauryl ether. While continuing to stir, cool to 35°C and successively add the ethyl alcohol, citric acid, and benzoyl peroxide (70%) aqueous slurry. Continue to stir for an additional 10 minutes and mill to obtain a smooth suspension of finely divided benzoyl peroxide.

Mixing may be accomplished in a stainless steel tank equipped with a propeller mixer, or preferably in a processing tank equipped with a rotorstator and paddle sweep that can be independently operated. Homogenization may be substituted for milling to obtain the final smooth dispersion.

Young's patent also illustrates the use of several other suspending agents in formulating a topical benzoyl peroxide suspension. The following are examples.

Formula No. 2	% by weight
Benzoyl peroxide (on an anhydrous basis)	15.00
Water	49.35
Ethyl alcohol	25.00
Polyoxyethylene (40) stearate	8.50
Colloidal magnesium aluminum silicate	1.50
Sodium carboxymethylcellulose	0.60
Citric acid	0.05

Formula No. 3	% by weight
Benzoyl peroxide (on an anhydrous basis)	5.00
Water	76.97
Ispropyl alcohol	10.00
Polysorbate 20	5.00
Hydroxypropyl methylcellulose	1.50
Xanthan gum	1.50
Phosphoric acid	0.03

Formula No. 4	% by weight
Benzoyl peroxide (on an anhydrous basis)	3.00
Water	68.94
Ethyl alcohol	15.00
Poloxamer 188	10.00
Hydroxypropyl methylcellulose	1.50
Guar gum	1.50
Tartaric acid	0.06

Formula No. 5	% by weight
Benzoyl peroxide (on an anhydrous basis)	15.00
Water	46.93
Ethyl alcohol	15.00
Polyoxyethylene laurate	20.00
Hydroxyethyl cellulose	2.50
Sodium carboxymethylcellulose	0.50
Citric acid	0.07

Formula No. 6	% by weight
Benzoyl peroxide (on an anhydrous basis)	7.50
Water	62.95
Isopropyl alcohol	15.00
Polyoxyethylene (20) oleyl ether	3.00
Colloidal aluminum magnesium silicate	1.00
PEG/PPG-18/4 copolymer	10.50
Citric acid	0.05

The following is an example of a topical suspension of benzoyl peroxide in an aqueous gel base in which a carbomer resin is the suspending agent.

Formula No. 7	% by weight
Water	81.50
Carbomer 940	2.00
Di-isopropanolamine	1.50
Propylene glycol	5.00
Benzoyl peroxide (on an anhydrous basis)	10.00

PROCEDURE: Heat the water to approximately 70°C in a stainless steel processing tank equipped with a propeller or rotor-stator mixer. Add the Carbomer 940 to the water through the eductor while mixing and continue mixing for approximately 1 hour until a lump-free suspension is obtained.

Successively add the di-isopropanolamine and propylene glycol while continuing to mix. Cool the batch to 35 to 40°C. Add the benzoyl peroxide (70%) slurry and mill or homogenize to obtain a smooth suspension.

Because this suspension does not contain alcohol, some air entrapment may occur. It is desirable to utilize a processing tank in which a vacuum can be drawn.

Although the active ingredient in this formulation has antibacterial properties it would be prudent to conduct a microbial challenge test on the finished formulation. Addition of preservative may be required.

Another carbomer resin (934) has been used to formulate a smooth nongreasy aqueous suspension of zinc oxide [98]

Formula No. 8	% by weight
Water, purified	76.0
Carbomer, 934	0.8
Sodium hydroxide (10% solution)	3.2
Zinc oxide	20.0

PROCEDURE: With the use of an eductor disperse the carbomer in the water. Add the sodium hydroxide solution with slow-speed agitation to minimize air-entrapment. Add the zinc oxide in the same manner. Continue mixing until homogeneous.

In order to avoid flocculation of the zinc oxide it is important to neutralize the carbomer aqueous dispersion prior to the addition of the zinc oxide.

Zinc pyrithione is the most commonly used antidandruff agent. It has very low solubility in water and therefore it is usually suspended and formulated as a cream or lotion shampoo.

Magnesium aluminum silicate is the suspending agent of choice for zinc pyrithione formulations.

Neutralized carbomer, hydroxypropyl methylcellulose, methylhydroxy ethylcellulose, cellulose gum, sodium chloride, and alkanolamides, alone or in combination, have been effectively used as thickeners in zinc pyrithione formulations.

The inclusion of EDTA and amphoteric or cationic surfactants in zinc pyrithione formulations may cause chemical instability.

If color additives are to be included in the formulation, it is desirable to use a combination that will impart a blue color, because zinc pyrithione will react with any ferric ion present to impart a blue-gray color to the formulation.

The following is a suggested formulation for a zinc pyrithione lotion shampoo:

Formula No 9	% by weight
A. Water, purified	25.40
Magnesium aluminum silicate	0.25
Cellulose gum	0.10
Zinc pyrithione (48%)	2.10
B. Disodium oleamido PEG-2 sulfosuccinate (30%)	29.00
Lanolin oil	1.00
Sodium lauryl sulfate (29%)	34.00
Lauramide DEA	7.50
C. Citric acid (0.4%)	0.25
FD&C Blue No. 1 (0.5%)	0.40
Fragrance	qs

PROCEDURE: Heat water to 70°C. While rapidly stirring successively add magnesium aluminum silicate, cellulose gum, and zinc pyrithione at intervals of approximately 15 minutes. Cool to approximately 45°C and return to weight by adding back any water lost by evaporation. In a separate suitable vessel, successively add the ingredients in B. While stirring heat to 40 to 45°C and stir until uniform. Add A to B while stirring and cool to 25 to 30°C. Add fragrance and color solution and stir until uniform. Add citric acid to adjust pH to approximately 7.9.

The following is a suggested formulation for a zinc pyrithione cream shampoo:

Formula No. 10	% by weight
A. Sodium lauryl sulfate paste (30%)	40.00
Lanolin oil	1.00
Glyceryl stearate	5.00
B. Water, purified	50.15
Sodium chloride	1.35
C. Zinc pyrithione (48%)	2.10
FD&C Blue No. 1 (0.5%)	0.40
Fragrance	qs

PROCEDURE: While stirring slowly, heat the ingredients of A to 70°C. Add the sodium chloride to the water (B) and heat to 70°C. When the sodium chloride is dissolved add A to B while stirring slowly. Add the zinc pyrithione (C) and continue to stir while cooling to approximately 40°C. Add color solution and fragrance and continue to stir while cooling to approximately 25°C.

Selenium sulfide is another widely used antidandruff ingredient. Because it is also virtually insoluble in water it is customarily formulated as a suspension in shampoo bases.

The following is a suggested formulation from a Baldwin and Young patent [99].

Formula No. 11	% w/v
Composition of equal parts of selenium sulfide and bentonite	5.0
Bentonite	4.0
Monobasic sodium phosphate	1.0
Glyceryl monoricinoleate	1.0
Triethanolamine lauryl sulfate	17.0
Citric acid	0.2–0.5
Fragrance	0.5
Water, purified	qs to 100.0

PROCEDURE: Wet the bentonite with water and add the triethanolamine lauryl sulfate while stirring. Successively add the glyceryl monoricinoleate and monosodium phosphate while continuing to stir. After the solution has become uniform add the selenium sulfide–bentonite powder in small increments. Continue stirring until a uniform suspension is obtained. Add the citric acid in sufficient quantity to adjust the pH of the composition to about 4.5. While continuing to stir add fragrance and bring water up to volume.

The following formulation is another example of a selenium sulfide suspension:

Formula No. 12	% by weight
Ammonium laureth sulfate (29%)	15.0
Ammonium lauryl sulfate (29%)	15.0
Citric acid	0.4
Cocamide DEA	4.0
Cocamidopropyl betaine (30%)	0.25
DMDM hydantoin (50%)	0.25
FD&C Blue No. 1 (1%)	0.04
Hydroxypropyl methylcellulose	0.4
Magnesium aluminum silicate	0.4
Fragrance	0.4
Sodium chloride	0.4
Titanium dioxide	0.5
Selenium sulfide	1.0
Water, purified	qs 100.0

PROCEDURE: Heat water to approximately 60°C. While stirring, add and disperse the magnesium aluminum silicate. When completely hydrated, slowly add the hydroxypropyl methylcellulose with continued stirring. Maintain temperature of approximately 60°C and continue to stir while successively adding the cocamide DEA, ammonium laureth sulfate, ammonium lauryl sulfate, cocamidopropyl betaine, DMDM hydantoin, citric acid, sodium chloride, and FD&C No. 1 solution.

Premix the titanium dioxide and the selenium sulfide. Cool batch to approximately 45°C and add the titanium dioxide–selenium sulfide blend while stirring rapidly. Add fragrance. Process through a colloid mill.

The following is an example of an antiacne suspension.

Formula No. 13		% by weight
A.	Water	80.0
	Sodium carboxymethyl cellulose, LP	0.2
	Sodium benzoate	0.1
	Carbowax 400	3.0
B.	Oleic acid	2.0
	Resorcinol	1.25
C.	Triethanolamine	1.5
D.	Sulfur, sublimed	2.5
	Color blend	5.0
E.	Propylene glycol	2.0
	Perfume	0.25
	Antifoam 60	0.2
	Sulfuric acid	2.0
F.	Alcohol	11.0

PROCEDURE: Heat water to 70°C. While stirring, rapidly add ingredients A (sodium CMC, Carbowax 400, and sodium benzoate). Heat ingredients B to 70°C and add to A while stirring rapidly. Add C (triethanolamine) and slowly cool to 30°C. Add D and mix. Presolubilize perfume in propylene glycol and add to bulk. Adjust pH to 3.5 Add F at about 25 to 28°C. Homogenize or mill to form a smooth suspension.

The following is a formulation for an antidandruff suspension shampoo.

Formula No. 14		% by weight
A.	Water	75.725
	Disodium EDTA	0.075
	Xanthan gum	0.05
	Sodium lauryl ether sulfate	7.5
	Disodium monolauryl ether sulfo-succinate	7.5
	Coconut fatty acid diethanolamine	3.0
	Imidurea	0.3
	Sodium chloride	0.5
B.	Propylene glycol	3.0
	Perfume	0.25
	Propylparaben	0.03
	Methylparaben	0.1
C.	Ketoconazole	2.0

PROCEDURE: Heat water to 70°C. While rapidly stirring, add xanthan gum. Cool to 50°C. While stirring slowly, add remaining ingredients of A, one after the other. Cool to 35°C. In a separate container, heat propylene glycol to 35°C and add propylparaben. Mix until a clear solution is formed. Add perfume and then add

other ingredients of B to A. Adjust pH to 6.2 to 6.8 with HCl or sodium hydrox-
ide. Add C to the bulk and mix slowly. Homogenize to make smooth suspension.
   Adapted from U. S. Patent #4,335,125 [100].
   The following is an example of a sunscreen suspension.

Formula No. 15		% by weight
A.	Octyl dimethyl PABA	7.0
	Benzophenone	3.5
	Mineral oil–lanolin alcohol	7.0
	C_{12}–C_{15} alcohol benzoate	7.5
	Stearic acid, triple pressed	2.0
B.	Water	61.2
	Glycerin	3.0
C.	Propylene glycol	3.0
	Methyl paraben	0.1
	Propyl paraben	0.03
	Perfume	0.25
D.	Zinc oxide, micronized	2.5
	Titanium dioxide, micronized	3.0

   PROCEDURE: While stirring slowly, heat the ingredients of A to 70°C. Add
ingredients of B, heating to 72°C, and stir vigorously for 10 minutes. Slowly cool
to 35°C. Add phase C while mixing slowly. Add ingredients of D one after the
other and mix for 10 minutes. Homogenize or mill to obtain smooth suspension.

ACKNOWLEDGMENTS

The authors wish to thank Ms. Patricia Leonard for her numerous helpful discussions and editorial assistance, and Elgie Ginsburgh and Cheryl Flynn for typing
the manuscript.

APPENDIX

Instruments Discussed and Their Manufacturers

Serial No.	Description of instrument	Manufacturer
1	[a]Light-scattering Royco	HIAC/Royco, Ins., Pacific Scientific Silver Spring, MD
2	[b]Light blockage Hiac	HIAC/Royco, Ins., Pacific Scientific Silver Spring, MD
3	[c]Electrical conductivity Coulter Counter	Coulter Electronics, Hialeah, FL
4	[d]Quantasorb	Quantachrome, Inc. Syosset, NY
5	[e]Carbopol resins	B. F. Goodrich Cleveland, OH
6	[f]Colloid mill	APV Gaulin Wilmington, MA

Serial No.	Description of instrument	Manufacturer
7	gLightnin mixer	Mixing Equipment Co. Rochester, NY
8	hDeaerator	Cornell Machine Co. Springfield, NJ
9	iRotostator homogenizer	Cherry Burrel, Inc. Louisville, KY
10	jViscometer, Haake	Haake, Inc. Paramus, NJ
11	kZetameter	Zetameter, Inc. New York, NY

REFERENCES

1. T. R. Bates, D. A. Lambert, and W. H. Johns, *J. Pharm. Sci.*, 58:1468 (1969).
2. M. C. Meyer, A. B. Straughn, and G. Ramchander, J. C. Cavagnol, and A. F. Biola Mabadeje, *J. Pharm. Sci.*, 67:1659 (1978).
3. N. Weiner, *Drug Dev. Ind. Pharm.*, 12(7):933 (1986).
4. G. Zografi, et al. Interfacial phenomena. In: *Remington's Pharmaceutical Sciences* (A. Gennaro, ed.), 18th ed., Mack Publishing Co., Easton, PA, 1990, pp. 257–270.
5. J. Rosen, Wetting and its modification by surfactants. In: *Surfactant and Interfacial Phenomenon*, John Wiley & Sons, New York, 1978, pp. 174–176, 262–269.
6. W. A. Zisman, *Advances in Chemistry*, #43, American Chemical Society, Washington, D.C., 1964, pp. 33–37.
7. E. G. Sharfin and W. A. Zisman, *J. Phys. Chem.*, 64:519 (1960).
8. J. L. Zatz, *J. Cosmet. Chem.*, 36:393 (1985).
9. *Use of Contact Angle in Surface Science*, Rame-hart Inc., Technical Bulletin, TB100, Mountainlake, N.J., 1983, p. 1.
10. A. W. Adamson, *Physical Chemistry of Surfaces*, 3rd ed., John Wiley & Sons, New York, 1976, p. 342.
11. E. F. Bartell and H. H. Zuidema, *J. Am. Chem. Soc.*, 58:1449 (1936).
12. A. N. Martin, *J. Pharm. Sci.*, 50:513 (1961).
13. B. A. Haines and A. N. Martin, *J. Pharm. Sci.*, 50:228 (1961).
14. M. J. Akers and R. L. Robinson, *J. Pharm. Sci. Tech.*, 41(3):88 (1987).
15. C. T. Rhodes, Disperse systems. In: *Modern Pharmaceutics*, (G. S. Banker and C. T. Rhodes, eds.) 2nd ed., Marcel Dekker, New York, 1990, pp. 327–354.
16. B. Derjaguin and L. Landau, *Acta Physiol. Chem.*, 14:633 (1941).
17. E. J. Verwey and T. T. G. Overbeek, *Theory of Stability of Lyophobic Colloids*, Elsevier, New York (1948).
18. B. A. Matthews and C. T. Rhodes, *J. Pharm. Sci.*, 59:518 (1970).
19. W. Schneider, S. Starchansky, and A. N. Martin, *Am. J. Pharm. Educ.*, 42:280 (1978).
20. B. A. Matthews and C. T. Rhodes, *J. Pharm. Pharmacol.*, 20:204S (1968).
21. B. A. Matthews and C. T. Rhodes, *Pharm. Acta Helv.*, 45:52 (1969).
22. B. A. Matthews and C. T. Rhodes, *J. Pharm. Sci.*, 59:521 (1970).
23. B. A. Matthews and C. T. Rhodes, *J. Pharm. Sci.*, 59:1360 (1970).
24. M. P. Short and C. T. Rhodes, *Can. J. Pharm. Sci.*, 8:46 (1973).
25. B. A. Matthews, *J. Pharm. Sci.*, 62:172 (1973).
26. R. G. Wilson and B. Ecanow, *J. Pharm. Sci.*, 52:757 (1963).
27. N. K. Patel, L. Kennon, and R. S. Levinson, Pharmaceutical suspensions. In: *The Theory and Practice of Industrial Pharmacy* (H. A. Lieberman, L. Lachman and J. Kanig, eds.), 3rd ed., Lea & Febiger, Philadelphia, 1986, pp. 479–482.

28. E. N. Hiestand, *J. Pharm. Sci.*, 53:1 (1964).
29. E. N. Hiestand, *J. Pharm. Sci.*, 61:268 (1972).
30. A. Otsuka, H. Sunada, and Y. Yonezawa, *J. Pharm. Sci.*, 62:751 (1973).
31. W. C. Liao and J. L. Zatz, *J. Soc. Cosmet. Chem.*, 31:107 (1980).
32. W. C. Liao, *J. Soc. Cosmet. Chem.*, 31:123 (1980).
33. J. L. Zatz, L. Schnitzer, and P. Sarpotdar, *J. Pharm. Sci.*, 68:1491 (1979).
34. A. Felmeister, G. M. Kuchtyak, S. Kozioi, and C. J. Felmeister, *J. Pharm. Sci.*, 62:2026 (1973).
35. H. E. Reiss, Jr. and B. L. Meyer, *Science* 160:1449 (1968).
36. T. W. Healy and V. K. Lamer, *J. Phys. Chem.*, 33:149 (1982).
37. J. S. Tempio and J. L. Zatz, *J. Pharm. Sci.*, 69:1209 (1980).
38. J. S. Tempio and J. L. Zatz, *J. Pharm. Sci.*, 70:554 (1981).
39. J. L. Zatz, et al., *Int. J. Pharm.*, 9:315 (1981).
40. A. Martin, J. Swarbrick, and A. Cammarata, Rheology. In: *Physical Pharmacy*, 4th ed., Lea & Febiger, Philadelphia, 1993, pp. 387, 455–458
41. D. A. Wadke, T. M. Serajuddin, and H. Jacobson, Preformulation testing. In: *Pharmaceutical Dosage Forms: Tablets,* Vol. 1, (H. A. Lieberman, and L. Lachman, eds.), 2nd ed., Marcel Dekker, New York, 1986, pp. 1–73.
42. E. F. Fiese and T. A. Hagen, Preformulation. In: *Theory and Practice of Industrial Pharmacy* (L. Lachman, H. A. Lieberman, and J. L. Kanig, eds.), 3rd ed., Lea & Febiger, Philadelphia, 1986, pp. 171–195.
43. T. J. Macek, *Am. J. Pharm.*, 137:217 (1965).
44. H. P. Fletcher, et al., *J. Pharm. Sci.*, 57:2101 (1968).
45. R. A. Nash, *Drug Cosmet. Ind.*, 65:97 (1965).
46. H. M. Abdou, Dissolution. In: *Remington's Pharmaceutical Sciences* (A. Gennaro, ed.), 18th ed., Mack Publishing Co., Easton, PA, 1990, pp. 600–601.
47. S. A. Kaplan, *Drug Metab. Rev.*, 1:15 (1972).
48. N. Pipel, *Chem. Process. Eng.*, 46:167 (1965).
49. United States Pharmacopeia XXIII and National Formulary XVIII, U.S. Pharmacopeial Convention, Inc., Rockville, 1995, pp. 1681, 2207.
50. *Cellulose Gums Chemical and Physical Properties*, Hercules, Inc., Wilmington (1984).
51. B. Idson and A. J. Scheer, Suspensions. In: *Problem Solver and Reference Manual*, FMC Corp., Philadelphia (1984).
52. *Methocel Cellulose Ether*, Dow Chemical Co., Midland (1988).
53. *Xanthan Gum/Keltrol/Kelzan—A Natural Biopolysaccharide for Scientific Water Control*, 5th ed., Kelco, Division of Merck & Co., Inc., San Diego.
54. J. L. Zatz, *Ind. Eng. Prod. Res. Dev.* 23:12 (1984).
55. *Carbopol® Water Soluble Resin Service Bulletin*, CP25, BF Goodrich, Cleveland (1993).
56. B. W. Barry, *Dermatological Formulations*, Marcel Dekker, New York, 1983, pp. 301–304.
57. R. J. Meyer and L. Cohen, *J. Soc. Cosmet. Chem.*, 10:143 (1959).
58. B. M. Berney and P. B. Deasy, *Int. J. Pharm.*, 3:73 (1979).
59. W. B. Swafford and W. L. Nobles, *J. Am. Pharm. Assoc.*, 16:171 (1955).
60. *Pemulen Polymeric Emulsifier* #TDS114–118, BF Goodrich Company, Cleveland (1990).
61. *Veegum Booklet*, R. T. Vanderbilt Co., Norwalk, CT (1993).
62. J. C. Symyn, *J. Pharm. Sci.*, 50(6):517 (1961).
63. G. E. Schumacher, *Am. J. Hosp. Pharm.*, 26:70 (1979).
64. P. A. Ciullo, *J. Soc. Cosmet. Chem.*, 32:275 (1981).
65. J. W. McGinity and J. L. Lach, *J. Pharm. Sci.*, 65:896 (1976).
66. J. C. Boylan, Liquids. In: *Theory and Practice of Industrial Pharmacy* (L. Lachman, H. A. Lieberman, and J. L. Kanig, eds.), 3rd ed., Lea & Febiger, Philadelphia, 1986, pp. 457–460.
67. J. Windheuser, *Bull. Parenteral Drug Assoc.*, 17:1 (1963).
68. H. N. Bhargava and A. Anaebonam, *Soap Cosmet. Chem.*, Specialties, 59(10):39 (1983).

69. *Keys to Chelation*, Dow Chemical Co., Midland, 1979, pp. 49–69.

70. S. Das and B. N. Dutta, *Eastern Pharmacist*, 8:31 (1964).

71. *CTFA International Color Handbook*, 2nd ed., Cosmetic Toiletries and Fragrance Association, Washington, DC (1992).

72. S. Harder and G. Van Buskirk, Pilot plant scale-up. In: *Theory and Practice of Industrial Pharmacy* (L. Lachman, et al, eds.), 3rd ed., Lea & Febiger, Philadelphia, 1986, pp. 681–689.

73. D. T. Hansford, *Powder Tech.*, 26:119 (1980).

74. I. Tabibi, Production of dispersed delivery systems. In: *Specialized Drug Delivery Systems* (P. Tyle, ed), Marcel Dekker, New York, 1990, pp. 321–323.

75. G. A. Van Buskirk, et al., *Pharm. Res.*, 11(8):1217 (1994).

76. G. L. Stanko and H. G. Dekay, *J. Am. Pharm., Assoc., Sci. Ed.*, 47:104 (1958).

77. B. A. Matthews and C. T. Rhodes, *J. Pharm. Sci.*, 57:569 (1968).

78. C. T. Lesschaft and H. G. Dekay, *Drug Standards*, 22:155 (1954).

79. A. P. Black and A. L. Smith, *Water Works Assoc.*, 58:445 (1966).

80. A. C. Shah, C. B. Peot, and J. F. Ochs, *J. Pharm. Sci.*, 62:671 (1973).

81. *CTFA Technical Guidelines*, Cosmetics, Toiletries and Fragrance Assn., Washington, DC (1992).

82. B. Idson, *J. Pharm. Sci.*, 57:1 (1967).

83. L. Lachman, P. Deluca, and M. J. Akens, Kinetic principles and stability testing. In: *Theory and Practice of Industrial Pharmacy* (L. Lachman et al, eds.), 3rd ed., Lea & Febiger, Philadelphia, 1986, p. 778.

84. P. Guirag, AAPS Workshop on Stability Guidelines for Testing Pharmaceutical Products, Washington, DC (1994).

85. International Conference on Harmonization Steering Committee Guidelines on Stability Testing of Pharmceuticals (1993).

86. FDA Guidelines for Submitting Documentation for the Stability of Human Drugs and Biologics, February 1987, p. 15.

87. J. T. Carstensen, Overview. In: *Drug Stability Principles and Practice*, Marcel Dekker, New York, 1990. pp. 7–9.

88. Stability of Drug Dosage Forms: World Health Organization Report, Pharm 88.82, 1988.

89. G. R. Duke, General considerations for stability testing of topical pharmaceutical formulations. In: *Topical Drug Delivery Formulations* (D. W. Osborne and A. H. Amann, eds.), Marcel Dekker, New York, 1990, pp 197–211.

90. Stability Concepts, PMA Joint OC-PDC Stability Committee Report, *Pharm. Tech.*, 8(6):42, (1984).

91. D. M. Winship and R. McCormack, Manufacturing and control requirements of the NDA and ANDA. In: *New Drug Approved Process* (RA Guarino ed.), Marcel Dekker, New York, 1993, p. 346.

92. "Guidelines on Stability Testing of Pharmaceutical Product," WHO Expert Committee 31st Report, Technical Report Series #790 (1990).

93. J. Tingstad, et al., *J. Pharm. Sci.*, 63:1361 (1973).

94. PMA's Joint OC-PDC Stability Committee, *Pharm. Tech.*, 15, (9):92–96 (1991).

95. C. J. Lintner, et al., *Am. Perfum. Cosmet.*, 85:31 (1970).

96. L. Chafetz, *Pharm. Res.*, 5(4):249 (1988).

97. H. Young, U.S. Patent #4,056,611 (1977).

98. *Carbopol Water Soluble Resin Service Bulletin* GC 36, Revised 1993, BF Goodrich, Cleveland.

99. Baldwin & Young, US Patent 2,694,669 (1954).

100. J. Heeves, L. J. J. Backx, and J. H. Mostmanf, U.S. Patent #4,335,125 (1992).

6

Reconstitutable Oral Suspensions

Clyde M. Ofner III, Roger L. Schnaare, and Joseph B. Schwartz

Philadelphia College of Pharmacy and Science, Philadelphia, Pennsylvania

I. INTRODUCTION

Although conventional oral suspensions can be administered immediately, there is an important category of suspensions that requires mixing prior to administration. These suspensions are commercial dry mixtures that require the addition of water at the time of dispensing and have a title designated in the United States Pharmacopeia (USP) of the form ". . . for Oral Suspension."

The reconstituted suspension is the formulation of choice when drug stability is a major concern. After reconstitution, these suspensions have a short but acceptable shelf life if stored at refrigerator temperatures. This chapter describes the ingredients, different physical types, the preparation, some problems, and typical formulas of suspensions for reconstitution.

II. CHARACTERISTICS OF SUSPENSIONS FOR RECONSTITUTION

A. Rationale

The most common reason for formulation of suspensions for reconstitution is inadequate chemical stability of the drug in an aqueous vehicle. In these cases, dissolution or even suspension of the drug results in a very short shelf life. For example, reconstituted suspensions of penicillin have a maximum shelf life of 14 days. The manufactured dry mixture, however, has a shelf life of at least 2 years.

Another reason for formulating suspensions for reconstitution is to avoid the physical stability problems often encountered in conventional suspensions. These problems include possible increased drug solubility due to pH changes from chemical degradation, incompatibility of ingredients, viscosity changes, conversion of polymorphic form and crystal growth, and caking.

Formulation for reconstitution reduces the weight of the final product because the aqueous vehicle is absent and, consequently, transportation expenses may be reduced.

The dry mixture may be shipped without regard to seasonal temperatures because its physical stability is less susceptible to temperature extremes as compared with conventional suspensions.

B. Desired Attributes

Suspensions for reconstitution require special considerations. Many antibiotics are formulated for reconstitution and are intended for a pediatric patient population. In addition, acceptable properties must be maintained before, during, and after reconstitution. Finally, the formulator must realize that the last step in the preparation of the product will be conducted beyond the control of the manufacturer.

Table 1 lists the required characteristics of suspensions for reconstitution. During manufacture, the dry blend, or mixture, must not segregate into a nonuniform mix because errors in dosage may result. Appropriate ingredients that disperse quickly must be employed. After reconstitution the high viscosity caused by refrigerated storage temperatures should not obstruct dose administration by the patient. The formulator must be aware that a final pediatric product must be acceptable to children who are ill and often uncooperative with administration of medication. If the patient will not swallow the medication, the product is useless.

III. COMMONLY USED INGREDIENTS

There are usually fewer ingredients in suspensions for reconstitution than in conventional suspensions. The criteria for selecting ingredients are based both on suitability for reconstitution and on the physical type of powder mixture desired. General guidelines can aid the formulator in the selection of ingredients, but every formulation of a different drug is unique, and the exact ingredients must be determined by the formulator.

A. General Considerations

Table 2 lists the functional excipients employed in suspensions for reconstitution. The ingredients are separated into categories of frequent and infrequent use. Not all formulators agree on the necessary excipients. Although it is listed here as an infrequent excipient, some formulators believe that an anticaking agent is mandatory [1]. Other formulators question the necessity of a dye [2]. Some dry mixtures are prepared by granulation, and the ingredients used in this process are listed in Table 2.

Table 1 Required Characteristics of Suspensions for Reconstitution

1. The powder blend must be a uniform mixture of the appropriate concentration of each ingredient.
2. During reconstitution the powder blend must disperse quickly and completely in the aqueous vehicle.
3. The reconstituted suspension must be easily redispersed and poured by the patient to provide an accurate and uniform dose.
4. The final product must have an acceptable appearance, odor, and taste.

Table 2 Frequent and Infrequent Excipients
Used in Suspensions for Reconstitution

Frequent	Infrequent
Suspending agent	Anticaking Agent
Wetting agent	Flocculating agent
Sweetener	Solid diluent
Preservative	Antifoaming agent
Flavor	Granule binder
Buffer	Granule disintegrant
Color	Antioxidant
	Lubricant

The number of ingredients should be kept to a minimum; the more ingredients in a formulation, the greater the possibility of problems. For example, the chances of compatibility problems are increased as more ingredients are used. Greater processing is required to incorporate more ingredients. More ingredients will require sampling and testing for quality control. The chances are increased that a regulatory agency will ban an ingredient or that a source will disappear.

The formulator should determine that each excipient is actually necessary. Every excipient should perform a necessary function for that particular product. A common method of reducing the number of ingredients is to use an ingredient that performs more than one function. Sucrose, for example, may perform two or three functions—as a sweetener, suspending agent, or solid diluent.

Some general guidelines have been suggested to aid in the selection of ingredients [2]. All ingredients should disperse rapidly on reconstitution. This criterion eliminates several suspending agents. Many preservatives are also not suitable. Liquids or sticky ingredients should be used at low levels.

B. Drug

There are 30 monographs of oral suspensions for reconstitution in the *United States Pharmacopeia,* 23rd edition (USP 23) [3]. This is approximately one-half the number of monographs of conventional oral suspensions. Some typical suspensions for reconstitution, their manufacturers, and drug concentration after reconstitution are listed in Table 3.

Nearly all drugs formulated as reconstitutable oral suspensions are antibiotics (see Table 3). The drug concentrations are usually intended for a pediatric dosage. Both the anhydrate and trihydrates of ampicillin are commonly used. Erythromycin ethylsuccinate is also formulated for reconstitution in dropper bottles for infants at a lower dosage. Although sodium dicloxacillin is water soluble, it is formulated as an insoluble form in suspension to help mask the odor and taste. Penicillin V potassium is also water soluble, but after reconstitution it is a suspension for the short time prior to complete dissolution. Since this drug dissolves soon after reconstitution the product is actually a solution and does not require a suspending agent. This product is classified as an oral solution in the *USP.* The combination product of probenicid and ampicillin is intended for adults; the entire preparation is consumed as one dose.

Table 3 Typical Reconstitutable Oral Suspensions

Drug	Some manufacturers	Drug concentration after reconstitution
Amoxicillin trihydrate	SmithKline Beecham, Mylan, Wyeth-Ayerst	125, 250mg/ 5 mL
Ampicillin	Warner-Chilcott, Biocraft	125, 250mg/ 5 mL
Cephalexin	Dista, Lederle	125, 250 mg/5 mL
Dicloxacillin sodium	Apothecon, Wyeth-Ayerst	62.5 mg/ 5 mL
Erythromycin ethylsuccinate	Abbott	100 mg/2.5 mL
	Barr, Schein, Major	200, 400 mg/ 5 mL
Penicillin V potassium	Lilly, Wyeth-Ayerst, URL	125, 250 mg/ 5 mL
Ampicillin and probenecid	Biocraft	3.5 g, 1 g/60 mL[a]

[a]Amount of each ingredient, respectively, per dose that is the total volume of the product.

C. Suspending Agent

Suspending agents should be easily dispersed by vigorous hand shaking during reconstitution. This rules out several common suspending agents because many require hydration, elevated temperatures, or high shear mixing for adequate dispersion. Some suspending agents that are not recommended include agar, carbomer, and methylcellulose [2]. Although both methylcellulose and aluminum magnesium silicate are not recommended [2], they have been used successfully in a cephalexin [4] and erythromycin ethylsuccinate [5] formulation, respectively.

Table 4 lists suspending agents recommended for use in suspensions for reconstitution [1,2]. The ionic charges of the agents are included for purposes of avoiding chemical incompatibilities with other ingredients.

The combination of microcrystalline cellulose and sodium carboxymethylcellulose is a common suspending agent. Total concentrations of the combination greater than 1% in the reconstituted product can result in thixotropic gels. This agent, and sodium carboxymethylcellulose alone, are anionic; they are incompatible with many cationic ingredients.

The natural gums are usually anionic and include exudates of tree and extracts from seaweed. Acacia and tragacanth have been used as suspending agents for many years. Tragacanth solutions are very viscous and have been used to suspend dense particles. The carrageenan and alginate suspending agents are seaweed extracts. The alginates produce highly viscous solutions and the iota-carrageenans produce thixotropic dispersions. A disadvantage of these natural products is batch variation in color, viscosity, gel strength, and hydration rate.

Xanthan gum is a common suspending agent in suspensions for reconstitution. Because it is produced by microbial fermentation there is good batch-to-batch uniformity and few microbial problems. Its solution viscosity is practically independent of pH and temperature.

The required concentrations for rapid dispersion during reconstitution must be determined for each suspending agent. Combinations of suspending agents have also been used. Additional information about these and other suspending agents is available in Chapter 4 of this volume [6].

Table 4 Suspending Agents Suitable for Use in Suspensions for Reconstitution

Agent	Ionic charge
Acacia	–
Carboxymethylcellulose sodium	–
Iota carrageenan	–
Microcrystalline cellulose with carboxymethylcellulose sodium	–
Povidone	0
Propylene glycol alginate	–
Silicon dioxide, colloidal	0
Sodium starch glycolate	–
Tragacanth	–
Xanthan gum	–

Source: Refs. 1 and 2.

D. Sweetener

The sweetener is a significant component of suspensions for reconstitution. Drugs frequently have a bitter taste, and suspending agents, particularly clays, may have a bland taste. Sweeteners can mask the unfavorable taste and enhance patient acceptance in the pediatric population that uses this product. Any increased viscosity as a result of the sweetener aids suspension of the drug particles.

Sucrose can perform both above functions of sweetener and suspending agent, and serve as a diluent in the dry mixture. In addition, sucrose can be milled to increase its surface area and be used as a carrier of liquid excipients such as volatile oils. Other sweeteners include mannitol, dextrose, aspartame, and sodium saccharin. Aspartame has fair acid stability but poor heat stability. Saccharin may become restricted by the Food and Drug Administration because of its carcinogenic potential.

E. Wetting Agents

Hydrophilic drugs are readily wetted by an aqueous vehicle. These drugs can usually be incorporated into suspensions without the use of a wetting agent. Many drugs in suspension, however, are hydrophobic; they repel water and are not easily wetted.

Surfactants are commonly used to aid in the dispersion of hydrophobic drugs. The *USP 23* lists 24 possible surfactants for use as wetting or solubilizing agents [7]. The formulator selects the appropriate wetting agent for optimum dispersion of the drug at the lowest effective concentration. Excess wetting agent can produce foaming and impart an unpleasant taste. The Hiestand method [8] of comparing wetting ability between surfactants can be used for the determination of the appropriate agent. A narrow hydrophobic trough holds the powder at one end while a solution of the wetting agent is placed at the other end. The better agents will have a fast rate of penetration through the powder.

Polysorbate 80 is a common wetting agent. It is nonionic and is chemically compatible with both cationic and anionic excipients and drugs. It is used in concentrations $\leq 0.1\%$. Another common wetting agent is sodium lauryl sulfate. This agent is anionic and may be incompatible with cationic drugs.

F. Other Ingredients

The ingredients described in this section include buffers, preservatives, flavors, and colors. Flocculating agents are not commonly used in suspensions for reconstitution because these products are usually redispersed frequently enough to prevent caking.

Buffers are used to maintain the optimum pH for all ingredients. Suspension pH is often adjusted to ensure that the drug remains insoluble. The polymeric suspending agents, however, have the greatest viscosity at the pH of their maximum solubility. The suspending agent should be stable at the pH of the system for the shelf life of the product. Certain preservatives, such as sodium benzoate, are most effective at low pH values in which the molecule is un-ionized. Sodium citrate is a common buffer used in suspensions for reconstitution.

Preservatives are required in most suspensions because the suspending agents and sweetener are often good growth media for microorganisms. The choice of preservatives in suspensions for reconstitution is limited because most of these ingredients require extended time periods for dissolution at room temperature. Examples of these "poorly soluble" preservatives that are not recommended include sorbic acid and the methyl or propyl hydroxybenzoates (parabens).

Sucrose in sufficient concentrations (ca. 60% w/w) can aid in the prevention of microbial growth. The resulting osmotic pressure of the aqueous vehicle is 16 times greater than an iso-osmotic, or isotonic, solution and is very unfavorable for microbial growth. Other common preservatives include sodium benzoate and sodium propionate.

Flavors also enhance patient acceptability of product. They are very important in the products that are intended for pediatric patients. Both natural and artificial flavors are used. Additional flavors used include raspberry, pineapple, and bubble gum. In some cases, refrigeration after reconstitution is required for the stability of the flavoring agent rather than for the stability of the drug [5].

Colorants are intended to provide a more aesthetic appearance to the final suspension. As relatively large cations or anions, these agents may be chemically incompatible with other ingredients. For example, FD&C Red No. 3 is a disodium salt, is anionic, and would be incompatible with a cationic wetting agent. Other common water-soluble colorants include FD&C Red No. 40 and FD &C Yellow No. 6. Additional information is available regarding the description, use, and analysis of colorants [9].

Anticaking agents, such as amorphous silica gel, have several functions in suspensions for reconstitution [1]. A common problem in dry mixtures is poor powder flow and caking. This is often caused by powder agglomeration due to moisture uptake. As a desiccant, these agents remove moisture from the dry mixture to facilitate good powder flow and prevent caking. In addition, anticaking agents separate the dry particles to inhibit fusion. They also provide thermal insulation, screen and insulate static charge conditions, and are chemically inert.

IV. PREPARATION OF DRY MIXTURE

Three types of dry mixture preparations are possible: powder blend, granulated products, and combination products. The preparation, advantages, and disadvantages of each type will be discussed in this section.

A. Powder Blends

Powder blends, sometimes called powder mixtures, are prepared by mixing the ingredients of the dry mixture in powder form. Ingredients present in small quantities may require a two-stage mixing operation. Such ingredients can be mixed with a portion of a major ingredient to aid in their dispersion. For example, milled sucrose provides a large surface area for the adsorption of the small quantities of flavor oils. The second stage comprises the mixing of the remaining ingredients.

The selection of the appropriate mixer involves several considerations, the most significant of which is that the mixer should rapidly and reliably produce a homogeneous mixture. Other practical considerations are the availability versus cost of a new mixer, ease of cleaning, and desirability of a completely closed system for operator protection.

There are three advantages of powder blends compared to granulated products [2]. Powder blends require the least capital equipment and energy. They are least likely to have chemical and stability problems because no heat or solvents are used in the granulating process. A low moisture content can be achieved in the dry mixture.

The primary disadvantage of powder blends is that they are prone to homogeneity problems. Two very important properties for the mixing of these powders are particle size and powder flow. The insoluble drug is usually milled to a smaller size than the sweetener or suspending agent and a difference in particle size of ingredients results. Too broad a size range of such particles can induce segregation into layers of different sizes. Poor flow can cause demixing. At the least, the consequence of these adverse conditions is a variation in dosage. For additional information on mixing, the reader is referred to other texts on solid processing [10–12].

Another potential problem in powder blends is the systematic loss of the active ingredient during mixing. This loss is illustrated by the report of an experiment [2]. After the mixing of the powder blend, 0.2% of the batch weight was lost. The lost material, however, was enriched with the active ingredient so that the drug content of the bulk mixture was depleted by 1.3%. The material lost during powder blending will have even greater significance if the active ingredient is a potent drug used in very low concentrations.

B. Granulated Products

All the ingredients in granulated products are processed by granulation. Wet granulation is the usual process and the granulating fluid is water or an aqueous binder solution. There are two methods of incorporating the drug. The drug can be dry-blended with the other ingredients or it can be dissolved or suspended in the granulating fluid.

Wet granulation usually consists of the following steps. The solid ingredients are blended and massed with the granulating fluid in a planetary mixer. The wet mass is formed into granules in one of the following before drying: vibratory sieve, oscillating granulator, grater, or mill. For drugs subject to hydrolysis, nonaqueous granulating fluids can be used. Fairly dry sucrose-based masses may divide down sufficiently in the airstream of a fluid bed drier without the use of a wet screening step [2]. Most often, however, wet massing and screening is the preferred method. The formed granules are dried in a tray oven or fluid bed drier. The dried granules are then screened in a vibratory sieve or oscillating granulator to break up or remove aggregates of granules.

The granulated product has some advantages over the powder product. These advantages are an improved appearance, improved flow characteristics, less segregation problems, and less generation of dust during filling operations.

There are, however, several disadvantages of the granulated product compared with the powder product. The granulated product requires more capital equipment and energy to process each batch. It is very difficult to remove the last traces of granulating fluid from the interior of granules. The residual fluid may reduce the stability of the product [13]. Another disadvantage is that the excipients as well as drug must be stable to the granulation process. For example, a large variation in flavor stability was reported upon wet massing and oven drying of several flavors [2]. Finally, uniform granulation is necessary because an excess of very small particles, or fines, will result in rapid segregation.

C. Combination Product

Powdered and granulated ingredients can be combined to overcome some disadvantages of granulated products. Less energy and equipment for granulation may be required if the majority of the diluent can be added after granulation. Also, heat-sensitive ingredients, such as flavors, can be added after drying of the granulation to avoid exposure to elevated temperatures.

The general method is first to granulate some of the ingredients, then blend the remaining ingredients with the dried granules before filling the container. Usually, the drug and other ingredients of a fine particle size are granulated with or without a portion of the diluent. The presence of the diluent helps to improve flow and reduces both segregation and dust formation [2].

In addition to the usual methods, the granules can be made by spray coating in a spray dryer [14]. As a special case, drug taste can be masked by microencapsulation [15] or coating with a water insoluble resin before blending with the remaining ingredients. This can be accomplished by spray coating, coacervation, or high-shear mixing of drug with the coating solution [2].

The disadvantage of the combination product is the increased risk of nonuniformity. The mix of granules and nongranular ingredients must not segregate into layers of different particle sizes. To achieve the necessary degree of homogeneity, the particle sizes of the various fractions should be carefully controlled. The allowed batch-to-batch variation, as a result of this concern, may be more stringent than the variation of the wholy granulated product.

The end result of preparing the dry mixture, regardless of the type, is to achieve physical uniformity. This ensures uniform potency during processing, bulk storage, and packaging. Table 5 summarizes the advantages and disadvantages of the above three types of dry mixtures used in suspensions for reconstitution.

D. Processing the Dry Mixture

The following guidelines have been recommended [1] for processing the dry mixture:

1. Use efficient mixing. Evaluate processing performance of batches on pilot scale-up equipment, not laboratory scale equipment.
2. Determine an adequate duration of mixing time.
3. Avoid accumulation of heat and moisture during mixing.
4. Limit temperature/humidity variations. A general rule is 70°C at $\leq 40\%$ relative humidity.

Table 5 Advantages and Disadvantages of Types of Dry Mixtures in Suspensions for Reconstitution

Type	Advantage	Disadvantage
Powder blend products	Economy; low incidence of instability	Mixing and segregation problems; losses of drug
Granulated products	Appearance; flow characteristics; less segregation; less dust	Cost; effects of heat and granulating fluids on drug and excipients
Combination of powder and granulation	Reduced cost; use of heat-sensitive ingredients	Ensuring nonsegregating mix of granular and non granular ingredients

Source: Ref. 2.

5. The finished batch should be protected from moisture. Store in lined containers with silica desiccant bags.
6. Sample for batch uniformity. Test at the top, middle, and bottom levels of dry mixture.

There are potential problems from changes in flowability of the dry mixture. The same flowability problems possible with powder blends, such as demixing, segregation, and moisture accumulation, can also occur during processing or in the completed dry mixture. Poor flowability or caking often occurs when individual particles fuse together. There are several reported causes, which include [1]:

1. Poor high-temperature stability
2. Surface charges
3. Variation of relative humidity
4. Crystallization
5. Packing due to weight of powder.

A common method of measuring flowability is by determining the angle of repose. When a powder or mixture is poured onto a horizontal surface, the powder mass builds up to a conical shape. The acute angle between the surface of the cone and the horizontal base is the angle of repose. A powder with good flowability will flow down the cone rather than build it up to produce a low angle of repose. Three general types of flow have been described [1]. An angle of repose of $\leq 38°$ indicates good flow. If the angle is $38°$ to $42°$ the powder has fair flow. An angle $\geq 42°$ indicates poor flow.

Some specific problems occurring after reconstitution illustrate the importance of uniformity and particle size [2]. A silicone antifoam agent was inadequately dispersed in the dry mixture. After reconstitution, droplets of the antifoam agent were observed at the surface, instead of a nearly invisible film. In another case, unmilled sodium carboxymethylcellulose having a particle size up to 500 μm was used in a dry mixture. After reconstitution, gelatinous lumps of slowly dissolving sodium carboxymethylcellulose were observed to adhere to the shoulder and neck of the bottle. Finally, an unmilled red dye having a particle size up to 500 μm was used in a dry mixture. After reconstitution, red streaks were observed as a result of slowly dissolving particles settling through the suspension.

V. STABILITY

Chemical stability is usually of more concern in suspensions for reconstitution than in conventional suspensions because the drug has poor stability in the presence of water. While there are usually only 14 days after reconstitution for separation problems to occur, physical stability before and after reconstitution is still a concern. Stability testing should include prototype formulas and full-scale stability tests. Carstensen discusses both chemical [16] and physical stability [17] testing of suspensions in his recent text on drug stability.

A. Chemical Stability

Drugs that degrade by hydrolysis, such as the penicillins, are common candidates for reconstitution. Drugs highly susceptible to oxidation or photolysis in solution may also be considered. In this case, degradation in the dry mixture would be limited to the surface of the solid particles and the interior would generally be protected from degradation.

Chemical stability should be determined in both the dry mixture and reconstituted suspension. Both should be examined not only at controlled room temperature but also at temperatures of potential exposure such as during shipment or storage of the product. Reconstituted antibiotic suspensions have been described as having a shelf life of 14 days at refrigerator temperatures in which the drug concentration does not fall below 90% of the original concentration. Several reconstituted antibiotic suspensions, however, demonstrate stabilities greater than this. For example, reconstituted suspensions of ampicillin trihydrate [18] and cefadroxil [19] retained 90% of their original concentrations after 6 weeks of refrigeration at 4°C; samples of ampicillin trihydrate maintained this 90% potency at room temperature for 30 days. In addition, reconstituted cephalexin monohydrate suspensions exhibited no appreciable degradation at –20, 4, and 25°C for 90 days [20] Amoxicillin, also, was reported to retain 90% activity at room temperature to remain stable for 1 week after reconstitution [21].

Stability evaluations of reconstituted oral suspensions should be conducted in a container of the same material and size in which the product is marketed. The repackaging of reconstituted suspensions may accelerate degradation. For example, reconstituted dicloxacillin sodium repackaged into unit-dose polypropylene oral syringes demonstrated an accelerated degradation at all temperatures compared to degradation in the manufacturer's original container [22]. Repackaging of the reconstituted combination product of amoxicillin trihydrate and potassium clavulanate oral suspension produced similar results. For this product it was concluded that the manufacturer's storage guidelines in the original containers should not be applied to dosages repackaged in unit-dose oral syringes [23]. An ampicillin suspension that was reconstituted in the original container, but stored in amber screw-cap unit-dose containers at refrigerator temperatures, contained only 89% of the drug after 5 days [24].

Not all repackaging of reconstituted oral suspensions adversely affects stability. The reconstituted cephalexin monohydrate oral suspension mentioned above that was stable at ambient temperatures and below for 90 days [20] had been repackaged in clear polypropylene oral syringes. The reconstituted ampicillin trihydrate suspensions described above that maintained 90% potency after 6 weeks at 4°C, and after 30 days at room temperature, also had been repackaged in plastic oral syringes. The investigators concluded that the expiration dates recommended by the manufacturer for this reconstituted suspension stored in its original container can also be used for storage in amber plastic oral syringes [18].

Some excipients may require chemical analysis. A notable example is the preservative. Degradation of the preservative is acceptable as long as sufficient preservative is present to maintain effectiveness. The effectiveness of the preservative is determined by challenge tests. Some flavors may also need analysis. An erythromycin ethylsuccinate suspension requires refrigeration to preserve taste, not to preserve drug stability [5].

Drug products are often exposed to elevated temperatures for the determination of a shelf-life (i.e., accelerated stability studies). This approach is, at best, risky for disperse systems. Testing at elevated temperatures causes large changes in physical properties such as viscosity. Irreversible changes may occur from precipitation or degradation of polymers in the dispersion. Higher temperatures can significantly change the solubility of the suspended drug.

Changes in degradation at elevated temperatures can be sufficient to alter the order of degradation kinetics. For example, reconstituted suspensions of ampicillin trihydrate [18], dicloxacillin sodium [22], and cephalexin [20] exhibited first-order degradation kinetics at 60° and 80°C, but exhibited zero-order degradation at temperatures ≤ 25°C.

Even in cases of zero-order degradation exhibited by a suspension at elevated temperatures, the apparent rate constant of degradation will change as the result of both the temperature-induced degradation of the small fraction in solution and the drug solubility in the solution. One method of accounting for both changes is to determine drug solubility at the various test temperatures, solve for degradation in solution given the measurements of the apparent zero-order rate constant and solubility, then calculate an estimate of stability at 25°C in the manner described by Swintosky et al. [25].

A method is available, however, that under certain conditions allows estimation of drug concentrations at room temperature based on degradation at elevated temperatures without the determination of drug solubility [26]. These conditions are: (a) degradation takes place only in solution and is first order, (b) the effect of temperature on drug solubility conforms to classical theory, and (c) dissolution is not rate limiting for degradation. The formulator should bear in mind that this method evaluates only the chemical stability of the suspension.

B. Physical Stability

Tests of physical stability should evaluate both the dry mixture and reconstituted suspension. Common evaluations on reconstituted suspensions include measurements of sedimentation volume and the ease of redispersion.

Sedimentation volume is obtained by measuring the height of settled drug particles in undisturbed bottles at intervals of time and expressing this height as a fraction of the initial height. Graduated cylinders are not currently used because the sedimentation height in small-diameter containers, such as 100-mL cylinders, can differ from that in wider bottles [1]. A high fraction, or sedimentation, volume, indicates good suspending ability. The worst case is the formation of a compact sediment of drug particles that cannot be redispersed. This cake would have a small sedimentation volume.

Ease of redispersion is a qualitative evaluation. It can be expressed in terms such as easy, moderate, difficult, or caked. Numeric scales have also been used. One evaluation used the number of inversions required to redisperse a 3-day-old suspension as the measurement of redispersibility [27].

Exposure to a cycle of temperature changes during which the suspension is frozen and thawed is another common method of evaluating physical stability. After a number of cycles, parameters such as sedimentation volume, distribution of particle size, and crystal changes can be measured. The last two parameters are followed by microscopic examination. Samples of the suspension are diluted and counted with the aid of an ocular grid. Photomicrographs can be used as permanent records for comparisons.

The physical stability of the dry mixture must be assessed. Potential problems include particle segregation from vibration during shipping. Temperature and humidity fluctuations during storage may reduce flowability or cake the dry mixture. Particles may fuse together and resist redispersion. High temperatures may even cause melting. Crystallization is also reported as a potential problem [1].

These potential problems should be examined. The possibility and extent of particle segregation can be examined with a vibrating bed. Tests at the anticipated extremes of temperature and humidity can illustrate the effect of flowability. Poor flow, incidentally, is reported as not uncommon at low relative humidities [1].

C. Guidelines for Stability Testing

This section briefly describes suggested guidelines [28] for prototype formula and full-scale stability testing. More extensive guidelines are available from the Food and Drug Administration [29]. Tests of the active drug are omitted because they are not usually required of the formulator. Both chemical and physical tests are conducted in these evaluations.

1. *Prototype Formulas*

Various formulations are subjected to extreme conditions in order to evaluate and compare their basic stability. Extremes of temperature, light, and humidity can be used. It should be mentioned that although these are screening tests, even good formulations may exhibit a poor response to some tests. Selection of the appropriate formulation for the final product should be made with some practical considerations. For example, particle separation may occur within the dry mixture during conditions of simulated shipping and storage, but the suspension may be easily reconstituted and administered without consequence. A reconstituted suspension may separate; however, the suspension may be easily redispersed and the appropriate dose administered. In both examples the obvious, undesired physical characteristics have no significant consequences, and in these situations the poor characteristics may be overlooked.

A screen based on temperature is a common test. Samples of the reconstituted suspension are stored in containers at room temperature, 37°, and 45°C. They are evaluated monthly for up to 4 months. These evaluations should include:

1. Chemical analysis for drug and preservative
2. Preservative challenge test at the initiation and conclusion of the study
3. Appearance compared to that of sample stored at 2° to 5°C
4. Viscosity
5. Homogeneity
6. pH
7. Sedimentation volume
8. Ease of redispersion

Such a screen test on the dry mixture should include higher temperatures and only the pertinent tests listed above should be performed. Additional tests may include flowability, examination for melting or fusing of particles, and changes in particle size distribution.

A screen based on light can be conducted on samples of formulas placed in containers that are exposed to a sunlamp at a constant distance, such as 12 inches, for 72 hours. The samples are inspected visually at appropriate intervals. The anticipated container of the marketed product should be used.

A screen based on humidity consists of storing samples in containers at 80% relative humidity and room temperature and 37°C. Controls should be stored at ambient humidity and the same temperatures. Samples should be taken and appropriate chemical and physical tests performed after 1, 2, and 3 months.

The freeze-thaw test may be conducted by placing the sample in a freezer for 18 hours followed by thawing at room temperature for 4 to 6 hours. Evaluate the appearance and conduct any other appropriate tests at this time. Repeat the freeze-thaw cycle up to 10 times. Conduct a chemical analysis at the conclusion of the test.

A temperature cycle exposes the formulation to both oven and refrigerator temperatures. Samples are placed in an oven at 45°C for 18 hours, removed and equilibrated to room temperature, and rated for appearance. The samples are then stored in a refrigerator for 18 hours, after which they are removed, warmed to room temperature, and again rated for appearance. The process may be repeated for 10 cycles and a chemical analysis should be performed at the end of the test.

2. *Full-Scale Stability*

The final formulation should be placed in the container for marketing and should be stored at 2° to 5°, room temperature, 37°, and 45°C. Samples should be taken and the appropriate chemical and physical tests conducted at specified intervals up to a maximum of 5 years. These times are listed in Table 6. The most reliable data for stability testing are from storage at room temperature, and consequently most tests are conducted on samples stored at this temperature. Tests at 6 months on samples stored at 45°C may provide a reasonable prediction of the chemical stability for 2 or 3 years, but the prediction must be confirmed by tests on room-temperature samples because of the potential problems at elevated temperatures described earlier. Actual samples must be available for assay at the date of expiration to confirm that predictions are true.

VI. TYPICAL FORMULAS

Published formulas of suspensions for reconstitution are listed in this section as examples, and for purposes of comparison. The antibiotic formulas are the most common of these suspensions and should serve as starting points for the formulator. It is unlikely that identical formulas can be used for different drugs or even for the same drugs. Excipients and their concentrations may vary depending on their individual specifications and the processing of the product.

A. Antibiotic Formulas

Four formulas are listed in this section. Detailed information on the specific preparation using these formulas [30] is not available and some of the reported information is

Table 6 Suggested Sample Times and Temperatures for Full-Scale Stability Testing

Time (months)	Temperature (°C)		
	25	37	45
0	X		
3	X	X	X
6	X	X	X
9	X		
12	X	X	
18	X		
24	X		
Each year to maximum of 5 years	X		

Source: Ref. 28.

based on interpretation by the authors. These formulas, however, contain a relatively small number of ingredients, and evaluation, with or without modification, should be uncomplicated. The percentages are based on reconstituted volume.

1. Sulfamethazine

Sulfamethazine	5 %
Sucrose	60 %
Sodium alginate	1.75 %
Sodium citrate	0.88 %
Citric acid	0.4 %
Sodium benzoate	0.2 %
Tween 80	0.08 %

The concentration of sulfamethazine after reconstitution is equivalent to 250 mg/5 mL. Sucrose is used as the solid diluent and sweetener. The suspending agent is sodium alginate. This formula uses citric acid and sodium citrate to buffer the reconstituted suspension to pH 5.0. The preservative is sodium benzoate. Tween 80, as as wetting agent, aids in the dispersion of the sulfamethazine. The sedimentation volume of this suspension after standing for 10 days at 30°C was 0.95.

2. Ampicillin Trihydrate

Ampicillin trihydrate	5.77 %
Sucrose	60 %
Sodium alginate	1.5 %
Sodium benzoate	0.2 %
Sodium citrate	0.125 %
Citric acid	0.051 %
Tween 80	0.08 %

When reconstituted, the concentration of ampicillin trihydrate provides 250 mg of ampicillin per 5 mL teaspoon. Ampicillin degradation products lower the pH of an unbuffered medium, which catalyzes degradation; maximum stability at pH 4.85 [31] is maintained with a citrate buffer. Less suspending agent, sodium alginate, is required in this formula than in the above formula. The wetting agent is Tween 80. The sedimentation value obtained under the same conditions as above (i.e., 10 days at 30°C) was 0.97.

3. Erythromycin Stearate

Erythromycin stearate	6.94 %
Sucrose	60 %
Sodium alginate	1.5 %
Sodium benzoate	0.2 %
Tween 80	0.12 %

When reconstituted, the concentration of erythromycin stearate provides 250 mg of erythromycin per 5 mL. The ethylsuccinate salt [5] is more common than the stearate salt in suspensions for reconstitution. Sucrose is the diluent and sweetener. The suspending agent and preservative are sodium alginate and sodium benzoate, respectively. A higher concentration of the wetting agent, Tween 80, is required in this formula than in the above formulas. The pH of the reconstituted suspension was 7, which is in the

Table 7 Comparison of Ingredients in Two Commercial Amoxicillin Suspensions for Reconstitution

Ingredient function	Product 1[a]	Product 2[b]
Active ingredient	Amoxicillin trihydrate	Amoxicillin trihydrate
Sweetener	Sucrose	Sucrose, mannitol
Suspending agent	Xanthan gum	Cellulose, CMC Na[c]
Dessicant	Silica gel	
Buffer	Sodium citrate	Sodium citrate, citric acid
Preservative	Sodium benzoate	—
Colorant	FD&C Red No. 3	D&C Red No. 28, FD&C Red No. 40
Flavor	Flavorings	Artificial flavors

[a]SmithKline Beecham Laboratories [33].
[b]Wyeth Laboratories [34].
[c]Carboxymethylcellulose sodium.

reported 7.0 to 8.0 pH range of excellent stability [32] and consequently a buffer was not used. The sedimentation volume after 10 days was 0.84.

4. *Tetracycline Hydrochloride*

Tetracycline hydrochloride	5.41 %
Sucrose	60 %
Sterculia gum	1 %
Sodium bicarbonate	0.76 %
Sodium benzoate	0.2 %
Tween 80	0.08 %

The reconstituted suspension contains tetracycline hydrochloride in each 5 mL equivalent to 250 mg of tetracycline. Sucrose is the solid diluent and sweetener. Sterculia gum is the suspending agent. Sodium bicarbonate is used to attain the recommended pH of 5.0 on reconstitution. The preservative is sodium benzoate and the wetting agent is Tween 80. The sedimentation volume after 10 days was 0.95.

B. Formula Comparison

The ingredients in two amoxicillin suspensions for reconstitution can be examined for comparisons and differences. Table 7 lists the ingredients in two commercial products [33, 34] that have similar formulas. Product 2 contains two sweeteners, sucrose and mannitol, whereas product 1 contains only sucrose. Product 2 uses a combination suspending agent of cellulose, perhaps microcrystalline, and carboxymethylcellulose sodium. Product 1 uses only xanthan gum. Product 1 uses silica gel as the desiccant but product 2 contains no such ingredient. Adjustment of pH is accomplished in product 1 with sodium citrate. Product 2 uses both sodium citrate and citric acid to adjust pH. Product 2 contains no preservative. Both products use colorants.

REFERENCES

1. B. I. Idson and A. J. Scheer, Suspensions. In: *Problem Solver* (J. Wallace, ed.), FMC Corporation, Princeton, NJ, 1984, pp. 14–15.

2. J. Ryder, *Int. J. Pharm. Technol. Prod. Manuf.*, 1:14–25 (1979).
3. *United States Pharmacopeia*, 23rd ed., United States Pharmacopeial Convention, Rockville, MD, 1995, p. 2364.
4. Keflex Package Insert, Dista Products Company, Division of Eli Lilly Industries, Inc., Carolina, Puerto Rico, Subsidiary of Eli Lilly and Company, Indianapolis, IN, February 1993.
5. E.E.S. Granules Package Insert, Abbott Laboratories, North Chicago, IL, Aug. 1991.
6. C. M. Ofner III, R. L. Schnaare, and J. B. Schwartz, Oral aqueous suspensions. In: *Pharmaceutical Dosage Forms: Disperse Systems*, 2nd ed., Vol. 2 (H. Lieberman, M. Rieger, and G. Banker, eds.) Marcel Dekker, New York, Chapter 4.
7. *United States Pharmacopeia*, 23rd ed., United States Pharmacopeial Convention., Rockville, MD, 1995, p. 2207.
8. E. N. Hiestand, *J. Pharm. Sci.*, 61:268–272 (1972).
9. D. M. Marmion, *Handbook of U.S. Colorants for Foods, Drugs, and Cosmetics*, 2nd ed. Wiley-Interscience, New York, 1984.
10. R. J. Lantz and J. B. Schwartz, Mixing. In: *Pharmaceutical Dosage Forms: Tablets*, Vol. 2 (H. A. Lieberman, L. Lachman, J. B. Schwartz, eds.), Marcel Dekker, New York, 1990, pp. 1–71.
11. E. G. Rippie, Mixing. In: *The Theory and Practice of Industrial Pharmacy* (L. Lachman, H. A. Lieberman, J. L. Kanig, eds.), Lea & Febiger, Philadelphia, 1986, pp. 3–20.
12. R. E. O'Connor, J. B. Schwartz, and E. G. Rippie, Powders. In: *Remington: The Science and Practice of Pharmacy* (A. R. Gennaro, ed.), Mack, Easton, PA, 1995, pp. 1598–1614.
13. D. Ball, T. Lee, J. Ryder, H. Seager, and D. Sharland, *J. Pharm. Pharmacol.*, 30:Suppl. 43P, 1978.
14. H. Seager, *Manuf. Chem.*, 48:25–35 (1977).
15. H. Seager and C. Taskis, *Manuf. Chem.*, 47:27 (1976).
16. J. T. Carstensen, *Drug Stability*, Marcel Dekker, New York, 1995 pp. 180–193.
17. J. T. Carstensen, *Drug Stability*, Marcel Dekker, New York, 1995, pp. 417–422.
18. M. F. Sylvestri and M. C. Makoid, *Am. J. Hosp. Pharm.*, 43:1496–1498 (1986).
19. M. C. Nahata and D. S. Jackson, *Am. J. Hosp. Pharm.*, 48:992–993 (1991).
20. M. F. Sylvestri, M. C. Makoid, B. E. Cox, *Am. J. Hosp. Pharm.*, 45:1353–1356 (1988).
21. M. A. Camacho Sanches, R. M. Saez Pastor, A. I. Torres Suarez, *An. R. Acad. Farm.*, 57:553–561 (1991).
22. M. F. Sylvestri, Makoid, M. C., and Adams. S. C., Am. J. Hosp. Pharm., 44:1401–1405 (1987).
23. Y. H. Tu, M. L. Stiles, L. V. Allen, K. M. Olsen, R. B. Greenwood, *Am. J. Hosp. Pharm.*, 45:1092–1099 (1988).
24. L. V. Allen, Jr., and P. Lo, *Am. J. Hosp. Pharm.*, 36:209–211 (1979).
25. J. V. Swintosky, E. Rosen, M. J. Robinson, R. E. Chamberlain, and J. R. Guarini, *J. Am. Pharm. Assoc., Sci. Ed.*, 45:37 (1956).
26. J. Tingstad, J. Dudzinski, L. Lachman, and E. Shami, *J. Pharm. Sci.*, 62:1361–1363 (1973).
27. C. A. Farley, *Pharm. J.*, 216:562–566 (1976).
28. P. J. Niebergall, personal communication.
29. *Guideline for Submitting Documentation for the Stability of Human Drugs and Biologics*, Food and Drug Administration, Center for Drug Evaluation and Research, Rockville, MD, 1987.
30. S. K. Baveja and K. C. Jindal, *Indian J. Pharm. Sci.*, 41:20–24 (1979).
31. J. P. Hou and J. W. Poole, *J. Pharm. Sci.*, 58:447–454 (1969).
32. R. F. Bergstron and A. L. Fites, *Am. J. Hosp. Pharm.*, 32:241 (1975).
33. Amoxil Package Insert, SmithKline Beecham Pharmaceuticals, Philadelphia, PA, December 1994.
34. Wymox Package Insert, Wyeth Laboratories Inc., Wyeth-Ayerst Co., Philadelphia, PA, February 1994.

7

Injectable Emulsions and Suspensions

Alison Green Floyd and Sunil Jain

Glaxo Wellcome, Inc., Greenville, North Carolina

I. INJECTABLE EMULSIONS

A. Introduction

Injectable emulsions have been successfully utilized as a source of calories and essential fatty acids for patients requiring long-term parenteral nutrition [1-6]. Most notable are the commercially available injectable fat emulsions used to prevent or treat essential fatty acid deficiency (EFAD) in various illnesses as well as in premature or low-birthweight infants [7,8]. Most products contain soybean or safflower oil and egg yolk derived phospholipid emulsifiers. Typical therapy includes a slow infusion of the emulsion via a peripheral vein or by central venous infusion over a 4- to 8-hour period [9]. Frequently, the fat emulsions are administered intravenously in combination with compatible amino acids, dextrose, and electrolyte solutions to provide for a total parenteral nutrition (TPN) or a three-in-one total nutrient admixture (TNA) [10-18]. Although it is generally not recommended, some patients require the extemporaneous addition of drugs to their fat emulsions or TNAs for delivery [19-29].

Parenteral emulsions are increasingly being used as carriers of drug substances because of their ability to incorporate drugs within their innermost phase, thus allowing for solubility and stability constraints of the drug to be minimized or bypassed altogether [29-33]. Because the drug is not in direct contact with the body fluids, the partitioning of drug from the internal to the external phase may contribute to a sustained release of drug. A more prolonged delivery can be achieved through the use of multiple emulsions by introducing an extra partitioning step before release to the body [34]. Formation of either water in oil in water (W/O/W) or oil in water in oil (O/W/O) multiple emulsions has allowed for prolonged release of various antineoplastic agents [35,36]. Additionally, emulsions may be used as a means of site-specific delivery; for example, delivering drugs to phagocytic cells of the reticuloendothelial system for treatment of a variety of parasitic and infectious diseases [30].

Many researchers have sought to produce an emulsion, free of undesirable side effects, that will meet these therapeutic needs. This presents a challenge to the formulating scientist because of the variable nature and stability of starting materials, such as the natural oils, and animal- or plant-derived emulsifying agents, such as lecithin. Additionally, required manufacturing steps—such as terminal sterilization in the case of large-volume parenterals—contribute to further formation of degradation products in these formulations. Unfortunately, the hydrolysis products of the phospholipids, lyso-phosphatidylcholine and lyso-phosphatidylethanolamine, are known to produce lysis of erythrocytes, although clinical toxicities due to this are rare [37]. However, with tight quality control over the entire process from selection of raw materials and equipment to the final manufacturing steps, the technology has advanced to the point of overcoming these obstacles.

It is the intent of this chapter to provide general knowledge and highly current background regarding the pharmaceutical aspects of injectable emulsions from a formulation development and manufacturing point of view.

B. Characteristics

The main feature common to all injectable emulsions is their strict particle size requirement. Products containing particles greater than 4 to 6 μm can result in emboli in the lungs, liver, kidneys, or brain [38,39]. The material responsible for lipid absorption and transport through the body, termed chyle, consists of particles that are remarkably uniform in size, varying in diameter from 0.2 to 3 μm. Chyle is composed of triglyceride in a central core surrounded by phospholipids and other surface-active agents [40]. In the case of the fat emulsions, attempts are made to mimic the composition and size of the chylomicra. Most commercial emulsions contain essential long chain triglycerides (LCT) (soybean or safflower oil); a newer emulsion [41] has a portion of the LCT replaced by medium chain triglycerides (MCT) (re-esterified fractionated coconut oil), providing a more readily metabolized regimen for compromised patients [4]. Injectable fat emulsions are stated to have a narrow particle size distribution with the average mean diameter ranging from 0.33 to 0.5 μm [4]; however, the particle size distribution for two commercially available fat emulsions was within the range of 0.4 to 1.0 μm, with some additional particles in the range of 2 to 5 μm [42].

Fat emulsions and any other injectable emulsion (water-in-oil, oil-in-water, and multiple emulsion systems) used for the delivery of drugs must meet the following requirements:

Physicochemical—physically and chemically stable, endotoxin free, sterilizable; maximum particle size less than 1 or 2 μm
Biological—low incidence of side effects, nonantigenic, and all components metabolized or excreted
Practical—stable to temperature extremes, reasonable cost (to the manufacturer and customer)

When used as a nutritional source, the commercially available fat emulsions provide a more concentrated source of calories as compared to carbohydrate or protein mixtures [6]. Because the oil component is insoluble in water, it does not exert an osmotic effect and thus can be used in vivo at higher concentrations. In addition to being an excellent source of calories, lipid supplies essential fatty acids (EFA), the fatty acids the body cannot derive from other sources.

Intravenous administration of fat emulsions in past years has been associated with many adverse physiological effects, such as back pain, fever, chills, headache, dizziness, blood pressure fluctuations, liver damage, and the "overloading syndrome" [43]. This syndrome may be manifested by a severe life-threatening reaction characterized by fever, blood disorders, hepatosplenomegaly, liver dysfunction, hyperlipidemia, seizures, and shock. Current therapies rarely result in these adverse effects because of improvements in purity of starting materials and knowledge of the distribution of emulsions in the body [6,31]. For example, fat emulsions are known to contain not only oil droplets, but free liposomes as the result of excess available surfactants present in the formulation [44]. Liposomes are known to be sequestered by the reticuloendothelial system (RES) [30]. Although some therapies may utilize this phagocytosis for site-specific delivery, chronic administration of long chain triglycerides may be deleterious to optimal RES function [45]. Stability and purity of the final formulation is thus a strict requirement in assuring its safety and efficacy by the parenteral route of administration.

Other adverse effects noted during lipid emulsion administration include tumor growth stimulation during administration of TPNs [46], hyperglycemia, hypertriglyceridemia [47], and effect on pulmonary function when administered to infants [48].

More recently the applications of these emulsions have increased in number, and many disadvantages have been overcome, so that the development of an emulsion formulation for parenteral administration is no longer one of trial and error but rather a scientific choice to fulfill a specific therapeutic need. This discussion is particularly concerned with the pharmaceutical aspects of injectable emulsions and their usage; therefore, it will be helpful to first consider each part of the formulation separately and then discuss how emulsions are processed.

C. Emulsion Ingredients

1. Oils

Numerous triglyceride oils have been investigated in the search for a stable, nontoxic oil for use in injectable emulsions. A wide variety of natural oils, including cottonseed, soybean, safflower, sesame, cod liver, linseed, coconut, corn, peanut, olive, coca butter, and butter oil have been studied [3]. Synthetic or semisynthetic substances such as triolein, ethyl oleate, dibutyl sebacate, and iso-amyl salicylate have been investigated with little success [1]. The oils most commonly used today are long chain triglycerides (LCTs) from vegetable sources (soybean or safflower oil) that contain a significant percent of linoleic acid, an essential fatty acid. Other fatty acids are typically present, along with trace amounts of impurities and degradation products [49]. One product containing cottonseed oil (Lipomul) was withdrawn from parenteral use following reports of toxic side effects associated with contamination of the oil with trace quantities of gossypol [49]. This was the first lipid product marketed in the United States. Since that time, enhanced purification techniques have concentrated on the commercialization of lipid emulsions containing soybean and safflower oil.

Medium chain triglycerides (MCTs) are being used more frequently in combination with LCTs (Lipofundin MCT/LCT 10% and 20%, B. Braun, Melsungen, West Germany) because they provide a more readily available source of energy [50]. MCTs are obtained from the re-esterification of fractionated coconut oil fatty acids (mainly caprylic and capric) and glycerin [51]. These fatty acids contain between 6 and 12 carbon atoms. MCTs are reported to be 100 times more soluble in water than are LCTs. Thus, they may have an increased ability to solubilize liposoluble drugs.

The purity of the oil is critical when applied to parenteral products and the presence of undesirable substances must be minimized. Purification may involve treatment with silicic acid or silica gel to remove undesirable components such as peroxides, pigments, thermal and oxidative decomposition products, and certain unsaponifiable matter (e.g., sterols and polymers) [52]. Solvent-based extraction processes are also designed to eliminate or reduce these substances. "Winterization" or storage at low temperatures for a prolonged period prior to filtration allows removal of components that may precipitate, such as the unsaponifiable components [49]. Natural oils must also be checked for the presence of aflatoxins, herbicides, and pesticides, which may be present due to inadvertent contamination.

High-quality food grade oils are a good source of starting materials for the preparation of injectable emulsions [49]. However, the manufacture of Intralipid (10% or 20% soybean oil) extract the oil from fresh soybeans. In addition to the purity of the oil, care must be taken to minimize or eliminate oxidation during processing of the oil and subsequent emulsion. Addition of antioxidants, such as α-tocopherol, to prevent oxidation of the oil may be employed [52].

As can be seen in Table 1, there are some differences in the fatty acid composition of cottonseed, soybean, and safflower oils. Because the absence of γ-linolenic acid has been associated with better thermal and oxidative stability [52] and linoleic acid is an essential fatty acid, high content of linoleic acid and low content of γ-linolenic acid are thus desirable features of these oils. However, linolenic acid has an important role in the development of the central nervous system in infants [4]. Thus, soybean oil–based emulsions should be used predominantly for infants. Soybean and safflower are the only oils that have continued long-term commercial acceptability in parenteral emulsions and can be found in several products. The composition and characteristics of some commercial fat emulsions are summarized in Table 2.

Additional oils have received recent attention in the development arena. Triacetin [53] a slightly water soluble oil (1 part triacetin in 14 parts water) has been used to solubilize taxol; because of its water solubility, it is expected to dissolve rapidly in the body, thus preventing phagocytosis and accumulation in the RES [51]. Squalane [31,54] is a saturated derivative of squalene [30], and both have shown solubilizing properties when used in emulsion formulations. Castor oil was successful in solubilizing two lipophilic anticancer drugs and resultant emulsions were monodispersed with a small average particle diameter of only 50 nm [31].

Table 1 Distribution of Fatty Acids in Cottonseed, Soybean, and Safflower Oils

Fatty acid	Cottonseed	Soybean	Safflower
Linoleic	45	51	77
Oleic	29	24	13
Palmitic	21	12	7
γ-Linolenic	2	9	—
Stearic	2	4	3

Table 2 Composition of Intravenous Fat Emulsions (in grams)

	Intralipid[a]	Liposyn[b]	Liposyn II[b]	Liporul[c] Infonutrol[d]	Lipofundin[e]	Lipofundin S[e]	Trivé 1000[f]	Nutrafundin[e]
Soybean oil	100,200	–	50,100	–	–	100,200	38	38
Safflower oil	–	100,200	50,100	–	–	–	–	–
Cottonseed oil	–	–	–	150	100	–	–	–
Egg phospholipids	12	12	12	–	–	–	–	–
Soybean phosphatides	–	–	–	12	7.5	7.5, 15	7.0	3.8
Glycerol	22.5	25	25	40	–	–	–	–
Glucose	–	–	–	40	–	–	–	–
Xylitol	–	–	–	–	–	–	–	100
Sorbitol	–	–	–	–	50	50	100	–
Pluronic F-68	–	–	–	3	–	–	–	–
DL-α-tocopherol	–	–	–	–	0.585	–	0.4	–
Maleic acid	–	–	–	–	–	–	10	–
Amino acid mixture	–	–	–	–	–	–	60	60
Water for injection to	1000	1000	1000	1000	1000	1000	1000	1000

[a]Clintec, U.S. *Note:* Similar formulas are marketed by Vitrum, Sweden; Travenol, U.S.; Alpha Therapeutic, U.S.; Green Cross, Japan; and Daigo, Japan.
[b]Abbott, U.S.
[c]Upjohn, U.S. (withdrawn from market).
[d]Astra-Hewlett, Sweden (withdrawn from market).
[e]Braun, West Germany.
[f]Egic, France.
Source: Adapted from *J. Parenteral Sci. Technol.*, 37:146 (1983), and updated.

2. Emulsifiers

Natural and synthetic agents have been considered as possible emulsifying agents because neither of the commonly used oils forms spontaneous emulsions when mixed with water [1]. Natural lecithin is defined as a mixture of phosphatides (Fig. 1), and has been obtained from both animal (egg yolk) and vegetable (soybean) sources. An advantage of using natural lecithin is that it is metabolized in the same way as fat and is not excreted via the kidneys, as are many synthetic agents [3]. Another advantage is that some phosphatide emulsions are very stable, resisting hydrolysis and oxidation if processed under inert atmosphere [40].

However, preliminary toxicological studies with the natural lecithins resulted in discouraging effects. These studies with soybean lecithin showed that this emulsifier was the principle cause of granulomatous lesions in rats given infusions of olive oil emulsions [55]. In addition, concentrations of soybean lecithin greater than 1% were associated with increased blood pressure. These lecithin-associated adverse reactions were attributed to impurities in the lecithin; totally purified lecithins, however, were less satisfactory as emulsifiers [56]. Until egg lecithin was chromatographically purified, emulsions made with this emulsifier could not be used clinically because they were too toxic [57]. Other studies employing both natural and purified egg lecithin produced hemolytic and other toxic effects after emulsion storage [58]. This was attributed to the hydrolysis of lecithin to lyso-lecithin, more commonly known as lyso-phosphatidylcholine (lyso-PC).

Consideration of parenteral toxicity has eliminated many of the otherwise excellent emulsifying agents that might be used in an injectable emulsion, mainly as a result of hemolytic reactions [49]. Also, stringent requirements must be met regarding emulsifier stability. For example, synthetic lecithins are more readily hydrolyzed in aqueous solution, and thus the resulting emulsion is not stable [40]. Natural lecithins undergo similar hydrolysis to form lyso-derivatives; however, it is known that phosphatidylcholine (PC) and lyso-PC form a complex that may reduce the toxic potential as well as improve the emulsion stability [49]. A stabilizing effect due to the mixture of lyso-derivatives present after terminal sterilization has also been demonstrated [37].

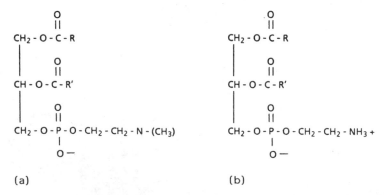

(a)   (b)

Fig. 1 Lecithin is defined as a mixture of phosphatides or fat-like compounds containing a phosphoric acid radical. R and R' are fatty acids. (a) Phosphatidyl choline (chemical lecithin) and (b) phosphatidyl ethanolamine (cephalin).

Even after purification, natural lecithin still contains a distribution of related substances [59]. While the major components of egg-derived lecithin, phosphatidylcholine and phosphatidylethanolamine (total approximately 90%) are uncharged at physiological pH, small amounts of phosphatidylserine and phosphatidylglycerol (2% to 5%) are present in an ionized form [60]. This distribution of phospholipids results in a droplet surface charge of approximately −40 to −50 mV. This charge is an important property of the emulsion and it is well known that additives altering this charge can significantly affect the emulsion stability [6,10–12,61]. Stability-related aspects regarding the surface charge will be further discussed later in this section.

Although highly purified lecithins reduce the incidence of side effects, they are not optimal emulsifiers [57]. Because the combination of phosphatides has been shown to be important to the stability of the emulsion formed, auxiliary emulsifying agents have been added to increase stability by forming "complex interfacial films" [1,31,33]. A wide range of *nonionic materials* has been investigated as potential auxiliary emulsifying agents: polyethylene glycol stearate, TEM (diacetyltartrate ester of monoglyceride), Drewmulse, (partially esterified polyglyercol), Myrj (polyoxyethylene monostearate), Carbowax (polyethyleneglycol), and Tergitol (nonyl phenyl ethers of macrogol ethers) [1]. However, these materials had given rise to toxic reactions of one form or another [1]. More recently, emulsifiers such as fatty acid esters of sorbitans (various types of Spans) and polyoxyethylene sorbitans (various types of Tweens) are now approved by the various pharmacopoeias for parenteral administration and can therefore be included in parenteral emulsion formulations [33].

One group of nonionic materials that has shown promise as emulsifiers for parenteral emulsions is the Pluronics (poloxamers or polyoxyethylene-polyoxypropylene derivatives) [62]. Emulsions containing Pluronic F-68 have been well tolerated over a short period of time; however, long administration led to the so-called "overloading syndrome." Further clinical investigation of this emulsion was restricted, resulting in inadequate data concerning incidences of pathophysiologic cause of the reaction [63]. Investigators continue to study the poloxamers as a nonionic emulsifer because of its ability to increase the zeta potential and thus contribute to the stability of the emulsion [64]. Cholesterol has also been utilized to increase emulsion stability [65]. Natural chyle is stabilized by lecithin complexed with protein; however, adding protein to injectable emulsions is contraindicated because of the foreign body reaction.

One study reported the emulsifying properties of F-alkylated phosphorylated surfactants with different polar heads for the emulsification of fluorocarbons, currently being investigated for oxygen-carriage and delivery [66]. The pharmaceutical and ultimate clinical acceptability awaits further experimentation and required in vivo tolerance.

In general, because of the relative safety and stability of the naturally derived, purified lecithins, they continue to be the most frequently employed emulsifiers in injectable emulsion formulations.

3. *Aqueous Phase*

Various substances have been added to the aqueous phase to adjust or control osmolarity, pH, oxidation, and microbial growth [1]. Because emulsified oil exerts no osmotic effect, additives are required to produce isotonic conditions in large-volume parenterals such as the injectable fat emulsions. Both ionic agents (sodium chloride) and reducing sugars (glucose, dextrose) are unsatisfactory because of interaction with the lecithin-emulsifying agent, resulting in brown discoloration and/or phase separation of the emulsion [1]. Glycerol has been preferred by the manufacturers of commercial soybean oil emulsion Intralipid, Soyacal, and Travamulsion) and a commercial safflower oil emulsion (Liposyn); other manufacturers have used sorbitol (Lipofundin, Trive 1000) or xylitol (Lipofundin S, Nutrafundin). The compositions of several intravenous fat emulsions are presented in Table 2. In addition to its contribution to tonicity, glycerol, in combination with proplyene glycol, has been shown to reduce the particle size and improve the creaming stability of oil-in-water emulsions [67].

Optimal stability of fat emulsions has been found to be pH dependent with an optimum in the range of 6.6 to 6.8 [58] or, more generally, 6 to 7 [49]. Various factors can alter the final pH of the emulsion product, such as addition of amino acids, dextrose, electrolytes, or drugs [61]. Additionally, hydrolysis of the parent phospholipids and in turn their lyso-compounds produces free fatty acids that will lower the pH [37]. Sterilization processes—inevitably accelerating the hydrolysis reactions—may also lower the pH of the formulation. During manufacture, therefore, the pH of the aqueous phase is usually adjusted slightly above physiological pH with a sodium hydroxide solution. Fat emulsions typically have a pH in the range of 8.0 to 8.3 [68].

Antioxidants such as alpha-tocopherol, deferoxamine mesylate, or ascorbic acid may be added to prevent peroxidation of unsaturated fatty acids [33,69]. Preservatives such as p-hydroxybenzoic acid (methyl and butyl derivatives) can be dissolved in the aqueous phase prior to emulsification [69].

D. Emulsion Manufacture

The manufacture of sterile injectable emulsions involves several steps, each of which play an important role in assuring a quality finished product. Of extreme importance is the maintenance of low bioburden during manufacture and sterility assurance in the final product, because the lipid component renders the formulation growth-promoting to microbiological insult. A typical flow diagram is provided for the manufacture of a hypothetical intravenous emulsion (Fig. 2).

1. *Compounding or Formulation Preparation*

The emulsifier, an osmotic agent, and any preservatives are usually dissolved or dispersed in the aqueous phase [49]. The phospholipids, antioxidants, and any lipophilic drugs to be incorporated are usually dissolved or dispersed in the oil phase. Filtration of every component of the emulsion is required to ensure low foreign particulate levels and bioburden before further processing. Hydrophilic membrane filtration is suitable for the aqueous phase. Hydrophobic filters are suitable for the oil and ethanol solution of the phosphatides, if used. Both phases are then heated to 70 to 85 °C with agitation. Conducting these processes under inert atmosphere is preferred, to minimize oxidation.

The addition of the phosphatides can be facilitated by dispersion in warm water by using a high-speed mixer fitted with a high-shear impeller. Another possible solution to this problem is to dissolve the phosphatide in anhydrous ethanol followed by transfer to the stirred aqueous phase. Precautions must be taken to guard against an obvious fire hazard. If nitrogen gas is bubbled through the hot aqueous phase, the phosphatide is dispersed under protective conditions and the alcohol is flushed off. The coarse emulsion is then formed by vigorous stirring or mixing. The final pH adjustment takes place after the emulsion is prepared before the batch is brought to final volume and homogenized.

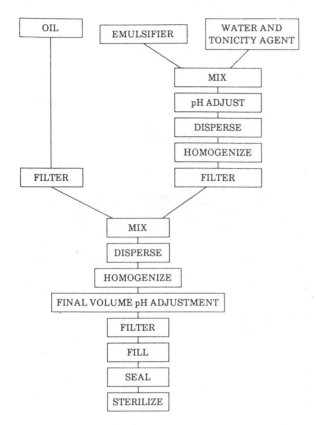

Fig. 2 Production flow diagram for hypothetical intravenous emulsion. (From J. J. Groves, *Parenteral Technology Manual,* Interpharm Press, Inc., Illinois, 1985, p. 36.)

2. *Homogenization and Particle Size Reduction*

Once the coarse dispersion is formed, it is necessary to reduce the particle size even further by homogenization [49]. As discussed previously, an essential requirement for injectable lipid emulsions is a small particle size (ideally not greater than 2 μm). Small particle size promotes good physical stability because creaming is prevented by Brownian movement [1]. In addition, large oil droplets (greater than 4 to 6 μm) can cause emboli. The required particle size can be achieved using various homogenizers or micro-fluidizers. Their utility on either laboratory or industrial scale must be acknowledged because equipment changes during scale-up may affect the physical and chemical stability and may affect the pharmacological efficacy as well. This step should be carefully controlled by taking sufficient in-process particle-size measurements to determine the end point of homogenization.

Colloid mills are effective only at reducing the average oil droplet size to approximately 5 μm and are thus not suitable for the preparation of injectable emulsions [49]. Ultrasonic homogenizers have successfully been utilized to produce injectable emulsions on a laboratory scale. However, no documentation was found to indicate that this process has been scaled up for manufacture of emulsions on a commercial scale.

The use of a high-pressure piston homogenizer of the type available from manufacturers such as the Gaulin Corporation[a] or Cherry-Burrell[b] is illustrated in Fig. 3. (A

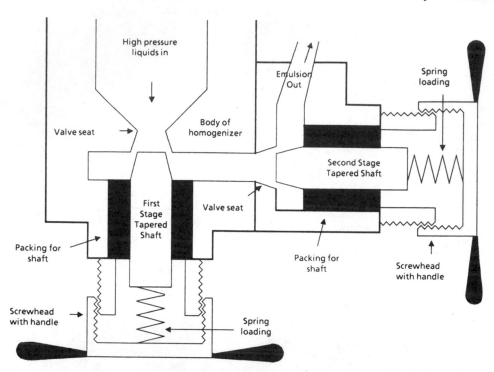

Fig. 3 One type of two-stage high-pressure homogenizer. (Adapted from *J. Parenteral. Sci. Tech.*, 37:148, 1983.)

list of suppliers/manufacturers of products listed throughout can be found in the Appendix). In these homogenization devices, the crude emulsion is forced under pressure through the annular space between a spring-loaded valve and the valve seat. The second stage is in tandem with the first, so that the emulsion is subjected to two very rapid dispersion processes. Pressures ranging from 3000 to 5000 psi are applied to the emulsion, usually under nitrogen protection [49,62]. The emulsion may be homogenized a number of times in order to achieve the necessary particle size.

A major concern of the homogenization process is the inevitable contamination produced from gasket materials, packing, and metal parts. These contaminants also originate from pumps and other metal surfaces. Pumps may be eliminated by transferring from vessel to vessel under nitrogen pressure if closed systems are used. One technology that has demonstrated good performance while minimizing the contamination is microfluidization.

Microfluidization, a relatively new proprietary technology (U.S. Patent 4,533,254), has been used very successfully to produce parenteral emulsions [70–73]. Microfluidizer^c processing is based on a submerged jet principle in which two fluidized streams interact at ultrahigh velocities in precisely defined microchannels within an interaction chamber, as illustrated in Fig. 4. The interaction field does not vary with time or location and has no moving parts. Process pressure can be varied from 500 to 20,000 psi and the process stream is accelerated to velocities of up to 1500 ft/sec. A combination of shear, turbulence, and cavitation forces results in the energy-efficient production of consistently fine droplets with a narrow size distribution. A typical set of particle-size

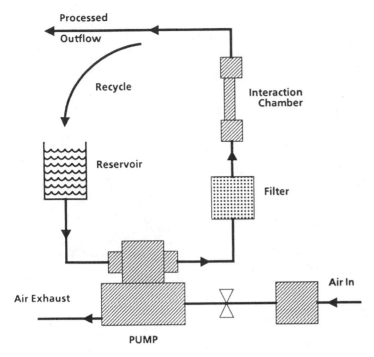

Fig. 4 Diagram of the microfluidizer. (Courtesy of Microfluidics Corporation, Newton, Massachusetts.)

data is presented in Table 3, demonstrating how repeated passage through the Microfluidizer reduces the mean droplet size and narrows the size range [73].

Comparison of the Microfluidizer to various conventional methods (such as standard vortexing, blade mixing, and homomixing) has demonstrated that greater emulsion stability may be achieved with microfluidization because of its superior ability to decrease the mean particle size and provide a narrower size distribution [54]. Oil in water emulsions with the desired particle size can thus easily be prepared by the use of a Microfluidizer.

Table 3 Prefiltration Particle Size Analysis After Microfluidization at 16,000–17,000 psi

No. of Processing cycles	Mean size (nm)	Size range (nm)
1	187	115–1000
2	157	81–405
4	164	118–315
5	164	90–308
7	165	81–270
7 filtered	163	37–189

Source: Adapted from *Pharm. Res.*, 9(7):860–863 (1992).

3. *Filtration*

After homogenization, the complete emulsion requires final filtration to remove large particles, but cannot remove particles with dimensions close to those of the oil droplets themselves. Consideration should also be given to the flow rate through the final filter because the presence of the small oil droplets will lower throughput of the membrane filter.

4. *Packaging*

Injectable emulsions provided in volumes of 100 to 1000 mL are packaged in USP type I or II glass bottles [49]. Some manufacturers appear to siliconize their bottles to provide a hydrophobic surface in contact with the emulsion. Plastic containers are generally unsuitable because they are permeable to oxygen and contain oil-soluble plasticizers, which may be extracted by the emulsion. Although no adverse clinical effects from small amounts of plasticizers have been reported, non-polyvinylchloride (PVC) administration sets and bags are available for use with lipid emulsions in clinical settings [21,28,74,75].

The stoppers used to package injectable emulsions are also carefully selected. The stopper must not be permeable to oxygen or become softened by contact with the oil phase of the emulsion. Coated stoppers are available and provide an inert barrier between the rubber compound and the product. The headspace of the final container may be flushed with nitrogen or evacuated prior to sealing to minimize oxidation of the emulsion.

5. *Sterilization*

For large-volume (100 to 1000 mL) injectable fat emulsions, sterilization is achieved by autoclaving. Sterilization conditions must be selected carefully to ensure a sterile product but minimize degradation of the thermolabile product [49]. An essential requirement is a low initial or low presterilization bioburden in the emulsion to allow the minimum heat input to the final product. Sterilization causes some hydrolysis of lipids and lecithins resulting in the liberation of free fatty acids (FFA), which are known to lower the pH of the emulsion [37].

As an alternative to terminal sterilization, it may be possible to sterilize the individual components and aseptically assemble the final emulsion [49]. Alternatively, the first published example of sterile filtration through a 0.22 μm cartridge filter for a parenteral emulsion is described for a microfluidized emulsion [73]. This approach minimizes or eliminates the heat input into the emulsion but does not provide the degree of sterility assurance provided by terminal sterilization.

E. Properties

1. *pH*

The pH of the emulsion is usually adjusted with a small quantity of sodium hydroxide to approximately 8.0 prior to sterilization. This is preferred because the pH of the emulsion falls on autoclaving, and also as a function of time during storage, as the result of glyceride and phosphatide hydrolysis liberating free fatty acids (FFA). The rate of FFA production is minimal if the pH of the emulsion is between 6 and 7 after sterilization [76]. However, the reported final pH of intravenous lipid emulsion varies. Values reported range from approximately 4.5 up to 7.2 [1].

The pH is important for maintenance of the desired particle size because of its effect on the surface charge of the particle [42]. This effect is demonstrated by an increase in electrophoretic mobility over a pH range of 6.5 to 9.0. This rise in mobility can be associated with the ionization of the phosphate groups in the surface film of lecithin. A breakpoint in the profile occurs at the isoelectric point for lecithin at pH 6.7 $\pm$ 0.2 [57]. A low pH (<5) can reduce the electrostatic repulsion between emulsified oil particles, thus resulting in coalescence and generation of large particles. The effect on emulsion stability as related to surface charge is discussed in more detail later in this section.

2. *Particle Size*

Particle size of the lipid globules has a direct effect on both toxicity and stability. Particles greater than 4 to 6 μm are known to increase the incidence of emboli and blood pressure changes [39]. Studies using electron microscopy have shown that the particles in commercial lipid emulsions are very similar to those in natural chylomicrons [1,77]. In both cases, particles consist of a core of triglyceride surrounded by a layer of phospholipid. There is also evidence that emulsion particle size directly affects the rate at which an emulsion is utilized by the body [78]. Emulsions with particles ranging from 0.5 to 1.0 μm are utilized more rapidly by the body than emulsions with 3 to 5 μm particles.

Manufacturing processes and variables producing the smallest particle size (usually 200 to 500 nm for fat emulsions) also lead to the formation of the most physically stable emulsions [70]. In one study, the mean particle size has been shown to decrease to approximately 250 nm upon an increase of egg phospholipid emulsifier concentration up to 1.2% (w/w) [79]. The particle size is also affected by the oil concentration, whereby increases in oil concentration greater than 10% may significantly increase the particle size.

Smaller particle sizes in the range of 1 to 100 nm can be achieved by the formation of microemulsions [80]. These systems consist of an oil phase, an aqueous phase, a primary surfactant (which will be adsorbed at the oil/water interface and determines whether the emulsion is O/W or W/O) and a secondary surfactant, known as a cosurfactant. The cosurfactant interacts with high specificity at the interface and forms a mixed duplex film. The microemulsion has the advantage of very small disperse phase diameter, which may impart thermodynamic stability.

3. *Surface Charge*

The distribution of neutral and ionized phospholipids present in purified lecithin results in a droplet surface charge (zeta potential) of approximately –40 to –50 mV. The surface potential plays an important role in the stability of emulsions through electrostatic repulsions. Ionized lipids are thought to have a favorable effect on emulsion particle size and stability through an increase in the surface charge and bilayer thickness of phospholipid films [81]. A reduction in the electrical charge is known to increase the rate of flocculation and coalescence, and thus its measurement is useful in stability assessment [82].

However, emulsions of equal zeta potential were found to have different flocculation behaviors in the presence of added electrolyte, thus indicating factors other than zeta potential alone can influence the physical stability [81]. It was further demonstrated that phosphatidic acid was the most important component of the mixed phosphatides for maintaining stability of the system in the presence of electrolytes. Surface charge could be optimized by choosing lecithins with varying amounts of negatively charged phosphatides such as phosphatidic acid, phosphatidylserine, or phosphatidylinositol [49,83].

Preliminary studies suggest that lipid particles with significant surface charge, either positive or negative, are more stable and are cleared from the bloodstream more rapidly than those with neutral charge [1]. Intralipid and Lipiphysan were found to consist of negatively charged particles. The cottonseed oil emulsion (Lipiphysan) was found to carry a higher particle charge than the soybean oil emulsion (Intralipid).

Electrokinetic properties of phospholipid-stabilized fat emulsions in the presence of various additives have been extensively studied [84–89]. In a fat emulsion consisting of model phospholipids, increasing amounts of negatively charged phospholipids (e.g. phosphatidylglycerol [PG]) cause an increase in the droplet charge, and the critical flocculation concentration to shift to higher electrolyte (calcium) concentrations [84]. The calcium concentration at which the droplet charge was zero (PZC, point of zero charge) also increased with increasing PG concentration. From this study, it appears that a *critical* zeta potential is required for stability; that is, the zeta potential at the critical flocculation concentration. A semiempirical theory based on the adsorption of ions to the phospholipids has been described that allows the accurate modeling and prediction of droplet zeta potential in mixed electrolyte solutions [85]. Another theoretical approach demonstrates that hydration forces are at least as important as the electrostatic forces in emulsion stability [86]. From this theory, it is postulated that the stabilizing effect of amino acids is due to their influence on the hydration forces. Further studies demonstrated that calcium-induced flocculation may be reduced by either addition of glucose [87] or amino acids [88]. More recently, electric sonic analysis (ESA) measurements of full strength TPNs demonstrated zeta potentials between +4 and –6 mV [89], which is significantly less than for the undiluted fat emulsions.

Zeta potential measurements are typically performed using a Doppler electrophoresis apparatus such as the Zetasizer,[d] or determined by the moving-boundary electrophoresis technique, where the electrophoretic mobility is measured and used to calculate the zeta potential [33]. A new technique for measuring zeta potential—electric sonic analysis or ESA [89]—can be performed using a Matec ESA 8000.[e] This technique allows the zeta potential to be determined for a concentrated dispersion without the typical necessary dilutions that could affect the emulsion stability.

F. Stability and Evaluation of Emulsions

As previously mentioned, the stability of emulsions is influenced by electrolytes, additives, or any change to the continuous phase composition. The stability of the formulation during storage as well as during administration is discussed below.

1. *Stability of the Formulation*

Stability of emulsions can be influenced by processing conditions, autoclaving, storage conditions, excessive shaking, or the addition of electrolytes or drugs. Most stability programs evaluate the short- and long-term stability of the formulation under typical and stressed conditions. Researchers utilizing stressed conditions for accelerated stability testing, such as shaking, freeze-thawing, or autoclaving [33], may not be able to correlate results to long-term or shelf-life storage because of the profound effect on the stability of the emulsion. A change in stability may be manifested in a number of ways.

These changes have been classified for discussion in the following categories: physical stability, chemical stability, and microbiological stability.

a. *Physical Stability.* Physical instability is indicated by particle size changes, flocculation, creaming, coalescence, and oil separation. Because the first indication of physical instability is usually an increase in particle size, this measurement is monitored routinely. Extreme temperature fluctuation such as freezing can result in an increased oil droplet size, leading to aggregation, coalescence, and ultimate separation [90]. Particle size determination is technically very difficult because the particle sizes usually extend beyond the limit of detection of any one given instrument. Thus, at least two complementary techniques should be employed. Many advanced instruments for determining particle size are available. For particle sizes less than 1 μm, photon correlation spectroscopy[f] (PCS) or quasi-elastic laser light scattering (QELS) is useful. For particles greater than 1 μm, coulter counter,[g] laser inspection system,[h] and electron microscopy[i] may be used. Detailed reviews of the application of these techniques to injectable emulsions have been given elsewhere [27,31,33,60]. The conventional light microscope is still invaluable for subjective observations on the degree of dispersion. However, it is important to emphasize that most of the techniques require significant sample dilution and thus flocculation may not be detected. Additionally, more than one method should always be employed because of the specific size ranges of detection and the sample preparation bias that may result.

b. *Chemical Stability.* Chemical instability is indicated by oxidation and hydrolysis of the oil and/or emulsifier, change in emulsion pH, and increase in free fatty acid content or rancidity of the oil. Additionally, the chemical stability of any incorporated drugs must be monitored.

Exposure to excessive heat accelerates the hydrolytic degradation. Initially, refrigerated storage was required for emulsion products sold in the United States [49]. This storage restriction has been lifted, allowing room temperature (<25°C for most products, <30°C for Liposyn) for a shelf life of at least 18 months.

Emulsions stored under nitrogen and not exposed to direct sunlight are unlikely to exhibit oxidative degradation. The stability of the emulsion is thus affected when the intact container is entered [68]. The integrity of the nitrogen layer in the sealed container is essential for long-term room temperature stability. For example, exposure of Intralipid 10% to the atmosphere results in gradual changes in the emulsion. No changes in the particle size distribution occurred during the first 36 hours at room temperature, but after 48 hours globule coalescence was noticeable and by 72 hours had become significant. Shelf life of subdivided emulsions may be increased by using refrigerated storage conditions.

c. *Microbiological Stability.* Support of bacterial and fungal growth by commercial fat emulsions has been demonstrated by inoculation of Intralipid, Liposyn, and Travamulsion [91,92]. Growth rates in the fat emulsion in most cases matched the growth rate in trypticase soy broth. Therefore, every precaution should be taken to prevent microbial contamination during processing and maintain sterility of these emulsions in clinical situations. A maximum hang time of 12 hours is recommended for administration of fat emulsions [93]. Small-volume parenteral emulsions should be recommended for single use only and may contain a preservative.

d. *Stability Protocol.* As in any stability evaluation, the product under evaluation must be thoroughly characterized physically and chemically at the start of the study. Initial observations and analysis ensure that the product was properly processed and establish baseline values for comparison with data from aged samples. Initial testing should include but not necessarily be limited to the following:

Physical examination—visual observation for creaming, coalescence, and oil separation

Chemical analysis—determination and characterization of drug substance, oil, phosphatide, and excipients present, including free fatty acids, lyso-lecithin, and oxidative degradation products

pH determination

Particle size and surface charge

Preservative test

Sterility test

Pyrogen test

The three critical aspects of emulsions with regard to toxicity are lyso-lecithin, free fatty acid content, and oil droplet size. Therefore, stability studies should closely monitor these aspects, while other aspects can be tested at less frequent intervals. In long-term studies, the sterility and pyrogen tests needs to be conducted initially, and at the expiry date. Yearly sterility and pyrogen testing may be conducted until a good predictor of the shelf life is available. A typical long-term stability protocol for a product of unknown stability is presented in Fig. 5. Accelerated stability evaluation for 6 months at 40°C or 12 months at 30°C is proposed by the International Conference on Harmonization (ICH) Tripartite guidelines. If the formulation remains stable under these accelerated conditions, the formulation is likely to survive a 2-year or greater shelf life at controlled room temperature (15 to 30°C). However, this may not be a good prediction for lipid emulsions because of the adverse effect stressed conditions such as heat may have on the physical and chemical stability. In these cases, real-time data would be the only suitable indicator, as required by the FDA for approval of expiry dates. As data are gathered and the stability of the product is better understood, the protocol can be modified to delete unnecessary assays and/or storage conditions.

2. Stability and Compatibility During Administration

a. *Injection Site.* Stability concerns of injectable emulsions continue throughout the duration of administration. Precipitation of the drug following injection of an emulsion formulation is unlikely to occur in the same way as after injection and dilution of a cosolvent-based formulation [27]. Thus, local irritation due to precipitated drug should also be reduced or eliminated. Although rare, instability at the injection site may be evident by aggregation or coalescence of the dispersed phase resulting in serious adverse effects to the patient or possible influence on drug availability.

b. *Stability at the Y-Site of a Free-Flowing Infusion.* Most commonly, fat emulsions are administered into the same peripheral vein as amino acid–dextrose solutions by a "piggy back" or "Y-site" infusion [94]. Mixing of the two preparations occurs just before entering the peripheral vein. Two primary factors affect stability of the emulsion. The first is the presence of electrolytes, either mono- or divalent cations. Monovalent cations cause progressive coalescence whereas divalent cations cause immediate flocculation [95]. For example, flocculation of Intralipid occurred in the Y-connector of a main line during infusion of Intralipid, calcium gluconate, and heparin [96]. Fortunately, there was no clinical evidence of fat embolism and the infusion was immediately discontin-

Conditions	Time Period										
	Initial	7 days	14 days	1 mos.	3 mos.	6 mos.	9 mos.	12 mos.	18 mos.	24 mos.	36 mos.
At Storage	%SPyP										
5 °C[1]					X	X	X	%	X	%	%S
25 °C					%	%P	%	%P SPy	%	%P SPy	%P SPy
30 °C					%	%P	%	%P			
40 °C				%	%	%P					
Fluorescent Light[2]				%	%						
Ultraviolet Light[3]		%	%								

[1] Only initial studies to determine temperature sensitivity

[2] Fluorescent light equivalent to 1000 foot candles

Note: Proposed ICH guidelines suggest exposure to 1380 foot candles fluorescent light for 3 and 8 days.

[3] Ultraviolet light equivalent to 1000 μwatts/cm^2

Fig. 5 Sample protocol for injectable emulsions.
Key:
- X appearance (color, clarity, phase separation, packaging) odor, viscosity, physical testing (viscosity, other physical tests), pH
- % X, active ingredient(s)/degradation products assay, free fatty acids, particle size distribution, particle surface charge
- P Preservative
- S Sterility test
- Py Pyrogen testing

ued. The second factor is the pH of the system, which if significantly altered could result in particle size changes, coalescence, and separation [4].

  c. *Compatibility with Administration Sets and Admixtures.* Potential for incompatibilities with the intravenous administration sets as the result of oxidation of the nutrients [8,76], absorption to the plastic [97], or extraction of plasticizers such as DEHP [98] has been reported. A multilayered bag with reduced permeability to oxygen (Mixieva Ultrastab^j) is available in Italy [75]. The bag is composed of a new triple-layer plastic, produced as a coextruded combination of ethyl vinyl acetate (EVA) and modified EVA–ethylvinyl alcohol (EVOH). The multilayered plastic has an oxygen permeability of 9 mL/m/24 hr/atm at 100% relative humidity, which is approximately 100 times less than a single layer of EVA plastic film [75]. Because DEHP release is more likely with hydrophobic solutions, lipid emulsions are more likely to extract it from the plastic bags. In an effort to eliminate extraction of plasticizers, a dual-chamber flexible container (Nutrimix, Abbott) is available that separately packages both amino acids and dextrose injection in one container [99]. The plastic contains a specially formulated nonplasticized thermoplastic copolyester (CR3) with no diethylhexylphthalate (DEHP); safety in animals according to USP biological standards has been confirmed. Empty 2- or 3-liter ethyl vinyl acetate containers[j] (EVA-Mix,[k] Infusobags[l]) are frequently used to prepare extemporaneously desired admixtures of lipid emulsions because they do not contain DEHP.

The combination of nutrients (fat emulsion, amino acids, dextrose, electrolytes, trace elements, multivitamins, and other additives) in a single container for subsequent infusion (termed total parenteral nutrition [TPN] or total nutrient admixture [TNA]) requires particular attention to the order of mixing. This is a critical consideration to the stability of the admixture [15,16]. Electrolytes should not be added directly to the fat emulsion. For best results, the electrolytes should either be added last or mixed with the amino acid injection and/or dextrose injection or transferred simultaneously with amino acids into the fat emulsion container.

Incompatibilities between fat emulsions and various additives are well understood. Additives such as calcium and magnesium as well as monovalent cations capable of altering the surface charge can significantly affect emulsion stability. Addition of amino acids, however, appears to prevent flocculation and coalescence that occurs in presence of these ions or dextrose [6]. It has been further demonstrated that this protective effect may be related to the relationship of the isoelectric point (pI) of the amino acids, the pH of the external media affecting the electrolytic association of the phospholipid, and the amino acid molecules adsorbed at the oil-water interface [12]. It is possible that the amino acids confer stability by reducing the critical zeta potential in the mixture [88] It was further demonstrated that three amino acid prodrugs, N-α-acetyl-L-arginine (Ac-Arg), N-α-acetyl-L-histidine (Ac-His), and N-α-acetyl-L-lysine (Ac-Lys), have been shown to have an excellent stabilizing effect on the emulsion compared with amino acids without acetyl groups. This is thought to be due to the weak electric effect of Ac-Arg, Ac-His, and Ac-Lys, which exist as neutral molecules in an aqueous solution [23].

G. Recent Applications of Intravenous Emulsions

Emulsion formulations of drugs may be employed to overcome solubility or stability limitations that are not otherwise resolved by pH control (if the drug has an ionizable group) or co solvents such as ethanol, glycols, dimethylacetamide (DMA), or dimethylsulfoxide (DMSO). The limitations of these solvents include precipitation of the drug on injection, pain or phlebitis, and inherent toxicities due to the solvent itself. Application of injectable emulsions as a vehicle for the administration of poorly water soluble drugs has been increasing over the years. Two approaches have been used to incorporate drugs into an emulsion: de novo preparation and extemporaneous addition of drugs to formulated emulsions.

1. *Emulsions Formulated to Contain Specific Drugs—de novo Preparation*

Numerous examples in the literature demonstrate injectable emulsion formulations of anticancer agents, vaccines, oxygen carriers, and other pharmaceutically active compounds. The drugs studied have been incorporated into an emulsion system to afford greater solubilization, stabilization, physical compatibility with administration sets, and reduction of irritation or toxicity, and to afford sustained or targeted drug delivery. Some examples of these application are presented below.

a. *Enhancement of Solubility or Stability.* Several de novo emulsion formulations of penclomedine [32], a practically insoluble (approximately 1 µg/mL) antitumor agent, were prepared using soybean oil emulsified with water using various lecithins (egg yolk lecithin: 60% and 99% α-phosphatidylcholine and soybean lecithin: 60% α-phosphatidylcholine) and glycerol, in the proportions listed in Table 4. Concentration of penclomedine in soybean oil was 183 mg/mL at room temperature, thus emulsions containing 5 or 10 mg/mL were easily obtained. All the emulsions had hydrodynamic particle sizes less than 500 nm. The emulsion prepared with the 99% α-phosphatidylcholine had initially the smallest particles, with an average of approximately 250 nm; however, it was the only emulsion studied that demonstrated an increase in particle size over the study period. No significant change or trend was observed in the physical or chemical stability of the other emulsion formulations after 12 months. Preliminary cytotoxicity results indicated that penclomedine emulsions showed better cytotoxic activity after both intraperitoneal and intravenous administration than a comparable dose from a suspension of the solid.

Taxol is an example of an anticancer agent that is formulated in a 1:1 mixture of ethanol:cremophor EL because of solubility and stability constraints [53]. This cosolvent mixture is diluted before to administration in isotonic saline and remains stable for only 3 hours. The solubility of Taxol in soybean oil was only 0.3 mg/mL; therefore, extemporaneous preparations using commercial fat emulsions were not feasible. A triacetin emulsion was prepared that contained 50% triacetin oil, 1.5% soy lecithin, 1.5% pluronic F 68, 2.0% ethyloleate, and 1.0% Taxol. (See Table 5.) Although chemical stability remained > 96% after 6 months at 22°C, physical instability was present. The addition of glycerol in concentrations up to 10% was beneficial to prevent creaming, but overall improvement in physical stability was minimal, thus glycerol was not in the final formulation for further toxicity testing. The authors concluded the observed emulsion instability was probably due to inadequate manufacturing equipment. The triacetin emulsion proved to be less hemolytic than 20% Intralipid alone, and acute toxicity in mice indicated an LD_{50} of 1.2 mL/kg. The typical dose of 30 mg Taxol or 3 mL of the triacetin emulsion in a 70-kg adult would correspond to only 0.043 mL/kg.

Diazepam is also poorly soluble in water, and the marketed formulation (Valium Injection), containing propylene glycol, ethanol, and benzyl alcohol, is believed to cause tissue irritation and thrombophlebitis. This cosolvent formulation was compared with an emulsion formulation (Diazemuls) consisting of 0.5 gram diazepam, 15.0 gram soybean oil, 5.0 gram acetylated monoglycerides, 1.2 gram egg yolk phosphatides, 2.5 gram glycerol made up to 100 mL with water [100,101] (Table 6). A significant difference was found in acute intravenous toxicity (LD_{50}) and tissue damage following intraarterial injection between the two formulations; in mice, however, the anticonvulsant activity

Table 4 Penclomedine Emulsions

Penclomedine (mg/mL)	Soybean oil (%)	Lecithin		Glycerin (%)
		Type	(%)	
5	10	99% Egg yolk	1.2	2.4
5	10	60% Soybean	1.2	2.4
10	10	60% Egg yolk	1.2	2.4
0 (placebo)	10	60% Soybean	1.2	2.4
0 (placebo)	10	60% Egg yolk	1.2	2.4

Source: Adapted from *J. Paren. Sci. Tech.* 42(3): 76–81 (1988).

Table 5 Taxol Cosolvent and Emulsion Formulations

Current formulation		Emulsion formulation	
Ingredient	Content (%)	Ingredient	Content (%)
Taxol	0.06	Taxol	1.0
Ethanol	5.0	Triacetin oil	50.0
Cremophor EL	5.0	Soy lecithin	1.5
Isotonic saline	90.0	Pluronic F68	1.5
		Ethyl oleate	2.0

Source: Adapted from *Pharm. Res.*, 4(2): 162–165 (1987).

was about equal. Diazemuls was administered to 9492 patients between 1975 and 1980 without serious side effects [102]. Only 9 (0.4%) of the 2435 patients given Diazemuls intravenously experienced pain. The clinical effect was found satisfactory in 2409 patients (99%). There was no reddening of the skin or tenderness along the vein related to the injection in any patient. Following intramuscular injection, only 7% of 30 patients receiving Diazemuls experienced pain compared to 43% of 30 patients receiving the conventional formulation. Pharmacokinetic studies indicated distribution and elimination of diazepam after intravenous injection were the same with both formlations.

In a subsequent study, a submicronized emulsion delivery system for diazepam was developed and evaluated for short- and long-term stability [64,69]. This formulation is also described in Table 6. Parameters contributing to enhanced stability included: initial pH of 7.4 or 8.0, oil phase of less than 25%, poloxamer (nonionic emulsifier) concentration between 1% and 2%, and phospholipid concentration between 1% and 1.25%. Changes in concentration of diazepam near the therapeutic concentration did not appear to affect emulsion stability.

Table 6 Diazepam Emulsion Formulations

Diazemuls emulsion formulation[a]		Submicronized emulsion formulation[b]	
Ingredient	Content (%)	Ingredient	Content (%)
Diazepam	0.5	Diazepam	0.5
Soybean oil	15.0	Soybean oil	20.0
Acetylated monoglycerides	5.0	Egg yolk phospholipids	1.2
Egg yolk phosphatides	1.2	Poloxamer	2.0
Glycerol	2.5	Glycerin	2.25
Water	q.s.	α-Tocopherol	0.02
		Methylparaben	0.2
		Butylparaben	0.075
		Water	q.s.

[a]*Source*: Adapted from *Acta Pharm. Suec.*, 20:389–396 (1983).
[b]*Source*: Adapted from *Int. J. Pharm.*, 54:103–112 (1989).

Propofol, a potent CNS depressant, is used intravenously for the induction and maintenance of anesthesia or sedation [103]. It is chemically unrelated to other marketed anesthetic agents. Propofol exists as an oil of low water solubility and therefore must be formulated as an emulsion for parenteral administration. The marketed emulsion is isotonic and has a pH of 7.0 to 8.5 (adjusted with sodium hydroxide), and contains propofol (10 mg/mL), soybean oil (100 mg/mL), glycerol (22.5 mg/mL), and egg lecithin (12 mg/mL). Propofol emulsion is diluted in dextrose solution before administration. Because of its lipophilicity (octanol/water partition coefficient is 5012:1), propofol readily crosses the blood-brain barrier, with a mean equilibrium half-life of 2.9 minutes. The potential advantage of propofol is rapid recovery and low incidence of postoperative nausea and vomiting.

b. *Physical Compatibility with Administration Sets.* In addition to the formulation difficulties, hydrophobic drugs are frequently taken up by standard intravenous infusion sets and bags composed of polyvinyl chloride or other materials. There is the additional possibility of extraction of plasticizers from intravenous administration components. Alternate materials composed of polyethylene or ethyl vinyl acetate are used for hydrophobic compounds such as nitroglycerin- and lipid-containing total parenteral administrations. The high affinity of hydrophobic drugs for the oil phase of an emulsion may decrease in affinity for the plastic of the bags. The absorption of a model compound, rhodamine B, into TPN plastics was studied and found to be decreased by the addition of albumin, egg phospholipids, and parenteral fat emulsions [97].

c. *Lipid Emulsions for Sustained-Release or Drug Delivery.* Two reports explored the possibility of using emulsions for prolonged release of barbiturate injections [104,105]. Formulations investigated are presented in Table 7. It was not possible for stability reasons to dissolve the barbituric acids in soybean oil and emulsify using egg phosphatides, necessitating the addition of other emulsifiers. Placebo emulsions, however, were considered well tolerated in these studies and unlikely to interfere with the effects of the barbiturates. The emulsions formulated acted as sustained-release systems, which prolonged the duration of action of the barbiturates. The oil droplets apparently serve as a depot from which the drug was released either to the blood or to the cell membranes of the brain capillaries by direct contact. In simple emulsion systems, the fraction of the drug available for absorption depends on two factors: the phase volume

Table 7 Barbiturate Emulsions

Barbiturate	(%)	Soybean oil (%)	Acetylated mono- glycerides (%)	Pluronic Type	Pluronic (%)	Glycerol (%)
Hexobarbitol	0.75	20	7.5	L–42	1.0	2.5
Thiopental	0.75	20	7.5	L–81	1.0	2.5
Cyclobarbital	1.5	20	10.0	F–88	1.0	2.5
Pentobital	0.75	20	7.5	F–88	0.25	2.5
				F–77	0.75	
Secobarbital	0.75	20	2.5	F–108	1.0	2.5

Source: Adapted from *Acta Pharm. Suecia,* 9:83 (1972).

ratio and the partition coefficient of the drug between aqueous and lipid phases in the delivery system [106]. A larger value for the partition coefficient will delay absorption of the total dose from the emulsion. The phase volume ratio affects the way in which the partition coefficient relates to the fraction of the dose available for absorption. If the aqueous phase is much larger than the oil phase, then large partition coefficient values will result in a small fraction available for absorption. If the oil phase is much larger than the aqueous phase, then the fraction available for absorption is inversely proportional to the partition coefficient. In addition, protein binding and hydrolytic degradation of barbiturates do not occur when the drug is in the oil phase, thus contributing to higher efficacy of the emulsion formulations compared to aqueous solutions.

Endoscopic injection of emulsified methyl-CCNU (lomustine) dissolved in sesame oil in rabbits led to enhanced drug uptake by the regional lymph nodes [107]. A clinical trial was then carried out by endoscopic injection of the emulsion containing 20 to 50 mg of lomustine in 24 patients with gastric cancer. In 5 of 11 cases, metastasized lymph nodes were apparently degenerated histologically. Thus, endoscopic injection may be beneficial for adjuvant cancer chemotherapy of lymph node metastases in gastric cancer.

Similar transport of cytotoxic agents to the lymphatic system has been demonstrated for bleomycin [108]. Intratumoral injection of emulsified bleomycin significantly increased the antitumor effects of the drug on AH-66 rat carcinoma. Also promising results with topical application of emulsified chemotherapy has been obtained. The antineoplastic effects might result from both the lymphotropic nature and the slow-release property of fat emulsions.

Fluosol, a stable perfluorochemical emulsion, is indicated to prevent or diminish myocardial ischemia by transportation of oxygen [109]. The perfluorochemical phase of the emulsion dissolves oxygen and carbon dioxide. Fluosol 400 mL frozen emulsion is stored frozen until use and then thawed and combined with two additional parts that adjust the pH, ionic strength, and isotonicity. The product cannot be given more than once in 6 months because of the perfluorochemical accumulation in the organs of the RES.

Another report describing concentrated fluorocarbon emulsions as an oxygen carrier [110] emphasizes that replacement of a small amount of the egg yolk phospholipids (EYP) by [2-(perfluorooctyl) ethyl] (6-D-glucosyl) (sodium) phosphate, in perfluorooctyl bromide (PFOB)/EYP emulsions, facilitates the emulsification process, reduces the average particle size, and achieves strong stabilization of the emulsion.

Preparation of drug-carrier emulsions for prednimustine, the 21-chlorambucil ester of prednisolone, consisting of particles with a mean diameter near 50 nm, was achieved using phosphatidylcholine-surfactant mixtures [31]. In all, 20 nonionic and four zwitterionic surfactants were tested. The results showed that the nonionic surfactants have varying degrees of effectiveness as coemulsifiers, with the polysorbate, Brij, and ethylene glycol ether groups performing the best. The zwitterionic species tended to reduce the emulsifying properties of egg phosphatidylcholine (EPC). The optimum formulation in terms of physical stability and biocompatibility consisted of castor oil:EPC:polysorbate 80 (1:0.4:0.12, weight ratios). This emulsion has the potential use as a targetable carrier for site-specific drug delivery of prednimustine and other lipophilic anticancer drugs.

Contrast agents have been delivered in ethiodized oil emulsion formulations for use in intravenous hepatography [111,112]. Emulsions with different emulsifiers and particle sizes were prepared and evaluated in rabbits and monkeys. The optimum formulation was based on 0.45% ethanol-soluble egg lecithin and 53% ethiodized oil and was most effective in reproducible opacification of the liver. The general emulsion preparation included dissolving water-soluble ingredients and emulsifiers in water and oil-soluble emulsifiers in oil. For the optimum formulation, an alcoholic extract of lecithin was added to the oil phase. Each phase was heated separately, with stirring, to 60°C. The oil phase was then added slowly to the aqueous phase followed by homogenization. The emulsions were then aseptically filtered through a 0.22 μm filter into previously sterilized vials, which were stoppered and crimped. The optimum emulsion was stable after storage at 2 to 6°C for 6 months with respect to its particle size distribution and hepatographic capacity. Superior liver scans were obtained when the particle sizes were in the range of 2 to 3 μm.

Naturally occurring polysaccharides, such as mannan, amylopectin, and pullulan, were coated on the surface of emulsion oil droplets in an O/W emulsion [113]. After intravenous injection into guinea pigs, the coated oil droplets were cleared from the bloodstream more slowly than the uncoated droplets. In this study, lung uptake of a mannan derivative–coated droplet emulsion, at 30 minutes after intravenous injection, was approximately 15 times higher than that of the conventional emulsions without the polysaccharide coat. This finding reveals that the surface of the droplets with polysaccharide derivatives can alter the metabolic fate of the emulsions, and thus drugs incorporated into these emulsions may be delivered to an inflamed site, a lymph node, or other phagocytic tissues and cells.

Physically stable and bioactive adjuvant vehicles for vaccine emulsions were prepared for [thr^1]-Muramyldipeptide (MDP) [54]. This emulsion vehicle contained 5% poloxamer 401 and 0.4% polysorbate 80, in phosphate-buffered saline, as cosurfactants and 10.0% squalene as the oil phase. The vehicle was prepared by four manufacturing methods for comparison of physical stability and biological activity. While the physical stability of the resultant emulsion increased in the order of standard vortexing method < blade mixing < homomixing < microfluidization, there were no significant differences when comparing antibody titer and delayed hypersensitivity.

Most drug-containing emulsions have previously described the use of high-pressure homogenization or microfluidization for emulsification; a recent study, however, has formulated three drug-containing emulsions by a spontaneous emulsification process [114]. Submicron emulsions of muramyltripeptide-cholesterol (MTP-Chol), diazepam, and amphotericin B were prepared using an original and simple method. This process included preparation of an oily alcoholic phase containing emulsifier, into which the drug was dissolved. The oily alcoholic solution was then slowly injected in the aqueous phase with moderate mixing. The appearance of a bluish opalescence was evident immediately. The ethanol was then removed under reduced pressure at 45 to 50°C, followed by concentration to the desired volume by removal of water at the same conditions. The mean particle diameter was approximately 200 to 300 nm for the diazepam and MTP-Chol emulsions; the amphotericin B–containing emulsion had a bimodal distribution with one population having particle size in the range of 315 ± 83 nm (81%) and the other 908 ± 210 nm (19%). The formulations containing diazepam or MTP-Chol were stable over the pH range of 4 to 10, after sterilization at 121 °C for 20 minutes; and although ultracentrifugation at 37,000 g produced phase separation, the emulsions were readily dispersed by stirring. Potential uses of these emulsions include reduced pain on injection for diazepam emulsion, reduced toxicity and improved uptake by macrophages for amphotericin B emulsions, and enhanced antitumor activity for MTP-Chol–containing emulsions.

2. *Extemporaneous Addition of Drugs to Formulated Emulsions*

The second approach used to incorporate drug additives into an emulsion is the extemporaneous aseptic addition of drugs into another product, such as Intralipid, Liposyn, or TNAs. This usually involves preparation of a concentrated solution of the drug in a solvent such as dimethylacetamide or ethanol. The addition must be carefully performed to prevent precipitation of the drug or cracking of the emulsion. Manufacturers of intravenous lipid emulsions specifically warn against this type of addition because of unknown effects on emulsion stability and drug availability. However, interest in using commercially available emulsions as vehicles has dramatically increased over the years and numerous studies have been conducted to determine the physical and chemical stability of these combinations.

   a. *Drugs Added to Fat Emulsions.*   Numerous compatibility studies have been reported on the admixture of various parenteral agents into Intralipid [19,20,115,116]. An excellent compilation of these studies has been provided by Trissel [9]. This review provides, in many cases, a concentration or time dependence to the physical compatibility by means of comparing results from independent studies. For example, aminophylline is reported to be physically compatible at a concentration of 1 gram per liter for up to 48 hours at 4°C and room temperature, but another study demonstrates microscopic globule coalescence at 500 mg per liter in 24 hours under similar storage conditions. Compounds found to be consistently incompatible with Intralipid are ampicillin sodium, calcium chloride ($\leq$ 1 gram per liter), calcium gluconate, carbenicillin, cloxacillin, and methicillin sodium.

   Satisfactory incorporation of some agents has been possible only by first solubilizing the agent prior to incorporation into the fat emulsion. One study reported the addition of 1-(2-chloroethyl)-3-(4 methyl cyclohexyl)-1-nitrosourea (NSC 95441, methyl-CCNU [lomustine]) to Intralipid by first dissolving the drug in absolute alcohol, followed by slow addition to the emulsion [19]. This preparation was found to be stable for 8 hours at room temperature and 7 days under refrigeration.

   A poorly water soluble and unstable anticancer agent, carbamic acid (1-methylethyl)-[5-(3,4-dichlorophenyl)-2,3-dihydro-1H-pyrrolizine-6,7-diyl] bis (methylene) ester (NSC 278214), was added to Intralipid and Liposyn [20]. The drug was dissolved in a dimethylacetamide/Cremophor solution that was sterile-filtered prior to aseptic addition to the commercially available lipid emulsions. Liposyn was found not as effective as the 10% and 20% Intralipid emulsions in stabilizing the drug. The reasons for this apparent discrepancy were not determined. It was further emphasized that the use of oil-in-water emulsions could be used as vehicles in the screening and evaluation of investigational drug substances that are poorly water soluble and would otherwise require extensive formulation development to produce a bioavailable dosage form.

   b. *Drugs Added to Total Nutrient Admixtures.*   Similarly, a compilation of compatibility results of various drugs added to total nutrient admixtures (TNA) is also presented by Trissel [9]. Within this review is the study by Baptista and Lawrence [117] on secondary antibiotic infusions and their effect on the physical stability of TNAs. The TNA contained the typical fat emulsion (20% lipid), amino acids 10%, dextrose 70%, electrolytes, heparin, minerals, and multivitamins in sterile water for injection.

All of the antibiotics studied resulted in acceptable stability except for the preparation containing tetracycline hydrochloride, which exhibited signs of creaming, oiling out, and phase separation. The incompatibility of tetracycline hydrochloride on the lipids in the TNA was attributed to the highly acidic pH of the ascorbic acid present in the tetracycline product.

The compatibility of theophylline in fat-containing TPN was studied at two dosages, one for smokers (0.9 mg/kg/h) and the other for patients with cor pulmonale (0.4 mg/kg/h) [30]. The theophylline concentrations and fat-droplet particle size measurements were constant in the TPN admixtures stored for 24 hours at room temperature.

H_2-receptor antagonists such as cimetidine, ranitidine, famotidine, and nizatidine are commonly incorporated in the formulation of parenteral nutrient admixtures. Their compatibility has been studied and found to be suitable over a wide range of concentrations [21,22,25–28].

The stability of famotidine (H_2-receptor antagonist) has been studied in TNAs containing dextrose, lipid, and amino acids: one TNA contained fat emulsions of LCT, and the other a mixture of both LCT and MCT [25–27]. Famotidine remained stable for up to 72 hours at room temperature in all TNAs studied and did not alter the physical or chemical integrity of the two lipid emulsions.

A fourth H_2-receptor antagonist, nizatidine [28], was also found to be compatible with TNA solutions containing 3 and 5 Intralipid or Liposyn II and did not appear to affect the emulsion stability.

II. INJECTABLE SUSPENSIONS

A. Introduction

Injectable suspensions are heterogeneous systems consisting of a solid phase dispersed in a liquid phase that may be either aqueous or nonaqueous. They should be sterile, pyrogen free, stable, resuspendable, syringeable, injectable, isotonic, and nonirritating. Because of these requirements injectable suspensions are one of the most difficult dosage forms to develop in terms of their stability, manufacture, and usage. These suspensions may be formulated as a ready-to-use injection or require a reconstitution step prior to use. They are usually administered by either subcutaneous (S.C.) or intramuscular (I.M.) route. Injectable suspensions usually contain between 0.5% and 5.0% solids and should have a particle size less than 5 μm for I.M. or S.C. administration [118]. Certain antibiotic preparations—for example, procaine penicillin G—may contain up to 30% solids [119]. Development of novel delivery systems for suspensions containing drug in the microparticulate forms have made it feasible to inject parenteral suspensions by the intravenous or intra-arterial route. The advantages and disadvantages of injectable suspensions are as follows.

1. *Advantages*

Therapeutic use of drugs that are insoluble in conventional solvents
Increased resistance to hydrolysis and oxidation as drug is present in the solid form
Possible controlled-release or depot action
Elimination of hepatic first-pass effect

2. *Disadvantages*

Difficulty in formulation
Difficulty in manufacturing
Discomfort to patient
Uniformity and accuracy of dose at time of administration
Maintenance of physical stability

B. Formulation Considerations

An overview of certain theoretical principles of suspension technology is essential to apply these concepts toward formulation development. Suspension are difficult to formulate because they are inherently thermodynamically unstable heterogeneous systems [120]. Interfacial properties of dispersed particles—such as the increase in the specific surface area with reduction in particle size and the presence of electrical charge on the surface of the particles—play an important role in the stability of suspensions. Equation (1) illustrates the principle that as the interfacial tension and the surface area approach zero, the surface free energy is minimized, thus enhancing physical stability of the system. Generally, particle size of the solids is reduced in suspensions to prevent settling of dispersed particles; however, this results in clumping of particles in an attempt to reduce the surface free energy. A stable suspension, therefore, uses surface-active agents (wetting agents) that minimize the interfacial tension and lower the surface free energy.

$$\Delta G = \gamma_{s/l} \cdot \Delta A \tag{1}$$

where

ΔG = change in the surface free energy in ergs
$\gamma_{s/l}$ = interfacial tension in dynes/cm^2 between dispersed particles and the dispersion medium
ΔA = change in surface area in cm^2

The charge at the shear plane associated with the particle surface is described as the zeta potential; when the value of the zeta potential is high, the electrostatic repulsive forces between two particles exceed the attractive London forces, resulting in deflocculation of particles [121]. Although, deflocculated particles settle at a slow rate, they form a hard cake on settling that is not redispersible. Flocculating agents are added to reduce the electrical forces of repulsion and at certain concentrations result in predominance of the attractive forces, causing loose aggregates or flocs to form. These aggregates settle quickly, do not bond tightly to each other, and are redispersible.

The rate of sedimentation of particles in a suspension is given by Stokes' Law [Eq. 2], which indicates that as the particle size decreases, the sedimentation rate (settling) decreases. Stokes' law also indicates that an increase in the viscosity of the liquid phase and/or minimal differences in the density of solid/liquid phases will minimize the sedimentation rate and thus enhance the physical stability of suspension.

$$s = \frac{d^2(\rho_s - \rho_l)g}{18\eta} \tag{2}$$

where

s = sedimentation rate in cm/sec
d = diameter of the particle in cm

ρ_s = density of the dispersed phase (solid phase)
ρ_l = density of the dispersion medium (liquid phase)
g = acceleration due to gravity
η = viscosity of the dispersion medium in poise

The formulation of a stable suspension mainly involves use of high solids content and/or increased viscosity of the system. However, most parenteral suspensions are usually dilute and have practical limitations for viscosity because of syringeability and injectability constraints. The limited number of parenterally acceptable excipients further accentuates the challenge to formulate an injectable suspension.

In addition to the above-mentioned limitations, the factors affecting the release of drug from the suspension and absorption from the intramuscular or subcutaneous injection site should be considered while developing suspension formulations. The rate of drug release from a suspension can be affected by different steps involved in the process [122]. These include dissolution of drug particles, perfusion of the area by blood, oil-water partition coefficient, and diffusion through the highly viscous adipose layer to the vascular system. The specific histological structure of the muscle and adipose tissue and the differences in their lipoidal character also influence the lipid solubility, protein binding and release rate of the drug. In addition, the injection depth is an important variable because the mean absorption times are considerably longer when the drug is shallowly injected in the adipose layer.

Therefore, the following properties of the parenteral suspension should be considered during the formulation development:

Solubility of drug in biological fluids at the injection site
Lipid solubility and oil-water partition coefficient of the drug
pKa of the drug
Dissolution rate of the solid drug from its dosage form
pH of the vehicle and tonicity of suspension
Particle size of the drug in suspension
Compatibility of other ingredients in the dosage form

Preformulation data regarding particle size and particle size distribution, dissolution and recrystallization, pKa, solvates and polymorphs, solubility, and pH stability/solubility profiles are needed for the formulation development. These physicochemical properties profoundly influence the formulation and stability of suspensions. For example, the rate of drug release from injected subcutaneous formulations of 17β-esters of norethisterone is controlled by the crystal form [123]. The lower melting point, more soluble crystal form A of the 4-(butoxy) phenylacetate ester prolonged the length of estrus suppression in rats to 31 days, whereas the B form produced suppression for about one day and is ineffective. Similarly, by controlling the crystallinity of insulin in the presence of zinc chloride, different long-acting insulin preparations (Ultralente, Lente, and Semilente Insulin) were obtained that differ in terms of onset, peak, and duration of action [124]. In another study, the dissolution performance of commercially available prednisolone acetate suspensions was related to particle size distribution and dissolution rate constant [125]. A diffusion-based model was proposed that incorporates physicochemical properties of the drug and the particle size characteristics. Similarly, differences in the particle size of two commercially available medroxyprogesterone acetate sterile suspensions contributed toward variation in their rate of absorption, peak serum concentrations, and bioavailability [126].

In addition to the physicochemical properties, product-related problems such as crystal growth, cake formations, and the possibility of product-package interactions should be considered during the development of parenteral suspensions [127]. Because the surface free energy of fine particles is greater than that of coarse particles, fine particles will be more soluble. For such systems, fluctuations in temperature will result in crystal growth as the fine particles dissolve with increase in temperature and the coarse crystals will grow at the expense of the fine particles. Certain agents like Tween and TritonX-100 at very low concentrations (0.005%), gelatin and polyvinylpyrrolidone (PVP) at concentrations <0.1%, adsorb on crystal surface and retard the crystal growth [121]. Freeze-thaw and elevated temperature tests can be useful in evaluating the crystal growth and crystal growth inhibitors.

C. Suspension Ingredients

Injectable suspensions usually contain both active ingredient(s) and excipients. Excipients used in the parenteral preparations must be nonpyrogenic, nontoxic, nonhemolytic and nonirritating; should be physically and chemically compatible with active ingredient(s); must not interfere with the therapeutic effect of the active ingredient(s); must maintain stability during sterilization and during the shelf life of the product; should be effective at low concentration; and should be acceptable from a regulatory point of view. International regulatory requirements should be considered for products intended for international marketing. Such stringent requirements limit the actual number of parenterally acceptable formulation additives used in parenteral suspensions, and most formulations contain relatively few ingredients. Typical excipients used in parenteral suspensions include the following:

    Flocculating/suspending agents
    Wetting agents
    Solvent systems
    Preservatives
    Antioxidants
    Chelating agents
    Buffering agents
    Tonicity agents

1. *Flocculating/Suspending Agents*

There are basically three techniques used to formulate a suspension: (a) controlled flocculation, (b) structured vehicle, or (c) a combination of a and b. The choice depends on whether the particles in a suspension are to remain flocculated or deflocculated. The controlled flocculation approach uses a flocculating agent(s) to form loosely bound aggregate or flocs in a controlled manner that settles rapidly but redisperses easily upon agitation. An appropriate amount of flocculating agent is added that results in maximum sedimentation volume and prevents cake formation. Electrolytes, surfactants, and hydrophilic colloids have been typically used as flocculating agents (Table 8). Electrolytes and surfactants reduce the electrical forces of repulsion between particles and allow the flocs to form, which in turn is influenced by the surface charge on the particles. The surface charge of the system can be measured by the zeta potential. The zeta potential must be controlled so as to lie within a range (generally less than 25 mV) to obtain a flocculated, noncaking suspension with maximum sedimentation volume [4]. Hydrophilic

Table 8 Typical Flocculating
Agents Used in Injectable
Suspensions

Surfactants
    Lecithin
    Polysorbate 20
    Polysorbate 40
    Polysorbate 80
    Pluronic F–68
    Sorbitan trioleate (Span 85)
Hydrophilic colloids
    Sodium carboxymethylcellulose
    Acacia
    Gelatin
    Methylcellulose
    Polyvinylpyrrolidone
Electrolytes
    Potassium/sodium chloride
    Potassium/sodium citrate
    Potassium/sodium acetate

colloids (generally negatively charged) not only affect the repulsive forces, but also provide a mechanical barrier to the particles. For example, a 25% PVP solution is used in combination with polysorbate 80 (2%) as a stabilizer to provide a stable injectable 30% osseous powder suspension [128].

An alternate formulation approach is to use structured vehicles (suspending or thickening agents) to keep the dispersed particles in the suspension in a deflocculated state. These agents function as viscosity-imparting agents and reduce the rate of sedimentation of the dispersed particles. Various hydrophilic colloids previously listed in Table 8 are used as structured vehicles. Ideally, these form pseudoplastic or plastic systems that undergo shear-thinning with some degree of thixotropy. However, the high viscosity and poor syringeability of such systems limit their use in parenteral suspensions. The deflocculated approach is used for oleaginous suspensions and for suspensions containing relatively high concentration of solids—for example, in the formulation of procaine penicillin G suspension. In another case, critical ratios of flocculating and deflocculating agents were employed to form a parenteral suspension of an anti-inflammatory compound [129].

2. *Wetting Agents*

Wetting of the suspended ingredient(s) is one of the most important aspects of the injectable suspension because the hydrophobic powders are often suspended in aqueous systems. Wetting, as described by Young's equation [Eq. (3)] illustrates that a θ (contact angle) less than 90° is observed in the case of hydrophobic powders, which usually require an adjuvant to aid in their dispersion. Various nonionic surfactants and nonaqueous solvents (glycerin, alcohol, and propylene glycol) are types of wetting agents commonly used in injectable suspensions.

$$\gamma_s = \gamma_{s/1} + \gamma_1 \cos \theta \tag{3}$$

where

γ_s = surface tension of solid
$\gamma_{s/1}$ = solid/liquid interfacial tension
γ_1 = surface tension of liquid

Wetting agents reduce the contact angle between the surface of the particle and the wetting liquid. To obtain maximum wetting efficiency, surfactants with hydrophilic-lipophilic balance (HLB) value in the range of 7 to 9 should be selected. The usual concentration of surfactant varies from 0.05% to 0.5% depending on the solid content of the suspension. Care should be taken in terms of the amount used; excessive amounts may cause foaming or caking or provide an undesirable taste/odor to the product. For example, in a nonaqueous suspension of cefazolin sodium in peanut oil, addition of polysorbate 80 at concentrations greater than 0.17% resulted in deflocculated suspensions that were difficult to redisperse [130]. Microscopic examination revealed extensive agglomeration and crystal growth of cefazolin sodium in the presence of polysorbate 80.

3. *Solvent System*

Solvent systems used in parenteral suspension are classified as either aqueous or nonaqueous vehicles. Choice of a typical solvent system depends on solubility, stability, and the desired release characteristics of the drug. Nonaqueous vehicles include both water-miscible and water-immiscible vehicles.

Water for injection is generally the preferred solvent system; however, nonaqueous water-miscible agents are used as cosolvents with water for injection to promote the solubility and stability in parenteral preparations. Examples of water-miscible nonaqueous vehicles include ethanol, glycerin, propylene glycol, and N-(β-hydroxyethyl)-lactamide [131]. The use of water-miscible cosolvents can lead to undesirable side effects. For example, intramuscular injection of propylene glycol–water, ethyl alcohol–water and polyethylene glycol (PEG) 400–water mixtures was found to cause muscle damage as measured by in vitro release of creatinine kinase from isolated rat skeletal muscle [132]. At moderate concentrations (20% to 40% v/v) of organic cosolvent, PEG 400 is less myotoxic than propylene glycol and ethanol. Myotoxicity was not correlated exclusively to a single physicochemical property of the cosolvent-water mixtures such as dielectric constants, apparent pH, surface tension, viscosity, or a combination of these for a series of cosolvents [133]. Based on these results, it was suggested that biochemical interactions between organic cosolvents and skeletal muscle fibers may be involved in the cosolvent-induced toxicity [134]. Additionally, lysis of human red blood cells in the presence of cosolvents such as propylene glycol; glycerol; PEG 200, 300, and 400; and ethanol have been reported [135]. In the presence of 0.9% to 2.7% sodium chloride, cosolvents other than PEG 300 and 400 were less hemolytic than when mixed with water. Hemolysis caused by cosolvents may be related to their possible binding with red blood cell membranes. Hemolytic potential of ethyl alcohol, PEG 400, is low whereas propylene glycol has a high hemolytic potential [136].

Nonaqueous water-immiscible vehicles used in parenteral suspensions include fixed oils as well as ethyl oleate, isopropyl myristate, and benzyl benzoate [137]. Fixed oils must be fluid at room temperature, and vegetable in origin, and should have good thermal stability at both high and low temperatures. Generally, an antioxidant is needed to ensure the stability of fixed oils over the shelf life of the drug product. Examples of various fixed oils used in suspension formulations include sesame oil, peanut oil, and castor oil [138]. Some other oils being studied in the development of parenteral suspensions [128] include almond oil, sunflower oil, iodinated poppy seed oil, cottonseed oil, and corn oil. Excessive unsaturation of an oil can cause tissue irritation. Some patients may have allergic reactions to the vegetable oils, hence specific oils used in the product should be listed on the product label. The type of oil and its volume have been found to affect the release rate of the drug from the suspensions. For example, the androgenic activity of testosterone and androsterone in oleaginous solution is dependent on the type of oil vehicle used [139]. Additionally, the subcutaneous activity of testosterone depends on volume of oil injected for the same amount of testosterone. By forming a long-acting ester such as testosterone propionate, the androgenic activity is greatly enhanced and is further increased by three times if the injection volume is increased from 0.2 to 0.8 mL.

4. *Tonicity Agents*

Isotonicity of the parenteral preparations for subcutaneous or intramuscular administration is desired to prevent pain, irritation, and tissue damage at the site of administration. The British Pharmacopoeia states that aqueous solutions for S.C., I.M., or intradermal injection should be made isotonic if possible. Examples of tonicity agents used in parenteral suspensions include dextrose and various electrolytes (e.g., sodium chloride).

5. *Preservatives*

Antimicrobial agents are required for parenteral products that are intended for multiple dosing to protect the product from accidental microbial contamination during clinical usage and to maintain sterility. Similarly, preservatives should be added to formulations aseptically packaged in single-dose vials if the active ingredient(s) does not have bactericidal or bacteriostatic properties or is growth promoting. A growth-promoting study should be conducted to determine the microbiological properties of the preservative-free formulation.

Antimicrobial preservative efficacy tests are required by the USP and EP to demonstrate effectiveness of the preservative during the shelf life of the product. The British Pharmacopoeia requires a 10^3 reduction in the surviving bacterial cells within 24 hours following inoculation of each milliliter or gram of the product with at least 10^6 bacterial cells [140]. The United States Pharmacopeia requires the same 10^3 reduction in bacterial cells within 14 days [141].

Some typical preservatives used in parenteral suspensions and their commonly used concentrations are as follows: benzyl alcohol (0.9% to 1.5%), methylparaben (0.18% to 0.2%), propylparaben (0.02%), benzalkonium chloride (0.01% to 0.02%), and thimerosal (0.001% to 0.01%) [142]. Benzalkonium chloride is used in ophthalmic dosage forms and not in injectable dosage forms. Propyl- and methylparabens are referred to chemically as propyl and methyl esters of *p*-hydroxy benzoic acids. Because of the inherent chemically reactive nature of preservatives, stability and compatibility problems of preservatives need to be evaluated for their usage in the final formulation. The low aqueous solubility of parabens and a decrease in stability with increasing pH complicates their use in the parenteral formulation [143]. Generally, parabens are solubilized by adding them to Alcohol USP or to a small volume of water heated to approximately 80°C. The heated solution requires further dilution to prevent precipitation of parabens before it cools significantly. Parabens are sensitive to excessive light exposure and are incompatible with alkaline excipients and polysorbate 80. Benzyl alcohol can cause convulsions in neonates and should be avoided in certain drug products with neonatal indications [144]. Most antimicrobial preservatives and antioxidants are known to volatilize or adsorb to rubber closures and can cause loss of sterility and stability and potential problems with flocculation and resuspendability of the product [127]. A USP Antimicrobial Preservative Effectiveness test should be conducted on preparations formulated with, for example, 90%, 75%, and 50% of the initial preservative concentration to determine the minimally effective concentration of the preservative over the shelf life of the drug product.

6. *Antioxidants/Chelating Agents*

Oxidation can lead to unacceptable discoloration of the drug product without necessarily causing significant potency loss. Drugs formulated in the reduced form have low oxidation potential and are susceptible to oxidation. Oxidative degradation of drugs in solutions is mediated either by free radicals or by molecular oxygen and can be catalyzed by metals, heat, light, hydroxy ions, or hydrogen ions. Antioxidants are added in the formulation to minimize this degradation by preferentially undergoing oxidation as the result of their lower oxidation potential or by terminating the propagation step in the free radical oxidation mechanism [145]. Antioxidants are either used alone or in combination with a chelating agent or other antioxidants. Certain compounds (e.g., ascorbic acid and citric acid) have been found to act as synergists and increase the effectiveness of antioxidants that block oxidative reactions. Chelating agents sequester heavy metals, thereby preventing the catalysis of oxidation reaction. Examples of suitable antioxidants and chelating agents and their typical concentrations for injectable dosage forms are listed in Table 9.

Auto-oxidation is defined as oxidative degradation by molecular oxygen. In such cases the exposure of active ingredient(s) to oxygen during the manufacturing process should be avoided. This can be accomplished by the following processes:

Table 9 Typical Antioxidants/Chelating Agents for Parenteral Preparations

Compound	Typical concentration (%)
Antioxidants (preferential oxidation, water soluble)	
Ascorbic acid	0.02–0.1
Sodium bisulfite	0.1–0.15
Sodium metabisulfite	0.1–0.15
Sodium formaldehyde sulfoxylate	0.1–0.15
Thiourea	0.005
Antioxidants (propagation termination, oil soluble)	
Ascorbic acid esters	0.01–0.15
Butylated hydroxytoluene (BHT)	0.005–0.02
Tocopherols	0.05–0.075
Chelating agents	
Ethylenediaminetetraacetic acid salts	0.01–0.075

Source: Ref. 7.

1. Purging the solvent system (i.e., Water for Injection USP) and bulk drug product with filtered (0.22 μm) nitrogen during the manufacturing process. By controlling the mixing speed and the nitrogen flow rate, the rate of oxygen removal can be improved.
2. Blanketing the bulk drug product with filtered (0.22 μm) nitrogen/argon during the filling operation.
3. Displacing oxygen from the head space of the filled container with filtered (0.22 μm) nitrogen.

7. *Other Stabilizers*

Various other stabilizers have been used in different specific parenteral suspensions of drugs. For examples, sugars such as sorbitol, sucrose, or fructose have been associated with enhanced stability of procaine benzylpenicillin and sodium benzylpenicillin parenteral suspensions [146]. Oil-based injectable suspensions of tetracycline in Miglyol are stabilized by the addition of maleic acid or a maleate salt [147]. D-Glucose, polyethylene glycol, or adenine inhibits the aggregation of aqueous suspension of nitrazepam during freezing and defrost to allow smooth passage through the syringe needle [148]. Aluminum monostearate is a water repellant used mostly in long-acting parenteral suspensions; it acts by reducing the interfacial tension.

Colloidal polymeric particles made from biodegradable materials such as polyhydroxybutyrate (PHB) are possible carrier systems for controlled delivery of drugs. These PHB carriers possess a low zeta potential, and that is further reduced by incorporation of oppositely charged drugs. Antiflocculants such as sodium pyrophosphate, sodium citrate, and sodium dihydrogen phosphate adsorb on the suspension particles and increase the electrostatic repulsions of the similarly charged particles and enhance the physical stability by increasing the zeta potential [149]. The antiflocculants should be selected by considering the effect of pH shifts, maximum net charge increase, and their toxicological acceptance.

Various types of injectable suspensions and the type and amount of each component are illustrated in Examples 1 through 4 [150–153].

D. Manufacturing Considerations

The manufacture of sterile suspensions is a complicated process that typically requires the sterilization and aseptic milling of the active ingredient(s), sterilization of the vehicle system (generally by sterile filtration), aseptic wetting and dispersion of the active ingredient(s), aseptic milling of the bulk suspensions, and aseptic filling of the bulk suspension into suitable sterile containers.

The vehicle may be sterilized through a sterilizing filter if the components are soluble and the viscosity is acceptable. A typical sterilizing filter system for vehicle sterilization is composed of a membrane filter placed in a stainless steel housing unit. For example Millipore[o] "Disk" (stacked) and "cartridge" (pleated) membrane systems on polymer supports provide significantly increased surface area compared to conventional flat membranes. Millipore Durapore membrane filters (hydrophobic modified polyvinylidenedifluoride) are used for both water-miscible and water-immiscible solvents. Other filter suppliers include Gelman[p], Pall,[q] and Sartorius.[r] The vehicle may also be sterilized by autoclaving.

The solid active ingredient may be sterilized prior to compounding into the suspension in a number of ways, such as sterile precipitation and/or crystallization, spray drying, lyophilization, dry heat, autoclaving, ethylene oxide, and radiation.

1. *Sterile Recrystallization*

The active ingredient(s) are dissolved in an appropriate solvent (usually organic solvent because of the hydrophobic nature of the active ingredient) and sterilized by filtration. A sterile "counter" solvent is aseptically added to the sterile drug solution or pH is significantly changed to generate the sterile crystalline material. The process requires strict controls to maintain batch-to-batch uniformity in particle characteristics. Factors such as stirring rates, temperature, pH, and concentration must be controlled during sterile crystallization. The crystals are aseptically collected, washed and dried to remove residual solvents, and milled to the appropriate particle size. Significant aseptic manipulation is required and the choice of solvents is limited. Examples of commonly used solvents are acetone, chloroform, and methylene chloride.

2. *Spray-Drying*

A sterile solution of the drug or slurry is sprayed through an atomizer with a fine orifice into a drying chamber where it is exposed to a stream of extremely hot sterile air for a very short interval to yield a sterile powder. The drug powder is collected as hollow spheres and filled into vials as a dry powder. If the required particle size is achieved during spray-drying, milling may not be required. This method is applicable to heat-labile materials because solvent evaporation from the solid surface maintains the temperature at less than ambient temperature. An overview of the spray-drying of pharmaceuticals is presented by Broadhead and coworkers [154].

3. *Lyophilization (Freeze-Drying)*

Freeze-drying is a technique for removing the solvent from a solution of active ingredient; it results in a cake/powder that is readily reconstituted upon addition of solvent because of high surface area. The process of freeze-drying involves freezing a sterile-filtered solution of active ingredient(s) and excipient(s) in bulk by lowering the temperature below the eutectic temperature of the solution. The solvent is removed during primary drying by sublimation by using controlled application of vacuum and heat below the eutectic temperature. This is followed by desorption of adsorbed water during secondary drying, resulting in a dry powder or cake.

If the lyophilization of the bulk material is done in trays as opposed to products packaged in individual vials, then the dried material is typically milled under aseptic conditions to the desired particle size. Advantages of lyophilization include accurate dose of high surface area solid, increased stability, pharmaceutically elegant product, reduced transportation costs, minimized interaction between product and packaging and minimized potential for particulate development. Disadvantages include lengthy process time, expensive process, facilities, equipment and labor, milling difficulties from the possible formation of light friable or dense hard material. Williams and Poli have presented an overview of the lyophilization process of pharmaceuticals [155].

4. *Sterilization*

Ethylene oxide (EtO) gas sterilization requires a 2- to 4-hour exposure, depending on the gas composition, temperature (ranging from 50 to 60°C), and the relative humidity (approx. 70%) in order to sterilize previously milled material. The sterilized material requires up to 3 days to degas following EtO exposure and should be monitored for ethylene oxide, ethylene glycol, and chlorhydrin residues [156]. This method is useful for heat-sensitive materials; however, ethylene oxide exposure poses a significant occupational hazard. The Occupational Health and Safety Administration has changed personal EtO exposure limits from 50 to 0.5 parts per million for an 8-hour time weighted average shift and to 5 parts per million for short exposure of 15 minutes.

Dry heat sterilization is one of the easiest and safest methods to use. However, very few active ingredient(s) can withstand the temperature and time periods required to ensure sterilization. Previously milled material is generally exposed to heat above 140°C for various time periods, depending on temperature.

Gamma irradiation can be used to sterilize bulk drug and/or finished product. Relatively low temperatures are required, no residual matter is deposited in the product, and maximum sterility assurance is achieved. Gamma irradiation can cause physical and/or chemical degradation of the product and/or the packaging components; therefore, preliminary experiments should be conducted to determine if stability is affected. The primary source used for gamma irradiation is cobalt-60.

5. Processing

Two basic methods are used to prepare parenteral suspensions:

(a) Aseptically combining sterile powder and vehicle. A schematic is shown in Fig. 6. This method involves aseptically dispersing the sterile, milled active ingredient(s) into a sterile vehicle system (solvent plus necessary excipients); aseptically milling the resulting suspension as required, and aseptically filling the milled suspension into suitable sterile containers. For example, this process is used for preparation of parenteral procaine penicillin G suspension.

(b) In situ crystal formation by combining sterile solutions. A schematic is shown in Fig. 7. In this method active ingredient(s) are solubilized in a suitable solvent system, a sterile vehicle system or counter solvent is added that causes the active ingredient to crystallize, the organic solvent is aseptically removed, the resulting suspension is asceptically milled as necessary, and then filled into suitable containers. For example, this process is used for testosterone and insulin parenteral suspensions.

In addition, several other methods are described for preparation of specific parenteral suspensions. Lyophilization of the product or direct fill of the dry powder in the final package can be used for parenteral suspension. Another approach is described for preparing an injectable suspension of a low melting compound, butyl-p-aminobenzoate, which forms solid lumps on cooling after dry heat sterilization [157]. The drug particles are dispersed in a solvent containing polysorbate 80 and normal saline. The suspension is then sterilized for 20 min at 120°C without cooling. The suspension is cooled while being shaken vigorously and then frozen to −18°C. Special milling procedures involving frequent defrosting/shaking of the frozen suspension are used to obtain acceptable particle size.

In another example, monodisperse insulin suspension is prepared by seeding the swine insulin solutions with insulin crystals of 3 to 5 μm and allowing it to crystallize till 70:30 crystal/amorphous ratio is obtained. At this point an aqueous solution containing $ZnCl_2$ and methylparaben is added and the pH is adjusted to 7.1 to 7.3 [158].

Another approach to preparing injectable suspensions as described by Portnoff and others consists of sterilizing by autoclaving the active component that has been dispersed

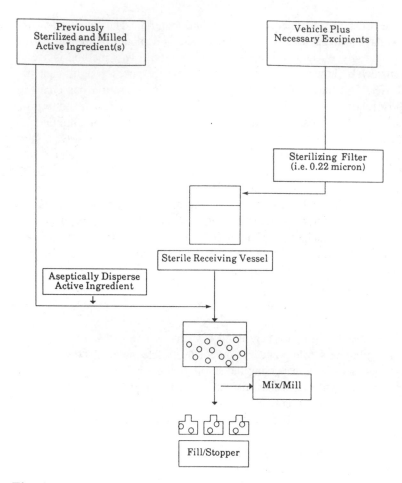

Fig. 6 A schematic of sterile manufacturing of injectable suspensions using aseptic technique.

as a slurry in a saturated aqueous solution of sodium chloride [159]. A schematic is shown in Fig. 8. Because the solubility of sodium chloride does not change significantly with temperature and the solution remains saturated during the autoclave cycle, the activity of water is not significantly increased at sterilizing temperatures. This allows a slurry of solid in this system to be autoclaved with a minimum risk of dissolving. The slurry is then aseptically combined with the remaining excipients to form the suspension. This method is used for sterile aqueous suspension of dexamethasone acetate. The advantages to this method are that solid material can be milled under clean but nonsterile conditions, the active ingredients are easily sterilized, and a suitable suspension manufactured without significant manipulations.

Nash and Haeger have described another method of preparing stable syringeable suspensions of parenteral drugs in complex flocculated forms [160]. These suspensions are prepared by adding drugs to a suspension formed by reacting an aqueous dilution of a polyether nonionic surfactant (polyoxyethylene sorbitan monooleate and carboxymethyl cellulose) with an aqueous solution of a hydroxylated preservative (phenol). The slurry is then passed through a colloid mill, pH adjusted, and made up to

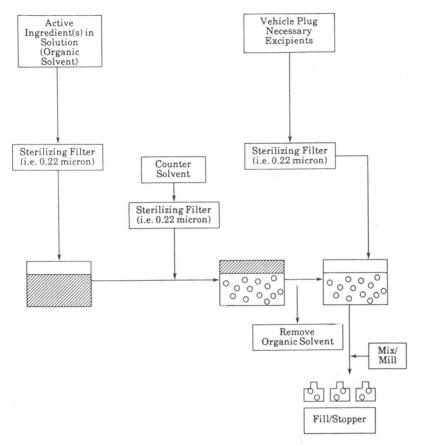

Fig. 7 A schematic of sterile recrystallization process for the manufacturing of injectable suspensions.

volume. This process is used for preparation of parenteral suspensions of triamcinolone hexacetonide, 21-deoxytriamcinolone acetonide, 1,4-dimethyl-1,4-diphenyl-2-tetrazene, and sulfadiazine.

If the suspension requires milling, Nash recommends using an Eppenbach Model NV-6-6204 micromill (colloid mill) that allows easy removal of the mill head for easier cleaning and sterilization [161]. The colloid mill mechanically shears the suspension as it passes through an adjustable clearance between a high-speed rotor and stator. Colloid mills are jacketed to allow cold water circulation and to prevent excessive heat buildup in the suspension. The suspension is generally recirculated for a period of time through the colloid mill to ensure complete dispersion.

Homogenizers consist of a pump and a valve containing a small orifice. The pump increases the pressure of the suspension, which forces it through the small orifice causing turbulence and hydraulic shear. The homogenizer generally produces a smaller particle size, less heat buildup, and less foaming than a colloid mill. However, homogenizers are more difficult to clean and sterilize than colloid mills.

Microfluidizers are available for preparation of dispersed systems on both laboratory and production size scale. In this process, liquid is pumped through microchannels

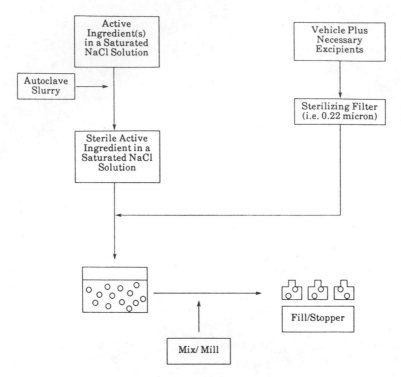

Fig. 8 A schematic showing use of saturated sodium chloride solution in the manufacturing of injectable suspensions.

to an impingement area at high operating pressures. The forces of shear, impact and cavitation reduce the particle size in the interaction chamber. Because the temperature of the interaction chamber may increase during microfluidization, the tubings can be cooled externally by immersing in ice bags or immersion into a ice slurry. A microfluidization-solvent evaporation method was utilized to prepare polymeric nanosuspensions containing indomethacin [162].

E. Stability and Evaluation of Parenteral Suspensions

Because suspensions are thermodynamically unstable systems, physical stability of suspensions becomes as important as the chemical and biological stability. In addition, injectable suspensions require evaluation of characteristics such as syringeability, injectability, isotonicity, sterility, and preservative effectiveness. Parenteral suspensions are frequently administered through 19 to 22 gauge needles, about 1 to 2 inches long, that have internal diameter in the range of only 300 to 600 microns. Rheological properties of an injectable suspension can provide some formidable challenge in their administration and delivery. Therefore, flow properties such as syringeability and injectability are necessary to evaluate and control.

1. *Syringeability* describes the ability of the suspension to pass easily through a hypodermic needle on transfer from the vial prior to injection. It includes characteristics such as the ease of withdrawal, clogging and foaming tendencies, and accuracy of

dose measurements. Increase in the viscosity, density, particle size, and concentration of solids in suspension hinders the syringeability of suspension. A suitable test is to ensure that the entire suspension passes through a 25-gauge needle of internal diameter 0.3 mm.

2. *Injectability* refers to the performance of suspension during injection and includes factors such as pressure or force required for injection, evenness of flow, aspiration qualities, and freedom from clogging [127]. The syringeability and injectability of suspension are closely related to the viscosity and particle characteristics of the suspension. A simple ejection of the suspension into the open, if done very slowly with intermittent application of pressure to the plunger can provide certain information about suspension. Most methods used for injectability are qualitative in nature. A force monitoring device such as Instron can be used to determine ejection and injection pressures, and test results can be recorded on a X-Y recorder. Another instrument to assess the injectability of parenterals measures the time required to smoothly inject a solution or suspension into meat under specified pressure from a syringe through a needle [163]. When a test solution is injected through glass and plastic syringes of various sizes, regression equations are obtained for a given syringe type and diameters using needles of various gauges. These equations permit the calculation of the expected injection time for a given syringe-needle system and for a given vehicle of a certain viscosity.

3. *Clogging* or blockage of syringe needles while administering a suspension may occur because of a single large particle or an aggregate that blocks the lumen of the needle or because of a bridging effect of the particles. It is advisable to avoid particles greater than one-third of the internal diameter of the needle to prevent clogging. Clogging, if observed at or near the needle end, is usually caused by restrictions to flow from the suspension and may involve combination of factors such as vehicle, wetting of particles, particle size, shape and distribution, viscosity, and flow characteristics of the suspension [161].

3. *Drainage* refers to the ability of the suspension to break cleanly away from the inner walls of the primary container-closure system and is another characteristic of a well-formulated parenteral suspension. Silicone coating of containers, vials, and plugs with dimethicone can improve the drainage of slightly overflocculated systems as well as of good suspensions.

4. *Resuspendibility* describes the ability of the suspension to uniformly disperse with minimal shaking after it has stood for some time. Qualitatively, light transmittance through the upper solution in a cylinder after it has been spun for about 2 minutes at 75 rpm can be used to detect the redispersion properties of the system [120]. Resuspendibility becomes a problem for suspensions that form cakes on standing due to settling of the deflocculated particles. Caking describes a process by which the particles undergo growth and fusion to form a nondispersible mass of material.

5. *Sedimentation Volume* is a qualitative term used to describe the amount of settling that has occurred in a suspension. The sedimentation volume is defined as the ratio of the final volume of the sediment, v_u, to the original volume, v_o, of the suspension [164]. The larger the fraction, the better is the suspendibility. Sedimentation volume is used to evaluate the changes in suspension characteristics with time and also to compare different suspension formulations. When the ratios are plotted against time, the more horizontal the slopes, the more flocculated the suspension. Generally, the sedimentation volume is direclty proportional to the size of the flocs, and the rate of settling is inversely proportional to the amount of deflocculation.

6. *Freeze-Thaw Cycles* are important for determining the ability of the suspension to withstand thermal shock, retard crystal growth, and maintain chemical stability of the active ingredient and overall physical stability. The freeze-thaw cycle promotes particle growth and may predict the results of long-term storage at room temperature. A total of three complete cycles with each cycle consisting of 24 hours at 40°C followed by 24 hours at 0°C is suggested, although various cycles are suitable.

7. *Crystal Growth* in suspensions is affected by the particle size distribution, changes in pH, temperature, crystal form, and solvate formation and by dissolution and recrystallization of the particles [127]. Crystal growth should be monitored by examining changes in particle size over time and comparing that with the initial particle size distribution. The tendency for crystal growth in a suspension can be diminished by using a narrow particle size range, decreasing interfacial tension (to reduce the free energy of particles), increasing the viscosity of suspending medium (may be difficult with parenteral suspensions as it affects the syringeability and flow), use of hydrophilic gums like polyvinylpyrrolidone, polysorbates (adsorb at particle surface and retard crystal growth), and choosing a different chemical form of the drug.

8. *Particle Size Measurements.* Variable particle size distribution in suspensions results from different factors, including preparation of suspension by precipitation methods where the degree of saturation and rate of nucleation are greatest at the beginning of the process, resulting in large particles initially and smaller particles subsequently; changes in pH caused by drug decomposition; changes in temperature; and changes during processing in several types of equipment and transfer steps. Particle size measurements are useful in that they allow aggregation or crystal growth to be evaluated. There are a number of methods used for particle size analysis; microscopic determination and coulter counter methods of particle size determination are preferred over Andresen pipette or subsieve sizer and turbidimetry. For particle size determinations below 1 μm, proton correlation spectroscopy may be employed using a Malvern Spectrophotometer. For example, Coulter Multisizer and HIAC/Royco particulate counter is used for the size characterization of reconstituted, lyophilized, attenuated *Mycobacterium bovis* Bacillus Calmette-Guerin (BCG) vaccine, Tice substrain, formulated as suspension [165]. The cumulative size distribution of the suspension fits the log-probit plot, and this information is used to determine the total number of organisms per ampule that is equivalent to the number of colony-forming units.

9. *Zeta Potential* determinations can be of great value in the development of suspensions, particularly if the controlled flocculation approach is used to formulate the suspension. The electrokinetic method measures the migration velocity of the suspension particles with respect to the net effective charges on the surface. The zeta meter is a microelectrophoretic mobility apparatus used to characterize flocculated and dispersed suspensions and to follow changes in physical stability with time. The electrophoretic velocity can be measured by laser Doppler anemometry using a Malvern Zetasizer[d] or by amplitude weighted phase structuration. Visually observed caking can be related to the changes in the zeta potential as well as to the changes upon addition of additives like electrolytes and surfactants.

10. *Compatibility with Diluents and other Parenterals.* Parenteral suspensions may require dilution prior to use if small concentrations of the drug are needed or may be mixed and injected with local anesthetics to reduce the pain associated with their administration. Even though dilution with water or normal saline will often cause the system to deflocculate, it may not be necessarily detrimental in the light of the time frame

of suspension administration, because of slow settling of deflocculated particles. However, agglomeration or coagulation of suspension on mixing with other parenterals may cause serious incompatibilities [161].

11. *Shipping Characteristics* of suspensions under various stresses of shipping such as vibration, impaction, and shaking determine the suspension's ability to retain its required attributes during transit. Ideally, the test should expose the suspension to both realistic climate and handling conditions. Common laboratory test methods used to evaluate shipping characteristics include vibrators, shakers, and impact devices.

12. *Product-Package Interactions.* Antimicrobial preservatives and antioxidants present in the suspension formulation are known to volatilize or adsorb to the stopper resulting in the formation of more monodispersed and less resuspendable suspension [159]. Also, the extractables from rubber closures are often masked in suspension. Agglomeration of fine particles on the surface of glass is another type of interaction and becomes particularly evident after the shipping test. The probability of particle agglomeration can be reduced by uniform siliconization of the vial, which also promotes efficient drainage of the suspension.

13. *Viscosity* describes the resistance to flow with applied stress for a particular system; a more viscous system requires greater force or stress to make it flow at the same rate as a less viscous system. An ideal suspension should exhibit a high viscosity at low shear (storage) with significant yield value and a low viscosity at high shear (agitation and syringeability) [166]. A fluid system will exhibit either Newtonian or non-Newtonian flow based on linear or nonlinear increase in the rate of shear with the shearing stress. The suspension viscosity can change due to concentration of active ingredient(s), particle shape, size, and distribution [167]. In addition, the actual manufacturing process, equipment and the length and type of exposure to mixing and/or homogenization shear can have a profound effect on the final suspension product.

Structured vehicles used in suspensions exhibit non-Newtonian flow and are either plastic, pseudoplastic, or shear-thinning with some thixotropy [168]. For example, sodium carboxymethylcellulose (CMC) and methylcellulose (MC) or methocel, most commonly used in parenteral suspensions, have pseudoplastic properties. Certain grades of CMC at high levels act as pesudoplastic thixotropes. The viscosity of CMC systems is dependent upon temperature, and storage at accelerated temperature may irreversibly degrade CMC. Sodium carboxymethylcellulose is compatible with most water-soluble nonionic and anionic polymers and gums but is incompatible with di- and trivalent salts. Viscosity of MC decreases on exposure to elevated temperatures. High levels of electrolytes and surfactants affect the methocel systems. Methocel is normally used in conjunction with other suspending agents and not as a primary suspending agent. For example, MC in combination with CMC is used as a suspending agent in aqueous suspension of desoxycorticosterone pivalate.

1. Stability Protocols

The active ingredient(s), excipients, and packaging components all play a role in the stability of injectable suspensions. Physical, chemical and biological stability of the product should be monitored routinely (see Table 10). Chemical and biological assays should determine the amount of active ingredient(s) remaining and quantitate any degradation product(s) or related substances. According to the new International Conference on Harmonization Tripartite Guidelines on stability, a minimum of 12 months' data in filing for three definitive batches, 2 of 3 pilot scale, is needed for long-term stabil-

Table 10 Stability Classifications

Chemical
    Active ingredient(s)
    Degradation product(s)
    Preservative(s)
Physical
    Resuspendibility
    Sedimentation volume
    Syringeability
    Crystal growth
    pH
    Freeze/thaw cycles
    Shipping test
    Moisture
    Particle size distribution
    Zeta potential
    Dissolution
    Rheology
Biological
    Sterility test
    Pyrogen test
    Biological assays
    Preservative effectiveness

ity indication. Sterility testing is recommended initially and at yearly time intervals till the proposed expiry date. Pyrogen testing is recommended only initially and at the proposed expiry date. The stability protocol can be designed based on the type of dosage form (i.e., injection or reconstitutable powder) and the sample protocols are presented in Fig. 9. Data generated by exposing samples to stress conditions can be used to decipher long-term stability of the product at ambient conditions. Such information at early stages of development is helpful in evaluating different formulations. Low-temperature storage data is needed for suspension formulations to evaluate crystal growth potential and thermal sensitivity. Comments on Fig. 9 are:

1. Parenteral suspensions should be stored at 25°C and at 25°C/60% relative humidity (RH) for lyophilized powders to generate real time data.
2. Storage at 5°C is crucial to determine thermal sensitivity and crystal growth potential of the product and may be done for the first three development batches.
3. Powder samples should be stored at 40°C/75% RH to determine the product integrity at high humidity. Should significant change occur at 40°C/75% RH, a minimum of 6 months' stability data from an ongoing 1-year study at 30°C/60% RH is required for initial registration application.
4. Generally, ready-to-use injectables should be limited to 24 to 36 months' shelf life; powders, 48 to 60 months.
5. Samples should be stored under UV light of intensity 1000 μwatts/cm^2 for 2 weeks and under fluorescent light of 1000 foot-candles for 3 months in final containers to approximate 2 years' exposure on the shelf. Proposed ICH guidelines suggest 1380 foot-candles for 3 and 8 days for monitoring fluorescent light sensitivity.

Conditions	Time Period											
	Initial	7 day	14 day	1 mos.	3 mos.	6 mos.	9 mos.	12 mos.	18 mos.	24 mos.	36 mos.	48 mos.
At Storage	%SPyPD											
5°C					x	x	x	%	x	%	%	%
25°C					%	%P	%	%PS	%	%PS	%PS	%PSPy
30°C					%	%P	%	%P				
40°C					%	%P						
Fluorescent Light				%	%							
Ultraviolet Light		%	%									

(a)

Conditions	Time Period											
	Initial	7 day	14 day	1 mos.	3 mos.	6 mos.	9 mos.	12 mos.	18 mos.	24 mos.	36 mos.	48 mos.
At Storage	%SPyM											
5°C						x		%		%	%	%
25°C/60%RH					%	%	%	%MS	%M	%MS	%SM	%SMPy
30°C					%M	%M	%	%M				
40°C/75%RH					%M	%M						
Fluorescent Light				%	%							
Ultraviolet Light		%	%									

(b)

Fig. 9 Sample protocols for injectable suspensions. (a) Ready-to-use and (b) reconstitutable powder.

Key:

- x   appearance, physical testing of reconstituted product (if applicable), packaging appearance, other appropriate physical tests.
- %   x, active ingredient(s)/degradation products assay, pH, redispersibility, sedimentation volume, particle size distribution, dissolution
- RH   Relative humidity
- M   Moisture analysis
- S   Sterility test
- Py   Pyrogen testing
- P   Preservative assay

The physical testing needed for parenteral suspension will depend on the type of dosage form. A ready-to-use suspension should be monitored for the following physical parameters as specified by protocol in Fig. 9a: resuspendibility, sedimentation volume, pH, syringeability and crystal growth, zeta potential, particle size distribution, and dissolution. A one-time freeze/thaw and shipping test is also necessary.

A reconstitutable cake/powder requires moisture analysis. Only short-term resuspendibility and sedimentation volume tests are needed because preparations are generally used within 8 to 12 hours after reconstitution. Crystal growth studies on the cake are recommended to monitor changes in particle size due to intrinsic moisture. Microbiological parameters should also be considered on extended storage of a reconstitutable powder.

F. Advances in Applications of Parenteral Suspensions

Parenteral suspensions are typically administered by intramuscular or subcutaneous route. The potential to administer suspensions by intravenous or other routes is being investigated to deliver drugs in the treatment of cancer [169,170], central nervous system disorders, and [171] viral diseases [172]. Suspensions are being studied as a potential dosage form to administer drugs present in microparticulate carrier systems (e.g., nanoparticles, microspheres, polymeric carrier systems) [173,174]. Parenteral suspensions have gained application for controlled/prolonged release of hormones, proteins, and other biologicals [175]. Some of these advances in applications of parenteral suspensions are described in this section.

1. Intratumoral Administration of Suspensions

Intratumoral injection of cisplatin-lipiodal suspensions (CL) in normal rabbit lung was investigated to assess the safety and feasibility of intratumoral injection of CL suspensions for lung cancer [169]. Some intrathoracic and intrabronchial leakage of CL suspensions was observed, but no noxious parenchymal damage to the lung or surrounding tissue was reported. The accumulation of lipiodal in mediastinal lymph nodes may provide a therapy for controlling mediastinal lymph nodes lesions either metastasized from lung cancer or manifested as the primary tumor. In another study, injection of nimustine-lipiodal suspension into tumors that had been implanted in mice was found effective for the primary cancerous lesions and lymph node metastatic lesions [170].

Lipiodal, an oily lymphographic agent, is an ethyl ester of the fatty acid of poppy seed oil (38% iodine by weight) and has been found to remain selectively in the hepatic tissue tumor site for a long time after injection into the hepatic artery. Administration of CL suspensions in hepatic arteries was found effective in the treatment of rat hepatic carcinoma [176]. Addition of increasing amounts of phosphatidylcholine to CL suspensions resulted in increased delivery of drug to the tumor tissue after hepatic arterial injection and decreased delivery to nontarget tissues in rabbits carrying VX-2 hepatic carcinoma [177].

2. Intravenous Administration of Suspensions

Because of the danger of vasoocclusion and pulmonary embolism with particle sizes greater than 5 μm, use of the intravenous route for the administration of parenteral suspensions has been limited. Various novel delivery systems containing drug in microparticulate forms are being investigated for intravenous delivery of parenteral suspensions. This has been particularly useful for central nervous system (CNS) active agents, diagnostic agents, and compounds slightly soluble in water and oil. For example, the pharmacological actions of CNS depressants such as methohexital sodium, midazolam maleate, and flunitrazepam, when given intravenously to rabbits in equimolar doses as suspensions and solutions elicited similar responses in terms of onset, duration, and maximal intensity of action between the two dosage forms [171]. The mean particle diameter of these suspensions ranged from 460 to 770 nm and the suspensions were well tolerated by animals. Because most of the CNS active compounds are lipophilic, these parenteral suspensions facilitate the use of intravenous route for water-insoluble CNS-active drugs in pharmacological screening experiments. Additionally, the use of co-solvents known to produce various side effects in formulations can be avoided.

An intravenous suspension for diagnostic imaging (e.g., magnetic resonance imaging) is described [178]. These suspensions are composed of magnetic particles and a chelating agent, or bioprecursor, which is a chelating agent bound by a biodegradable bond to a biomolecule or a biologically inert macromolecular matrix or carrier. A suspension containing superparamagnetic particles and starch gel beads (1.5 μm) containing DTPA 100 mg/ml suspended in sterile aqueous 0.9% sodium chloride solution is described.

Drugs that are very slightly soluble in water and oil (e.g., spironolactone and antineoplastic agents 1-4,-bis-(dl-2,3-oxidoporpoxi)-anthraquinone, 1,4 dihydroxy anthraquinone) provide additional challenge for parenteral formulation development because of solubility constraints. A suspension-emulsion system is reported for intravenous administration to mice and rats for use in early developmental experiments for the above-mentioned drugs [179]. The drug is ground in medium chain triglycerides using a wet ball milling process. The resulting suspension is then incorporated in an O/W emulsion using soybean lecithin and cholesterol as emulsifiers and then homogenized by a high-pressure homogenization process [180]. Lecithins with low phosphatidylcholine contents allowed formation of more stable emulsions because of high zeta potential but resulted in greater droplet sizes. A combination of poloxamer 188 and lecithin S75 used as emulsifier reduced the particle size of this suspension emulsion system to within the range of 1 to 2 μm. Hence, the choice of emulsifier is based on the balance between the required particle size and stability. These suspension-emulsions are well tolerated by animals and provide a new method to administer drugs with low solubility in both water and oil.

In another application, epidural injection of 10% butamben suspension for cancer pain in dogs and in two cancer patients did not appear to cause any local tissue damage or neurolysis [181]. Epidural administration provided a depot analgesic effect lasting up to several months. No significant pathology in spinal cord, meninges, or spinal nerves of dogs or cancer patients was observed with epidural administration. Subarachnoid butamben administration should be avoided, as it is associated with side effects such as adhesive arachnoiditis.

3. Microparticulate Drug Carriers Administered as Intravenous Suspensions

Various microparticulate drug carriers such as microspheres, nanoparticulates, and liposomes are being investigated for intravenous administration as suspensions. Nanoparts are polymerized solidified micelles (spherical particles less than 80 nm in size) of nontoxic polymeric material with entrapped bioactive materials [173]. Partitioning of drugs into nanoparts offers promise as parenteral delivery systems for proteins and labile drugs such as tetanus toxoid, urease, and human IgG in suspension form—with no loss of biological activity. Their use as adjuvants in immunological application can provide stable antigen fixation and higher antibody titers.

Subacute toxicity studies were performed in rabbits to evaluate intravenous use of thalidasine polyphase liposomes in the form of suspension for antitumor agents. No pathological changes were reported and no adverse effects on the rabbit leukocytes were observed [174].

Erythrocyte membranes were investigated as biodegradable carriers for intravenous injection of doxorubicin [182]. Two different preparations of doxorubin in rats were used: (a) erythrocyte-ghosts-doxorubicin (EGD), where doxorubicin was taken up by erythrocyte ghosts suspension during incubation at 37°C, and (b) erythrocyte-vesicles-doxorubicin (EVD), where doxorubicin was incubated with erythrocyte ghosts suspension after it was sonicated to produce vehicles smaller in size than the erythrocytes. EVDs were found particularly effective in preventing the accumulation of doxorubicin in heart tissue, thereby minimizing the cardiotoxicity associated with doxorubicin.

4. *Delivery of Drugs Used in Infectious and Viral Diseases*

Azidothymidine (5%) adsorbed on cyanoacrylate nanoparticles with particle size of 0.2 μm was suspended in water, and the suspension was administered to patients infected with human immunodeficiency virus [172]. Similarly, a suspension of ansamycin adsorbed to cyanoacrylate nanoparticles was used to treat AIDS patients infected with *Myobacterium avium intracellulare.*

5. *Controlled-Release Delivery Systems*

Parenteral suspensions are ideal dosage forms for prolonged and controlled therapy. A number of injectable depot suspension products are available that utilize different formulation approaches to provide constant and sustained therapeutic drug levels with reduced frequency of injection [175]. These can be further classified based on the approach used to provide sustained release.

a. *Formulations containing water-insoluble drug derivatives such as salts, complexes, and esters with low aqueous solubility.* For example, aqueous suspensions of penicillin G benzathine (Bicillin L-A, Wyeth-Ayerst), of penicillin G procaine (Crysticillin A.S., Squibb), of penicillin G benzathine-penicillin G procaine combination (Bicillin C-R, Wyeth-Ayerst), oleagenous suspensions of penicillin G procaine, and of naloxone pamoate. More recently, stabilization of prolonged-release intramuscular suspension containing penicillin G salts in the presence of lecithins, Kollidon 17 PF, and glyceryl monooleate is reported [183] In another case, to obtain a long-lasting parenteral opioid analgesic, the hydrochloride salt of nalbuphine was formulated as suspension in methylcellulose, sodium carboxymethylcellulose, and polyethylene glycol [184]. The resulting suspension produced a twofold increase in the drugs half-life after intramuscular injection in rats and dogs.

Long-acting insulin preparations have been developed either by complexing insulin with protamine or globin in zinc chloride or by controlling the crystallinity of the insulin in the presence of zinc chloride. For example, Ultralente, Semilente, and Lente preparations of insulin have different onset, peak, and duration of action.

Complexation of drugs with cyclodextrin and the delivery of such complexes in the form of a suspension is being investigated to provide prolonged release. For example, Heptakis (2,6 -di-O-ethyl)-β-Cyclodextrin(DE-β-CyD), which is slightly soluble in water, can serve as a sustained release type carrier for water-soluble drugs with short biological half-lives. DE-β-CyD was investigated as a parenteral sustained-release carrier in rats for buserelin acetate, a luteinizing hormone–releasing hormone superagonist, from an injectable oily suspension in arachis oil containing the drug or its DE-β-CyD complex [185]. The poor water solubility of the drug-CyD complex significantly retarded the in vitro release. Effective continuous plasma levels of buserelin were maintained for 1 month after a single subcutaneous injection indicating a potential therapeutic efficacy for the treatment of endocrine-dependent metastatic prostate carcinoma or endometriosis.

Water-insoluble but oil-soluble prodrugs in the forms of esters for different steroids have been developed for the desired prolonged duration of action. The suspension formulations of some of these steroid esters are used for the desired depot effect. For example, aqueous suspensions of micronized medroxyprogesterone acetate crystals (Depo-Provera, Upjohn), estradiol valerate oleaginous suspension (Delestrogen, Squibb; Duratrad, Ascher), microcrystalline desoxycortisone pivalate in oleagenous suspension (Percorten Pivalate, Ciba), betamethasone acetate suspension (Celestone Soluspan suspension, Schering) and triamcinolone acetonide (diacetate or hexacetonide) (Aristospan, Fujisawa) are currently available for depot effect.

b. *Formulations that utilize water immiscible vehicles such as vegetable oils with water-repelling agents such as aluminum monostearate.* For example, oleagenous suspension of micronized penicillin G procaine (with particle size 50% or more over 50 μm) in sesame oil or peanut oil gelled with 2% aluminum monostearate produces a longer depot action than in ungelled peanut oil [186]. The similar concept has been utilized in the development of parenteral controlled-release suspension formulations for relaxin, naloxone, and naltrexone pamoate [187]; naltrexone–aluminum tannate and naltrexone–zinc tannate [188]; and aurothioglucose (Solganal, Schering). Long-acting vitamin B_{12} product, Depinar (Armour) is a combination of readily absorbable vitamin B_{12} and a sustained-release cyanocobalamin–zinc tannate in sesame oil gelled with 2% aluminum monostearate.

c. *Complexation of insoluble salts with polybasic-organic acids and of insoluble complexes with polyvalent metallic ions.* For example, an insoluble interferon-α–protamine–zinc complex also containing human serum albumin (HSA) for maximum insoluble complex formation and glycine as a chelator of zinc [189]. Addition of protamine before zinc to the solution of interferon-α solution in phosphate buffer containing HSA and glycine ensures formation of an insoluble protein complex that exists as colloidal particles and remains in the dispersion for an extended period of time. Other examples are adenocorticotropin hormone (ACTH)–zinc tannate, naloxone–zinc tannate suspensions.

d. *Dispersion in polymer beads or microcapsules such as lactide/glycolide copolymers or homopolymers.* For example, a subcutaneous suspension formulation for sustained release of lobeline consisted of a physical-constraint modulation system containing 35% lobeline in lactic acid–glycolic acid copolymer microparticles for treating drug dependency or aiding in cessation of smoking [190]. Similarly, a long-acting, injectable contraceptive norethindrone formulation has been developed by preparing biodegradable norethindrone-dispersing polymer beads (90 to 180 μm in particle size) of 90% lactide/ 10% glycolide copolymer and then suspending them in 1% w/v aqueous methylcellulose solution [191].

e. *Adsorption-type depot formulations.* A long-acting injectable dosage form for a somatostatin analogue to improve glucose control in patients with type I diabetes is prepared by adsorbing somatostatin analogue on zinc phosphate suspension [192]. The binding of histidyl-histidine residues present on the somatostatin analogue to zinc phosphate particles is responsible for obtaining a stable flocculated suspension.

6. *Miscellaneous Applications*

A gelatin suspension (GS) prepared by mixing gelatin powder with saline was used to detect the clinical usefulness of endoscopic injection therapy for gastrointestinal hemorrhage [193]. No abnormal histological changes, including inflammation and ulceration, were observed in dogs after endoscopic injection, and ulcer healing was significantly accelerated by the gelatin suspension. These results suggested that endoscopic injection therapy using GS seems to be safe, simple, and useful for gastrointestinal hemorrhage.

Atelocollagen microcapsules suspended in viscous aqueous support media may be injected for sustained-release drug delivery or as a filler for soft or bone tissue [194]. These microcapsules optimally comprise a polysaccharide, glycosaminoglycan, suspended in an aqueous support medium containing 1% sodium hydroxide dereticulated atelocollagen. The microcapsule composition is released as a continuous thread from an injection needle.

An insoluble calcium salt of bisphosphonic acid was formulated as an aqueous suspension for intramuscular or subcutaneous administration in the prevention or treatment of calcium metabolic disorders [195]. The suspension provided a slow release of bisphosphonic acid and reduced the tissue damage and localized pain and irritation at the site of injection in rats; it also reduced the bone loss.

Example 1 Sterile Triamcinolone Diacetate Aqueous Suspension

Ingredient	Amount (mg)	Type
Triamcinolone diacetate, micronized	40.00	Active ingredient
Polysorbate 80 NF	0.2%	Surfactant
Polyethylene glycol 3350 NF	3.0%	Suspending vehicle
Sodium chloride	0.85%	Tonicity agent
Benzyl alcohol	0.90%	Preservative
Water for Injection	q.s.	
Total	1.0 mL	

Source: Ref. 150.

Example 2 Sustained Release Medroxyprogesterone Aqueous Suspension

Ingredient	Amount (mg)	Type
Medroxyprogesterone acetate	100.00	Active ingredient
Polyethylen glycol 3350	27.6	Suspending vehicle
Polysorbate 80	1.84	Surfactant
Sodium chloride	8.30	Tonicity agent
Methyl paraben	1.75	Preservative
Propyl paraben	0.194	Preservative
Water for Injection	q.s.	Vehicle
Total	1.0 mL	

Source: Ref. 151.

Example 3 Oleaginous Suspension Formulation: Aurothioglucose Suspension

Ingredient	Amount (mg)	Type
Aurothioglucose	50.0	Active ingredient
Aluminum monostearate	2.0	Suspending agent
Propylparaben	1.0	Preservative
Sesame oil	q.s.	Vehicle
Total	1.0 mL	

Source: Ref. 152.

Example 4 Suspension Upon Reconstitution Formulation: Spectinomycin Hydrochloride Sterile Powder

Ingredient	Amount (g)	Type
Spectinomycin hydrochloride	2.0	Active ingredient

Source: Ref. 156.

ACKNOWLEDGMENTS

The authors wish to thank the previous contributors, Drs. J. Bruce Boyett and Craig W. Davis, for the opportunity to update this chapter. We also acknowledge their technical expertise in reviewing this manuscript.

APPENDIX

List of Materials/Instruments and Their Suppliers/Manufacturers

[a]Manton-Gaulin homogenizer — Gaulin Corporation, Everett, Massachusetts

[b]Junior 125 Viscolizer — Cherry-Burrell, Cedar Rapids, Iowa

[c]Microfluidizer — Microfluidics Corporation, Newton, Massachusetts

[d]Zeta Sizer 2 or 4 — Malvern Instruments, Ltd. Malvern, England

[e]Matec ESA 8000 — Matec Applied Sciences, Hopkinton, Massachusetts

[f]Malvern Photo Correlation Spectrometer — Malvern Instruments, Ltd. Malvern, England

[g]Coulter Nan-Sizer — Coulter Electronics, Inc. Hialeah, Florida

[h]Galai Cis-1 — Galai Co. Migdol Haemek, Israel

[i]Model EM 109 — Carl Zeiss F. R. G.

[j]Abbott Laboratories, North Chicago, Illinois

[k]Miramed, Mirandola, Italy

[l]Travenol Laboratories, Inc., Deerfield, Illinois, and Abbott Laboratories, North Chicago, Illinois

[m]EVA-Mix, GilMed Industries, Northbrook, Illinois

[n]Infusobags, Geistlich

[o]Disk Cartridge, Millipore Corporation, Bedford, Massachusetts

[p]Gelman Sciences, Filtration Division, Ann Arbor, Michigan

[q]Pall Corporation, Glen Cove, New York

[r]Sartorius Filters, Inc., Hayward, California

REFERENCES

1. S. S. Davis, Pharmaceutical aspects of intravenous fat emulsions, *J. Hosp. Pharm.,* 32(8&9):149–171 (1974).
2. L. P. Jeffrey, P. N. Johnson, D. J. Slonka, and H. T. Randall, Intravenous fat emulsion: An innovative concept, *Hosp. Form.* 12(11):772–773 (1977).
3. A. Wretlind, Development of fat emulsions, *J. Parent. Enter. Nutr.,* 5(3):230–235 (1981).
4. M. Roesner and J. P. Grant, Intravenous lipid emulsions, *Nutr. Clin. Pract.,* 2:96–107 (1987).
5. J. M. Long, Safe and effective fat emulsions, *Nutr. Clin. Pract.* 2:92–93 (1987).
6. K. Y. Warshawsky, Techniques and procedures; intravenous fat emulsions in clinical practice, *Nutr. Clin. Pract.* 7:187–196 (1992).
7. R. J. Cooke, Y. Y. Yeh, D. Gibson, D. Debo, and G. L. Bell, Soybean oil emulsion administration during parenteral nutrition in the preterm infant: Effect on essential fatty acid, lipid, and glucose metabolism, *J. Pediatr.,* 111:767–773 (1987).
8. K. C. Higbee and P. P. Lamy, The use of intralipid in neonates and infants, *Hosp. Form.,* 15:117–119, 122, 127 (1980).
9. L. A. Trissel, *Handbook of Injectable Drugs,* 8th ed., American Society of Hospital Pharmacists, Inc., Maryland, 1994, p. 420.
10. G. Hardy, R. Cotter, and R. Dawe, The stability and comparative clearance of TPN mixtures with lipid, *Adv. Clin. Nutr.,* Proc. Int. Symp., 2nd, (I. D. A. Johnston, ed.) Meeting Date 1982, 241–60. MTP: Lancaster, UK (1983).
11. R. S. Henry, R. W. Jurgens, R. Sturgeon, N. Athanikar, A. Welco, and M. Van Leuven, Compatibility of calcium chloride and calcium gluconate with sodium phosphate in a mixed TPN solution, *Am. J. Hosp. Pharm.,* 37:673–674 (1980).
12. A. Takumura, F. Ishii, S. Noro, M. Tanifuji, and S. Nakajima, Study of intravenous hyperalimentation: Effect of selected amino acids on the stability of intravenous fat emulsions, *J. Pharm. Sci.,* 73 (1):91–94 (1984).
13. S. A. Turner, Stability and clinical use of intravenous admixtures containing lipid emulsion, *Pharm., J.,* 234:799–800 (1985).
14. V. A. Parry, K. R. Harrie, and N. L. McIntosh-Lowe, Effect of various nutrient ratios on the emulsion stability of total nutrient admixtures, *Am. J. Hosp. Pharm.,* 43:3017–3022 (1986).
15. F. A. Sayeed, H. W. Johnson, K. B. Sukumaran, J. A. Raihle, D. L. Mowles, H. A. Stelmach, and K. R. Majors, Stability of liposyn II fat emulsion in total nutrient admixtures. *Am. J. Hosp. Pharm.,* 43:1230–1235 (1986).
16. F. A. Sayeed, M. G. Tripp, K. B. Sukumaran, B. A. Mikrut, H. A. Stelmach, and J. A. Raihle, Stability of total nutrient admixtures using various intravenous fat emulsions, *Am. J. Hosp. Pharm.* , 44:2271–2280 (1987).
17. B. E. Rabinow, S. Ericson, and T. Shelborne, Aluminum in parenteral products: Analysis, reduction, and implications for pediatric TPN, *J. Parent. Sci. Technol.* 43(3):132–139 (1989).
18. C. Washington and T. Sizer, Stability of TPN mixtures compounded from lipofundin S and aminoplex amino-acid solutions: Comparison of laser diffraction and Coulter Counter droplet size analysis, *Int. J. Pharm.,* 83:227–231 (1992).
19. C. L. Fortner, W. R. Grove, D. Bowie, and M. D. Walker, Fat emulsion vehicle for intravenous administration of an aqueous insoluble drug, *Am. J. Hosp. Pharm.,* 32:582–584 (1975).
20. A. A. El-Sayed and A. J. Repta, Solubilization and stabilization of an investigational antineoplastic drug (NSC no. 278214) in an intravenous formulation using an emulsion vehicle, *Int. J. Pharm.,* 13:303–312 (1983).
21. R. J. Baptista, J. D. Palombo, S. R. Tahan, A. J. Valicenti, B. R. Bistrian, C. F. Arkin, and G. L. Blackburn, Stability of cimetidine hydrochloride in a total nutrient admixture, *Am. J. Hosp. Pharm.,* 42:2208–2210 (1985).
22. S. M. Cano, J. B. Montoro, C. Pastor, L. Pou, and P. Sabín, Stability of ranitidine hydrochloride in total nutrient admixtures, *Am. J. Hosp. Pharm.,* 45:1100–1102 (1988).

23. F. Ishii, A. Takamura, and H. Ogata, Compatibility of intravenous fat emulsions with prodrug amino acids, *J. Pharm. Pharmacol.*, 40:89–92 (1988).

24. L. Bullock, J. F. Fitzgerald, and M. R. Glick, Stability of famotidine 20 and 50 mg/L in total nutrient admixtures, *Am. J. Hosp. Pharm.*, 46:2326–2328 (1989).

25. J. B. Montoro, L. Pou, P. Salvador, C. Pastor, and S. M. Cano, Stability of famotidine 20 and 40 mg/L in total nutrient admixtures, *Am. J. Hosp. Pharm.*, 46:2329–2332 (1989).

26. B. F. Shea and P. F. Souney, Stability of famotidine in a 3-in-1 total nutrient admixture, *DICP Ann. Pharmacother.*, 24:232–235 (1990).

27. R. J. Prankerd, and V. J. Stella, The use of oil-in-water emulsions as a vehicle for parenteral drug administration, *J. Parenter. Sci. Technol.*, 44(3):139–149 (1990).

28. J. Hatton, S. G. Holstad, A. D. Rosenbloom, T. Westrich, and J. Hirsch, Stability of nizatidine in total nutrient admixtures, *Am. J. Hosp. Pharm.*, 48:1507–1510 (1991).

29. A. Andreu, D. Cardona, C. Pastor, and J. Bonal, Intravenous aminophylline: In vitro stability in fat-containing TPN, *Ann. Pharmacother.*, 26(1):127–128 (1992).

30. M. Singh and L. J. Ravin, Parenteral emulsions as drug carrier systems, *J. Parenter. Sci. Technol.*, 40:34–41 (1986).

31. B. Lundberg, Preparation of drug-carrier emulsions stabilized with phosphatidylcholine-surfactant mixtures, *J. Pharm. Sci.*, 83(1):72 (1994).

32. R. J. Prankerd, S. G. Frank, and V. J. Stella, Preliminary development and evaluation of a parenteral emulsion formulation of penclomedine (NSC-338720) a novel, practically water insoluble cytotoxic agent, *J. Parenter. Sci. Technol.*, 42(3):76–81 (1988).

33. S. Benita and M. L. Levy, Submicron emulsions as colloidal drug carriers for intravenous administration: Comprehensive physicochemical characterization, *J. Pharm. Sci.*, 82(11).1069–1079 (1993).

34. A. F. Brodin, D. R. Kavaliunas, and S. G. Frank, Prolonged drug release from multiple emulsions, *Acta Pharm. Suec.*, 15 (1):1–12 (1978).

35. C. J. Benoy, L. A. Elson, and R. Schneider, Multiple emulsions, a suitable vehicle to provide sustained release of cancer chemotherapeutic agents, *Br. J. Pharmacol.*, 45:135– (1972).

36. T. Yoshioka, K. Ikeuchi, M. Hashida, S. Muranishi, and H. Sezaki, Prolonged release of bleomycin from parenteral gelatin sphere-in-oil emulsion, *Chem. Pharm. Bull.*, 30(4)1408–1415 (1982).

37. C. J. Herman and M. J. Groves, Hydrolysis kinetics of phospholipids in thermally stressed intravenous lipid emulsion formulations, *J. Pharm. Pharmacol.* 44:539–542 (1992).

38. R. P. Geyer, D. M. Watkin, L. W. Matthews, and J. Store, Parenteral nutrition. XI. Studies with stable and unstable fat emulsions administered intravenously, *Proc. Exp. Biol.*, 77:872–876 (1951).

39. T. Fugita, T. Sumaya, K. Yokohama, Fluorocarbon emulsion as a candidate for artificial blood: Correlation between particle size of the emulsion and acute toxicity, *Eur. Surg. Res.*, 3:436–453 (1971).

40. M. J. Groves, *Parenteral Products*, William Heirmann Medical Books, LTD, London, 1973, pp. 30–40.

41. R. H. Müller and S. Heinemann, Fat emulsions for parenteral nutrition. III: Lipofundin MCT/LCT regimens for total parenteral nutrition (TPN) with low electrolyte load, *Int. J. Pharm.*, 101:175–189 (1994).

42. R. C. Mehta, L. F. Head, A. M. Hazrati, M. Parr, R. P. Rapp, and P. P. DeLuca, Fat emulsion particle-size distribution in total nutrient admixtures, *Am. J. Hosp. Pharm.*, 49:2749–2755 (1992).

43. J. E. F. Reynolds, ed., *Martindale: The Extra Pharmacopoeia*, 30th ed, The Pharmaceutical Press, London, England, 1988, p. 1048.

44. M. J. Groves, M. Wineburg, A. P. R. Brain, Presence of liposomal material in phosphatide stabilized emulsions, *J. Disp. Sci. Technol.* 6(2) 237–243 (1985).

45. D. L. Seinder, E. A. Mascioli, N. W. Istfan, K. A. Porter, K. Selleck, G. L. Blackburn, and B. R. Bistrian, Effects of long-chain triglyercide emulsions on reticuloendothelial system function in humans, *J. Parenter. Enter. Nutr.,* 13(6):614–619 (1989).

46. W. T. Chance, L. Cao, J. I. Nelson, T. Foley-Nelson, and J. E. Fischer, Acivicin reduces tumor growth during total parenteral nutrition (TPN), *Surgery,* 102(2):386–394 (1987).

47. R. J. Cooke, Y. Y. Yeh, D. Gibson, D. Debo, and G. L. Bell, Soybean oil emulsion administration during parenteral nutrition in the preterm infant: Effect on essential fatty acid, lipid, and glucose metabolism, *J. Pediatr.,* 111:767–773 (1987).

48. Z. Friedman, K. H. Marks, M. J. Maisels, R. Thorson, and R. Naeye, Effect of parenteral fat emulsion on the pulmonary and reticuloendothelial systems in the newborn infant. *Pediatrics,* 61:694–698 (1978).

49. P. K. Hansrani, S. S. Davis, and M. J. Groves, The preparation and properties of sterile intravenous emulsions, *J. Parenter. Sci. Technol.,* 37(4):145–150 (1983).

50. M. Rubin, D. Harell, N. Naor, A. Moser, E. Wielunsky, P. Merlob, and D. Lichtenberg, Lipid infusion with different triglyceride cores (long-chain vs medium-chain/long-chain triglyercides): Effect on plasma lipids and bilirubin binding in premature infants, *J. Parenter. Enter. Nutr.,* 15(6):642–646 (1991).

51. Karlshams USA Inc., Technical Bulletin CAS# [65381–09–1], Columbus, OH 1992.

52. S. S. Chang, Purification of Nutritive Oils, U.S. Patent No. 74–498568 (1978).

53. B. D. Tarr, T. G. Sambandan, and S. H. Yalkowsky, A new parenteral emulsion for the administration of taxol. *Pharm. Res.,* 4(2):162–165 (1987).

54. D. M. Lidgate, R. C. Fu, N. E. Byars, L. C. Foster, and J. S. Fleitman, Formulation of vaccine adjuvant muramyldipeptides. 3. Processing optimization, characterization, and bioactivity of an emulsion vehicle, *Pharm. Res.,* 6 (9):748–751 (1989).

55. R. P. Geyer, G. V. Mann, J. Young, T. D. Kinney, and J. F. Stare, Parenteral nutrition V. Studies on soybean phosphatides as emulsifiers for intravenous fat emulsions, *J. Lab. Clin. Med.,* 33:163–174 (1948).

56. D. A. Yeadon, L. A. Goldblatt, and A. M. Altschull, Lecithin in oil-in-water emulsions, *J. Am. Oil Chem. Soc.,* 35:435–438 (1958).

57. H. J. Zeringue, M. L. Brown, and W. S. Singleton, Chromatographically homogenous egg lecithin as stabilizer of emulsions for intravenous nutrition, *J. Am. Oil Chem. Soc.,* 41:688–691 (1964).

58. F. F. Lambert, J. P. Miller, and D. V. Frost, Deposition of lecithin in parenteral fat emulsions, *Am. J. Physiol.,* 186:397 (1957).

59. M. L. Schneider, Achieving purer lecithin, *Drug. Cosmet. Ind.,* Feb. 54 (1992).

60. C. Washington, The stability of intravenous fat emulsions in total parenteral nutrition mixtures, *Int. J. Pharm.,* 66:1–21 (1990).

61. C. D. Black and N. G. Popovich, A study of intravenous emulsion compatibility: Effects of dextrose, amino acids, and selected electrolytes, *Drug Intell. Clin. Pharm.,* 15(3):184–193 (1981).

62. P. E. Schurr, Composition and preparation of experimental intravenous emulsions, *Can. Res.,* 29:258–260 (1969).

63. J. F. Muller, Intravenous fat emulsions—an enigma, *Bull. Parenter. Drug. Assoc.,* 21(6):226–228 (1967).

64. M. Y. Levy and S. Benita, Design and characterization of a submicronized O/W emulsion of diazepam for parenteral use, *Int. J. Pharm.,* 54:103–112 (1989).

65. C. Horowitz, L. Krutz, and L. S. Kaminsky, The emulsifying properties of egg yolk phosphatidylcholine, *Lipids,* 7:234–239 (1972).

66. M. P. Krafft, P. Vierling, and J. G. Riess, Synthesis and preliminary data on the biocompatibility and emulsifying properties of perfluoroalkylated phosphoramidates as injectable surfactants, *Eur. J. Med. Chem.,* 26:545–550 (1991).

67. G. D. Chanana and B. B. Sheth, Particle size reduction of emulsions by formulation design 1: Effect of polyhydroxy alcohols, *J. Parent. Sci. Technol.,* 47(3):130–134 (1993).

68. L. A. Trissel, *Handbook of Injectable Drugs*, 8th ed., American Society of Hospital Pharmacists, Inc., Maryland, 1994, p. 419.

69. M. Y. Levy and S. Benita, Short- and long-term stability assessment of a new injectable diazepam submicron emulsion, *J. Parent. Sci. Technol.*, 45(2):101–107 (1991).

70. D. M. Lidgate, R. C. Fu, and J. S. Fleitman, Using a mcirofluidizer to manufacture parenteral emulsions, *BioPharm.*, 2:28–33 (1989).

71. C. Washington and S. S. Davis, The production of parenteral feeding emulsions by microfluidizer, *Int. J. Pharm.*, 44:169–176 (1988).

72. C. Washington, New technology for emulsion production, *Manuf. Chemist*, March: 49, 52, 55 (1988).

73. D. M. Lidgate, T. Trattner, M. S. Richard, and R. Maskiewicz, Sterile filtration of a parenteral emulsion, *Pharm. Res.*, 9(7):860–863 (1992).

74. L. D. Pelham, Rational use of intravenous fat emulsions, *Am. J. Hosp. Pharm.*, 38:198–208 (1981).

75. M. C. Allwood, P. W. Brown, C. Ghedini, and G. Hardy, The stability of ascorbic acid in TPN mixtures stored in a multilayered bag, *Clin. Nutr.*, 11:284–288 (1992).

76. J. Boberg and I. Hakansson, Physical and biological changes in an artificial fat emulsion during storage, *J. Pharm. Pharmacol.*, 16:641–646 (1964).

77. A. Wretlind, *Parenteral Nutrition in Acute Metabolic Illness*, Academic, Orlando, Florida, 1974, Chapter 5.

78. A. M. Laval-Jeantet, M. Laval-Jeantet, and C. Bergot, Effect of particle size on tissue distribution of iodized emulsified fat following intravenous administration, *Invest. Radiol.*, 17:617–620 (1982).

79. F. Ishii, I. Sasaki, and H. Ogata, Effect of phospholipid emulsifiers on physicochemical properties of intravenous fat emulsions and/or drug carrier emulsions, *J. Pharm. Pharmacol.*, 42:513–515, (1990).

80. N. J. Kale and L. V. Allen, Studies on microemulsions using Brij 96 as surfactant and glycerin, ethylene glycol and propylene glycol as cosurfactants. *Int. J. Pharm.*, 57:87–93 (1989).

81. J. T. Rubino, The influence of charged lipids on the flocculation and coalescence of oil-in-water emulsions. I: Kinetic assessment of emulsion stability, *J. Parenter. Sci. Technol.* 44(4):210–215 (1990).

82. H. S. Yalabik-Kas, S. Eryilmaz, and A. A. Hincal, Stability assessment of emulsion systems, *S.T.P. Pharma.*, 1:978–984 (1985).

83. J. T. Rubino, The influence of charged lipids on the flocculation and coalescence of oil-in-water emulsions. II: Electrophoretic properties and monolayer film studies, *J. Parenter. Sci. Technol.*, 44(5):247–252 (1990).

84. C. Washington, A. Chawla, N. Christy, and S. S. Davis, The electrokinetic properties of phospholipid-stabilized fat emulsions, *Int. J. Pharm.*, 54:191–197 (1989).

85. C. Washington, The electrokinetic properties of phospholipid-stabilized fat emulsions. II. Droplet mobility in mixed electrolytes, *Int. J. Pharm.*, 58:13–17 (1990).

86. C. Washington, The Electrokinetic properties of phospholipid-stabilized fat emulsions. III. Interdroplet potentials and stability ratios in monovalent electrolytes, *Int. J. Pharm.*, 64:67–73 (1990).

87. C. Washington, A. Athersuch, and D. J. Kynoch, The electrokinetic properties of phospholipid-stabilized fat emulsions. IV. The effect of glucose and of pH, *Int. J. Pharm.*, 64:217–222 (1990).

88. C. Washington, M. A. Connolly, R. Manning, and M. C. L. Skerratt, The electrokinetic properties of phospholipid-stabilized fat emulsions. V. The Effect of amino acids on emulsion stability, *Int. J. Pharm.*, 77:57–63 (1991).

89. C. Washington, The electrokinetic properties of phospholipid-stabilized fat emulsions. VI. Zeta Potentials of Intralipid 20% in TPN Mixtures, *Int. J. Pharm.*, 87:167–174 (1992).

90. M. R. Cutie, Effects of cold and freezing temperatures on pharmaceutical dosage forms, *U.S. Pharmacist*, Oct. 35–48 (1979).

91. K. S. Crocker, R. Noga, D. J. Filibeck, S. H. Krey, M. Markovic, and W. P. Steffee, Microbial growth comparisons of five commercial parenteral lipid emulsions, *J. Parenter. Ent. Nutr.*, 8:391–395 (1984).

92. C. H. Kim, D. E Lewis, and A. Kumar, Bacterial and fungal growth in intravenous fat emulsions, *Am. J. Hosp. Pharm.* 40:2159–61 (1983).

93. D. H. Brown, R. A. Simkover, Maximum hang times for I.V. fat emulsions, *Am. J. Hosp. Pharm.*, 44:284–285 (1987).

94. L. A. Trissel, *Handbook of Injectable Drugs*, American Society of Hospital Pharmacists, Inc., Maryland, 1994, p. 430.

95. L. A. Trissel, *Handbook of Injectable Drugs,* American Society of Hospital Pharmacists, Inc., Maryland, 1994, p. 426.

96. P. Raupp, R. von Kries, E. Schmidt, H.-G. Pfahl, and O. Günther, Incompatibility between fat emulsion and calcium plus heparin in parenteral nutrition of premature babies, *Lancet*, p. 700 (1988).

97. C. Washington and C. J. Briggs, Reduction of absorption of drugs into TPN plastic containers by phospholipids and fat emulsions, *Int. J. Pharm.*, 48: 133–139 (1988).

98. M. C. Allwood, Release of DEHP plasticiser into fat emulsion from IV administration sets, *Pharm. J.*, p. 600 (1985).

99. M. G. Tripp, S. K. Menon, and B. A. Mikrut, Stability of total nutrient admixtures in a dual-chamber flexible container, *Am. J. Hosp. Pharm.*, 47:2496–2503 (1990).

100. R. Jeppsson and S. Ljungberg, Anticonvulsant activity in mice of diazepam in an emulsion formulation for intravenous administration, *Acta Pharmacol. Toxicol.*, 36:312–320 (1975).

101. T. Kronevi and S. Ljungberg, Sequelae following intra-arterially injected diazepam formulations, *Acta Pharm. Suec.*, 20:389–396 (1983).

102. O. Von Dardel, C. Mebius, T. Mossberg, and B. Svensson, Fat emulsions as a vehicle for diazepam: A study of 9492 patients. *Br. J. Anaesth.*, 55:41–47 (1983).

103. T. N. Riley, R. G. Fischer, and A. L. Paysinger, New drugs 1989, *U. S. Pharm.*, 15: 33–57 (1990).

104. S. Ljungberg and R. Jeppsson, Intravenous injection of lipid soluble drugs, *Acta Pharm. Suec.*, 7:435–440 (1970).

105. R. Jeppsson, Effects of barbituric acids using an emulsion form intravenously, *Acta Pharm. Suec.*, 9:81–90 (1972).

106. P. L. Madan, Sustained-release drug delivery systems: Part V, parenteral products, *Pharm. Mfg.*, 2(6):51–57 (1985).

107. H. Fujiwara, Fundamental study of endoscopic injection of emulsified anticancer drug for lymph node metastases of gastic cancer using a stable fat emulsion containing methyl-CCNU, *Akita Igaku*, 10(4): 567–592 (1984).

108. T. Takahashi, S. Ueda, K. Kono, and S. Majima, Attempt at local administration of anticancer agents in the form of fat emulsions, *Cancer*, 38:1507–1514 (1976).

109. FDC Reports, January 1990, p.8.

110. A. Milius, J. Greiner, and J. G. Riess, Improvement in emulsification ease, particle size reduction and stabilization of concentrated fluorocarbon emulsions by small amounts of (D-glucosyl)[2-(perfluoroalkyl)ethyl] phosphates as surfactants. *Coll. Surf.*, 63(3–4):281–9 (1992).

111. G. Grimes, M. Vermess, J. F. Gallelli, M. Girton, and D. C. Chatterji, Formulation and evaluation of ethiodized oil emulsion for intravenous hepatography, *J. Pharm. Sci.*, 68(1): 52–56 (1979).

112. M. Vermess, D. C. Chatterji, G. J. Grimes, and J. F. Gallelli, Ethiodized oil emulsion for intravenous hepatography. U.S. Patent No. 110293 810327, 23 pp. (1980).

113. K. Iwamoto, T. Kato, M. Kawahara, N. Koyama, S. Watanabe, Y. Miyake, and J. Sunamoto, Polysaccharide-coated oil droplets in oil-in-water emulsions as targetable carriers for lipophilic drugs, *J. Pharm. Sci.*, 80(3):219–224 (1991).

114. W. Yu, E. S. Tabosa do Egito, G. Barrat, H. Fessi, J. P. Devissaguet, and F. Puisieux, A

novel approach to the preparation of injectable emulsions by a spontaneous emulsification process, *Int. J. Pharm.,* 89:139–146 (1993).

115. J. T. Frank, Intralipid compatibility study, *Drug. Intell. Clin. Pharm.,* 7:351–352 (1973).
116. B. Lynn, Intralipid compatibility study, *Drug. Intell. Clin. Pharm.,* 8:75–76 (1974).
117. R. J. Baptista and R. W. Lawrence, Compatibility of total nutrient admixtures and secondary antibiotic infusions, *Am. J. Hosp. Pharm.,* 42:362–363 (1985).
118. E. L. Parrot, Fluid pharmaceutical suspensions and emulsions. In: *Pharmaceutical Technology,* Burgess Publishing Co., Minneapolis, 1971, p. 346.
119. R. A. Nash, Pharmaceutical suspensions. *Drug Cosmet. Ind.,* 97:843 (1965).
120. A. Delgado, G. A. Parera, and F. Gonzalez-Caballero, A study of the electrokinetic and stability properties of nitrofurantoin suspensions. II: Flocculation and redispersion properties as compared with theoretical interaction energy curves, *J. Pharm. Sci.,* 79(8): 709–715 (1990).
121. W. I. Higuchi, J. S. Swarbrick, N. F. F. Ho, A. P. Simonelli, and A. Martin, Particle phenomenon and coarse dispersions. In: *Remington's Pharmaceutical Sciences* (A. Osol, ed.), 16th ed., Mack Publishing Co. Easton, PA, 1980, p. 294.
122. J. Zuidema, F. A. J. M. Pieters, and G. S. M. J. E. Duchateau, Release and absorption rate aspects of intramuscularly injected pharmaceuticals, *Int. J. Pharm.,* 47:1–12 (1988).
123. R. P. Enever and G. A. Lewis, Long acting contraceptive agents: The influence of pharmaceutical formulation upon biological activity of esters of norethisterone, *Steroids,* 41(3):369–379 (1983).
124. K. Hallas-Moller, K. Peterson, and J. Schlichtkrull, Crystalline and amorphous insulin-zinc compounds with prolonged action, *Science,* 116:394 (1952).
125. P. J. M. Stout, N. Khoury, S. A. Howard, and J. W. Mauger, Dissolution performance related to particle size distribution for commercially available prednisolone acetate suspensions, *Drug. Dev. Ind. Pharm.,* 18(4):395–408 (1992).
126. E. J. Antal, C. F. Dick, C. E. Wright, I. R. Welshman, and E. M. Block, Comparative bioavailability of two medroxyprogesterone acetate suspensions, *Int. J. Pharm.,* 54:33–39 (1989).
127. M. J. Akers, A. L. Fites, and R. L. Robison, Formulation design and development of parenteral suspensions, *J. Parenter. Sci. Technol.,* 41(3):88–96 (1987).
128. O. V. Rastopchina, T. S. Kondrat'eva, V. A. Sokolov, and A. F. Kalashnik, Development of stable injectable osseous powder suspension (in Russian) *Farmotsiya* (Moscow), 41(4):14–18. (1992).
129. J. B. Portnoff, Parenteral suspensions comprising 1-(p-chlorobenzoyl)-2-methyl-5-methoxy-3indolyl acetic acid as active ingredient, U.S. 4093733 780606, 4 pp. (1978).
130. K. S. E. Su, J. F. Quay, K. M. Campanale, and J. F. Stucky, Nonaqueous cephalosporin suspension for parenteral administration: Cefazolin sodium, *J. Pharm. Sci.,* 73(11):1602–1606 (1984).
131. F. J. Careleton, Aqueous and non-aqueous solvents in parenteral preparations, *Bull. Parenter. Drug Assoc.,* 21:142–146 (1967).
132. G. A. Brazeau and H. L. Fung, Use of an in vitro model for the assessment of muscle damage from intramuscular injections: In vitro–in vivo correlation and predictability with mixed solvent systems, *Pharm. Res.,* 6:776–771 (1989).
133. G. A. Brazaeu and H. L. Fung, Physicochemical properties of binary organic cosolvent-water mixtures and their relationships to muscle damage following intramuscular injection, *J. Parenter. Sci. Technol.,* 43:144–149 (1989).
134. G. A. Brazeau and H. L. Fung, Mechanisms of creatinine kinase release from isolated rat skeletal muscles damaged by propylene glycol and ethanol, *J. Pharm. Sci.,* 79:393–397 (1990).
135. K. W. Reed and S. H. Yalkowski, Lysis of human red blood cells in the presence of various cosolvents. Part 3. Effect of Differing NaCl Concentrations, *J. Parenter. Sci. Technol.* 40:88–94 (1986).

136. K. W. Reed and S. H. Yalkowski, Lysis of human red blood cells in the presence of various cosolvents, *J. Parenter. Sci. Technol.*, 39:64–69 (1985).

137. A. J. Spiegel and M. M. Noseworthy, Use of nonaqueous solvents in parenteral products, *J. Pharm. Sci.*, 52(8):917–927 (1963).

138. K. E. Avis, Parenteral preparations. In: *Remington's Pharmaceutical Sciences* (A. Osol, ed.), 16th edition, Mack Publishing Company, Easton, PA, 1980, p. 1467.

139. B. E. Ballard and E. Nelson, Prolonged-action pharmaceuticals. In: *Remington's Pharmaceutical Sciences* (A. Osol, ed.), 15th ed., Mack Publishing Company, Easton, PA, 1975, Chap. 91.

140. *British Pharmacopoeia*, London, Her Majesty's Stationery Office, 1993, Appendix XVIC, pp. A191–192.

141. *The United States Pharmacopeia*, 23rd rev., United States Pharmaceutical Convention, Inc., Rockville, MD, 1995, p. 1681.

142. M. J. Akers, Considerations in selecting antimicrobial preservatives agents for parenteral product development, *Pharmaceut. Technol.*, 8(3):36–46 (1984).

143. M. Windholz, S. Budavari, R. F. Blumetti, and E. S. Otterbain, eds., *The Merck Index*, 11th ed., Merck and Company, Inc., Rahway, NJ, 1983, pp. 959, 1248.

144. J. J. Gershanik, G. Boecler, W. George, A. Sola, M. Leitner, and C. Kapadia, The gasping syndrome: Benzyl alcohol poisoning? *Clin. Res.*, 29:895A (1981).

145. L. Lachman, H. Lieberman, and J. Kanig, eds., *The Theory and Practice of Industrial Pharmacy*, 2nd ed., Lea & Febiger, Philadelphia, 1976, p. 589.

146. R. Huettenrauch, *Stabilization of suspensions* (in German), DD 209970 A1 840530, 8 pp. (1984).

147. J. Heidt, *Stabilized injectable suspensions* (in German) DE 3233661 A1 830324, 10 pp. (1983).

148. K. Tokkyo, Aggregation inhibitors of aqueous suspensions during defrost (in Japanese) JP 55006613 800208 Showa (1980).

149. J. S. Lucks, B. W. Muller, and R. H. Muller, Poymeric and emulsion carriers—interaction with antiflocculants and ionic surfactant, *Int. J. Pharm.*, 63:183–188 (1990).

150. R. Arky, *Physician's Desk Reference*, 48th ed., Medical Economics Data Production Company, Montvale, NJ, 1994, p. 959.

151. R. Arky, *Physician's Desk Reference*, 48th ed., Medical Economics Data Production Company, Montvale, NJ, 1994, p. 2417.

152. R. Arky, *Physician's Desk Reference*, 48th ed., Medical Economics Data Production Company, Montvale, NJ, 1994, p. 2170.

153. R. Arky, *Physician's Desk Reference*, 48th Ed., Medical Economics Data Production Company, Montvale, NJ, 1994, p. 2452.

154. J. Broadhead, S. K. Edmond Rouan, and C. T. Rhodes, The spray drying of pharmaceuticals, *Drug Dev. Ind. Pharm.* 18:1169–1206 (1992).

155. N. A. Williams, and G. P. Polli, The lyophilization of pharmaceuticals: A literature review, *J. Parent. Sci. Technol.*, 38(2):48–59 (1984).

156. G. S. Banker, and E. T. Rhodes, eds., *Modern Pharmaceutics*, Marcel Dekker, New York, 1979, p. 466.

157. R. J. E. Grouls, E. W. Ackerman, E. J. A. Machielsen, and H. H. M. Korsten, Butyl p-aminobenzoate. Preparation, characterization and quality control of a suspension injection for epidural analgesia, *Pharm. Weekbl. Sci. Ed.*, 13(1):13–17 (1991).

158. H. G. Feldmeier, Monodisperse insulin suspension injections (in German) DD 290134 A5 910523 (1991).

159. J. B. Portnoff, E. M. Cohen, and M. W. Henley, Development of parenteral and sterile ophthalmic suspensions—The R & D approach, *Bull. Parenter. Drug Assoc.*, 31(3):136–143 (1977).

160. R. A. Nash and B. E. Haeger, Stable syringeable suspensions of parenteral drugs in complex flocculated form. US3457348 690722, 3 pp. (1969).

161. R. A. Nash, Parenteral suspensions, *Bull. Parent. Drug Assoc.*, 26(2):91 (1972).

162. R. Bodmeier and H. Chen, Indomethacin polymeric nanosuspensions prepared by microfluidization, *J. Control. Rel.*, 12:223–233 (1990).

163. W. A. Ritschel and Suzuki, In vitro testing of injectability, *Pharm. Ind.*, 41(5):468–475 (1979).

164. E. N. Hiestand, Theory of coarse suspension formulation, *J. Pharm. Sci.*, 53(1):1–18 (1964).

165. A. Zhang and M. J. Groves, Size characterization of mycobacterium bovis BCG (Bacillus Calmette Guerin) vaccine, Tice substrain, *Pharm. Res.*, 5:607–610 (1988).

166. A. N. Martin, J. Swardbrick, and A. Commarata, eds., Coarse dispersions. In: *Physical Pharmacy*, Lea & Febiger, Philadelphia, 1983, pp. 551–553.

167. *The United States Pharmacopeia*, 23rd rev., United States Pharmaceutical Convention, Inc., Rockville, MD, 1995.

168. J. C. Boylan, The application of rheology to parenteral suspensions and emulsions, *Bull. Parenter. Drug. Assoc.*, 19:98–109 (1965).

169. S. Onohara, M. Nakajo, K. Abeyama, H. Shinmaki, K. Sagara, H. Mukai, N. Uchiyama, N. Miyaji, and O. Harada, Percutaneous injection of cisplatin lipiodol suspension (CLS) in rabbit lung, aiming at intratumoral injection therapy for lung cancer (in Japanese), *Nippon Igaku Hoshasen Gakkai Zasshi*, 52(10):1433–1442 (1992).

170. S. Otaki, H. Kaneko, E. Fukuma, and T. Yamakawa, Experimental study on the effect of injection with anticancer agent–oil suspension (in Japanese) *Gan To Kagaku Ryoho*, 19(10):1587–1589 (1992).

171. H. Viernstein and C. Stumpf, Similar central actions of intravenous methohexitone suspension and solution in the rabbit, *J. Pharm. Pharmacol.*, 44(1):66–68 (1992).

172. J. Kreuter, S. Wolfgang, and S. Troester, Pharmaceutical suspensions containing active agents adsorbed to particulate carriers for the treatment of infection with human immunodeficiency virus and related secondary infections (in German), Ger. Offen. DE 3717406 A1 881222, 3 pp. (1988).

173. G. Birrenbach and P. P. Speisser, Polymerized micelles and their use as adjuvants in immunology, *J. Pharm. Sci.*, 65(12):1763–1766 (1976).

174. X. Gu, Z. Ma, S. Xin, H. Li, S. Sun, S. Pei, X. Shen, M. Zhou, J. Tao, and D. Lin, Anticancer drugs. II. Study on intravenous injections of polyphase liposome 139 and 76 suspensions (in Chinese) *Zhongcaoyao* 13(5):15–20 (1982).

175. Y. W. Chien, Long-acting parenteral drug formulations, *J. Parenter. Sci. Technol.*, 35(3):106–139 (1981).

176. A. Kawakami, The effects of hepatic arterial administration of cisplatin suspended in lipiodol on rat hepatic carcinoma (in Japanese) *Kinki Diagaku Igaku Zasshi*, 15(2):209–224 (1990).

177. M. Nakasima, M. Nakano, Y. Ishii, K. Matsuyama, M. Ichikawa, H. Sasaki, J. Nakamura, and J. Shibasaki, Tissue distribution of cisplatin after hepatic arterial injection of a cisplatin-lipiodol suspension containing phosphatidylcholine to rabbits carrying VX-2 hepatic carcinoma, *Pharm. Res.* 6(4):342–345 (1989).

178. J. Kalveness and T. Thomassen, Chelating agent and magnetic particle-containing compositions and their use, PCT Int. Appl. WO 8911873 A1 891214, 27 pp. (1989).

179. K. J. Steffens, A. Lich, and H. Perschbacher, O/W emulsions as carriers for micronized drug particles, *Manuf. Chem.*, 63:23–26 (1992).

180. P. C. Schmidt, H. Perschbacher, K. J. Steffens, and H. P. Kraemer, Development of a suspension-emulsion system for parenteral application in animals, *Acta Pharm. Technol.*, 35(1):34–37 (1989).

181. M. Shulman, N. J. Joseph, and C. A. Haller, Effect of epidural and subarachnoid injections of a 10% butamphen suspension, *Reg. Anesth.*, 15(3):142–6 (1990).

182. A. Al-Achi and M. Bojoujerdi, Pharmacokinetics and tissue uptake of doxorubicin associated with erythrocyte-membrane: Erythrocyte-ghosts vs erythrocyte-vesicles, *Drug Dev. Ind. Pharm.*, 16:2199–2219 (1990).

183. E. Dimitrova and A. Dimitrova, Recent approaches to the development of injection dosage forms with antibiotics. III. Stabilization of prolonged release suspensions containing penicillin G salts, (in Bulgarian) *Farmatsiya* (Sofia) 37(6):36–40 (1987).

184. M. A. Hussain, B. J. Aungst, M. B. Maurin, and L. S. Wu, Injectable suspensions for prolonged release nalbuphine, *Drug Dev. Ind. Pharm.* 17(1):67–76 (1991).

185. K. Uekama, H. Arima, T. Irie, K. Matsubara, and T. Kuriki, Sustained release of buserelin acetate, a leutinizining hormone-releasing hormone agonist, from an injectable oily preparation utilizing ethylated β-Cyclodextrin, *J. Pharm. Pharmacol.*, 41:874–876 (1989).

186. F. H. Buckwater and H. L. Dickison, The effect of vehicle and particle size on the absorption, by the intramuscular route, of procaine penicillin G suspensions, *J. Am. Pharm. Assoc., Sci. Ed.*, 47:661 (1958).

187. L. Lachman, R. H. Reiner, E. Shami, and W. Spector, Long-Acting Narcotic Antagonist Formulations, U.S. Patent 3,676,557 (1972).

188. A. P. Gray and D. S. Robinson, Insoluble salts and complexes of cyclazocine and naloxone. In: *Narcotic Antagonists* (M. C. Braude, L. S. Harris, E. L. May, J. P. Smith, and J. E. Villareal, eds.) Raven Press, New York, 1974, p. 555.

189. Z. Yim, I. A. Chaudry, and M. A. Zupon, Sustained release parenteral pharmaceuticals containing α-interferon-protamine-Zn complexes (Schering Corp., USA) Eur. Pat. Appl. EP 281299 A1 880907, 5 pp. (1988).

190. J. P. Kitchen, I. A. Muni, and Y. N. Boyu, A controlled sustained release delivery system for targeting drug dependency (Dynagen, Inc., USA), PCT Int. Appl. WO 9219226 A1 921112, 67 pp. (1992).

191. J. D. Gresser, D. L. Wise, L. R. Beck, and J. F. Howes, Larger animal testing of an injectable sustained release fertility control system, *Contraception*, 17:253 (1978).

192. J. L. Deyoung and E. L. Lien, A long-acting injectable dosage form for a somatastatin analog, *J. Parent. Sci. Technol.*, 38(6):234–236 (1984).

193. S. Hotta, Studies on the endoscopic injection therapy using gelatin suspension for gastrointestinal hemorrhage (in Japanese) *Aichi Ika Daigaku Igakkai Zasshi*, 21(1):15–33 (1993).

194. I. Orly and A. Huc, Injectable composition containing collagen microcapsules, PCT. Int. Appl. WO 9313755 A1 930722, 26 pp. (1993).

195. G. S. Brumar and D. Ostonic, Use of bisphosphonic acid calcium salts for the treatment of calcium metabolism disorders (Merck & Co. Inc., USA), Eur. Pat. Appl. EP 449405 A2 911002, 11 pp. (1991).

8

Aerosol Suspensions and Emulsions

John J. Sciarra

Sciarra Laboratories, Inc., Hicksville, New York

I. CHARACTERISTICS OF DISPERSED AEROSOL SYSTEMS

The aerosol dosage form for oral and topical use was developed in the mid-1950s and ever since that time has found widespread acceptance because of its ease of use and therapeutic efficacy.

Pharmaceutical aerosols are dosage forms containing therapeutically active ingredients intended for topical administration, introduction into body cavities, or by inhalation via the respiratory tract. The dosage form is packaged in a metal or glass container and sealed with either a metered- or continuous-spray valve. The aerosol product itself consists of two components: (a) concentrate (containing the active ingredient(s) and (b) propellant(s). The propellant provides the internal pressure that forces the product out of the container when the valve is opened and delivers the product in its desired form. For metered-dose inhalers (MDIs) the product is delivered as a finely dispersed mist (particles less than 8 μm in diameter) and, for topicals, as a spray, foam, or semisolid.

A. Introduction

1. *Metered-Dose Inhalers*

Metered-dose inhalers have been used to deliver various active ingredients to the respiratory system and, to date, have included those drugs used in the treatment of asthma and other conditions. These compounds include steroids, β_2-agonists, and other similar compounds. These compounds include epinephrine hydrochloride or bitartrate, ergotamine tartrate, albuterol, metaproterenol sulfate, beclomethasone dipropionate, flunisolide hemihydrate, cromolyn sodium, nedocromil sodium, ipatropium bromide, salmeterol xinafoate, triamcinolone acetonide, pirbuterol acetate, bitolterol mesylate, dexamethasone sodium phosphate, terbutaline sulfate, nitroglycerin, and budesonide and are illustrative of some of the medicinal agents available as a metered-dose oral inhaler or nasal inhaler.

Most of the oral inhalers are intended to treat asthma symptomatically; the nasal inhalers are intended for management of symptoms of allergic rhinitis.

The aerosol dosage form enjoys a widespread acceptance for the administration of therapeutically active agents by oral or nasal inhalation. These products offer many advantages to patients. These advantages include packaging in a small, compact container that is convenient to use and easy to administer. A rapid therapeutic action is attained, and the availability of these preparations for use by asthmatics has allowed these patients to carry out normal daily activities. The medication is available for immediate use, thereby quickly alleviating the asthmatic attack when it occurs. Other medication is effective in preventing asthmatic attack and is used prophylactically.

Other advantages of metered-dose inhalers (MDIs) include (a) circumvention of the first pass effect, (b) avoidance of degradation in the G.I. tract, (c) lower dosage (which will minimize adverse reactions), (d) dose titration to meet individual needs of the patient, (e) presentation of an alternate route of administration when the therapeutic agent may chemically or physically interact with other medicinals needed concurrently, and (f) alleviation of interactions with meal content or timing. It is a viable alternative when the drug entity exhibits erratic pharmacokinetic properties upon oral or parenteral administration.

Drugs that are likely candidates for aerosol administration must be: (a) nonirritating to the respiratory and/or nasal airways, (b) reasonably soluble in respiratory fluids (drugs having poor solubility characteristics are more likely to be irritating), (c) effective in a relatively low dosage, and (d) exhibit passive transport (absorption) through respiratory and or nasal membranes.

Medicinal products having a high potential for use as metered-dose oral and/or nasal inhalations would include antianginal preparations; antiasthmatic preparations; steroids sympathomimetics; anticholinergics; antibiotics; antivirals; and immunizing agents. These represent only a few of the drug categories that have shown success when formulated as a metered-dose inhaler.

2. *Topical Aerosol Pharmaceuticals*

Topical pharmaceutical aerosols have been accepted by both patient and physician because of their esthetic properties, ease of application, maintainability of sterility (where the package is sterile), tamperproof system, prevention of contamination of the unused contents, and increased stability. Topical aerosols have been dispensed as sprays, foams, and semisolids. When applied to the body they reduce pain that may result from the mechanical rubbing of ointments and creams onto the skin. Through use of a metered-dose valve, an accurate amount of medication can be dispensed each time the valve is actuated. Topical products that have been formulated as an aerosol include first-aid products containing local anesthetics and antiseptics; adhesive tape removers and bandage adherants; athletic and sports applications; burn remedies; foot preparations; germicidal and disinfectant products; spray-on bandages, protectives; topical dermatologics, including antibiotics and steroids; veterinary applications; body liniments and rubs; vaginal applications, including contraceptive foams; rectal foams; edible foams; and saline solutions to cleanse contact lenses.

3. *Intranasal Delivery; Aerosols and Pumps*

This section is organized with the objective of providing basic information and, where applicable, technical background in the fundamentals of intranasal drug delivery and in the development of nasal drug delivery systems for the administration of local and systemic therapeutic agents (e.g., vasoconstrictors, hormones, polypeptides, etc.) [1].

Over the last three to four decades many categories of drugs were considered for intranasal use, but only when all other routes of administration failed. Today this method is being considered as a primary route of drug administration in the light of some major advances in evaluating a drug's pharmacokinetics via this route of administration as well as inordinate interest of researchers and marketers in this promising drug delivery system. Other factors contributing to both the interest and recent successes in intranasal delivery include improved technology in the area of metered pumps and aerosolized devices and recent advances and discoveries in drug adjuvants, carriers, and promoters.

Recently, several drugs have been administered intranasally in a gel form. Development programs are under way involving the dispensing of several protein products (including insulin) in the form of a nasal spray. Because these materials are generally dissolved in water, they are dispensed as a fine spray using a pump system rather than a true aerosol system. Newer technology in this area includes the use of barrier systems (bag-in-can) together with a metered valve to dispense nasal solutions [2].

Drugs that are most likely candidates for delivery via the nasal passages must be nonirritating to the respiratory airways and/or nasal mucosa and must be reasonably soluble in respiratory and nasal fluids. Because the medication must be accurately delivered in small doses, only those drugs that are therapeutically active in low dosages are likely candidates. Additionally, the compounds must exhibit passive transport (absorption) through respiratory membranes (carrier and active transport are possible, but this area is relatively unexplored at the present time). They must have minimal local or topical activity on nasal mucosa and should be stable and compatible in intranasal vehicles having a pH between 5.5 and 7.5.

It is also possible to develop a nasal aerosol that is similar to a metered-dose inhaler. In this case the drug must be soluble or dispersed in the vehicle and propellant. Several products are currently available in this form.

a. *Advantages and Disadvantages of Intranasal Delivery.* Without dealing with any specifics related to the physiochemical characteristics of the therapeutic agent, some of the major advantages cited for intranasal delivery include: (a) rapid onset of action, (b) circumvention of the first-pass effect, (c) avoidance of degradation in G.I. tract, (d) lower dosage (minimizes adverse reactions), (e) convenience, (f) simplicity of dosage delivery system, (e) dose titration to individual needs, and (f) alternative route when therapeutic agent may chemically or physically interact with other medicinals needed concurrently.

Those drugs not possessing the above-named characteristics may be successfully administered intranasally if the proper adjuvants (surface-active agents, bile salts, etc.) are administered concurrently. Use of local vasoconstrictors has also been employed to modify the absorption characteristics of drugs administered intranasally. Micronization may also be appropriate for intranasal delivery for poorly soluble drugs so as to increase their rate of dissolution when necessary.

4. *Oral Sprays*

Oral sprays are designed so that they can be sprayed either into the mouth or under the tongue. When sprayed under the tongue they are termed sublingual sprays. One such product, Nitro-Lingual, (Rhône-Poulenc Rorer), is currently available. A variety of oral sprays are marketed as mouth fresheners. Both types of these products are formulated in essentially the same manner. In order for drugs to be used in this type of system they must be soluble in both the vehicle and the propellant as well as therapeutically active in a low dosage. They must be capable of undergoing transmucosal adsorption. Nitroglycerin is a perfect drug for this system because it is active in low dosage, is quickly absorbed when administered under the tongue, and is quick acting. The aerosol system diminishes, if not eliminates, the loss of the drug through volatilization from nonaerosol containers.

B. Physicochemical Aspects of Aerosol Systems [3]

An aerosol system consists of a product concentrate, propellant, container, and suitable valve. The concentrate can be of the solution, dispersion, emulsion, or semisolid type; the propellant can be either a liquefied or a compressed gas. Depending on the nature of the propellant and product concentrate (as well as the combination of these two components with the appropriate valve and actuator), the product can be dispensed as a spray, foam, or semisolid. There are various ways in which the aerosol components can be brought together to form a finished aerosol product. The product concentrate can be dissolved or mixed with the propellant so that a true solution is formed. A cosolvent may be added in cases in which the propellant and concentrate are immiscible, although this is not always possible. The concentrate can also contain insoluble solids that can be dispersed throughout the propellant. If the propellant and concentrate phases are immiscible, it may also be possible to bring them together by means of an emulsifying agent or surfactant, resulting in the formation of an emulsion. This emulsion can be dispensed as a foam or as a spray, depending on the nature of each phase and the design of the valve and actuator. Additional systems that serve to simply push the contents out of the container or else to separate the propellant from the concentrate are also available (bag-in-can).

1. *Solution Systems*

This type of aerosol system consists of two distinct phases: liquid and vapor. The system may be defined as a "solution of active ingredients in pure propellant or a mixture of propellant and solvent." The solvent is used to dissolve the active ingredient and/or to retard the evaporation of the propellant. Solution aerosols are relatively easy to formulate, provided that the ingredients are soluble in the propellant. However, the liquefied gas propellants are nonpolar in nature and in most cases are poor solvents for some of the commonly used medicinal ingredients. Through use of a solvent that is miscible with the propellant, one can achieve varying degrees of solubility. Ethyl alcohol has found widespread use for this purpose. Other solvents finding use in pharmaceuticals can be used with topical aerosols.

When the valve of a solution aerosol is depressed, a mixture of active ingredients, solvents, and propellants is emitted into the atmosphere. As the liquid propellant encounters the warm surrounding air, it tends to vaporize and, in so doing, breaks up the active ingredients and solvents into fine particles. Depending on their size, the particles remain suspended in air for relatively long periods of time. The particles of spray can vary from as small as 5 to 10 μm or less to as large as 50 to 100 μm.

As the solution-type aerosol is dispensed, the product is forced up the dip tube, through the valve and actuator, and into the atmosphere. The propellant is trapped within the liquid concentrate, which has been partially dispersed in passing through the valve and actuator. The propellant starts to vaporize and, in doing so, reduces the size of the liquid droplets. The size of these droplets will depend on the nature of the propellant, the amount of propellant, the nature of the product concentrate, and the valve design. Metered-dose inhalers require particles of less than 8 μm whereas nasal aqueous aerosols generally have particles in the range of 50 to 75 μm. Topical sprays have a particle size of about 100 μm.

2. *Suspension Systems*

For substances that are insoluble in the propellant or the mixture of propellant and solvent, or in cases where a cosolvent is not desirable, the active ingredients can be suspended in the propellant vehicle. When the valve is depressed, the suspension is emitted, followed by rapid vaporization of the propellant, leaving behind the finely dispersed active ingredients. This system has been used successfully to dispense antiasthmatic aerosols as well as topical aerosols containing antibiotics. However, the formulation of this type of aerosol is not without difficulty. Problems involving caking, agglomeration, particle size growth, and clogging of the valve arise. Some of the more important factors that must be considered in formulating this type of system include:

Moisture content of ingredients
Particle size of the solid therapeutic agent
Solubility of active ingredients
Density of both propellant and active ingredients
Use of surfactant or dispensing agent

Both active ingredients and propellant when used with this type of system must be anhydrous. Particle size growth will occur that will have an adverse effect on the particle size distribution of the MDI as well as the dose uniformity. It is generally agreed that the total moisture content of the system should be below 300 ppm for topicals and below 100 ppm for metered-dose inhalers. The propellants can be dried by passing them through desiccants, and the other ingredients can be dried by the usual methods.

The initial particle size of the insoluble ingredients should be in the micron range, generally from 1 to 5 μm. A jet pulverizer or ball mill can be used to reduce the particle size.

The chemical salt of the active ingredient having minimum solubility in the propellant and solvents should be selected. It is the slight solubility of the active ingredients in the propellants and solvents that contributes to particle size growth. This phenomenon, known as Ostwald Ripening, will occur because the small particles have higher equilibrium solubilities than larger particles of the same substance. These small particles will gradually dissolve and deposit onto the surface of the larger particles, resulting in an increase in particle size of the originally micronized active drug substance.

By adjusting the density of the propellant and/or the insoluble material so that they are approximately equal, the rate of sedimentation can be reduced substantially. This can be accomplished by using a mixture of different propellants of varying densities as well as by addition of an inert powder to the active ingredients.

Final consideration should be given to the use of a surfactant or dispersing agent. Sorbitan oleate, lecithin, oleic acid, and oleyl alcohol have been used with oral and metered-dose inhalers; isopropyl myristate has been used primarily with topicals.

Although it may be easier to formulate a solution system compared to a suspension system, the latter is generally preferred because one can obtain closer control over the particle size distribution of droplets dispersed from the suspension aerosol. Suspensions generally show greater stability of the active ingredient as compared with solutions.

3. *Emulsion Systems [4]*

Water and hydrocarbon or fluorinated hydrocarbon propellants are not miscible. In order to formulate a suitable aerosol using these materials, various techniques can be used. An emulsion aerosol consists of active ingredients, an aqueous or nonaqueous vehicle, a surfactant, and a propellant. Depending on the choice of ingredients, the product can be emitted as a stable or quick-breaking foam or as a spray.

a. *Foam System.*   The propellant used in an emulsion is an important part of this system and determines the type of foam produced. The propellant is generally considered part of the immiscible phase and as such can be in the internal or external phase. When the propellant is included in the internal phase, a typical stable or quick-breaking foam is emitted. When the propellant is in the external phase, the product is dispensed as a spray. Figure 1 illustrates these two types of emulsions.

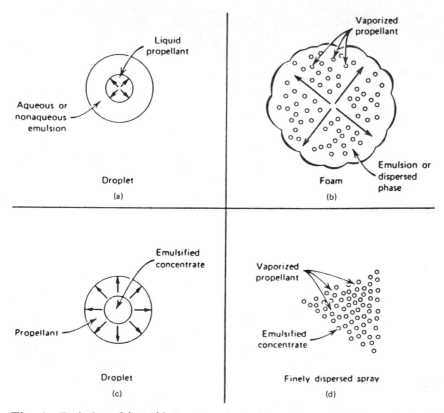

Fig. 1 Typical emulsion with propellant in the internal or external phase. (a) Propellant in internal phase, (b) formation of aerosol foam, (c) propellant in the external phase, and (d) formation of a wet spray. (From Ref. 3.)

As can be seen in Fig. 1a, when the propellant is in the internal phase the propellant vapor must pass through the emulsion formulation in order to escape into the atmosphere. In traveling through the emulsion, the trapped vaporized propellant forms a matrix for a foam to develop, as seen in Fig. 1b. Depending on the nature of the formulation and the propellant, the foam can be stable or quick-breaking.

Figure 1c illustrates a typical emulsion system in which the propellant is in the external or continuous phase. As the liquefied propellant vaporizes, it escapes directly into the atmosphere, leaving behind droplets of the formulation, which are emitted as a wet spray (Fig. 1d). This system is typical of many water-based aerosols.

b. *Stabilized Foams.* In an emulsion system where the propellant is in the internal phase (generally part of the oil phase of the emulsion), water makes up the external or dispersed phase, although nonaqueous solvents can also be used. The propellant is generally used to the extent of about 7% to 10% of the total weight. When a hydrocarbon propellant is used (such as isobutane/propane blends), as little as 3% to 4% is sufficient to produce a suitable foam. This propellant is emulsified with the aqueous or nonaqueous emulsion; however, some of the propellant will vaporize and be present in the head space to produce the necessary vapor pressure. The pressure will be approximately 40 psig, depending on the propellant that is used. When the valve is depressed, the pressure forces the emulsion up the dip tube and out the valve. A stable foam will result such as one used for shaving foams.

Typical of these topical foams will be certain steroid-containing foams and the edible foams. They are expected to maintain their rigid structure; in the case of a topical foam, until rubbed into the skin. Edible foams would be expected to remain rigid while on the measuring spoon or until taken orally.

c. *Quick-Breaking Foams.* These foams consist of ethyl alcohol, water, and a surfactant that is soluble in either alcohol or water but not in both. Other miscible solvents can be used in place of alcohol and water. The surfactant can be nonionic, anionic, or cationic. The product is dispensed as a foam but quickly collapses upon coming into contact with the skin. This is particularly advantageous in pharmaceutical aerosols for topical application, because the foam will reach the affected area and then collapse, so that there is no further injury by mechanical dispersion of the product. Steroid, burn, and other topical preparations can be applied in this manner.

One advantage of a foam system over a spray system is the fact that the area with which the product can come into contact is limited. Preparations containing irritating ingredients may also be dispensed in this manner. The incidence of airborne particles can be substantially reduced, thereby lowering the toxicity of spray products that cause irritation on release and may be inhaled.

d. *Spray Emulsions.* The base for this type of product is a water-in-oil emulsion. A fairly large amount of propellant (about 25% to 30%) is miscible with the outer oil phase so that the propellant remains in the external phase of the final emulsion. When this system is dispensed, the propellant vaporizes, leaving behind droplets of water-in-oil emulsion with no foaming, as shown in Figs. 1c and 1d. Because the propellant and concentrate phase tend to separate on standing, products formulated using this system must be shaken before use. A hydrocarbon propellant or a mixed hydrocarbon/fluorocarbon propellant is preferred for this system, because the specific gravity of the propellant is less than 1 and the propellant will float on the aqueous layer. In addition, such systems use a vapor tap valve, which tends to produce finely dispersed particles.

II. COMMONLY USED RAW MATERIALS

Aerosol products consist of a concentrate and propellant(s). The concentrate is made up of active ingredients, solvents, dispersing agents and, depending on the type of product, various inert ingredients used to prepare solutions, suspensions, and emulsions. These ingredients are no different from the ones used in nonaerosol products and will not be discussed in this chapter. Only those ingredients specifically required for the aerosol dosage form will be included.

A. Propellants [5,6]

The propellant is responsible for developing the proper pressure within the container and for expulsion of the product when the valve is opened. It also is responsible (together with the valve) for dispensing the product as a spray, foam, or semisolid. Various types of propellants are utilized. The fluorinated hydrocarbons such as trichloromonofluoromethane (Propellant 11), dichlorodifluoromethane (Propellant 12), and dichlorotetrafluoroethane (Propellant 114) find widespread use in most aerosols for oral, nasal, and inhalation use; topical pharmaceutical aerosols utilize hydrocarbons (propane, butane, and isobutane), a limited number of hydrofluorocarbons and hydrochlorofluorocarbons (142b, 152a, 22), and compressed gases such as nitrogen and carbon dioxide.

1. Chlorofluorocarbons (CFCs)

The use of chlorinated fluorocarbons for aerosols and other commercial uses has been seriously curtailed and, in certain cases, banned. These compounds have been implicated in causing a depletion of the ozone layer and partial showing responsibility for the "greenhouse" effect (increase in earth's temperature, rising sea levels, and altered rainfall patterns). Depletion of the ozone layer is alleged to have resulted in an increase in the incidence of skin cancer. This is due to a greater penetration of the ozone layer by the skin-cancer-causing ultraviolet radiation from the sun (ozone will prevent these rays from penetrating the earth's atmosphere). In 1974, the Environmental Protection Agency (EPA), the Consumer Protection Service Commission (CPSC), and the Food and Drug Administration (FDA) promulgated a "ban" on the use of chlorofluorocarbons, namely Propellants 11, 12, and 114, in most aerosols. Certain pharmaceutical aerosols for inhalation use were exempted from this ban. According to the Montreal Agreement reached in 1988, beginning in 1989, the production of these propellants was restricted worldwide. It is expected that by 1995, the production of CFCs will be reduced to only the amount needed for certain exempted uses, *including metered-dose inhalers*. At present, there is *no* reason to believe that the exemption for MDIs will be rescinded. It is estimated that less than 0.4% of the world's production of CFCs is used for MDIs. What will happen remains to be seen; however, alternatives to Propellants 11, 12, and 114 are now under development and study. At the present time Propellants 11, 12, and 114 are being used with metered-dose inhalers and it is highly unlikely that alternatives will be approved for this purpose much before the end of the first decade of the 21st century. In the meantime, metered-dose inhalers should still be formulated with chlorofluorocarbons (as there are no suitable alternatives available at the present time), but studies must be initiated using some of the currently available potential alternatives [7]. Topical pharmaceuticals can be reformulated or, in the case of new products, formulated with the currently available alternative propellants. These will be covered in detail.

The most commonly used propellants for metered-dose inhalers are trichloromono-fluoromethane (Propellant 11), dichlorodifluoromethane (Propellant 12), and dichloro-tetrafluoroethane (Propellant 114).

```
        Cl                      Cl                     F   F
        |                       |                      |   |
   Cl—C—F                  Cl—C—F               F—C—C—F
        |                       |                      |   |
        Cl                      F                      Cl  Cl

   Propellant  11          Propellant  12          Propellant  114
```

Propellant 11 has a vapor pressure of 13.4 psia at 21.1° and a boiling point of 23.7°. Therefore, it is not suitable for use as a propellant alone. It is normally combined with Propellant 12. Propellant 11 is stable in nonaqueous aerosols and is a good solvent for many drugs. It has a tendency to hydrolyze in the presence of water.

Propellant 12 is a very stable compound and is blended with Propellants 11 and 114 to achieve the proper pressure. Because it has a vapor pressure of 84.9 psia at 21.1° and a boiling point of −29.8°, it can be used without any other propellant.

Propellant 114 is a poor solvent for medicinal agents and is extremely stable. It has a vapor pressure of 27.6 psia at 21.1° and a boiling point of 3.6°. It is commonly blended with Propellant 12 to obtain higher vapor pressures of the aerosol product. It is also used in combination with Propellant 12 in order to achieve a proper balance among solubility of drugs or miscibility of cosolvent containing the drug, particle size, and pressure.

Listed in Table 1 are the commonly used propellants for metered-dose inhalants; several of their physicochemical properties are included. Propellant 12 or a blend of fluorocarbon propellants is generally used for pharmaceutical aerosols as indicated in Table 2. By varying the proportion of each component, any desired vapor pressure can be achieved within the limits of the vapor pressure of the individual propellants. In many instances, Propellant 11 is used as the vehicle for the drug, cosolvents, and other ingredients, and either Propellant 12 or a blend of Propellants 12 and 114 is added to bring the final product to the desired vapor pressure. As can be seen in Table 2, the vapor pressure can vary from about 37 psig to about 70 psig (vapor pressure of pure Propellant 12) depending on the actual composition of the final product. The addition of ethyl alcohol or other similar solvents will also lower the vapor pressure according to "Raoult's Law of Partial Pressures." The mixture will actually show a positive deviation from Raoult's Law because the attraction of propellant molecules for molecules of ethyl alcohol is less than the attraction between molecules of propellant or molecules of alcohol. This results in an increase in escaping tendency and, consequently, an increase in vapor pressure, as compared to the results expected from Raoult's Law. This can be seen in Fig. 2.

2. Hydrofluorocarbons (HFCs)

According to the Clean Air Act of 1990, as well as regulations of the FDA and the EPA, the use of CFCs in nonessential, nonexempted products will be prohibited by the year 2000. This date has subsequently been changed to 1995. The exempted products include metered-dose inhalers. While additional exemptions will be rare, it is possible to seek additional exemptions for medicinal products that are essential and cannot be made

Table 1 Properties of Chlorofluorocarbon Propellants[a] (for use with metered-dose inhalers—MDIs)

Propellant no.	Chemical name	Molecular weight	Boiling point °F (°C)	Vapor pressure (psig)		Liquid density g/mL/70°F (21.1°C)	Water solubility % w/w 70°F (21.1°C)	Flash point[b] (°F)
				70°F (21.1°C)	131°F (54.4°C)			
11	Trichloromonofluoromethane	137.4	74.8 (23.7)	-1.3	39.0	1.485	0.009	0
12	Dichlorodifluoromethane	120.9	-21.6 (-29.8)	70.3	196.0	1.325	0.008	0
114	Dichlorotetrafluoroethane	170.9	38.8 (3.6)	12.9	63.5	1.468	0.007	0

[a]Available as Dymel (E. I. du Pont de Nemours and Company, Inc.) and Genetron (Allied Signal Corporation) in the United States.
[b]These chlorofluorocarbon propellants are all nonflammable and will extinguish a flame.

Table 2 Blends of Chlorofluorocarbon Propellants for Metered-Dose Inhalers (MDIs)

Propellant blend[a]	Composition	Vapor pressure (psig) 70°F	Density (g/mL) 70°F
12/11	50:50	37.4	1.412
12/11	60:40	44.1	1.396
12/114	70:30	56.1	1.368
12/114	40:60	39.8	1.412
12/114	45:55	42.8	1.405
12/114	55:45	48.4	1.390
12/114/11	50:25:25	42.2	1.400

[a]It is generally understood that the designation "propellant 12/114 (70:30)" indicates a composition of 70% by weight of propellant 12 and 30% by weight of propellant 114.

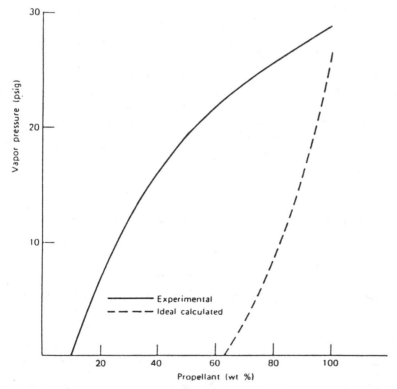

Fig. 2 Vapor pressure versus composition at 21°C for mixture Genetron 12/114 (20:80) and ethyl alcohol. (From L. Flanner, Vapor pressure of solvents and propellant mixture, Allied-Signal Corporation, Morristown, New Jersey.)

without a CFC. The manufacturer must show that the product is essential and that other propellants are not suitable, and must file a New Drug Application (NDA).

Two propellants have potential application for use with MDIs. They include trifluoromonofluoroethane (P-134a) and heptafluoropropane (R-227). Selected physicochemical properties of these substances are shown in Table 3. These compounds differ from CFCs in that they do not contain chlorine and have one or more hydrogens. They will break down in the atmosphere at a faster rate than the CFCs, resulting in a lower ozone-destroying effect. At present, these two potential replacements for Propellant 12 are undergoing safety and toxicological testing but still are a long way from receiving approval for use with MDIs. They also leave a tremendous void in that there is no alternative to Propellant 11. Propellant 11 has been used to make a slurry with the medicinal agent and then added to Propellant 12. Use of R-227 and P-134a would necessitate a change in manufacturing techniques as well as changes in formulation. Currently used dispersing agents may not be suitable because of their limited solubility in both of these propellants. However, because they do have a vapor pressure of about 70 psig (P-134a) and 43 psig (R-227), they can be used individually or combined to achieve a suitable vapor pressure.

3. *Other Liquefied Gas Propellants*

Topical pharmaceutical products must be formulated using a propellant other than the chlorofluorocarbons. For this purpose, a series of hydrochlorofluorocarbons and hydrofluorocarbons are available. These propellants do not present a hazard to the environment and can be used successfully to formulate topical pharmaceuticals. Table 4 illustrates these propellants along with some of their more useful physicochemical properties. As can be seen from Table 4, these propellants have suitable vapor pressures making them useful for a variety of different products. Propellants 152a and 142b may be blended to yield a vapor pressure within the useful range of from 35 to 50 psig. They may also be blended with Propellant 22 to give the desired nonflammability to the final mixture as well as to obtain a higher vapor pressure. The vapor pressure of various propellant blends is shown in Fig. 3.

A kauri-butanol value is used to estimate the relative solvent power of a liquid. The kauri-butanol value of a solvent is the number of milliliters required to produce a specific degree of turbidity when the solvent is added to 20 grams of a standard solution of kauri resin in *n*-butyl alcohol at 25°C. These values are useful only for relatively nonpolar solvents such as the hydrocarbon and fluorocarbon propellants. Table 4 and

Table 3 Selected Properties of Possible Alternative Propellants

Property	Trifluoromono- fluoroethane	Heptafluoro- propane
Molecular formula	CF_3CH_2F	CF_3CHFCF_3
Numerical designation	134a	R-227
Molecular weight	102	170
Boiling point (1 atm), °F (°C)	−15.7 (−26.5)	2.55 (−16.3)
Vapor pressure (psig), 70°F	70.0	44.1
Vapor pressure (psig), 130°F	198.7	135.1
Liquid density (g/ml) 20°C	1.21	1.41

Table 4 Propellants Useful for Topical Pharmaceutical Aerosols

Designation	Propellant 22	Propellant 142b	Propellant 152a
Formula	$CHClF_2$	CH_3CClF_2	CH_3CHF_2
Molecular weight	86.5	100.5	66.1
Boiling point, °F (°C)	−41.4 (−40.8)	14.4 (−9.44)	−11.2 (−23.0)
Vapor pressure (psig), 70°F	121	29	62
Vapor pressure (psig), 130°F	297	97	176
Density (g/mL), 70°F	1.21	1.12	0.91
Solubility in water (wt. %), 70°F	3.0	0.5	1.7
Kauri-butanol value	25	20	11
Flammability limits in air (vol. %)	Nonflammable	6.3–14.8	3.9–16.9
Flash point, °F	—	—	—

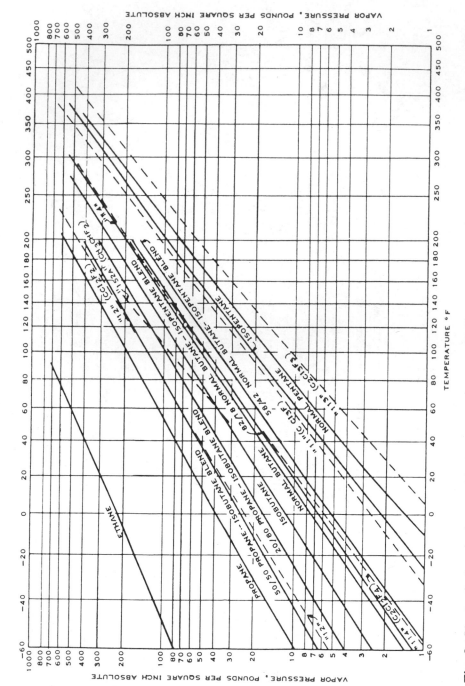

Fig. 3 Blends of selected mixtures of hydrocarbons, chlorofluorocarbons, and other propellants. (Courtesy of Phillips Petroleum Company, Bartlesville, Oklahoma.)

Table 5 Selected Properties of Hydrocarbons and Dimethyl Ether

	Propane	Isobutane	n-Butane	DME
Formula	C_3H_8	$i\text{-}C_4H_{10}$	$n\text{-}C_4H_{10}$	CH_3OCH_3
Molecular weight	44.1	58.1	58.1	46.07
Boiling point, °F (°C)	-43.7 (-42.0)	10.9 (-11.7)	31.1 (-0.56)	-12.7
Vapor pressure (psig), 70°F	109	31	17	63
Vapor pressure (psig), 130°F	257	97	67	174
Density (g/mL), 70°F	0.50	0.56	0.58	0.66
Solubility in water (wt. %), 70°F	0.01	0.01	0.01	34
Kauri-butanol value	15	17	20	60
Flammability limits in air (vol. %)	2.2-9.5	1.8-8.4	1.8-8.5	3.4-18
Flash point, °F	-156	-117	-101	-42

5 illustrate these values. Generally the higher the value, the greater the miscibility with nonpolar solvents.

4. Hydrocarbons

The hydrocarbon propellants butane, propane, and isobutane have replaced the chlorofluorocarbons as the propellant for most consumer aerosol products (other than MDIs). They have also been used for topical pharmaceuticals. They are ideal for use with foams because they are nontoxic, nonreactive, and relatively inexpensive; yield a satisfactory foam; and are environmentally acceptable. The chief drawback to their use is their flammability. However, this is of greater concern to the manufacturer than to the consumer. As can be seen in Table 5 they all have a density of about 0.5 to 0.6 g/mL and therefore less is required as compared to a fluorocarbon (generally 1.2 to 1.4 g/mL). They can also be blended with each other and with hydrochlorofluorocarbons and hydrochlorocarbons so as to obtain different vapor pressures, as seen in Fig. 3. These propellants are available preblended to vapor pressures of 17 to 108 psig. Figure 4 illustrates these compositions. Blends of Propellant 22 with hydrocarbons will produce mixtures having different flammability characteristics.

Recently dimethyl, ether has been used to formulate aerosols. As can be seen in Table 5, its main advantage over all other materials used in aerosol formulations is its rather high miscibility with water (about 34%). This allows the formulator greater flexibility in developing different types of aerosol systems. Table 6 includes the companies from which aerosol propellants are available.

5. Compressed Gases

With the introduction of saline solutions for cleaning contact lenses, the use of nitrogen as an aerosol propellant has increased [8]. The compressed gases nitrogen, nitrous oxide, and carbon dioxide are limited in use, but they are used in those cases where a large quantity of water is present and the product must be dispensed as a spray. Such is the case with contact lens cleaners. Nitrogen is used because its inertness and its lack of solubility and miscibility with water. It is used to push the contents out of the container and to dispense a fine stream of solution that can be directed to the contact lens. Nitrous oxide and carbon dioxide are used with products where solubility of the gas in the product is desirable. Their main use at the present time is with foams. Table 7 indicates some of the other properties of these gases. Unlike liquefied gases, there is a drop in pressure as the contents of a product with a compressed gas are dispensed. The formulator must ensure that there is sufficient gas remaining in the product as the container is emptied. Figure 5 illustrates this behavior.

B. Metered- and Continuous-Spray Valves

A valve is an important component of all aerosols and is responsible together with the propellant for the delivery of the product in the desired form whether it be as a spray, foam, semisolid, or as a fine mist having particles below 8 μm. suitable for inhalation.

1. Metered Valves

Metered valves, fitted with a 20 mm ferrule, are used with glass bottles and aluminum canisters for all metered-dose inhalers (MDIs). These same valves are also used for intranasal inhalers. The metered valve should accurately deliver a measured amount of

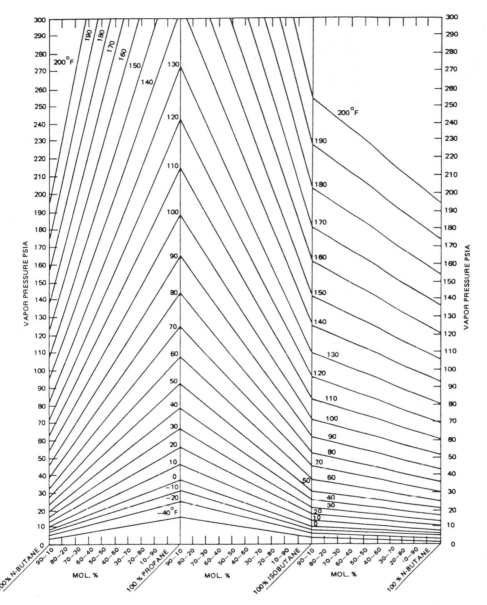

Fig. 4 Vapor pressure of hydrocarbon blends. (Courtesy of Phillips Petroleum Company, Bartlesville, Oklahoma.)

product and the amount should be reproducible, not only for the dose delivered from the same container but from different containers as well.

Two basic types of metered valves are available, one for inverted use and the other for upright use. Generally, valves for upright use contain a thin capillary tube and are used with solution type aerosols. On the other hand, suspension or dispersion aerosols utilize a valve for inverted use that does not contain a dip tube. However, either type of valve can be used with each of these products. Figure 6 illustrates a typical valve for inverted use; Fig. 7 illustrates a valve designed for upright use.

Table 6 Trademark Names for Propellants

Fluorocarbon propellants		Hydrocarbon propellants	
Trademark	Company	Trademark	Company
Dymel	E. I. duPont de Nemours & Co. Wilmington, Delaware	Phillips	Phillips Petroleum Co. Petrochemical Division Bartlesville, Oklahoma
Genetron	Allied-Signal Corp. Morristown, New Jersey	Aeron ("Aeropin")	Diversified Chemicals and Propellants Co. Westmont, Illinois
		Aeropres ("Aeropin")	Aeropres Corp. Shreveport, Louisiana
		TPI	Technical Petroleum Co. Chicago, Illinois

Table 7 Properties of the Compressed Gases

	Carbon dioxide	Nitrous oxide	Nitrogen
Formula	CO_2	N_2O	N_2
Molecular weight	44.0	44.0	28.0
Solubility in water (% w/w, 70°F, 100 psig)	1.5	0.7	—
Solubility in isobutane	5.3	7.3	—
Solubility in ethyl alcohol	5.6	5.7	—
Solubility in Propellant 11	3.5	4.9	—

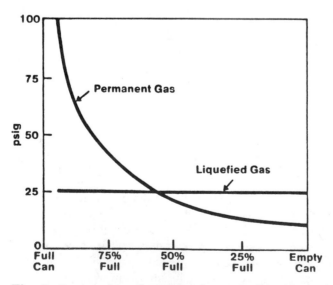

Fig. 5 Pressure drop of compressed gas propellant (nitrogen) as product is dispensed. (Courtesy E. I. duPont de Nemours and Co.)

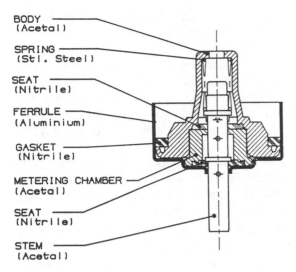

Fig. 6 Metered valve for inverted use. (Courtesy of Bespak, Inc., Cary, North Carolina.)

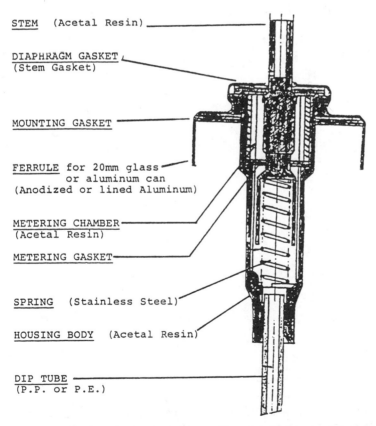

Fig. 7 Metered valve for upright use. (Courtesy of Valvois of America, Greenwich, Connecticut.)

An integral part of these valves is the metering chamber, which is directly responsible for the delivery of the desired amount of therapeutic agent. The degree of metering can be varied so that from about 25 to 150 microliters (μL) of product can be delivered per actuation. Most of the products now commercially available utilize dosages
in the range of 35 to 75 μL. The chamber is sealed via the metering gasket and the stem
gasket. In the actuated position, the stem gasket will allow the contents of the metering chamber to be dispensed while the metering gasket will seal off any additional product from entering the chamber. In this way the chamber is always filled (primed) and
ready to delivery the desired amount of therapeutic agent [9].

These valves should retain their prime over fairly long periods of time. However,
it is possible for some of the material in the chamber to slowly return to the main body
of the product in the event the container is stored upright (for those used in the upright
position). The degree to which this can occur varies with the nature of the product, the
construction of the valve, and the length of time between actuations of the valve. Loss
of prime can be reduced, as seen in Figs. 8a and 8b, through use of a drain tank. The

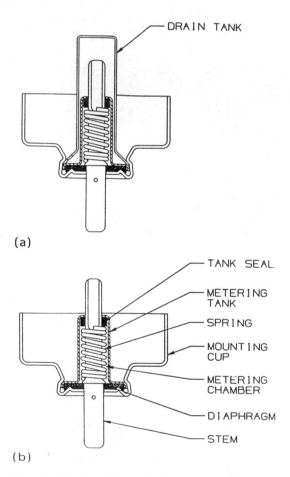

Fig. 8 Cutaway diagram of a metered-dose aerosol valve (a) with and (b) without drain tank
shown with stem down, or firing orientation. (Courtesy of Riker Laboratories, Inc./3M., Minneapolis, Minnesota.)

drain tank will retain any of the product that may revert back to the container. This amount is then dispensed along with the amount of product in the metering chamber so as to dispense a full dose of product. Another approach to providing a metering valve that will not lose its prime is illustrated in Fig. 9. This valve incorporates a "siphon" in its design that will keep the metering chamber full with product for substantially longer periods than the conventional capillary action/surface tension principle of retention.

Both types of valves are currently used on commercially available metered-dose inhaler aerosols. During the development stage, the compatibility of the valves should be determined with the exact formulation to be used so as to determine the accuracy of the metered dose developed in regard to doses delivered from the same container of product and from different containers. Additionally, it is important to ensure that there is no interaction between the various valve subcomponents and the formulation. If distortion or elongation of some of the plastic subcomponents occurs, this may result in leakage, inaccurate dosage, and/or decomposition of the active ingredients.

Metered dose valves suitable for use on nasal and inhaler aerosols are available from Valois, Riker (also Neotechnic), Spruhventile, VARI, and Bespak. These valves have been used on most of the aerosol inhalation products in the United States and in other

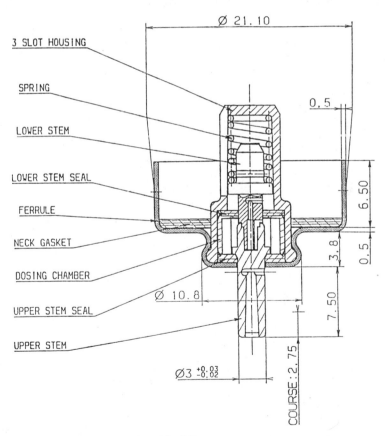

DOSE: 25-35-50-55-58-63-75

Fig. 9 Metering valve with increased retention of dose. (Courtesy of Valvois of America, Greenwich, Connecticut.)

countries of the world. It is estimated that almost a half billion of these valves are produced worldwide.

The specific valve used on each of the MDIs must be carefully selected as to size of metering chamber, stem and body orifices, and materials used in the manufacture of the stem, gasket(s), ferrule, metering chamber, spring, housing (body), and dip tube. Some of these materials are specified for use only with certain active ingredients and raw materials. In this instance, it is best to contact the manufacturer in order to determine which material is best with the specific product formulation. It is then necessary to carry out compatibility studies with each of the subcomponents in order to ascertain their usefulness. This is especially important when alternate propellants are used because there may be interaction between propellant and gaskets.

2. *Continuous-Spray Valves*

These valves are used primarily with topical pharmaceuticals. For the most part they consist of about seven subcomponents, as shown in Fig. 10. Each of these subcomponents can be made in a variety of different materials depending on the compatibility of the material with the formulation. Table 8 indicates some of the commonly used materials for each of the subcomponents. These materials must be tested with the specific

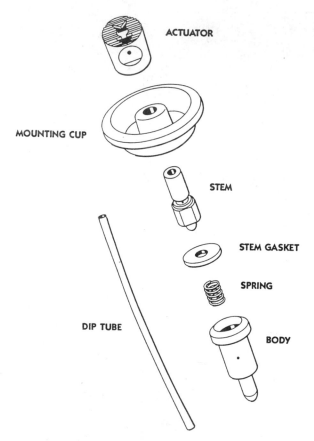

Fig. 10 Continuous-spray and foam-type valve. (Courtesy of Precision Valve Corporation, Yonkers, New York.)

Table 8 Materials Used in Valve Construction

Subcomponent	Material
Actuator (button, spout)	Polypropylene, polyethylene
Mounting cup	Tinplate, aluminum
Mounting cup gasket	Flowed-in or polyethylene sleeve
Stem	Nylon, Delrin, Acetal
Stem gasket	Buna N, Neoprene, Butyl
Spring	Stainless steel-passivated, stainless steel
Body	Nylon, Delrin, Acetal
Dip tube	Polyethylene, polypropylene

formulation in order to determine its compatibility with the formulation. Leakage and/ or absorption (or adsorption) of the active ingredient are sometimes noted with these valves and generally can be overcome through proper selection of the material of construction.

Depending on the design of the actuator or spout, the product can be dispensed as a spray, foam, or a semisolid. Additional valves are available for use with products that are extremely viscous or may require a high flow rate (creams, gels, lotions, ointments). In this case the valve consists of a mounting cup, sealing gasket, and a one-piece stem and body. These valves are designed to discharge the contents as the valve is tilted rather than depressed. The product is dispensed directly from the valve inner opening to the stem/body and is emitted as a foam or semisolid depending on the formulation.

There are several large-volume metered-dose valves designed for use with topical pharmaceuticals. One such design is shown in Fig. 11. As can be seen from this fig-

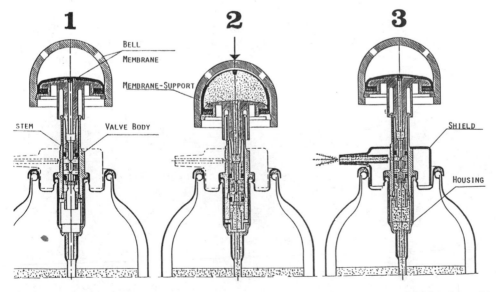

Fig. 11 Cutaway drawing of Lablabo large-volume metering valve. (1) Metering chamber with metering chamber membrane collapsed—valve closed, (2) membrane filled with product—valve depressed, and (3) product dispensed—valve released. (Courtesy of Lablabo, Montrogue, France.)

ure, the product will fill a metering chamber located in the actuator part of the valve system and the metered dose is dispensed as the button is released. Another metered valve is also available from Bespak that dispenses the product on the downstroke.

3. *Actuators, Buttons, Spouts, Oral Adapters, Mouthpiece, and Tube Extenders*

These units are fitted over the valve and are used to dispense the product in its desired form. These units must be considered as part of the formulation because they are ultimately responsible for the delivery of the product. In the case of metered-dose inhalers, the oral adapter (mouthpiece, tube spacer) must deliver the product in a particle size range of below 10 μm and in most cases between 2 and 6 μm. Changing the design of the unit will affect the particles dispensed. Figure 12 illustrates several different designs for these actuators.

C. Containers

1. *Glass*

Various containers have been used for these pharmaceutical aerosols. Because of esthetics and excellent compatibility with drugs, glass and aluminum containers have found widespread use in the pharmaceutical industry.

Plastic-coated glass bottles ranging in size from 10 ml to 30 mL have been used primarily with solution aerosols rather than suspension type, although there is no technical or scientific rationale for this other than the fact that one can note the amount of material left in the container by holding the bottle in the path of a strong light. Glass bottles are not recommended for suspension aerosols because of the visibility of the suspended particles, which may present an esthetic problem for the patient. Glass, being inert, has always been preferred for use with all types of pharmaceuticals, although with the advent and introduction of many newer materials of construction glass has been replaced by aluminum containers for most aerosols.

The plastic coating on the glass container serves to product the user from flying glass in the event the container is accidentally dropped and the glass breaks. The plastic coating around the neck of the container serves to absorb some of the shock from the crimping operation and decreases the danger of breaking around the neck area.

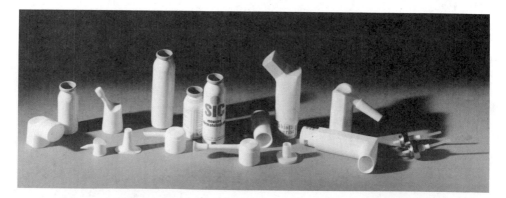

Fig. 12 Various applicators, oral and nasal adapters, etc., for use with pharmaceutical aerosols.

All commercially available bottles have a 20 mm neck finish and adapt easily to all of the metered aerosol valves presently available. In addition, the plastic coating also serves as an ultraviolet light absorber so that the contents are protected from the deleterious effects of light. These plastic coatings are available in a clear finish or in various colors. Glass is advantageous in its excellent compatibility with pharmaceuticals and in its ability to permit one to view the level of contents remaining in the container.

2. *Aluminum*

Aluminum is used as the material of construction for most other metered-dose aerosols. This material is extremely lightweight and also is essentially inert, although aluminum will react with certain solvents and chemicals. Aluminum can be used without an internal organic coating for certain aerosol formulations (especially those that contain only active ingredient and propellant) but many containers are available that have an internal coating made from an epon- or expoxy-type resin. The coating formulations are generally confidential; however, many of the container manufacturers have a Drug Master File at the Food and Drug Administration (FDA) that contains all pertinent information as to the exact formulation, safety evaluations, inertness, and so forth, of the coating material. Aluminum can also be anodized for added resistance.

These aluminum containers are also made with a 20 mm opening so as to receive the generally available metered valves. However, a variety of openings ranging from 15 to 20 mm are also available for special and customized applications. Because the aluminum container is made from a "slug" and fabricated by an extrusion or deep drawn process, there are no seams in the container, making it virtually leakproof (except for the area where the valve is crimped into place).

3. *Tin-Plated Steel*

These containers are used for most nonpharmaceutical aerosols and are the least expensive and most versatile of all containers. They are used for some topical pharmaceuticals if the size of the container exceeds 6 or 8 ounces. Today, however, aluminum is replacing these large-sized tinplate containers (8 to 12 ounce) wherever possible. For example, contact lens cleaner saline solutions are packaged in aluminum containers rather than tinplate.

4. *Other Containers*

Although the greater number of aerosol products utilize the typical aerosol container, there are many additional container systems available that allow for special dispensing of any product.

The viscosity of the product, incompatibility of the product concentrate and propellant, and desired dispensing characteristics of the finished product represent a few of the reasons why the typical aerosol systems may be unsuitable. For such cases, several additional systems characterized by provision for a physical separation of propellant and product are available.

Many designs have been submitted for these systems and several have found use in pharmaceuticals. Barrier packs utilize a plastic bag or piston to separate the product from the propellant. In barrier packs, only the product is delivered, and there is never any contact between product and propellant (unless the propellant or product permeates through the plastic bag or piston).

The following packages have been developed and are available [2,5]:

Piston type

Plastic bag

Collapsible metal tube

Laminated film

The use of these systems has been indicated in the cited publications. These systems are especially useful for semisolids and for foams. A post-foaming gel has been developed and packaged in this type of container. One such system is illustrated in Fig. 13.

III. TYPICAL FORMULATIONS

An aerosol formulation consists of two essential components: product concentrate and propellant. The product concentrate consists of active ingredients, or a mixture of active ingredients and other necessary agents such as solvents, antioxidants, and surfactants. The propellant may be a single propellant or a blend of various propellants and is selected to give the desired vapor pressure, compatibility, and dispensing characteristics (10).

A. Sublingual Aerosols (Oral)

These aerosols are formulated as solution system because they are generally administered sublingually or buccally and designed to obtain a rapid response. This system is

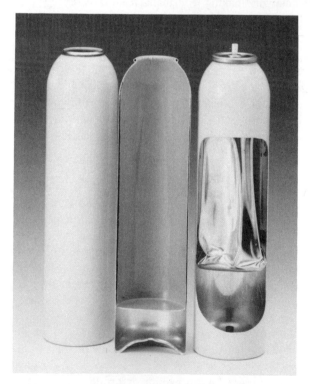

Fig. 13 Cross section of a "bag-in-can" system. (Courtesy of Lechner U.S.A. Ltd.)

used to dispense nitroglycerin and several aromatics used as a mouth freshener. A typical formulation for this type of product follows:

Nitroglycerin	0.41 mg
Dichlorodifluoromethane	10.66 mg
Dichlorotetrafluoroethane	16.01 mg
Inert flavors, stabilizers, etc.	22.92 mg
	50.00 mg

This system is packaged in an aluminum container and fitted with a metered-dose valve that will deliver 50 mg of total product per dose.

B. Metered-Dose Inhaler (MDI) [11–13]

These products may be formulated as either a solution or a suspension aerosol.

1. *Solution Aerosol*

The active ingredients are soluble directly in the propellant or in a mixture of water, ethyl alcohol, and propellant. They may also require the use of an antioxidant, preservative, and flavoring agents. This system can be exemplified by the following formula:

Isoproterenol HCl	0.25 g
Ascorbic acid	0.01 g
Ethyl alcohol	33.00 g
Dichlorodifluoromethane	33.37 g
Dichlorotetrafluoroethane	33.37 g
	100.00 g

This system is packaged in a plastic-coated glass bottle and fitted with a metered-dose valve having a dip tube.

2. *Suspension Aerosol*

Various methods have been used to overcome the difficulties encountered due to the use of a cosolvent. One such system involves a dispersion of active ingredients in the propellant or a mixture of propellants. To decrease the rate of settling of the dispersed particles and to decrease particle agglomeration, various surfactants or suspending agents have been added. This has now become the system of choice for dispensing metered-dose inhalers. This system can be formulated as follows:

Active ingredient:	Micronized
Dispersing agent or surfactant:	Sorbitan trioleate
	Lecithin and lecithin derivatives
	Oleic acid
	Oleyl alcohol
	Ethyl alcohol
Propellant(s):	12/11
	12/114
	12/114/11
	12

The physical stability of an aerosol dispersion can be increased by (a) control of moisture content, (b) use of derivatives of active ingredients having minimum solubility in propellant system, (c) reduction of initial particle size to less than 5 μm, (d) adjustment of density of propellant and/or suspensoid so that they are equalized, and (e) use of dispersing agents. A typical formulation would include:

	Weight %
Epinephrine bitartrate (within 1 to 5 μm)	0.50
Sorbitan trioleate	0.50
Propellant 114	49.50
Propellant 12	49.50

The epinephrine bitartrate has minimum solubility in the propellant system but is sufficiently soluble in fluids of the lungs to exert a therapeutic activity. A formulation for an MDI that contains a steroid would include:

Steroid compound	8.4 mg
Oleic acid	0.8 mg
Propellant 11	4.7 g
Propellant 12	12.2 g

The oleic acid is present as a dispersing agent for the steroid and is an aid in the prevention or reduction of particle growth or agglomeration. In addition, it serves as a valve lubricant and prevents the metered valve from "sticking" in the open position.

C. Intranasal Delivery (Aerosols and Pumps)

From a scientific standpoint, intranasal delivery should be evaluated for drugs that:

1. Require a rapid onset of action (similar to I.V. injection)
2. Are to be administered to patients who cannot swallow (unconscious, comatose, nauseated, tube fed, etc.)
3. Are erratically absorbed from the G.I. tract
4. Are considerably metabolized in the first liver pass
5. Are currently only administered by somewhat less convenient routes of administration (e.g., I.V., S.C., I.M., vaginally, and rectally)
6. Present administration problems to geriatric, pediatric, and physically impaired patients
7. Are given on a prn basis

The following list prioritizes some of the drugs that are currently being considered for intranasal delivery:

1. Polypeptides (oxytocin, synthetic lysine)
2. Insulin
3. Migraine headache formulas (propranolol, ergotamine)
4. Premenstrual tension formulas (progesterone)
5. Antihistamines (miscellaneous)
6. Vaccines (antivirals)
7. Cardiovascular agents (NTG)

8. Steroidal preparations (beclomethasone, flunisolide)
9. Antidotes

Metered pumps are seen in Fig. 14 and metered aerosol valves have received the most attention in the past 3 to 5 years for intranasal delivery. Pump technology has made enormous advances as a result of the fluorocarbon ban in 1976 [14]. Pumps are designed to accurately deliver volumes as low as 25 μL and as high as 0.5 to 1.0 mL. The larger volumes are delivered as streams of liquid, whereas low-volume pumps actually deliver fine mists. Improvements in the metered-valve pump now permit the pump to be utilized in any position. Aerosol delivery systems often are probably better suited for lower dose administration, but can be modified to deliver large volumes of liquid also. Actuators and adapters for both pump and aerosolized systems already exist and at present there is a trend to customize the adapter to the product [15].

The pump also permits the administration of a metered dose of steroid without utilizing propellants that often cause smarting and irritation by their cooling effects on the nasal mucosa. The metered aerosol pump also ensures accurate dosing and eliminates

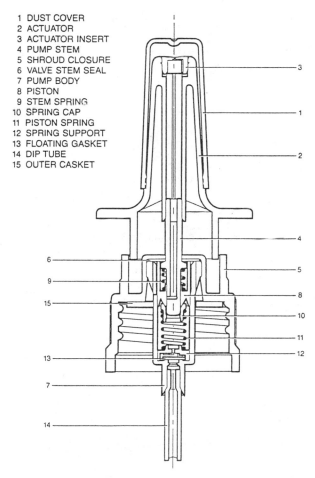

1 DUST COVER
2 ACTUATOR
3 ACTUATOR INSERT
4 PUMP STEM
5 SHROUD CLOSURE
6 VALVE STEM SEAL
7 PUMP BODY
8 PISTON
9 STEM SPRING
10 SPRING CAP
11 PISTON SPRING
12 SPRING SUPPORT
13 FLOATING GASKET
14 DIP TUBE
15 OUTER CASKET

Fig. 14 Valois VP3-18PH pump for nasal delivery systems. (Courtesy of Valvois of America, Greenwich, Connecticut.)

many of the administration problems associated with nose drops. The concept of propellant-free metered delivery offers a new dimension to intranasal delivery of potent therapeutic agents.

1. *Vehicle for Intranasal Delivery (Aqueous)*

The following are characteristics that must be incorporated into the vehicle that will contain the active ingredient:

A pH in the range of 5.5 to 7.5, (preferably less than 7.0)
A mild buffer capacity
An accepted physiological range of tonicity
Not modify the normal viscosity of mucus
Compatibility with normal ciliary motion and ionic constituents of the secretions
Compatibility with a large proportion of nasal medicaments
Sufficient stability to retain activity upon long standing on the patient's shelf
Contain, when necessary, sufficient antimicrobial agents to suppress growth of the
    bacteria being introduced by the device.

2. *Formulation (Aqueous)*

A typical phosphate buffer formula containing a water-soluble drug dispensed with an aerosol pump intended for nasal use (pH 6.5) is given below:

Adjuvant (if necessary)
    $NaH_2PO_4 \cdot H_2O$ 0.65
    $Na_2HPO_4 \cdot 7H_2O$ 0.54
    NaCl   0.45
Antioxidant (if necessary)
    Preservative   0.01–0.1%
    Distilled water qs ad   100 mL

3. *Aerosol Preparation*

Nasal aerosols can also be formulated as a metered-dose nasal inhaler in a manner similar to metered-dose oral inhalers. In fact, many of the commercial nasal preparations are the same formulation as the inhaler except that a nasal adapter is used in place of the oral adapter. Another formulation technique that can be used with nasal aerosols is to formulate an emulsion that would be dispensed as a fairly wet spray. A suggested starting formulation would include:

	% w/w
Active ingredient dissolved in oil vehicle	up to 10.0
Surfactant	up to 5.0
Cosolvent (if necessary)	up to 15.0
Propellant 12/114	up to 70.0

    This can be packaged in a conventional container and metered valve and fitted with a nasal adapter.

    The nasal cavity is covered by a mucous blanket. The mucous blanket extends over the surface of the nasal cavity, paranasal sinuses, trachea, pharynx, esophagus, and into the stomach. The mucous film is in continous motion, being moved along by ciliary action. The direction of flow of mucus is inward toward the nasopharynx. Mucus is a moderately viscous, pseudoplastic mucoprotein system. Under normal conditions, foreign bodies such as dust, bacteria, powders, and oil droplets are engulfed in the film and carried out of the nose into the nasopharynx. Drugs administered intranasally follow exactly the same passageway if the vehicle and/or drug do not upset the mucous blanket. Improperly formulated products, cold temperatures, viral invasion, dust, and allergens can alter normal ciliary action and may promote loss of drug through leakage.

4. *Intranasal Delivery of Peptides and Protein [16,17]*

Scientists have been examining the intranasal delivery of peptides since the early 1920s, but it is only recently that so much attention has been placed on this alternate route of administration. Clinical evaluations currently under study with peptides include the treatment of viral diseases, cancer, wounds and burns, dwarfism, immune disorders, and anovulation. Intranasal delivery of drugs such as thyrotropin-releasing hormone (TRH), enkephalin analogues, oxytocin, vasopressin analogues, luteinizing hormone–releasing hormone (LHRH) agonists and antagonists, glucagon, growth hormone–releasing film (GHRF), and insulin has been tested in humans.

D. Topical Aerosols

Topical pharmaceutical aerosols may be formulated by using the formulations included in this section.

1. *Prototype Topical Aerosol Solution*

Active ingredient: Dissolved in system
Solvents: Ethyl and isopropyl alcohol, glycols, isopropyl esters, surfactants
Antioxidants: Ascorbic acid
Preservatives: Methyl- and propylparaben
Propellant(s)*: Isobutane, propane/butane, propane/isobutane, Propellant 22, Propellant 152a/142b, Propellant 22/142a, dimethyl ether

These products are dispensed as fairly wet sprays. They are generally fitted with a continuous-spray valve and a spray actuator. Caution should be observed so that the emitted spray contains relatively large particles that will not be accidentally inhaled when sprayed.

2. *Prototype Topical Aerosol Suspension*

Active ingredient(s): Pass through a 325 mesh screen
Dispersing agents: Isopropyl myristate, mineral oil, sorbitan esters, polysorbates, glycol ethers, and derivatives
Propellant(s): Hydrocarbons; 142a, 152b, 22; dimethyl ether

---

*Other combinations of these propellants can also be used to obtain desired solubility and flammability characteristics (e.g., Propellant 22/isobutane).

Suspension aerosols can be used with antibiotics, steroids, and other insoluble active ingredients.

3. *Emulsions (Foams)*

Emulsion and foam aerosols consist of active ingredients, aqueous or nonaqueous vehicle, surfactant, and propellant and are dispensed as a stable or quick-breaking foam, depending on the nature of the ingredients and the formulation. The liquefied propellant is emulsified and is generally found in the internal phase. Nonaerosol emulsions are usually in lotion or viscous liquid form, but aerosol emulsions are dispensed as foams, and this can be advantageous for various applications involving irritating ingredients, or when the material is applied to a limited area. Foams may be formulated as aqueous stable foams, quick-breaking foams, and edible foams.

The formulations used for these systems are quite diverse and complex. However, the following can be used as a starting point for emulsions to be dispensed as a foam:

Active ingredient: Solubilized in fatty acid, vegetable oil, glycol
Emulsifying agents: Fatty acid soaps (triethanolamine stearate), polyoxyethylene sorbitan esters, emulsifiable waxes, surfactants
Other modifiers: Emollients, lubricants, preservatives, perfumes, etc.
Propellant(s): 12/114 (only if exempted), hydrocarbons, hydrofluorocarbons, hydrochlorofluorocarbons

Depending on the ingredients used to prepare the formulation, a stable to quick-breaking foam that can be used to dispense various active ingredients including steroids and other dermatological ingredients can be obtained.

A nonaqueous stable foam may be prepared from:

	% w/w
Glycol or oil base	91.0–92.5
Emulsifying agent	4.0
Hydrocarbon or other propellants	3.5–5.0

Glycerylmonostearate, S.E., is commonly used as the emulsifying agent for these foams. A modification of this foam that can be used to incorporate medicinal agents used orally, referred to as an "edible foam," consists of:

	% w/w
Vegetable oil	90.0
Emulsifier	5.0
Propellant	5.0

The oil is generally peanut oil, cottonseed oil, safflower oil, or soybean oil; the emulsifier is glyceryl monostearate, S.E. These ingredients can be safely used for oral products, as can propane, which is used as the propellant. Although these products are used with a continuous-spray valve, it might be desirable to meter the dosage. The metered valve shown in Fig. 11 is useful with these systems.

Quick-breaking foams can be formulated using the following:

	% w/w
Active ingredients	up to 25.0
Surfactant	0.5–5.0
Water	28.0–45.0
Ethyl alcohol	15.0–20.0
Isobutane	3.0–5.0

By varying the ratio of surfactant to alcohol/water, varying degrees of foam stability can be obtained.

IV. MANUFACTURING PROCEDURE

Both manufacturing procedures and packaging must be considered simultaneously, as part of the manufacturing operation takes place during the packaging of the product. The concentrate, which contains the active ingredients, solvents and cosolvents, and other inert ingredients and may even contain a small portion of the propellant, is compounded separately and then mixed with the remainder of the propellant. Two systems are available for use that include a cold- and a pressure-fill system. Present-day technology and the availability of good equipment give preference to the pressure method over the cold-fill method. Additionally, there is less propellant that escapes into the atmosphere from the pressure process, making the pressure process more environmentally friendly.

A. Cold Fill

1. *Laboratory*

The active ingredients are dissolved or suspended in part of the propellant and/or a cosolvent. This is then chilled to about –30°C and added to a cold container. The propellant is also chilled to –30°C and then added to the container. The valve is sealed in place.

2. *Production*

The same procedure is utilized except that the product may be made in a large stainless steel mixing tank fitted with a jacket capable of cooling the tank to below –60°C. The tank is fitted with a homogenizer as well as a mixer. The product is generally passed through a filter in order to break up agglomerates should they be present.

An alternate procedure has been developed and is referred to as "one-stage filling." The previous procedure is known as "two-stage filling." The compounding is carried out in a closed tank that is capable of being chilled to at least –45 to –60°C. Part of the Propellant 11 is added to the tank and, for suspensions, the dispersing agent is added. This is mixed well and followed by the addition of the micronized active ingredient. This is then mixed well using a homogenizer or dispersing mixer. The remainder of Propellant 11 is added. If solvents or other ingredients are present, they are also added at this stage. Then the other propellants are added. This is then dispersed and mixed well. The product is filled directly into cold cans and the valve sealed in place.

Regardless of the method used, each can is placed into a water bath to test for leaks or, alternatively, weighed and allowed to stand about 30 days and then reweighed. This will separate out any gross leakers.

B. Pressure Fill

The pressure-fill method is the method of choice in filling pharmaceutical aerosols. Pressure-fill equipment is available and is capable of producing upwards of 35 to 50 cans per minute to about 160 cans per minute.

1. *Laboratory*

The concentrate is prepared in a manner similar to the cold-fill method except that all ingredients are kept at room temperature. The concentrate is then added to the can and a valve is sealed into place. The propellant is added through the valve under pressure. A pressure burette can be used where a nonmetered valve is employed as seen in Fig. 15. However, metered valves require a pressure of about 300 to 600 psig to open the metered valve to its filling orifice. This will require special pressure-filling equipment, which is currently available. The finished aerosols are then check-weighed as indicated under the cold-fill method.

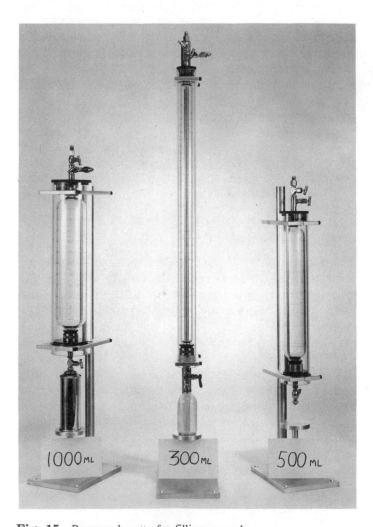

Fig. 15   Pressure burette for filling aerosols.

2. *Production*

The production procedure is essentially the same as the laboratory procedure. In order to minimize loss, the concentrate should be held at about $-15°C$ while it is being added to each container. Additionally, the mixture must be constantly mixed to ensure an even distribution of the concentrate in the mixing tank.

It is also possible to use the same alternate method as indicated under "Cold Fill" with the pressure method. However, a sealed pressure vessel must be used to compound the product. The product can then be filled under pressure into a container that has previously been fitted with a metered valve. The product is then forced through the valve stem of the metered or nonmetered valve. This method is useful only with metered-dose inhalers and thoes products with a relatively small fill (under one ounce). For larger volumes, the process would be too slow for commercial use.

Provisions must be made to purge the container of air as excess air trapped in the container would give excessive pressures and may cause decomposition of the active ingredient. This can be done by adding a drop of two of Propellant 11 or Propellant 12 to each can prior to adding the concentrate. The propellant will vaporize and expel most of the air from the can. Alternatively, this can also be accomplished at the end of the filling process by actuating each can several times (in the inverted position for dip tube products and upright for products without a dip tube). This will expel some of the air present and release the excess pressure. For metered-dose inhalers, all valves must be actuated several times in order to determine if the valve is operating properly and also to prime the valve so that when it is actuated by the user a full dose will be dispensed.

C. Quality Control

A quality control system for aerosols is no different from the system used for nonaerosol pharmaceuticals except that several in-process tests are necessary in order to ensure that the concentrate has been properly prepared [18]. In most cases this will include an assay to determine the level of active ingredient present. Other tests are dependent on the nature of the product. Because moisture is a critical parameter for suspension and dispersion aerosols, it should also be checked at this point.

Weights of both the concentrate and the propellant must be checked routinely throughout the manufacturing process. Any errors in these weights will affect the amount of active ingredient present in the final product and will result in the product's rejection. Automatic checkweighers are now available that will take a tare weight of the empty container, record the concentrate weight, and record the propellant weight and the final weight. Other essential tests that must be carried out on metered-dose inhalers include (a) particle size distribution, (b) dosage uniformity, (c) medication content, and (d) weight loss. The USP/NF lists many of these tests along with detailed test procedures [19]. Other procedures are also available [20,21].

D. Special Test Procedures

1. *Particle Size Distribution*

Particle size is an important characteristic for metered-dose inhalers. The formulation, valve, and mouthpiece are responsible for this criteria. It is determined by an impaction technic, microscopic technic or laser beam technic. Table 9 indicates these methods. The Cascade Impactor has been used to a great extent for this purpose [22–24].

Table 9 Summary of Particle Sizing Methods

Method	Size range (μm)	Major problems
Optical microscopy	0.2–300	0.2 μm limit of resolution: spreading of larger droplets
Cascade impactors	0.2–20	Wall losses/disaggregation; rebound/re-entrainment; limited size data
Light-scattering counters	0.1–20	Refractive index; shape sensitivity; coincidence; cross-sensitivity; calibration; isokinetic sampling
Holography	3–1000	Lower limit 3 μm; two stages in sizing; formation and reconstruction; analysis time
Photography	5–1000	Small depth of field; automation difficult but possible; difficulty in three dimensions

Another instrument finding use in determining the particle size distribution of metered-dose inhalers is the Malverne Particle Sizer. This instrument utilizes laser diffraction to determine particle size. When a particle scatters light it produces a unique light intensity that can be accurately measured using a computer. The intensity of the light is dependent upon the size of the particle.

One must take into consideration exactly what is being measured by the specific particle size measurement. For example, when one measures the particle size of a particle by a light-scattering or laser diffraction method, the relationship of the measurement to the amount of drug represented in the particle must be considered. It is possible that the particle or droplet will consist of solvent, propellant, dispersing agent, and little, if any, drug. Many of these optical methods are fast and accurate for determining the size of the particle, but are limited in indicating the amount of drug present. An impaction technic, using a Cascade Impactor, together with the analytical determination of the amount of drug collected at each stage, assures that the particle size distribution is related to the actual amount of drug contained in each particle.

2. *Dosage Uniformity*

Uniformity is generally measured by determining the actual weight of product dispensed each time the valve is opened. The dose dispensed must be within specifications from the first to the last dose. However, one must consider the problem of loss of prime with initial doses and tail-off with the last 10 to 12 doses. In order to ensure delivery of the labeled number of doses, an excess of product is added to each container.

It is necessary to check the weight of product delivered not only within each container but from container to container. In this regard the integrity of the valve is involved.

Related to this test is the amount of drug present in each dose dispensed. This is generally referred to as "content uniformity." As each dose is dispensed, it is collected in a suitable solvent and assayed. It is possible to obtain results where the total amount of product dispensed is within specifications but the amount of drug present is not. This can be due to particle agglomeration, drug sticking to the wall of the container, and absorption of the drug by the valve subcomponents.

IV. STABILITY

A stability program for aerosol pharmaceuticals consists of an examination of all materials used in the product both separately and collectively. The propellants do not present a stability problem, because they all are very stable materials when used with the usual pharmaceutical ingredients. The most important characteristic of the stability program, especially for metered-dose inhalers, is the compatibility of the active ingredient(s) with the propellants, container, and valve. Other than the chemical assay method for the active ingredient, most of the other test parameters are concerned with a physicochemical evaluation. The test protocol should include storage at two different temperatures, generally room temperature, 35 to 40°C and, depending on the nature of the product, either refrigeration temperature (about 4°C) or 50 to 55°C. The drug is generally not expected to be stable at this high temperature and, in many instances, will decompose, but the exceptionally high pressures place an undue stress on the container and the valve. The products are examined for certain characteristics initially upon preparation; after 30, 60, and 90 days; and then after 6 months and 1, 2, and 3 years. Accelerated temperature studies are discontinued after 1 year with the long-range room temperature study continuing for at least 2, and possibly 3, years.

A. Parameters to Be Evaluated

It is suggested that the following be evaluated during the stability study.

Metered-dose inhalers, oral and nasal aerosols: pressure, weight loss, total medication-can content, weight uniformity, moisture content, valve delivery, particle size, unit spray, degraded products, content uniformity, plume, particulate matter, microbiological content, interaction of product with valve, interaction of product with can

Topical sprays: pressure; weight loss; delivery-amount/second; specific gravity, density, viscosity, etc.; interaction of product with valve; interaction of product with container; others depending on nature of product

Foams: same as sprays; foam's density and characteristics; amount delivered if metered-dose, amount delivered if nonmetered

B. Test Procedures and Methods

Many of these test procedures have been discussed elsewhere and the reader is referred to the selected references for further information [3–5,9,10,18,19]. Specifications must be developed for each of the parameters studied.

REFERENCES

1. Y. W. Chien, Transnasal Systemic Medications, Elsevier Press, New York, 1985.
2. M. L. San Giovanni, New Developments in nasal sprayers, *Spray Technol. Marketing, 3*: 28–31 (1993).
3. J. J. Sciarra and Stoller, L., The Science and Technology of Aerosol Packaging, Wiley, New York, 1974.
4. P. Sanders, Handbook of Aerosol Technology, 2nd ed., R. E. Krieger Publishing Company, Malabar, Florida, 1987.

5. M. Johnsen, The Aerosol Handbook, 2nd ed., Wayne Dorland Co., Mendham, New Jersey, 1982.
6. Handbook of Pharmaceutical Excipients, 19, 99, 101, 145, 240, 333, American Pharmaceutical Association/The Pharmaceutical Society of Great Britain, Washington, D.C. and London, England, 1986.
7. J. J. Daly Jr. and M. L. San Giovanni, Replacements for CFC Propellants, *Spray Technol. Market., 3*:34–38 (1993).
8. T. G. Manners, Aerosolized saline solutions, Aerosol Age, 33:37 (1988).
9. E. F. Fiese, W. G. Gorman, D. Dolensky, R. J. Harwood, W. A. Hunke, N. C. Miller, H. Mintzer, and N. J. Harper, Test method for evaluation of loss of prime in metered dose aerosols, *J. Pharm. Sci., 77*:90–93 (1988).
10. J. J. Sciarra, Aerosols. In: *Remington's Pharmaceutical Sciences,* 19th ed., Mack Publishing Company, Easton, PA, (in press).
11. J. J. Sciarra, Pharmaceutical and cosmetic aerosols, *J. Pharm. Sci., 63*:1815–1836 (1974).
12. J. J. Sciarra, Pharmaceutical Aerosols. In: *Modern Pharmaceutics,* 3rd Ed., Marcel Dekker, New York (in press).
13. A. J. Hickey, *Pharmaceutical Inhalation Aerosol Technology,* Marcel Dekker, New York (1992).
14. J. J. Sciarra, Mechanical pumps for pharmaceutical aerosols, Aerosol Age, 21:16 (1976).
15. J. A. Ranucci, D. Cooper, and K. Sethachutkul, Effect of actuator design on metered dose inhaler plume/particle size, *Pharm. Technol., 16*: 84–91 (1992).
16. S. Lee and J. J. Sciarra, Development of an aerosol dosage form containing insulin, J. Pharm. Sci., 65:567–572 (1976).
17. R. A. Hudson and C. D. Black, Novel delivery methods for protein drugs, *Am. Pharm. NS33*:23–24 (1993).
18. J. J. Sciarra, Quality Control for Pharmaceutical and Cosmetic Aerosol Products in Quality Control in the Pharmaceutical Industry, Vol. 2 (Cooper, M. S., ed.), Academic Press, New York, 1973.
19. U. S. Pharmacopeia XXII/NFXVII, United States Pharmaopeial Convention, Rockville, Maryland, 1990, pp. 1556–1557, 1689–1690.
20. G. P. Burke, G. Poochikian, and P. Botstein, Regulatory science of inhalation aerosols, *J. Aerosol Med., 4*:3, 265–268 (1991).
21. Production and quality control of metered dose inhalers (MDIs), Pharmacopoeial Forum, 11:934–940 (1985).
22. J. J. Sciarra and A. J. Cutie, Simulated respiratory system for in-vitro evaluation of two inhalation delivery systems using selected steroids, J. Pharm. Sci., 67:1428–1431 (1978).
23. M. A. Johnsen, Properties of aerosol particles, *Spray Technol. Market., 2*: 46–55 (1992).
24. S. M. Milosovich, Particle size determination via cascade impaction, *Pharm. Technol., 16*: 82–86 (1992).
25. W. G. Gorman and F. A. Carroll, Aerosol particle size determination using laser holography, *Pharm. Technol., 17*: 34–37 (1993).

9

Ophthalmic Ointments and Suspensions

Krishna M. Bapatla and Gerald Hecht

Alcon Laboratories, Inc., Fort Worth, Texas

I. INTRODUCTION

Products used for the diagnosis and treatment of ocular diseases are formulated using the same scientific principles and technology as dosage forms intended for other target organs. Development of ophthalmic dosage forms requires the same considerations, such as safety, availability, efficacy, and pharmaceutical elegance, in addition to meeting applicable regulations on a worldwide basis. Many of the current ophthalmic preparations are available as sterile, buffered, isotonic solutions, because a majority of the ophthalmic drugs are water soluble. In fact, solution dosage forms are preferred, as drops are easier to administer. However, in situations where there are solubility limitations, or when a prolonged therapeutic action is desired, disperse systems such as suspensions, gelled systems, and ointments are indicated. In contrast to oral and topical products, ophthalmic dosage forms are required to be manufactured sterile and to maintain sterility during multiple applications or administration. Manufacturing facilities and equipment requirements for ophthalmic preparations are quite similar to those required for parenteral products.

II. CHARACTERISTICS OF OPHTHALMIC OINTMENTS, GELLED SYSTEMS, AND SUSPENSIONS

Ophthalmic ointments, gelled systems, and suspensions ideally should have the following desirable attributes:

Nonirritating to the ocular tissues
Homogeneous—particles uniformly dispersed, smooth and free from lumps or agglomerates
Relatively nongreasy
Should not cause blurred vision
Should not cause intolerable foreign body sensation
Sterile and adequately preserved, if intended for multiple use (multidose package)

Efficacious—provide adequate amount of drug for the required duration
Physically and chemically stable

Many of the commercially available ophthalmic ointments, suspensions, and gelled systems are safe, well tolerated, and accepted, although they do not meet all the desired attributes. The principal differences between them are that gelled systems and suspensions are primarily aqueous in nature, in contrast to ointments, which are oleaginous. Consequently, gelled systems are not greasy and do not cause blurred vision, depending on the concentration and type of polymers (viscolizers) and dispersing agents used. Many of the difficulties encountered in formulating dispersed systems for oral administration and for topical application are also encountered in developing ophthalmic dispersed systems. Crystal growth, caking, and inability to resuspend are some of the common problems encountered in suspensions. Formation of large suspended agglomerates in suspensions can cause severe eye irritation upon instillation.

Common problems encountered in formulating stable ophthalmic ointments are as follows:

Limited options available for the methods of sterilization
Difficulties in producing sterile micronized drug substances
Formation of agglomerates
Separation of the liquid phase from the semisolid ointment base on aging

III. ANATOMY OF THE EYE AND ADNEXA

No attempt will be made in this chapter to present an in-depth discussion of the anatomy of the eye and adnexa, as this subject is quite adequately covered by previous authors in the pharmaceutical literature [1,2]. For purposes of this discussion, however, an anatomical cross section of the human eye is presented (Fig. 1) to identify specific tissues, their functions, and their involvement in selected ophthalmic disease states as well as to locate specific sites of drug administration and action. Primarily, consideration will be given in this discussion to ointments, gel systems, and suspensions applied topically. Additionally, however, drugs are administered via parenteral-type dosage forms subconjunctivally, into the anterior and posterior chambers, the vitreous chamber, and Tenon's capsule, or via retrobulbar injection. For orientation, the student is encouraged to become familiar with the following anatomical members of the eye, some of which are shown in Fig. 1.

Conjunctiva
    Inferior conjunctival sac
    Superior conjunctival sac
Cornea
    Epithelium
    Stroma with its anterior modified zone of Bowman
    Descemet's membrane
    Endothelium
Anterior chamber
    Angle of anterior chamber
    Schlemm's canal
    Spaces of fontana

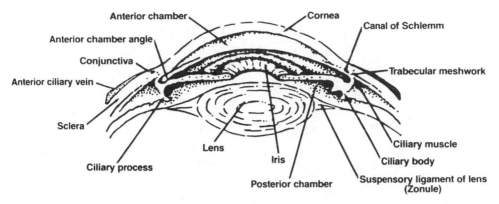

Fig. 1 Anatomical cross section of the anterior portion of the human eye.

Uveal tract
   Choroid
   Ciliary body
   Iris
Posterior chamber
Zonule of Zinn
Lens
Vitreous humor
Retina
Meibomian glands

Figure 2 presents an anatomical view of the lids and lacrimal system. This includes the lacrimal gland, excretory ducts, the superior and inferior lacrimal puncta and canalicula, and the lacrimal sac. Further reference will be made to both of these anatomical presentations later in this chapter.

IV. SAFETY CONSIDERATIONS: GENERAL

A. Sterility

Every ophthalmic product must be manufactured sterile and proved sterile on a lot-by-lot basis before release of the product to the marketplace. In general, the United States Pharmacopeia (USP 23), the British Pharmacopoeia, 1993, and the European Pharmacopoeia, 1983, recognize five methods of achieving sterilization:

1. Steam sterilization at 121°C
2. Dry-heat sterilization
3. Sterilization by filtration
4. Gas sterilization (ethylene oxide, propylene oxide)
5. Sterilization by ionizing radiation (electron accelerators, radioisotopes)

Because the vast majority of commercially available ophthalmic products are available in flexible plastic packaging, sterilization of the bulk product followed by aseptic

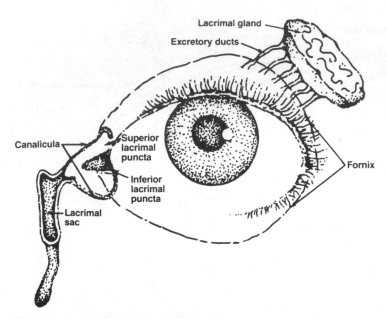

Fig. 2 Anatomical view of the lids and lacrimal system.

filling into presterilized containers is the method usually employed. It is the manufacturer's responsibility to ensure the safety and efficacy of the manufacturing process and the absence of any adverse effects of this process on the product such as the possible formation of toxic substances, which is an ever-present possibility with gas sterilization or when ionizing radiation is used.

The entire subject of process validation, which includes sterilization validation, must be accomplished for each product in order to lend "validity" to the presumptive sterility test of the official compendia. Sterility tests are conducted on random samples of the finished package. Suggested guidelines for the number of samples to be tested are dependent on whether or not sterilization has taken place in the sealed final container. The aforementioned pharmacopoeias set forth the proper method of sampling and the number of samples to be tested. In products that are rendered sterile in their final container by terminal heat sterilization methods the practice of Parametric Product Release is gaining acceptance. By this procedure, a lot of product that can be shown to have been exposed to a set of parameters (time and temperature) previously validated for a specific lot size and sterilizer lead configuration can be considered as having been sterilized, and the presumptive sterility test can be waived.

B. Ocular Toxicity and Irritation

Assessment of the ocular irritation potential of ophthalmic products represents an extremely important step in the development of both over-the-counter (OTC) and prescription ophthalmic ointments, gel systems, and suspensions.

Procedures used in evaluating ocular toxicity and irritation have appeared in excellent review articles [3–5]. Significant advances have been made resulting in greater reliability, reproducibility, and predictability.

The historical evaluation of these procedures can be traced through the literature [6–15], as can an understanding of the mechanisms of ocular response to irritants, based upon examination of the conjunctiva [16–18], cornea [7,19–21] and the iris [7,22,23].

Albino rabbits are currently used to test the ocular toxicity and irritation of ophthalmic formulations. Several articles relate to the use of rabbits as predictors for human responses. The rabbit has obvious advantages associated with its use. The rabbit is readily available, docile, easily handled, relatively inexpensive, easy to maintain, has a large eye, both corneal surface and bulbar conjunctival areas are large and easily observed, and the iris is unpigmented, allowing ready observation of the iridal vessels [4]. The primary differences between rabbits and humans in ophthalmic studies relate in rabbits to less tearing, lower blinking rate, loosely attached eyelids, presence of a nictitating membrane [16,17,24,25], differences in the structure of Bowman's membrane, and a slower re-epithelialization of the cornea [7]. The primate eye has also gained in popularity as an ocular model for the evaluation of drugs and chemicals because of its similarity to human ocular tissue structure and physiological functions [16, 24]. The use of corneal and conjunctival cell cultures has also been under consideration in recent years for the evaluation of ophthalmic product toxicity.

Various governmental agencies have published guidelines for eye irritancy studies [25,26]. These guidelines are directed toward ophthalmic formulations, chemicals, cosmetics, ophthalmic containers, and other materials that may accidentally or intentionally contact the eye during use. The USP presents guidelines for a 72-hour ocular irritation test in rabbits using saline and cottonseed oil extracts of plastic containers used for packaging ophthalmic products. Containers are conditioned (cleaned, sterilized) as in the final packaged product and extracted by submersion in saline and cottonseed oil. Ocular changes are examined using a biomicroscope following topical ocular instillation of the extracts and blanks in rabbits. If ocular changes between extracts and blanks are similar, the plastic component passes and is rated satisfactory.

As a part of the Federal Hazard Substances Act (FHSA), a modified Draize test was adopted [27–29] as the official method for eye irritancy evaluation [30]. Although a proposed change to include ocular irritation tests as part of the FHSA methods was made in 1972 [31], it was determined that the proposed method performed no better [32] than those already used.

It has been stated that the best way to determine the degree of irritation or differences between test materials may not be the FHSA or Draize methods, as these are pass/fail procedures [32]. Possibly a better judgment of irritancy is based on degree, frequency, and duration of ocular changes. These changes are graded by macroscopic examination and a provision allows for substitution of a slit-lamp (biomicroscope) examination and/or fluorescein staining of the cornea [4,28,29].

Current guidelines for toxicity evaluation of disperse systems involve both single and multiple applications. The multiple applications may extend over a 21-day period and involve both irritation and systemic toxicological studies.

During the application of these guidelines for ophthalmic disperse products, ocular examination and biomicroscopic examinations on rabbit eyes are completed with objective reproducible grading [4,33] for conjunctival congestion, conjunctival swelling, conjunctival discharge, aqueous flare, iris involvement, corneal cloudiness, severity, area of corneal opacity or cloudiness, pannus, and intensity of fluorescein staining.

In addition to in vivo testing of ophthalmic disperse systems, primarily in rabbit eyes and secondarily in primate eyes, numerous in vitro methods have been developed over the past few years as alternatives to in vivo ocular testing. Particular attention has recently been given to evaluation of preservative effects on corneal penetration [34,35], cytotoxicity [36–38], and effects on wound healing [39,40].

C. Preservation and Preservatives

In 1953 the FDA required that all ophthalmic products be manufactured sterile [41]. Preservatives are included as major components of multiple-dose ophthalmic suspensions for the primary purpose of maintaining sterility of the product after opening and during use unless prepared sterile in a unit-dose package. This is likewise the case with gel systems and ointments packaged in tubes, unless the presence of a preservative is contraindicated because of the special nature of the ophthalmic disease process being treated. The use of the popular plastic eyedrop container has reduced, but not completely eliminated, the chances of inadvertent contamination. There can be a "suck-back" of an unreleased drop when pressure on the bottles is released. If the tip is allowed to touch a nonsterile surface, microorganisms could be introduced. There is no suck-back with products packaged in tin or laminated plastic/paper tubes. It is therefore important that the pharmacist instruct the patient on the proper use of an ophthalmic dispensing container to minimize the hazards of contamination. The contamination hazard is magnified in the busy clinical practice of the ophthalmologist, where numerous diagnostic solutions of cycloplegics, mydriatics, and dyes are used—from the same container—in many patients. This cross-contamination hazard can be eliminated by the use of packages containing small volumes and designed for single application only. However, these single-use packages still contain (as a large-scale manufacturing necessity) an amount in excess of the several drops (0.05–0.20 mL) to be used. Unfortunately, there is a tendency to use the entire contents and thereby create a contamination hazard and defeat the purpose of any special packaging.

A procedure is described in the USP to test products for antimicrobial preservative effectiveness and to interpret the results [42]. The preservative effectiveness test is carried out as part of the formulation development sequence. Cultures of *Candida albicans, Aspergillus niger, Escherichia coli, Pseudomonas aeruginosa*, and *Staphylococcus aureus* are used: a standardized inoculum with organism counts of 100,000 to 1,000,000 per milliliter for each microorganism is prepared and tested against the preserved formula. The inoculated tubes or containers are incubated at 20°C or 25°C for 28 days with examination at days 7, 14, 21, and, under certain governmental guidelines, at day 28. The preservative is effective in the product if the concentrations of viable bacteria are reduced to not more than 0.1% of the initial concentrations by day 14, the concentrations of viable yeasts and molds remain at or below the initial concentrations during the first 14 days, and the concentration of each test microorganism remains at or below these designated levels during the remainder of the 28-day test period. Importantly, most ophthalmic product manufacturers utilize this as a *minimum* standard and attempt to formulate their products with a safety margin for preservation.

Considerable emphasis in the ophthalmic literature is placed on the effectiveness of preservatives against *Pseudomonas* because of reports of loss of vision through corneal ulcerations within 24 to 48 hours from eye products contaminated with *Ps. aeruginosa*. This organism is not the most prevalent cause of bacterial eye infections, even though it is a common inhabitant of human skin, but it is the most opportunistic and virulent. *Staphylococcus aureus* is responsible for the majority of bacterial infections of the eye.

The eye seems to be remarkably resistant to infection when the corneal epithelium is intact. When there is a corneal epithelial abrasion, organisms can enter freely and *Ps. aeruginosa* can readily grow in the cornea and rapidly produce an ulceration and loss of vision. This microorganism has been found as a contaminant in a number of studies evaluating the sterility of ophthalmic products and particularly in sodium fluorescein solutions used to detect corneal epithelial damage.

There is a group of ophthalmic products such as miotics, irrigating solutions, and enzyme products in which the use of preservatives is prohibited. These products are used intraocularly at the time of eye surgery. In this type of usage, there is a potential for toxicity if the products contain preservatives. These products should be packaged in sterile, single-use containers without preservatives.

1. Choice of Preservative

The choice of preservative is limited to only a few chemicals that have been found over the years to be safe and effective for this purpose. These are benzalkonium chloride, chlorobutanol, thimerosal, polyquat, methyl- and propylparaben, phenylethanol, chlorhexidine, polyaminobiguanide, and various combinations of these chemicals. The chelating agent disodium edetate (EDTA) is often used to increase the activity against certain *Pseudomonas* strains, particularly with benzalkonium chloride. Chlorhexidine as the hydrochloride, gluconate, or acetate is widely used in the United Kingdom and Australia but was not used in the United States until 1976—and then only in a soft contact lens disinfection solution. This limited choice of preservative agents is further narrowed when the requirements of chemical and physical stability and compatibility are considered for a particular formulation and package.

a. *Benzalkonium Chloride.* The most widely used preservative is benzalkonium chloride, generally used in combination with disodium edetate. The official benzalkonium chloride is a quaternary ammonium compound defined in USP 23 as an alkylbenzyldimethylammonium chloride mixture with alkyl chains beginning with n-C_8H_{17} and extending through higher homologues, with n-$C_{12}H_{25}$, n-$C_{14}H_{29}$, and n-$C_{16}H_{33}$ constituting the major portion. This compound's popularity is due to the fact that despite its compatibility limitations, it has generally been shown to be the most effective and rapid-acting preservative and has an excellent chemical stability profile. It is stable over a wide pH range and does not degrade, even under excessively hot storage conditions. It has pronounced surface-active properties. The antimicrobial activity can be reduced by adsorption to certain package components, large anions, surfactants, and so on. It is cationic and this unfortunately leads to a number of incompatibilities with large negatively charged molecules, either through production of a salt of lower solubility or actual precipitation. It is usually advisable to design the formulation to avoid these incompatible anions rather than substitute a less effective preservative. There are several listings of incompatibilities of benzalkonium chloride in the literature that are helpful but should not be totally relied on. Compatibility is determined by the total environment in which the drug or preservative molecules function; that is, the total product formula. The pharmaceutical manufacturer can sometimes design around what appears to be an incompatibility, whereas the extemporaneous compounder may not have these options or, more importantly, the ability to test the final product for its stability, safety, and efficacy.

The usual concentration of benzalkonium chloride used in topical eye drops is 0.01%, with a range of 0.004% to 0.02% [43]. Benzalkonium chloride has been found to enhance corneal penetration of certain compounds [34,44,45].

Richards [46] and Mullen et al. [47] summarized the literature on benzalkonium chloride. The conclusion drawn was that benzalkonium chloride up to 0.02% has been well substantiated as being suitable for use in topical ophthalmic drug products when the conditions of its use are properly controlled. McDonald [48] studied various concentrations in rabbit eyes via several dosing regimens, the most severe being a one-day acute regimen in which a 0.05 mL dose was instilled in the cul-de-sac at 20-minute intervals for 6 consecutive hours. Ocular changes were graded by macroscopic and biomicroscopic slit-lamp examination. A dose-response pattern for conjunctival congestion, swelling, discharge, and iritis was noted. He concluded that up to 0.02% benzalkonium chloride is a permissible level in ophthalmic solutions.

Numerous articles have appeared in the literature comparing the antibacterial activity of benzalkonium chloride with that of other preservatives. Many of the articles give conflicting results, which is not surprising considering that different test methods, formulas, and criteria were used to arrive at these diverse conclusions. Adequate data are available to conclude that the manufacturer can only rely on the test results for each particular product, using the USP 23 or a similar test, to decide on which preservative(s) to use and in what concentration(s), in order to achieve a satisfactory, effective, and stable new product.

Some strains of *Pseudomonas aeruginosa* have been found that are resistant to benzalkonium chloride and, in fact, can be grown in concentrated solutions of this agent. This has caused great concern because of the virulent nature of this organism in ocular infections, as discussed earlier. Thus, it was an important finding in 1958 that the acquired resistance could be eliminated by the presence of ethylenediaminetetraacetic acid (EDTA) in the solution. This action of EDTA has been correlated with its ability to chelate divalent cations, which appear to decrease the effectiveness of benzalkonium chloride. The use of disodium edetate, where it is compatible, is recommended in concentrations up to 0.1%.

b. *Organic Mercurials.* When benzalkonium chloride cannot be used in a particular formulation, thimerosal, an organic mercurial, may be used up to 0.01%. Although thimerosal can be used effectively in some products, it has been found to relatively weak and slow in its antimicrobial activity. This organic mercurial is generally more effective in neutral to alkaline solutions; however, it has been used successfully in slightly acid formulations. The FDA has issued a regulation restricting the mercurial preservative content of cosmetics applied around the eye. Several countries have banned use of mercurials entirely.

c. *Chlorobutanol.* This alcohol has been found to be an effective preservative and is used in several ophthalmic products. Over the years, it has proved to be a relatively safe preservative for ophthalmic products [49]. However, in addition to its relatively slower activity, it has a number of severe formulation and packaging limitations. It possesses adequate room temperature stability when used in an acidic solution, usually around pH 5 or below. About 30% of chlorobutanol will be lost during autoclave sterilization for 20 to 30 minutes at pH 5. The hydrolytic decomposition of chlorobutanol produces HCl, and the pH of the product decreases with time. Products containing chlorobutanol require the use of glass or other impervious packaging, because this volatile compound has been shown to readily permeate popular polyolefin plastic ophthalmic containers. Chlorobutanol is generally used at a concentration of 0.5%. Its maximum water solubility is only about 0.7%, with a slow dissolution rate. Heat can be used to increase its dissolution rate, but will also cause some decomposition and sublimation. Concentrations as low as 0.125% have shown antimicrobial activity under certain conditions. In spite of its limitations, chlorobutanol may be acceptable as a preservative if its concentration does not fall below 80% of label and the product meets the USP Antimicrobial Preservative Effectiveness criteria during the shelf life of the product.

d. *Methyl- and Propylparaben.* These esters of parahydroxybenzoic acid have been used primarily to prevent mold growth, but in higher concentrations do possess some weak antibacterial activity. Their effective use is limited by their low aqueous solubility and reports of causing of stinging and burning sensations in the eye. They have been found to bind to a number of nonionic surfactants and polymers, reducing their bioactivity. They are used primarily in ointments by combining the methyl ester at 0.03% to 0.1% with the propyl ester at 0.01% to 0.02%.

e. *Phenylethyl Alcohol.* This substituted alcohol has been used at a 0.5% concentration, but in addition to its weak activity it has a number of limitations. It is volatile and loses activity via permeation through a plastic package. It has limited water solubility, can be "salted out," and can produce burning and stinging sensations in the eye. It has been recommended primarily for use in combination preservative systems.

f. *Polyquat (Polyquaternium-1).* This polyquaternium compound is relatively new to ophthalmic preparations. Its advantage over other quaternary ammonium compounds seems to be in its inability to penetrate ocular tissues, especially the cornea. At clinically effective preservative levels, polyquat is approximately 10 times less toxic than benzalkonium chloride [50]. This preservative has been extremely useful for soft contact lens care products because of its insignificant adsorption or absorption by the lens, and its practically nonexistent sensitization potential.

g. *Chlorhexidine.* Chlorhexidine, a bis-biguanide, has been demonstrated to be somewhat less toxic than benzalkonium chloride and thimerosal at effective preservative concentrations [38, 50–52]. This finding was confirmed in a series of in vitro and in vivo experiments [53–55].

h. *Polyaminopropyl Biguanide.* This preservative is also relatively new to ophthalmic formulations and has been used primarily in contact lens solutions. At the concentrations used in these solutions, polyaminopropyl biguanide was found to have a low toxicity potential [56, 57].

V. EFFICACY CONSIDERATIONS

The efficacy of drugs administered orally or parenterally can be evaluated by measuring the concentration of the drug in plasma or urine as a measure of its bioavailability. However, the bioavailability of drugs administered as topical ophthalmic dosage forms cannot be evaluated by sampling ocular tissue fluids, such as aqueous humor, without causing severe ocular damage. In the case of drugs such as mydriatics or miotics, the efficacy can be evaluated by measuring changes in pupil diameters. In the case of antiglaucoma drugs, which are administered to control ocular hypertension, drug efficacy can be evaluated by monitoring the intraocular pressure (a noninvasive method). Absorption of drugs across the cornea is not an important requirement in external infections and inflammatory conditions of the eye such as conjunctivitis or blepharitis. However, in the case of a deep-seated inflammation such as iritis or uveitis, transcorneal and/or transconjunctival penetration does become an important therapeutic factor.

A.   Absorption Of Drugs From The Eye

It is often assumed that drugs administered topically to the eye are rapidly and totally absorbed and are available at a desirable site in the globe of the eye to exert their therapeutic effect. Indeed, this is generally not the case. Were this true, we would not see drug products containing as much as 5% to 10% of such systematically active drugs as atropine, homatropine, and pilocarpine marketed for ophthalmic use.

Absorption of drugs administered as topical ophthalmics is affected by several factors. These are: the nature of the eye itself, with its limited capacity to hold the administered dosage forms; tear fluid and aqueous humor dynamics (secretion and drainage rates); absorption by conjunctival tissues; penetration across cornea and sclera; residence time and spillage; blinking rate; reflex tearing caused by the administered product. The normal capacity of the lower cul-de-sac to hold tears is approximately 7 μL. A human eye can accommodate approximately 30 μL of a suspension or 30 μg of an ointment in the absence of blinking. At the present time, commercial suspensions are packaged in polyethylene or polypropylene bottles with plugs that deliver approximately 20 to 60 μL in each drop. Commercial ointments and gels, on the other hand, are packaged in ophthalmic tamper-evident tubes. Delivery of the ointment or gel from these containers is poorly controlled and subjective. Most manufacturers recommend a thin bead of ointment or gel 1/4 inch to 1/2 inch long be instilled into the lower cul-de-sac. For many years, better ways of administering ophthalmic ointments have substantially evaded the formulators of such dosage forms. New developments on the horizon may ameliorate this problem or eliminate it completely. The importance of controlling the drop size in ophthalmic products is being recognized by several recent publications [58–61]. Because of the limited capacity of the cul-de-sac of the eye, approximately 80% of the administered 50 μL drop is expelled by spillage and loss from the palpebral fissure into the nasolacrimal duct. If blinking occurs, the residual volume of 10 μL indicates that 90% of the administered volume of two drops will be expelled [62].

Drug absorption also depends on the residence time of the administered dose in the eye. Gamma detection techniques and fluorometric analyses were used to study residence time using a single channel analyzer coupled to a sodium iodide high-energy probe [63]. The precorneal residence time of an ophthalmic ointment radiolabeled by inclusion of technetium-99m tin colloid was found to be significantly greater than a 0.3% solution of hydroxypropyl methylcellulose (HPMC) in humans using gamma scintigraphy [64].

Drainage of the administered drop via the nasolacrimal system into the gastrointestinal tract begins immediately upon instillation. This takes place when reflex tearing causes the volume of fluid in the palpebral tissues to exceed the normal lacrimal volume of 7 to 10 μL. Reference to Fig. 2 indicates the pathway for this drainage. The excess fluid volume enters the superior and inferior lacrimal puncta, down the canalicula into the lacrimal sac, and then into the gastrointestinal tract. It is due to this mechanism that significant systemic effects from certain potent ophthalmic medications have been reported [65, 66]. It is also the mechanism by which a patient may occasionally sense a bitter or salty taste following use of eyedrops.

Another mechanism competing for drug absorption into the eye is the superficial absorption of the drug into the palpebral and bulbar conjunctiva with concomitant rapid removal from the ocular tissues by peripheral blood flow. Underlying the conjunctival mucous membrane is the sclera with its circulatory system. The sclera is the white part of the eye, which is a tough covering that forms the external protective coat of the eye along with the cornea.

In competition with the three foregoing forms of drug removal from the palpebral fissure is the transcorneal absorption of drug—that route most effective in bringing drug to the anterior chamber of the eye via absorption. The cornea is an avascular body and, with the precorneal tear film, is the first refracting mechanism operant in the physiological process of sight. It is composed of three general layers: the lipid-rich epithelium, the lipid-poor stroma, and the lipid-rich endothelium. Different studies on the relative lipid content of these three tissues have shown that the corneal epithelium and corneal endothelium each contain approximately 100 times as much lipid as the corneal stroma. This is a primary physiological factor influencing drug penetration through the cornea and into the aqueous humor. For a topically administered drug to traverse the intact cornea and to appear in the aqueous humor, it must possess both hydrophilic and lipophilic properties.

The transport of drugs across the cornea has been studied both in vivo and in vitro. The in vitro studies are simpler to analyze than the in vivo absorption studies, which are complicated by tear flow, tear drainage, corneal transport, and elimination from the aqueous humor, not to mention safety hazards to patients in sampling ocular fluids unlike sampling blood or urine. Pharmacokinetic modeling via this scheme (Fig. 3) has been successful in fitting the aqueous humor levels of pilocarpine following topical administration [67] (Fig. 4). Although this type of data fitting has been quite successful, there has not been a sufficient number of such systematic studies to determine the role of molecular properties in affecting the various pharmacokinetic parameters.

One of the key parameters in ocular absorption is the corneal permeability coefficient, and this transport process has been studied extensively in vitro [68–70]. For a series of molecules of similar size, it was shown that the permeability increases with octanol/water distribution (or partition) coefficient until a plateau is reached. Modeling of this type of data has led to the earlier statement that drugs need to be both oil and water soluble. The epithelium is modeled as a lipid barrier (possibly with aqueous pores) and the stroma as an aqueous barrier. The endothelium is very thin and porous compared to the epithelium [71].

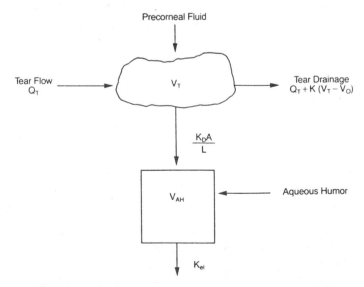

Fig. 3 Pharmacokinetic model for transport of drugs across the cornea. (From Ref. 67.)

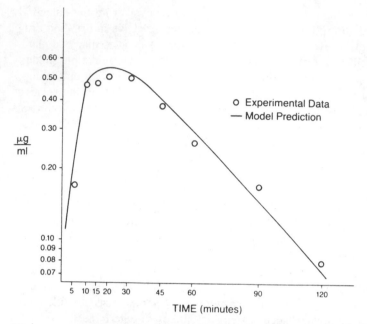

Fig. 4 Comparison of model-predicted (—) and experimental (O) aqueous humor concentrations following instillation of 5 μL of 1 × 10⁻² M pilocarpine in rabbits. (From Ref. 67.)

Mechanisms of corneal drug penetration have been studied recently by Grass and coworkers from kinetic [72], ultrastructural [73], and modeling [74] points of view. A model relating the parameters of permeability coefficient in the cornea with partition coefficient and molecular weight of the penetrating species was presented [74]. Their model assumes the availability of a "pore" pathway that was applied to small hydrophilic compounds and assumes that an aqueous diffusional space is available for transport of these compounds. They state that this is in contrast to an alternate "partitioning" mechanism, which is the most probable route of transport for larger or more lipophilic compounds.

This model represents the cornea as a laminated membrane with a lipid layer (epithelium) and an aqueous layer (stroma).

The equation for the permeability coefficient of this laminated membrane is given by:

$$K_{per} = 1/[(L_s/D_s) + L_e/(D_p + PD_e)] \qquad (1)$$

where K_{per} is the permeability coefficient, P is the partition coefficient, L_s and L_e are the thicknesses of stroma and epithelium, respectively, and D_s, D_e, and D_p are the apparent diffusion coefficients for the stroma, lipid epithelium, and the epithelial pores, respectively. The area fractions for the pore and nonpore regions have been included in the apparent diffusion coefficient.

Equation (1) was fit to a data set of approximately 50 molecules, including the published data from steroids [68], beta blockers [69], carbonic anhydrase inhibitors [75], and aniline derivatives [76], where diffusion through pores could be neglected ($D_p = 0$).

Equation (1) can be rearranged to give Eq. (2), when $D_p = 0$

$$K_{per} = \frac{P}{\dfrac{PL_s}{D_s} + \dfrac{L_e}{D_e}} \tag{2}$$

It is apparent from Eq. (2) that the permeability coefficient is linear with P for small partition coefficients and constant for large P. Thus, for small P the epithelium is the barrier and for large P the stroma is the barrier.

The role of molecular size in governing the magnitude of the diffusion coefficient has also been studied. Since the molecular weight dependence of the diffusion coefficients for polymers obeys a power law equation [77], a similar form was chosen by Grass and coworkers [74] for the corneal barriers. That is, the molecular weight dependence of the diffusion coefficients was written as:

$$D_e = D_e^{(0)} M^a \tag{3}$$

and that for the stroma was modeled as:

$$D_s = D_s^{(0)} M^d \tag{4}$$

where M is the molecular weight, a and d are power constants, and $D_e^{(0)}$, $D_s^{(0)}$ are constants obtained from data fitting.

Ocular Drug Delivery Systems

A number of approaches to the delivery of drugs for ocular treatment has been investigated and proposed. These range from simple systems such as aqueous suspensions where the viscosity, and hence the residence time, has been increased by cellulosic polymers to complex systems such as penetration enhancers, external devices (collagen shields, iontophoresis, pumps), ion-exchange resins, liposomes, microspheres/microparticles, polymeric films, inserts, prodrugs, mucoadhesives, and metabolism-based drug design.

The usefulness of penetration enhancers in promoting drug penetration across the cornea was investigated for drugs varying from hydrophilic to lipophilic characteristics [78]. Four purported penetration enhancers were studied. They were Azone (laurocapram), hexamethylenelauramide, hexamethyleneoctanamide, and decylmethylsulfoxide. The hydrophilic drugs tested were acetazolamide, cimetidine, guanethidine, and sulfacetamide. Moderately lipophilic drugs tested were bunolol and prednisolone. Flurbiprofen and its amide analogue were chosen as representative lipophilic drugs. These drugs were tested in the absence or in the presence of various concentrations of Azone. The corneal penetration of hydrophilic compounds was enhanced at least 20-fold at 0.1% Azone concentration. For prednisolone and bunolol, the maximal enhancement was at 0.025% to 0.1% Azone and was marginal (two- to fivefold). However, Azone inhibited rather than enhanced the corneal penetration of lipophilic flurbiprofen and its amide analogue. All four enhancers behaved similarly in enhancing corneal penetration of cimetidine. Corneal penetration enhancers may have clinical benefits in improving ocular drug delivery of hydrophilic compounds with the possibility of reducing the concentration of the drug in the administered dosage forms; however, their utility may depend on their toxicological profiles.

External devices such as collagen shields, iontophoresis, and pumps have been used to deliver ophthalmic medications and to enhance ocular drug delivery [79]. Collagen shields have been used to deliver drugs and promote corneal epithelial healing. The efficacy of collagen shields soaked with drugs was demonstrated in animal models of graft rejection and bacterial keratitis.

There are difficulties associated with the use of corneal shields such as difficulty of insertion and blurred vision. In fact, Kaufman and coworkes [80] report that for patients with conditions requiring chronic rather than acute therapy, the advantages of collagen shields in providing high and sustained levels of drugs and/or lubricants to the cornea are outweighed by the difficulty of insertion of the shield and problem of blurred vision. They developed a delivery system in which collagen pieces suspended in a viscous vehicle can be instilled into the lower forniceal space, thereby simplifying application and reducing blurring of vision. The collagen pieces (Collasomes) can be formulated with various constituents such as antibiotics or cyclosporine, or with chemical alterations such as the inclusion of a lipid (Lacrisome) for treatment of dry eye syndromes. Collasomes hydrated in a solution of fluorescein sodium and suspended in a methylcellulose vehicle produced fluorescein concentrations 17 to 42 times higher in the cornea and 6 to 8 times higher in the aqueous humor compared to fluorescein-containing solution alone. The authors suggest that the fluorescein is used as a model compound for water-soluble drugs. In a controlled clinical study, the authors report that 76% of patients with moderately severe keratoconjunctivitis sicca (KCS) preferred Lacrisomes to the vehicle control because of a more soothing effect and longer duration of comfort. The authors report that all preparations are well tolerated by all study subjects.

Iontophoresis uses an electrical current to carry an ionized drug across tissues. Transcorneal iontophoresis delivers high concentrations of a drug to the anterior segment of the eye. Transcorneal iontophoresis bypasses the lens-iris diaphragm and produces adequate vitreous levels. Pumps deliver fluid to the eye for extended periods of time via a tube with its distal opening in the conjunctival sac, corneal stroma, anterior chamber, or vitreous cavity. Clinical acceptance of the collagen shield for drug delivery to the anterior chamber is better than iontophoresis or pumps probably because the collagen shield is simpler and more convenient to use.

Ion-exchange resin technology was used in enhancing ocular bioavailability of a glaucoma drug in an ophthalmic suspension [81]. This product has been marketed successfully since 1990. According to the authors, the new delivery system involved both binding and release of drug from ion-exchange resin particles. The authors state that the ocular comfort of betaxolol was greatly enhanced by reducing the availability of free drug molecules in the precorneal tear film. The resin concentration was selected to obtain optimum binding of the drug. The zeta potential of the suspended particles was adjusted to produce a flocculated suspension. Drug-resin particles were then incorporated into a structured vehicle containing carbomer (Carbopol 934P, B. F. Goodrich) to enhance physical stability and ease of resuspendibility of the product. The delivery system also optimized the bioavailability of betaxolol, reducing the total drug concentration in half to 0.25% in betaxolol suspension as compared to the 0.5% betaxolol solution dosage form. Increased comfort of the 0.25% betaxolol suspension as well as its bioequivalence in animal models (rabbits) was confirmed in clinical trials.

Liposomes (phospholipid-based vesicles) have been investigated since the early 1970s as a delivery system to various target organs. Because of their structural versatility, liposomes have the potential to be tailor-made for specific targets in the body including the eye. Although the application of liposomes in developing ophthalmic formulations has not been commercially successful, investigations continue in this area. The disposition and pupillary effects of atropine and atropine sulfate in various liposomal formulations were compared to solutions after instillation in rabbit eyes [82]. Atropine entrapped in multilamellar lipid vesicles (MLVs) with positive surface charge displayed the most prolonged effect, lasting up to 12 hours. MLVs with neutral or negative charges maintained the effect for 9 hours; the aqueous solution of atropine was effective for only 7 hours. Preparations containing atropine sulfate displayed a similar pattern, although they were shorter-acting than the corresponding base products. Increased ocular bioavailability of atropine was attributed to enhancement of pulse entry with little evidence of sustained drug release. Barber and Shek [83] investigated the tear-induced release of liposome-entrapped agents. Rabbit tear fluid was shown to promote the release of entrapped 5-carboxy fluorescein and acetylcholinesterase. The authors attribute this destabilization of the liposomes to multifactorial mechanisms. Durrani and coworkers [84] evaluated the bioavailability of pilocarpine nitrate in rabbits from a mucoadhesive liposomal ophthalmic drug delivery system using carbomer 1342 (Carbopol 1342). The in vitro release of pilocarpine was extended by the presence of the polymer coating. The absorbed film was shown to provide a substantial barrier to drug release. Carbomer 1342 coated reversed-phase evaporation vesicles (REVs) showed a larger area under the miotic intensity curve and a longer duration of action compared with uncoated REVs. However, no significant differences were found between the area under miotic intensity curve and duration of action between coated REVs and a phosphate-buffered saline solution containing the same concentration of pilocarpine nitrate.

Microspheres or microparticles are drug-containing small polymeric particles that are suspended in a liquid carrier medium. The microspheres could be erodible or nonerodible. Several approaches have been used to formulate drugs for topical and intraocular drug delivery. Upon administration of the microparticle suspension in the eye, the drug is released into the precorneal tear film by diffusion, chemical reaction, polymer degradation, or ion-exchange [85]. Particles reside in the cul-de-sac of the eye and act as reservoir of the drug. Kinetics of in vitro release and pharmacokinetics of miotic response from gelatin and albumin microspheres of pilocarpine in rabbits has been reported [86]. The microspheres were loaded with an aqueous suspension of pilocarpine nitrate. The drug release was reported to be biphasic by the authors. Prolongation of therapeutic response was observed by comparison to aqueous or viscous solutions of the drug. The calculated pharmacokinetic parameters showed a lag time in the appearance of miosis, prolonged half-life of the input of response, delayed time of the peak response, but an enhanced intensity of the action when colloidal carriers are used. The applicability of a lipid microsphere drug delivery system using a lipid microsphere containing hydrocortisone 17-butyrate-21-propionate [87] was investigated. Tritium-labeled drug suspension was compared to tritium-labeled drug microsphere in rabbit eyes. The lipid microsphere was shown to deliver the drug to anterior ocular tissues more significantly than the aqueous suspension of the drug.

Disposition of dexamethasone in different ocular tissues was investigated following the application of the drug as ocular inserts of different polymer films in comparison to the suspension dosage form [88]. The disposition of dexamethasone in corneal tissue, which was rather poor relative to the conjunctiva and iris-ciliary body in the case of the suspension, was markedly enhanced through the application of the drug as films. Both Eudragit and cellulose acetate phthalate based films enhanced the disposition of the drug in aqueous humor at specific time intervals. Release of pilocarpine and salts of pilocarpine from compression-molded films was studied as delivery systems [89]. It was found that the choice of salt and molecular weight of hydroxypropyl cellulose significantly affected drug release. Pilocarpine hydrochloride was released faster than pilocarpine nitrate when the highest molecular weight grade of hydroxypropyl cellulose was used. Similarly, Saettone and coworkers [90] studied the release characteristics of pilocarpine nitrate from polymeric ophthalmic inserts coated with a mixture of Eudragit RL and RS prepared by extrusion. The release of the drug was evaluated in vitro and by measuring the miosis produced in rabbits. As expected, the coated inserts released the drug over an extended period of time compared to uncoated inserts. The uncoated inserts released 50% of the drug within 30 minutes, whereas the coated inserts released 50% of the drug in 3 to 5 hours depending on the type of material and thickness. Miosis in rabbits was observed over a 9- to 10-hour period with coated inserts compared to uncoated inserts, which showed no sustained-release characteristics as expected.

Patient acceptance of novel ophthalmic delivery systems (NODS) has been studied in Germany by Diestelhorst and coworkers [91]. NODS are ocular inserts of polymeric films containing drugs. Patients were asked to compare the ocular irritation of NODS with Isopto Naturale, an isotonic buffered tear-substitute product. The results indicated that in healthy volunteers NODS are not as well tolerated as conventional eyedrops when compared for ocular discomfort. However, NODS have a potential advantage in situations where a drug is unstable in aqueous media and the presence of an antimicrobial preservative is not desirable.

Stella and coworkers [92] investigated the sustained delivery of methylprednisolone from ocular inserts made of gellan gum (Gelrite). They compared the release of drug from films containing gellan covalently bound to methylprednisolone, gellan films with physical entrapment of methylprednisolone, and methylprednisolone suspended in a gellan dispersion in water in rabbits and in in vitro models. Results indicated that in vitro, the gellan-methylprednisolone films released the drug in a zero-order pattern. Compared with the suspension, the films yielded a four-times higher area under the tear fluid concentration versus time curve but showed a tendency to slip out of the eye because of a high degree of swelling. It was concluded by the authors that gellan-based drug delivery systems may be used to increase the residence time of methylprednisolone in the tear fluid.

The use of an absorbable gelatin sponge (Gelfoam) was investigated as an ocular drug delivery system by incorporating pilocarpine [93]. Prolonged in vitro release of pilocarpine was achieved through modification of the device by embedding a retardant to occlude the interstices in the Gelfoam matrix remaining after embedding the drug. Cetyl ester wax and polyethylene glycol 400 monostearate were evaluated as retardants by the authors. The device embedded with cetyl ester wax released pilocarpine in a zero-order pattern. The device impregnated with polyethylene glycol 400 monostearate exhibited anomalous drug transport. The absorption of water by this retardant and the formation of a gel layer on the surface slowed the penetration of the release medium into the deeper sections of the matrix, as well as the rapid outward diffusion of the drug, resulting in a prolonged release of pilocarpine.

Hydrogels of varying proportions of polyethylene glycol (PEG) 200 in polyvinyl alcohol (PVA) were examined as ocular inserts for sustained delivery of gentamicin [94]. Uniform sections of the PEG-PVA gel films were mounted in a modified diffusion cell containing isotonic phosphate buffer at 37°C. Release of gentamicin was monitored for up to 6 days. In vitro diffusion studies showed that 20% to 90% of the drug was released at the end of the study (144 hours) depending on PEG content, which ranged from 0% to 15% by volume—which increased with increasing PEG content. PVA with low concentrations of PEG or no PEG exhibited an initial lag period of up to 48 hours before a drug burst release of approximately 24 hours. Higher PEG concentrations in the PVA matrix reduced the lag periods.

Another approach was the formation of hydrogels in situ as delivery systems [95]. Aqueous compositions containing polymers that exhibit reversible phase transitions are reported to form gels in situ depending on the pH, temperature, and ionic strength of the environment. An aqueous solution containing 1.5% methylcellulose and 0.3% carbomer was found to form a gel under simulated physiological conditions of the eye. Such a system offers the convenience of delivering drops to the eye from a bottle; the drops turn into a gel on mixing with the tear fluid with a potential for increased residence time in the eye and increased ocular bioavailability.

Dipivefrin, a dipivalyl derivative of epinephrine, a prodrug, has been on the market for several years. Prodrug approach is beneficial in some cases where the drug might not be sufficiently stable or bioavailable, or has similar undesirable physicochemical properties. Four lipophilic derivatives of a beta blocker (tilisolol hydrochloride) were synthesized and evaluated for ocular delivery as prodrugs [96]. Results indicated that all prodrug candidates were gradually hydrolyzed to tilisolol in a pH 7.4 buffer solution and showed rapid enzymatic conversion to tilisolol in ocular tissue homogenates. Once converted to tilisolol, the penetration of the drug was enhanced through the corneal, conjunctival, and scleral membranes.

Saettone and coworkers [97] evaluated a series of low-viscosity polyanionic natural or semisynthetic polymers containing either cyclopentolate or pilocarpine in albino rabbits. Small but significant increases of the areas under activity versus time curves were found with some polymeric complexes. The authors believe that there is mucoadhesion with these polymers.

There are two major novel metabolism-based drug design concepts proposed by Bodor [98] that have significant advantages when used in the design of safe, specific ophthalmic drugs. According to Bodor, one is based on predictable enzymatic activation processes by enzymes found at the site of action, for example, the iris-ciliary body. The second major retrometabolic design involves a "soft drug" approach. Among the soft drug design strategies, Bodor states that the "inactive metabolite" and the "soft analog" approaches are the most useful for designing safe and selective ophthalmic drugs. In the first case, the design process starts with a known or predicted inactive metabolite of the drug. This inactive metabolite is then structurally modified in the "chemical activation" stage to the soft drug, which is isosteric and/or isoelectronic with the drug to produce the pharmacological activity at the target receptor sites. By design, however, the soft drug is also subject to a facile, predictable metabolism leading in one step to the starting inactive metabolite. Generally, this is accomplished by hydrolysis. Successful use of this general concept has led to soft beta blockers as antiglaucoma agents, short-acting anticholinergic agents (mydriatics), and corticosteroids (anti-inflammatory agents). The corticosteroids, because of their unique design, do not elevate intraocular pressure (IOP) and do not produce other systemic and local side effects, according to the author.

Chemical and physical instability, difficulties in manufacturing sterile products on a large scale, potential eye irritation by these external devices and lipid-based vehicles might have contributed to some of the reasons for the limited success of many of the liposome, microspheres, and other delivery systems.

The major task remaining for corneal penetration studies is to relate the in vitro data to the in vivo experiments. A considerable amount of in vivo experimental work remains to be done, however, before a sufficient database exists to build adequate predictive models from molecular properties such as partition coefficient and molecular size. When such data become available, good models should be forthcoming, and the design of molecules for improved corneal penetration will become much easier.

VI. COMMONLY USED RAW MATERIALS

A. Potential Actives

Drugs used for the topical treatment of various ocular diseases may be classified as follows:

1. Antiglaucoma drugs
2. Miotics
3. Mydriatics
4. Cycloplegics
5. Anti-inflammatory agents
6. Anti-infectives
7. Diagnostic agents
8. Miscellaneous drugs

It is beyond the scope of this book to present an in-depth discussion of these drugs. The reader is referred to textbooks on ocular pharmacology [99–101].

Glaucoma is a disease characterized by ocular hypertension and progressive visual loss that could result in blindness due to damage to the optic nerve and retina. Drugs used in controlling glaucoma by topical administration are pilocarpine, carbachol, echothiophate, demecarium, and beta blockers such as betaxolol, timolol, or bunolol. Osmotic agents such as 50% glycerine, 45% isosorbide in water or carbonic anhydrase inhibitors such as acetazolamide, methazolamide, or dichlorophenamide are administered orally for relieving intraocular pressure.

Miotics, such as pilocarpine and carbachol, reduce the pupil size by contraction of the iris sphincter muscles. In addition to their use in the treatment of glaucoma, they are also used, as is acetylcholine chloride, to reverse the mydriasis (dilation of the pupil) produced for diagnostic purposes or for surgical procedures to remove cataracts and subsequent implantation of intraocular lenses. Atropine, homatropine, scopolamine, tropicamide, and cyclopentolate are drugs that possess parasympathomimetic activity with both mydriasis and cycloplegia. Epinephrine and phenylephrine are drugs belonging to the class of drugs known as sympathomimetics having only mydriatic action. Cycloplegics are drugs that block the loss of accommodation of pupil size.

Corticosteroids are indicated for treating ocular inflammations. The concentration of the steroid chosen as an anti-inflammatory agent depends on the potency of the steroid and the ocular tissue that is inflamed. High-potency steroids such as prednisolone acetate, fluorometholone acetate, fluorometholone, and dexamethasone are used for inflammatory conditions of the uveal tract in concentrations ranging from 0.1% to 1.0%. Medrysone and hydrocortisone are steroids that have a lower potency and hence are used in mild ocular inflammations.

Anti-infective agents such as quinolones, tobramycin, gentamicin, neomycin, chloramphenicol, and polymyxin are used to treat ocular infections with a potential for severe ocular damage, such as loss of cornea. For less severe infections of the eye, such as conjunctivitis or blepharitis, sulfacetamide and sulfisoxazole are usually administered.

Because ocular infections and inflammations occur simultaneously in many cases, several commercial products are available as combinations of anti-infective and anti-inflammatory agents. In the latter case, the efficacy of these combination products is recognized by the Food and Drug Administration.

Very few drugs are available for combating fungal and viral infections of the eye. Idoxuridine has been shown to be useful against herpes simplex viral infections of the cornea. Erythromycin, chloramphenicol, and tetracyclines are used to control secondary infections caused by bacteria in viral infections such as trachoma. Superficial fungal keratitis is treated with the antifungal antibiotic natamycin and with nystatin.

Sodium fluorescein is administered as a diagnostic agent topically to determine whether the corneal epithelium is intact or not and intravenously for angiography and angioscopy of the retina, fundus, and of the iris vasculature.

Local anesthetics such as tetracaine, proparacaine, and benoxinate are used for inducing local anesthesia before certain diagnostic procedures.

B. Inactives in Ophthalmic Suspensions and Gelled Systems

Pharmacologically and therapeutically inactive ingredients such as buffers, stabilizers, surfactants, viscosity-increasing agents, and osmolality adjusters are used in formulating ophthalmic gel systems and suspensions. Coloring and flavoring agents are not permitted in ophthalmic products. The choice and the concentration of inactive ingredients depend on physical and chemical compatibilities and freedom from ocular irritation.

1. *Buffering and pH Adjustment*

The chemical stability of many ophthalmic drugs is controlled by the pH of the gel or suspension. It is particularly important to minimize drug product decomposition to obtain adequate shelf-life stability.

In addition to maximizing the chemical stability of the active ingredient(s), the comfort of ophthalmic suspensions is also influenced by the pH. Patient compliance is greatly enhanced when the products are very comfortable on instillation into the eyes. Comfort is usually identified by the lack of stinging, burning, or foreign body sensation upon instillation. Eye care products that produce ocular irritation lead to reflex tearing, which, in turn, will speed up the drainage of the ophthalmic dosage form and decrease bioavailability. The pH of ophthalmic gel systems and suspensions should be targeted to 7.4 ± 0.1, which is the pH of normal tears, to cause the least amount of disruption to the natural buffer system of the tear fluid. A suitable buffer system (e.g., borate, phosphate, citrate, bicarbonate, or acetate) is selected, such that it is compatible with the drug substance and the other components of the formulation. Ocular irritation potential is dependent on the pH of the product, type (weak or strong), and concentration of buffer chosen, and the nature of the drug substance itself. The buffer system selected should provide sufficient buffer capacity to maintain the pH of the product within the specified limits during its shelf-life storage but also allow the tear fluid to adjust the pH of the product to physiologic range upon instillation in the eye.

In general, buffer concentrations range from 50 to 200 millimolar; most frequently, below 100 millimolar. In the case of drug substances that are weak acids or bases, the intrinsic buffer capacity is adequate without additional buffers.

Selection of the buffer system to be used also depends on the pH at which the drug substance is optimally stable and soluble. The buffer system chosen should have a pK_a as close to the target pH as possible or practical because buffer capacity is maximum when pH is equal to pK_a. If one examines the Henderson-Hasselbalch equation for a weak acid,

$$pH = pK_a + \log \frac{[salt]}{[acid]}$$

maximum buffer capacity occurs when the concentrations of the salt and acid are equal. This is the case when the weak acid is 50% ionized or dissociated.

It follows that when the concentrations are equal,

$$\log \frac{[salt]}{[acid]} = \log 1$$

and since $\log 1 = 0$, $pH = pK_a$.

It is important to evaluate the effect of buffers on the stability of drugs because buffers can act as general acid or base catalysts causing degradation of drugs. Tears have some intrinsic buffer capacity, and it is likely that they can change the pH of the instilled product quickly to physiologic range if the buffer capacity of the product administered is low. In some instances, the pH of the products is formulated outside of the physiologic range for reasons of enhancing stability (e.g., pilocarpine and epinephrine) or solubility (weak acids or bases).

2. Stabilizers

Stabilizers are primarily antioxidants, used in ophthalmic formulations to retard the degradation of drugs such as epinephrine and phenylephrine, which are susceptible to oxidative degradation. The most commonly used antioxidants in ophthalmic dosage forms are sodium bisulfite or metabisulfite. Other antioxidants used are acetylcysteine, ascorbic acid, sodium thiosulfate, and 8-hydroxyquinoline. These antioxidants are used up to 0.3% level to provide adequate shelf-life stability. These agents are oxidized preferentially instead of the active component. Disodium edetate is used in many ophthalmic formulations to chelate metal ions that catalyze redox reactions.

3. Surfactants

Surfactants are used in relatively low concentrations to disperse drugs such as steroids in formulating ophthalmic suspensions. The surfactant selected should be free from potential for causing ocular irritation and toxicity. Nonionic surfactants are less toxic than cationic or anionic surfactants. Anionic surfactants act essentially like soaps upon instillation in the eye, producing severe ocular irritation. Cationic surfactants are less irritating than anionic surfactants. The concentration of surfactants in ophthalmic suspensions should be chosen at the lowest possible level, because surfactants are known to bind to preservatives and decrease their antimicrobial preservative effectiveness. Polysorbate 80, polysorbate 20, tyloxapol, polyoxyethylene fatty acid esters, and poloxamers are some of the commonly used surfactants in formulating ophthalmic suspension. In general, surfactants are used in concentrations ranging from 0.01% to 0.20%, with 0.1% being the usual concentration.

4. Viscosity-Increasing Agents

Polyvinyl alcohol, methylcellulose, hydroxypropyl methylcellulose, hydroxyethylcellulose and one of the several high molecular weight cross-linked polymers of acrylic acid known as carbomers [102] are commonly used to increase the viscosity of ophthalmic solutions and suspensions. Although these agents reduce surface tension significantly, their primary benefit is to increase the ocular contact time, thereby decreasing the drainage rate and increasing drug bioavailability. A secondary benefit of the polymer solutions is a lubricating effect that is largely subjective but noticeable to many patients. One disadvantage to the use of the polymers is their tendency to dry to a film on the eyelids and eyelashes; however, this can be easily removed by wiping with a damp tissue.

Numerous studies have shown that increasing the viscosity of ophthalmic products increases contact time and pharmacological effect, but there is a plateau reached where further increases in viscosity produce only slight or no increases in effect. Blaugh and Canada [103], using methylcellulose solutions, found increased contact time in rabbits up to 25 cp (centipoise) and a leveling off at 55 cp. Lynn and Jones [104] studied the rate of lacrimal excretion in humans using a dye solution in methylcellulose concentration from 0.25% to 2.5%, corresponding to viscosities of 6 to 30,000 cp, the latter being a thick gel. The results were as shown in the following tabulation.

Methylcellulose concentration	Time to dye appearance through nasolacrimal duct
0.0%	60 seconds
0.25%	90 seconds
0.50%	140 seconds
1.00%	210 seconds
2.50%	255 seconds

Chrai and Robinson [105] conducted studies in rabbits and found that over a range of 1.0 to 12.5 cp viscosity there is a threefold decrease in the drainage rate constant and a further threefold decrease over the viscosity range of 12.5 to 100 cp. This decrease in drainage rate increased the concentration of drug in the precorneal tear film at zero time and subsequent time periods, which resulted in a higher aqueous humor drug concentration. The magnitude of aqueous humor drug concentration increase was smaller than the increase in viscosity, about 1.7 times, for the range 1.0 to 12.5 cp and only a further 1.2-fold increase at 100 cp.

Because direct determination of ophthalmic bioavailability in humans is not possible without endangering the eye, investigators have used fluorescein to study factors affecting bioavailability: penetration of fluorescein can be quantitated in humans through the use of a slit-lamp fluorophotometer. Adler et al. [106], using this technology, found only small increases in dye penetration over a wide range of viscosities. The use of fluorescein data to extrapolate vehicle effects to ophthalmic drugs in general would be questionable because of the large differences in chemical structure, properties, and permeability existing between fluorescein and a majority of ophthalmic drugs.

The major commercial viscous vehicles are hydroxypropyl methylcellulose (Isopto) and polyvinyl alcohol (Liquifilm). Isopto products most often use 0.5% of the cellulosic and range from 10 to 30 cp in viscosity. Liquifilm products have viscosities of about 4 to 6 cp and use 1.4% polymer.

Carbomer 940 is used in a commercial ophthalmic gel product containing pilocarpine to provide a once-a-day application at bedtime. The carbomer is used in the formulation to produce a viscous gel that contributes to the prolonged availability of the drug. Comparative rheological studies were conducted on four types of carbomer viscous solutions at concentrations ranging from 0.01% to 0.025% [107]. The authors studied the effects of autoclaving, tonicity agents, and storage on rheological behavior. Carbomers 940, 941, and 910 had better thickening properties than carbomer 934. Sterilization data demonstrated that autoclaving was convenient for all types of carbomers studied. Mannitol was the most suitable tonicity adjusting agent. The authors concluded that carbomers 940, 941, and 910 are suitable for ophthalmic use, with carbomer 940 showing the best appearance and clarity.

5. Osmolarity-Adjusting Agents

In addition to selecting the optimum pH range and buffer system, it is important to adjust the tonicity (osmolarity) of ophthalmic products such as solutions, suspensions, and gels to minimize discomfort upon instillation in the eye. The word tonicity refers to the effect solutions have on maintaining the "tone" of red blood cells (erythrocytes) and tissues on prolonged contact with these solutions. The term tonicity has been used in medical practice for many years. A solution is said to be isotonic if red blood cells maintain their tone or shape in it. Isotonic solutions exert the same osmotic pressure as most body fluids. Both fluids such as blood plasma and lacrimal fluid normally exert an osmotic pressure corresponding to that of 0.9% w/v solution of sodium chloride. Solutions containing the equivalent of 0.9% w/v sodium chloride are said to be isotonic with respect to the red blood cells.

The terms isotonic and tonicity should always be used when referring to physiologic fluids. The term isosmotic refers to the physical property of the solution comparing the osmotic pressure of two fluids, neither one being physiologic.

Solutions containing significantly less than 0.9% sodium chloride are referred to as hypotonic solutions and exert less osmotic pressure. Red blood cells will swell and may burst (hemolysis) as the result of diffusion of water into cells when placed in hypotonic solutions. Solutions containing significantly more than 0.9% sodium chloride are called hypertonic solutions and will cause diffusion of water out of the red blood cells leading to shrinkage (crenation).

Classification of solutions based on their observed effects on red blood cells is not very practical in formulating products unless one can quantitate these tonicity values. The term osmol is used to express quantitatively the osmotic properties of aqueous solutions, suspensions, and gels. Measurement of tonicity is based on the colligative properties of solutions. Freezing point depression and boiling point elevation are generally used to measure the tonicity. An osmol is defined as the weight of a solute in grams existing in solution as molecules that is osmotically equivalent to the gram molecular weight of an ideally behaving nonelectrolyte. It is also defined as the amount of solute that will produce one Avogadro number, 6.02×10^{23} particles in solution. Thus, the osmol weight of a nonelectrolyte is equal to its gram molecular weight in dilute solutions.

Osmolality and osmolarity are terms used to express the tonicity values of solutions. Tonicity values are expressed as milliosmols rather than osmols for convenience. One can draw the analogy between osmolality/osmolarity relationship with molality/molarity relationship for solutions. An osmolal solution reflects a weight-to-weight relationship between the solute and the solvent. A solution has an osmolal concentration of one when it contains 1 osmol or 1000 milliosmols of solute per kilogram of water. Because osmolality is a weight-to-weight expression, the concentration of the solution is not influenced by temperature changes and one can get a more precise measurement of the colligative properties. On the other hand, osmolar solutions reflect a weight-to-volume relationship between solute and solvent. Thus, a solution has an osmolar concentration of one when it contains 1 osmol or 1000 milliosmols of solute per liter of solution. The two terms, osmolality and osmolarity, have been used interchangeably although they represent w/w versus w/v relationships. In dilute solutions, the error introduced by interchanging the two terms is not significant. However, in concentrated solutions, the error may become significant.

Osmolarity may be computed to obtain a theoretical value by using one of the following equations, if one knows the concentration, molecular weight, and—for electrolytes—the number of ions that it dissociates into, for each of the solutes in a formulation:

For nonelectrolytes:

$$\text{mOsm/liter} = \frac{\text{Concentration in g/L}}{\text{Molecular weight in g}} \times 1000$$

and for strong electrolytes:

$$\text{mOsm/liter} = \frac{\text{Concentration in g/L}}{\text{Molecular weight in g}} \times \text{number of ions formed} \times 1000$$

This is a rather simplistic approach that does not take into account the interparticle interactions and the degree of dissociation. Because of the complex nature of ophthalmic formulations, it is much easier, first, to prepare a formulation without osmolarity-adjusting agents and then measure the osmolality.* This is then followed by adusting the osmolality upward to isoosmotic value by adding the required quantity of an osmolarity adjusting agent. Subsequent lots are then manufactured with the osmolarity-adjusting agent incorporated into the formulation. Sometimes formulations will be hypertonic even without adding any osmolarity-adjusting agent because of the concentration of the drug substance required for therapeutic reasons. In such cases of hypertonic formulations, the potential ocular irritation and discomfort may be minimized by using the lowest possible concentrations of the other inactive ingredients in the formulations.

The reader is referred to other excellent publications for detailed discussions on osmotic pressure, osmolarity, osmolality, tonicity, and so forth [108–110].

6. Vehicles

Ophthalmic suspensions and gel systems are primarily water-based products. In the case of drugs that are not stable in an aqueous vehicle, nonaqueous vehicles such as vegetable oils, liquid petrolatum, and petrolatum are used. The oils used in preparing ophthalmic

---

*Freezing Point Method. Advanced Digimatic, Model 3 D-II or Advanced Microosmomoter, Model 3 MO. Both commercially available from Advanced Instruments, Inc., Needham Heights, MA 02194. Vapor Pressure Method. Vapor Pressure Osmometer, Wescor, Inc., Logan, Utah 84321.

products should be of the highest purity, similar to the vehicles used for parenteral administration. However, it is important to evaluate the ocular comfort of these products containing nonaqueous vehicles.

7. Packaging

Ophthalmic solution and suspension dosage forms have been packaged almost entirely in plastic dropper bottles since the introduction of the Drop-Tainer plastic dispenser in the 1950s. A few products still remain in glass dropper bottles because of special stability considerations. The main advantage of the Drop-Tainer and similarly designed plastic dropper bottles are convenience of usage by the patient, decreased contamination potential, lower weight, and lower cost. The plastic bottle has the dispensing tip as an integral part of the package. The patient simply removes the cap and turns the bottle upside down and squeezes gently to form a single drop that falls into the eye. The dispensing tip can be designed to deliver only one drop or a stream of fluid for irrigation, depending on the pressure applied. When used properly, the solution remaining in the bottle is only minimally exposed to airborne contaminants during administration and thus will maintain very low to nonexistent microbial content as compared with the old-style glass bottle with separate dropper assembly.

The plastic bottle and dispensing tip is made of low-density polyethylene (LDPE) resin, which provides the necessary flexibility and inertness. Because these components are in contact with the product during its shelf life, they must be carefully chosen and tested for their suitability for ophthalmic use. In addition to stability studies on the product in the container over a range of normal and accelerated temperatures, the plastic resins must pass the USP biological and chemical tests for suitability. The LDPE resins used have been found to be compatible with a very wide range of drugs and formulation components. Their disadvantages are their sorption and permeability characteristics. Volatile ingredients such as the preservatives chlorobutanol and phenylethyl alcohol can migrate into the plastic and eventually permeate through the walls of the container. The sorption and permeation can be detected by stability studies if it is significant. If the permeating component is a preservative, a repeat test of the preservative effectiveness with time will determine if the loss is significant. If necessary, a safe and reasonable excess of the permeable component may be added to balance the loss over the shelf life. Another means of overcoming permeation effects is to utilize a secondary package such as a peel-apart blister or pouch composed of nonpermeable materials (e.g., aluminum foil or vinyl). The plastic dropper bottles are also permeable to water, but weight loss by water vapor transmission has a decreasing significance as the size of the bottle increases. The consequences of water vapor transmission must be taken into consideration when assessing the stability of a product, and appropriate corrections for loss of water on the analysis of components must be applied. Because the LDPE resins are translucent, additional package protection may be required if the drug is light sensitive. This can be achieved by using a resin containing an opacifying agent such as titanium dioxide, by placing an opaque sleeve over the exterior of the container, or by placing the bottle in a cardboard carton. Extremely light-sensitive drugs such as epinephrine and proparacaine may require a combination of these protective measures. Colorants other than titanium dioxide are rarely used in plastic ophthalmic containers; however, the use of colorants is common for the cap for a very important purpose. Red is used to denote a mydriatic drug such as atropine, and green a miotic drug like pilocarpine. This is an aid to the physician and the dispensing pharmacist to prevent potentially serious mistakes. The pharmacist should dispense the ophthalmic product only in the original unopened container. A tamper-evidence feature such as a cellulose or metal band around the cap and bottle neck is provided by the manufacturer.

The LDPE resin used for the bottle and the dispensing tip cannot be autoclaved and they are sterilized either by [^{60}Co] gamma irradiation or ethylene oxide. The cap is designed such that when it is screwed tightly onto the bottle, it mates with the dispensing tip and forms a seal. The cap is usually made of a harder resin than the bottle, such as polystyrene or polypropylene, and is also sterilized by gamma radiation or ethylene oxide gas exposure.

A special plastic ophthalmic package has been introduced that uses a special grade of polypropylene that is resistant to deformation at autoclave temperatures. With this specialized packaging the bottle can be filled, the dispensing tip and cap applied, and the entire product sterilized by steam under pressure at 121°C.

The glass dropper bottle is still used for products that are extremely sensitive to oxygen or contain permeable components that are not sufficiently stable in plastic. Powders for reconstitution also utilize glass containers because of their heat transfer characteristics, which are necessary during the freeze-drying process. The glass used should be USP type I for maximum compatibility with the sterilization process and the product. The glass container is made sterile by dry-heat or steam autoclave sterilization., Amber glass is used for light resistance and is superior to green glass. A sterile dropper assembly is usually supplied separately. It is usually gas-sterilized in a blister composed of vinyl and Tyvek, a fused, porous polypropylene material. The dropper assembly is made of a glass or LDPE plastic pipette and a rubber dropper bulb. The manufacturer carefully tests the appropriate plastic and rubber materials suitable for use with the product, and therefore they should be dispensed with the product. The pharmacist should aseptically place the dropper assembly in the product before dispensing it and instruct the patient on precautions to be used to prevent contamination.

Ophthalmic ointments are packaged in small collapsible tin tubes usually holding 3.5 g. The pure tin tube has been found to be compatible with a wide range of drugs in petrolatum-based ointments. Aluminum tubes have been considered and may eventually be used because of their lower cost and as an alternative should the supply of tin become a problem. Until internal coating technology for these tubes advances, the aluminum tube will be a secondary packaging choice. Plastic tubes made from flexible LDPE resins have also been considered as an alternative material but do not collapse and tend to suck-back the ointment. Plastic tubes recently introduced as containers for toothpaste have been investigated and may offer the best alternative to tin. These tubes are laminates of plastic and various materials such as paper, foil, and so on. A tube can be designed by selection of the laminate materials and their arrangement and thickness to provide the necessary compatibility, stability, and barrier properties. The various types of metal tubes are sealed using an adhesive coating covering only the inner edges of the bottom of the open tube to form the crimp, which does not contact the product. Laminated tubes are usually heat-sealed. The crimp usually contains the lot code and expiration date. Filled tubes may be tested for leaks by storing them in a horizontal position in an oven at 60°C for at least 8 hours. No leakage should be evidenced except for a minute quantity that could come only from within the crimp of the tube or the end of the cap. The screw cap is made of polyethylene or polypropylene. Polypropylene must be used for autoclave sterilization, but either material may be used when the tubes are gas-sterilized. A tamper-evident feature is required for sterile ophthalmic ointments; this may be accomplished by sealing the tube or the carton holding the tube such that the contents cannot be used without providing visible evidence of destruction of the seal. The Teledyne Wirz tube used by most manufacturers has a flange on the cap that is visible only after the tube has been opened the first time.

The tube can be a source of metal particles and must be cleaned carefully prior to sterilization. The USP contains a test procedure and limits the level of metal particles in ophthalmic ointments. The total number of metal particles detected under 30 times magnification that are 50 μm or greater in any dimension is counted. The requirements are met if the total number of such particles counted in 10 tubes is not more than 50, and if not more than one tube is found to contain more than eight such particles.

C. Inactives in Ophthalmic Ointments

Ophthalmic ointments are prepared from oleaginous bases composed of white petrolatum, mineral oil, and a special liquid petrolatum/polyethylene base. Most ophthalmic ointments are suspension ointments in which the drug is suspended in a simple non-aqueous base; however, a few are marketed as emulsion-based ointments. Dispersing agents such as anhydrous lanolin, lanolin, polyoxyl 40 stearate, polyethylene glycol 300, polyethylene glycol 400, cetyl alcohol, and glyceryl monostearate are used to disperse the microfine powdered drug substances into the ointment base. Antimicrobial preservatives used in preserving ophthalmic ointments are methylparaben, propylparaben, phenylethyl alcohol, phenylmercuric acetate, and chlorobutanol. The antimicrobial preservatives are indicated for products packaged in multidose containers to prevent microbial growth should the product become contaminated during patient use. Ophthalmic ointments that contain broad-spectrum antimicrobial agents may be formulated without added preservatives, provided the product passes a simulated patient in-use test or an appropriate microbial challenge test for control of microbial growth. For products made with nonaqueous (anhydrous) bases, the United States Pharmacopeia (USP) states that a suitable antimicrobial preservative effectiveness test may be feasible only at a particular stage in manufacture [42].

The USP also provides for microbial limit tests for the estimation of the number of viable aerobic microorganisms and for freedom from designated microbial species in raw materials, in-process bulk, and finished product when the presence of such microorganisms poses a health and safety hazard.

VII. MANUFACTURING CONSIDERATIONS

Because the official compendia require all topical ophthalmic medications to be sterile, the manufacturer of such medications must consider all current approaches to the manufacture of sterile pharmaceuticals in designing a manufacturing procedure for sterile ophthalmic pharmaceutical ointments, gel systems, and suspensions. It is quite rare that the composition or the packaging of the ophthalmic pharmaceutical will lend itself to terminal sterilization, the simplest form of manufacture of sterile products. Only a few of those drugs formulated in simple aqueous vehicles are stable to normal autoclaving temperatures and times (121°C for 30 minutes); such drugs are packaged in glass or other heat deformation–resistant packaging and thus can be sterilized in this manner.

Most ophthalmic ointments, gel systems, and suspensions, however, do *not* fall into the foregoing category. In general, the active principle is not particularly stable either physically or chemically on heating. Further, to impart viscosity, aqueous products are generally formulated with the inclusion of high molecular weight polymers, which may likewise be adversely affected by heat physically and/or chemically. Lastly, the convenience of plastic dispensing bottles has led to the use of heat-deformable polyolefin packaging. Polyolefins of higher molecular weight, however, are beginning to emerge as autoclavable packaging.

Because of these product sensitivities, most ophthalmic pharmaceutical products are aseptically manufactured and filled into previously sterilized containers in aseptic environments using aseptic filling and capping techniques. This is the case for ophthalmic suspensions, gel systems, and ointments; and rather specialized technology is involved in their manufacture. In the case of suspensions, the drug substance to be suspended must be sterile when introduced into the aseptic manufacturing scheme. This will require that the insoluble (or sparingly soluble) drug substance be *presterilized* via a validated procedure using dry heat, steam under pressure, ethylene oxide gas, or ionizing radiation. These sterilization methods are described in detail with appropriate performance criteria in USP 23. Alternatively, it may be dissolved into organic solvents and filtered through inert, sterilizing microporous membranes into a sterile receiver and thereafter be aseptically precipitated from solution and maintained in a sterile condition through subsequent filtration and drying. When validated, these processes may be used to yield a sterile solid for aseptic incorporation into the manufacturing procedure. In general, however, the manufacture of sterile ophthalmic pharmaceutical products requires special attention to environment, manufacturing techniques, raw materials (including packaging components), and equipment. These will be dealt with individually herein for those products that cannot be terminally sterilized.

A. Environment

Aside from drug safety, stability, and efficacy, the major design criteria of ophthalmic ointments, gel systems, or suspensions is the additional safety criteria of sterility and freedom from extraneous foreign particulate matter. Current United States standards for good manufacturing practices (GMPs) provide for the use of specially designed, environmentally controlled areas for the manufacture of sterile large- and small-volume injectables for terminal sterilization. These environmentally controlled areas must meet the requirements of Class 100,000 space in all areas where open containers and closures are *not* exposed, or where product filling and capping operations are *not* taking place. Where open container and closures are exposed, or where product filling and capping operations are taking place, these areas must meet the requirements of Class 100 space [111]. As defined in Federal Standard 209, Class 100,000 and Class 100 spaces contain 100,000 and 100 particles, respectively, per cubic foot of air of a diameter of 0.5 μm or larger. Often, these design criteria are coupled with laminar airflow concepts [112,113]. This specification deals with total particle counts and does not differentiate between viable and nonviable particles. It should be kept in mind that Federal Standard 209 was promulgated as a "hardware" or mechanical specification for the aerospace industry and has found applications in the pharmaceutical industry as a tool for the design of aseptic and particle-free environments. Class 100,000 conditions can be achieved in the conventionally designed clean room where proper filtration of air supply and adequate volume turnover rates are provided. Class 100 conditions over open containers and over microbiological sampling sites can be achieved with properly sized HEPA (high efficiency particulate air) filtered laminar airflow sources. Depending on the product needs and funds available, some aseptic pharmaceutical manufacturing environments have been designed totally to Class 100 laminar flow specifications, although during actual product manufacture the generation of particulate matter by equipment, product, and (most importantly) people may cause these environments to demonstrate particulate matter levels two or more orders of magnitude greater than design. It is for this reason that specialists in the design of pharmaceutical manufacturing and hospital operating room environments are beginning to view these environments not from the standpoint of total particles per cubic foot or space *alone*, but from the standpoint of the ratio of viable to nonviable particles [114]. Such environmental concepts as *mass air transfer* may lead to meaningful specifications for the space in which a nonterminally sterilized product can be manufactured with confidence when properly validated [115].

When dealing with the environment in which a sterile product is manufactured, the materials used for construction of the facility, as well as personnel attire, training, and conduct in the space, and the entrance and egress of personnel, equipment, packaging, and product all bear heavily on the assurance of product sterility and minimization of extraneous foreign particulate matter. Walls, ceilings, and floors should be constructed of materials that are hard, nonchipping or nonflaking, smooth, and unaffected by surface cleaning agents and disinfectants. All lights and windows should be flush mounted in walls and ceilings for ease of cleaning and disinfection. Ultraviolet lamps may be provided in recessed, flush-mounted fixtures to maintain surface disinfection; however, their use may be difficult to validate and may lead clean-room personnel into a false sense of security as regards clean-room techniques. Separate entrances for personnel and equipment should be provided through specially designed air locks that are maintained at a negative pressure relative to the aseptic manufacturing area and at a positive pressure relative to nonenvironmentally controlled areas. Equipment should be designed for simplicity of operation and should be constructed for ease of disassembly, cleaning, and sterilization or sanitization.

The importance of personnel training and behavior cannot be overemphasized in the maintenance of an acceptable environment for the manufacture of sterile ophthalmic products or sterile pharmaceutical agents in general. Personnel should be trained in the proper mode of gowning with sterile, nonshedding garments, and also in the proper techniques and conduct for aseptic manufacturing. For the maximum in personnel comfort and to minimize sloughing of epidermal cells and hair, the environment should be maintained between 68 and 72°F and between 45% and 60% relative humidity.

B. Manufacturing Techniques

In general, and to contrast with the subject matter of this chapter, aqueous ophthalmic *solutions* are manufactured by methodology that calls for the dissolution of the active ingredient and all or a portion of the excipients into all or a portion of the water, and the sterilization of this solution by heat or by sterilizing filtration through sterile depth or membrane filter media into a sterile receptacle. If incomplete at this point, this sterile solution is then mixed with the additional required sterile components, such as previously sterilized solutions of viscosity-imparting agents or preservatives, and the batch is brought to final volume with additional sterile water.

Aqueous ophthalmic *suspensions* are handled in much the same manner, except that prior to bringing the batch to final volume with additional sterile water, the solid to be suspended is previously rendered sterile by heat, by exposure to ethylene oxide or ionizing radiation, or by dissolution in an appropriate solvent, sterile filtration, and aseptic crystallization. The sterile solid is then added to the batch either directly or by first dispersing the sterile solid in a small portion of the batch. After adequate dispersion, this small sterile portion can be readily added to the remainder of the batch, aseptically, with proper aseptic rinsing. The batch is then brought to final volume with sterile water. Because the eye is sensitive to particles as small as 20 to 25 μm in diameter, proper raw material specifications regarding particle size of the solid to be dispersed must be established and verified on each lot of raw material and final product. In general, particle size of suspended drug should be primarily 5 to 10 μm or smaller.

When an ophthalmic ointment is manufactured, all raw material components must be rendered sterile prior to compounding unless the ointment contains an aqueous fraction that can be sterilized by heat or filtration or unless the ointment is terminally sterilized by heat, filtration, or ionizing radiation. The ointment base is sterilized by heat and appropriately filtered while molten to remove extraneous foreign particulate matter. It is then placed into a sterile steam-jacketed kettle to maintain the ointment in a molten state under aseptic conditions, and the previously sterilized microfine active ingredient and excipients are added aseptically. While still molten, the entire ointment may then be passed through a previously sterilized colloid mill to adequately disperse the insoluble components.

After the product is compounded in an aseptic manner, it is filled into previously sterilized containers. Commonly employed methods of sterilization of packaging components include exposure to heat, ethylene oxide gas, and ultraviolet and [60Co] irradiation. Where a product is to be used in conjunction with ophthalmic surgical procedures and must enter the aseptic operating area, the exterior of the primary container must be rendered sterile by the manufacturer and maintained sterile with appropriate packaging. This is accomplished by aseptic packaging or by exposure of the completely packaged product to ethylene oxide gas, [60Co] irradiation, or heat.

C. Raw Materials

All raw materials used in compounding ophthalmic pharmaceutical products must be of the highest quality available. Complete raw material specifications for each component must be established and must be verified for each lot purchased. Where raw materials are rendered sterile prior to compounding, the reactivity of the raw material with the sterilizing medium must be completely evaluated and the sterilization must be completely validated to demonstrate its capability of sterilizing raw materials contaminated with large numbers (10^5 to 10^7 per gram) of microorganisms that have been demonstrated to be most resistant to the mode of sterilization appropriate for that raw material. As mentioned previously, particle size distribution must be carefully controlled for raw material components used in ophthalmic suspensions.

As is the case for most sterile (and nonsterile) aqueous pharmaceuticals, the largest portion of the composition, by far, is water. At present, USP 23 allows the use of "Purified water" as a pharmaceutical aid for all official aqueous products with the exception of preparations intended for parenteral administration [42]. For preparations intended for parenteral administration, the USP requires the use of "Water for Injection" (WFI), "Sterile Water for Injection," or "Bacteriostatic Water for Injection" as a pharmaceutical aid. Because some pharmaceutical manufacturers produce a line of parenteral ophthalmic drugs as well as topical ophthalmic drugs, the provision of WFI manufacturing capability is being redesigned into new and existing facilities in order to meet these requirements. In doing so, systems must be designed to meet all of the requirements for WFI currently listed in the USP and the guidelines listed for such systems by the FDA in their good manufacturing practices proposals for large- and small-volume parenterals [116]. Briefly, these proposals call for the generation of water by distillation or by reverse osmosis and its storage and circulation at 80°C (or, alternatively, its disposal every 24 hours) in all stainless steel equipment of the highest attainable corrosion-resistant quality.

D. Equipment

The design of equipment for use in controlled environment area follows similar principles whether for general injectable manufacturing or for the manufacture of sterile ophthalmic pharmaceuticals. All tanks, valves, pumps, and piping must be of the best available grade of corrosion-resistant stainless steel. In general, stainless steel type 304 or 316 is preferable. All product-contact surfaces should be finished either mechanically or by electropolishing to provide a surface as free as possible from scratches or defects that could serve as a nidus for the commencement of corrosion [117]. Care should be taken in the design of such equipment to provide adequate means of cleaning and sanitization. For equipment that will reside in aseptic filling areas, such as filling and capping machines, care should be taken in their design to yield equipment as free as possible from particle-generating mechanisms. Wherever possible, belt- or chain-drive concepts should be avoided in favor of sealed gear of hydraulic mechanisms. Further, equipment bulk should be held to an absolute minimum directly over open containers during filling and capping operations to minimize introduction of equipment-generated particulate matter and to minimize creation of air turbulence, particularly when laminar flow is used to control the immediate environment around the filling/capping operation.

In the design of equipment for the manufacture of sterile ophthalmic pharmaceuticals, manufacturers and equipment suppliers have turned to the relatively advanced technology in use in the dairy and aerospace industries—where such concepts as CIP (clean-in-place), COP (clean-out-of-place), automatic heliarc welding, and electropolishing have been in use for several years. As a guide in this regard, the reader is referred to the so-called 3A standards for the dairy industry issued by the U.S. Public Health Service [118].

For most ophthalmic suspensions and ointments, standard stainless steel, sterilizable manufacturing equipment is employed. This is not necessarily the case with aqueous gel systems where aseptic pH adjustment may be required or suspended solids must be added. A relatively new type of equipment was introduced in the pharmaceutical industry during the late 1970s and the 1980s called turboemulsifiers, which are supplied by several reputable specialty equipment manufacturers. In essence, this equipment must be capable of all compounding steps that may involve high-speed mixing or slower-sweep action mixing, addition of pH-adjusting media (sterile or nonsterile), and suspended solids (nonsterile or presterilized). The equipment must allow the mixture to be brought to volume with vehicle (sterile or nonsterile), deaerated (vacuum rated to 23 to 30 inches of water), and must be jacketed to allow steam-sterilization at pressures up to 20 psig.

VIII. FORMULATION OF TYPICAL OPHTHALMIC SUSPENSIONS AND OINTMENTS

A. Introduction

An attempt will be made in this segment to provide a checklist that would be helpful in developing ophthalmic products in general. The checklist is not intended to encompass all aspects of formulation development, but to cover major requirements. Development of ophthalmic dispersed systems requires knowledge and expertise in many scientific disciplines. Figure 5 shows a flowchart for developing formulations. The formulator must approach his or her task in a logical and systematic manner, applying sound scientific principles. The formulator should have sufficient justification for each of the ingredients incorporated into the formulation. The formulator should always try to develop simple but stable, elegant, safe, and effective formulations.

B. Preformulation Research

Preformulation research consists of generating a database for the drug substance, evaluating the compatibility of various excipients with the drug substance, developing a number of prototype formulations from which a final and, if required, one or two backup formulations are selected for further development.

The preformulation database should provide adequate information about the drug substance—including its potential shortcomings or limitations—to guide the formulators in developing acceptable dosage forms. All the ingredients used in ophthalmic preparations should meet official compendial standards and should be manufactured under

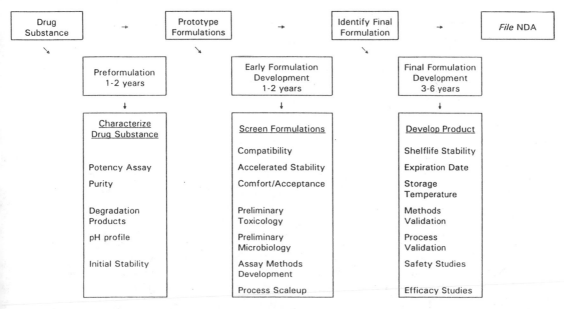

Fig. 5 Flowchart for developing formulations.

current Good Manufacturing Practice (cGMP) regulations in an approved facility. If an ingredient is not listed in any compendium, it should be characterized adequately and its safety established for its intended use.

The preformulation database for raw materials should consist of as many of the following criteria as applicable:

1. Compendial status of the ingredients. Does the raw material meet the compendial specifications? Are the analytical procedures adequate?
2. Is it commercially available from a reliable source?
3. Is it manufactured under cGMP regulations? Is the manufacturing facility an approved cGMP facility? Dose the manufacturer have a Drug Master File with the FDA?
4. Molecular structure and molecular weight.
5. Color, odor, melting point, particle size, shape, and distribution. Does it exhibit polymorphism?
6. Is it adequately characterized by differential thermal analysis (DTA), differential scanning calorimetry (DSC), and thermal gravimetric analysis (TGA)?
7. Is it adequately characterized by visible, UV, IR, NMR, and mass spectrometric methods?
8. Does it exhibit optical activity?
9. What is the solubility profile with respect to pH and dielectric constant?
10. What is the stability profile with respect to pH, temperature, oxygen, light, and moisture?
11. What is the compatibility profile of the drug substance with commonly used ophthalmic antimicrobial preservatives, chelating agents, antioxidants, buffers, viscosity-building agents, and osmolality-adjusting agents?
12. Which method of sterilization—dry heat, ethylene oxide, gamma irradiation, or other—is acceptable?
13. What are the preliminary toxicology, microbiology, and ADME (absorption, distribution, metabolism, and excretion) profiles?
14. Are there any safety hazards or special storage and handling requirements?

For more information, the reader is referred to a detailed discussion on the subject of preformulation research published elsewhere [119].

C. Early Formulation Development

Development of prototype formulations is built on the preformulation database generated for the drug substance and any new excipients planned for inclusion in the new formulation. During this phase of early formulation development, the emphasis is on screening a number of formulations to select a final formulation and possibly one or two backup formulations. The screening phase consists of evaluating the short-term accelerated stability and compatibility of several formulations. Accelerated studies are typically performed at high temperatures considered to be stress conditions.

Preliminary evaluation of the ocular irritation potential, preservative effectiveness, package compatibility, and stability are the key parameters evaluated during this stage of development. The formulator should address the following issues/questions:

1. Develop a plan and allocate resources.
2. Prepare as many prototype formulations as necessary to evaluate packaging compatibility, short-term stability, preservative effectiveness, and ocular irritation. Stability evaluation consists of the following parameters that are appropriate: appearance, homogeneity, osmolality, pH, particle size and distribution, freeze-thaw cycling studies, effect of light, and concentrations of the drug substance, and the antimicrobial preservative. During this phase, it is not necessary to have fully validated chemical assays; however, they should be stability indicating. Ocular irritation, preservative effectiveness, and chemical assays may be performed only on one or two representative formulations in view of the high costs associated with these tests.
3. Consult and communicate with Process Development/Pilot Plant personnel for an appropriate manufacturing method, including sterilization methods.
4. Evaluate the short-term (usually 1 to 2 years) stability data and obtain preliminary estimates of shelf life and storage temperature. Selection of primary package, final, and backup formulations should be possible at the end of this study period.
5. Establish preliminary specifications for in-process (bulk) and finished product. Include compendial requirements for the proposed dosage form, if any.
6. Identify any potential problems and develop an action plan to solve them.
7. Evaluate the suppliers of raw materials (drug substance and additives) to begin final formulation work.
8. The formulator should communicate his or her selection of final and backup formulations to Analytical Chemistry, Microbiology, Toxicology, Packaging, Process Development, and other appropriate departments. It is imperative to consult with personnel in these departments and obtain their concurrence for the selection of final and backup formulations.

D. Final Formulation Development

Development of a final product (formulation/package system) requires the input of many functional units, such as Marketing, Regulatory Affairs, and Manufacturing, outside of Research and Development. It is essential to consult these functional units for the selection of appropriate package sizes, number of lots to be put on stability, adequacy of real-time stability data for New Drug Application (NDA) to meet regulatory requirements, and adequacy of data on comfort, patient acceptance, safety and efficacy, and many other issues.

Key activities during this development phase are:

1. Preparation of pilot plant/process scale-up batches to evaluate and validate the manufacturing process. It is highly recommended that at least one lot should be prepared in the manufacturing plant using actual production size equipment to evaluate potential process problems associated with scale-up.
2. Long-term stability studies should be conducted to confirm shelf-life storage temperature, expiration date, and establish shelf-life stability specifications for the product. Long-term stability studies should be conducted on the formulation/primary package systems intended for marketing. At least one of the lots on long-

term stability should be representative of a production-size lot made with manufacturing equipment. Provide adequate support to testing groups (Analytical Chemistry and Microbiology) for validation of the assay procedures.

3. Provide adequate support to Toxicology, ADME (adsorption, distribution, metabolism, and excretion), and Clinical/Medical for evaluation of the long-term safety and efficacy of the final formulation.

The following checklist may be used to guide the formulator in developing a final formulation.

1. Has preformulation and early formulation work been completed? Are the data adequate to begin final formulation development?
2. Has a plan been drawn up, reviewed, and approved? Are sufficient resources allocated?
3. Has a final formulation been identified?
4. Are there any unresolved issues before initiating long-term shelf-life stability studies?
5. Are the data sufficient to support Phase I safety studies?
6. Have the final formulation and specifications been communicated to other functional units, such as Analytical Chemistry, Microbiology, Toxicology, Pilot Plant/ Process Development, Clinical Supplies Manufacture?
7. Have Analytical Chemistry, Microbiology, and other testing groups verified the assay procedures? Have appropriate samples and vehicles been provided to the testing groups?
8. Have the required lots been prepared for stability studies? Check with Regulatory Affairs for concurrence.
9. If the primary package components are sterilized by ethylene oxide, have the package components and the formulation been examined for ethylene oxide residues?
10. Is a backup formulation required for this product?
11. Has the manufacturing process been reviewed by Process Development?
12. Have clinical supplies/pilot batches been prepared? Are there any problems in scaling up the batch size?
13. Are the data for the final formulation sufficient to support Phase II clinical studies?
14. Are the lots on stability (number and package sizes) adequate for both scientific and regulatory requirements?
15. Are there any special stability studies indicated or required?
16. Are the data sufficient to initiate and support Phase III clinical studies?
17. Have product specifications been finalized?
18. Are storage temperature requirements and expiration data finalized?
19. Has the final formulation been endorsed by Analytical Chemistry, Toxicology, Microbiology, and Clinical/Medical Science?
20. Have all processing parameters been established and verified?
21. Has a summary of all key development data/activities been prepared?
22. Have all appropriate sections of the New Drug Application (NDA) been prepared for submission?
23. Is there any potential follow-up work that is required?

E. Formulation Development: Examples

1. *Suspensions*

The approximate composition of a typical ophthalmic suspension and its method of manufacture are shown in the following sections.

Prednisolone Acetate Ophthalmic Suspension

Prednisolone acetate, micronized	1.0%
Benzalkonium chloride (preservative)	0.01%
Disodium edetate (chelating agent)	qs
Phosphate buffer	qs
Hydroxypropylmethylcellulose (viscosity-increasing agent)	qs
Polysorbate 80 (dispersing agent)	qs
Sodium chloride (osmolality-adjusting agent)	qs
Sodium hydroxide (to adjust pH) and/or	qs
Hydrochloric acid (to adjust pH)	qs
Purified water	qs 100 mL

Manufacturing Process. Ophthalmic suspensions are manufactured by a process that is similar to that of ophthalmic solutions. All water-soluble ingredients (phosphate buffer, disodium edetate, sodium chloride, and benzalkonium chloride) are dissolved in a portion of the water, pH-adjusted to the target range of 6.8 to 7.2, and sterile-filtered into a sterile receiver. The hydroxypropylmethylcellulose is dispersed in another portion of water and sterilized in an autoclave and polish-filtered. The micronized prednisolone acetate powder is sterilized by a validated procedure (e.g., by ethylene oxide). The sterile powder is then dispersed under aseptic conditions in a high-shear mixer into a sterile-filtered solution of polysorbate in water. This prednisolone acetate dispersion is then added to the aqueous solution containing the buffer with continuous mixing under aseptic conditions. The sterile hydroxypropylmethylcellulose solution is then added with continuous mixing under aseptic conditions to be combined suspension of the drug and the buffer solution. The pH of the suspension should be checked and adjusted, if necessary, to the target range under aseptic conditions. The final volume is adjusted with sterile water, and the suspension is stirred until uniform. After in-process bulk testing, the suspension is filled into presterilized plastic bottles under aseptic conditions. The bulk suspension should be stirred continuously during filling to assure that settling of the particles does not occur. Similarly, it is also essential to keep the length of the filling lines as short as practical so that the suspended particles do not settle in the filling lines. These precautions are necessary to assure that the suspension meets the content uniformity requirements of the USP for the drug substance. The bottles are then plugged and capped with presterilized plugs and caps under aseptic conditions. Tamper-evident seals are then placed on the bottles.

2. *Gels*

At the present time, only one ophthalmic gel is on the market. This product contains pilocarpine in a clear aqueous carbomer gel formulation. The approximate composition of the gel is listed below.

Pilocarpine Gel

Pilocarpine hydrochloride	4.0%
Benzalkonium chloride (preservative)	0.008%
Disodium edetate (chelating agent)	
Carbomer 940 (gelling agent)	
Sodium hydroxide (to adjust pH)	qs
and/or	
Hydrochloric acid (to adjust pH)	QS
Purified water	qs 100 mL

Manufacturing Process.   The carbomer is dispersed in a portion of the water and sterilized in an autoclave. The pilocarpine hydrochoride, disodium edetate, and benzalkonium chloride are dissolved in another portion of water. The solution is sterilized by membrane filtration. The carbomer dispersion is then added to the solution of pilocarpine under aseptic conditions. The pH is checked and adjusted, if necessary, to the target range under aseptic conditions. The final volume is adjusted with sterile water under aseptic conditions. The product is then filled into presterilized ophthalmic gel tubes under aseptic conditions.

3.   Ointments

Gentamicin Ophthalmic Ointment

Gentamicin sulfate (as gentamicin base)	0.3%
Methylparaben (preservative)	0.05%
Propylparaben (preservative)	0.01%
White petrolatum	qs 100 g

Manufacturing Process.   The gentamicin sulfate is micronized in a jet mill or other suitable micronizer and sterilized by a validated sterilization process, such as with ethylene oxide. The methylparaben and propylparaben are dissolved in molten white petrolatum. The molten petrolatum base is then sterile-filtered through a suitable sterilizing membrane. The petrolatum is cooled to about 38 to 42°C with continuous mixing to assure that the parabens are distributed uniformly. The sterile gentamicin sulfate is then dispersed under aseptic conditions into the warm petrolatum base, with stirring, until the ointment is homogeneous. After the bulk ointment is tested and released, it is filled into presterilized ophthalmic tubes under aseptic conditions.

ACKNOWLEDGMENTS

The authors wish to acknowledge the assistance of Ms. Terry Praznick, Alcon Laboratories, Inc., for providing valuable literature and bibliography search for this manuscript. The authors also acknowledge the assistance of the R&D Word Processing Center for typing this manuscript.

REFERENCES

1. J. D. Mullins, *Remington's Pharmaceutical Sciences,* 17th ed., Mack Publishing Co., Easton, PA, 1985, p. 1558.

2. R. C. Tripathi and B. J. Tripathi, Anatomy, orbit and adnexa of the human eye. In: *The Eye*, vol. 1a, 3rd ed. (H. Davson, ed.), Academic Press, New York, 1984, pp. 1–268.

3. F. N. Marzulli and M. E. Simon, Eye irritation from topically applied drugs and cosmetics: Preclinical studies, *Am. J. Optom.*, 48:61 (1971).

4. T. McDonald and J. Shadduck, *Adv. Mod. Toxicol.*, 3:139 (1977).

5. P. K. Basu, Toxic effects of drugs on the corneal epithelium: A review, *J. Toxicol.- Cut. & Ocular Toxicol.*, 2:205–227 (1984).

6. J. S. Friedenwald, W. F. Hughes, Jr., and H. Hermann, *Arch. Ophthal.*, 31:379 (1944).

7. C. Carpenter and H. Smyth, *Am. J. Ophthal.*, 29:1363 (1946).

8. L. W. Hazelton, *Proc. Sci. Sect. Toilet Goods Assoc.*, 17:490 (1973).

9. L. M. Carter, G. Duncan, and G. K. Rennie, Effects of detergents on the ionic balance and permeability of isolated bovine cornea, *Exp. Eye Res.*, 17:5, 409–416 (1973).

10. J. H. Kay and J. C. Calandra, *J. Soc. Cosmet. Chem.*, 13:281 (1962).

11. K. L. Russell and S. G. Hoch, *Proc. Sci. Sect. Toilet Goods Assoc.*, 37:27 (1962).

12. I. Gaunt and K. H. Harper, The potential irritancy to the rabbit eye mucosa of certain commercially available shampoos, *J. Soc. Cosmet. Chem.*, 15:290 (1964).

13. S. P. Battista and E. S. McSweeney, Approaches to a quantitative method for testing eye irritation, *J. Soc. Cosmet. Chem.*, 16:119 (1965).

14. J. H. Beckley, *Am. Perfum. Cosmet.*, 80:51 (1965).

15. C. T. Bonfield and R. A. Scala, *Proc. Sci. Sect. Toilet Goods Assoc.*, 43:34 (1965).

16. E. V. Buehler and E. A. Newmann, A comparison of eye irritation in monkeys and rabbits, *Toxicol. Appl. Pharmacol.*, 6:701–710 (1964).

17. C. H. Dohlman, The function of the corneal epithelium in health and disease. The Jonas S. Friedenwald Memorial Lecture, *Invest. Ophthal.*, 10(6):383 (1971).

18. W. H. Spencer, ed., *Ophthalmic Pathology: An Atlas and Textbook*, 3rd ed., Saunders, Philadelphia, 1985.

19. R. R. Pfister, The normal surface of corneal epithelium: A scanning electron microscopic study, *Invest. Ophthal.*, 12:654 (1973).

20. D. M. Maurice, The cornea and sclera. In: *The Eye*, 2nd ed., Vol. 1 (H. Davson, ed.), Academic Press, New York, 1969, pp. 489–600.

21. J. H. Prince, C. D. Diesem, I. Eglitis, and G. L. Ruskell, *Anatomy and Histology of the Eye and Orbit in Domestic Animals*, Charles C. Thomas, Springfield, Illinois, 1960.

22. H. Davson, In: *The Eye*, 2nd ed., Vol. 1 (H. Davson, ed.), Academic Press, New York, 1969, pp. 217–218.

23. B. S. Fine and M. Yanoff, *Ocular Histology: A Text and Atlas*, Harper & Row, New York, 1972.

24. W. R. Green, J. B. Sullivan, R. M. Hehir, L. G. Scharpf, and A. W. Dickinson, *A Systematic Comparison of Chemically Induced Eye Injury in the Albino Rabbit and Rhesus Monkey*, The Soap and Detergent Association, New York, 1978, pp. 405–415.

25. Committee for the Revision of NAS Publication 1138, National Research Council, *Principles and Procedures for Evaluating the Toxicity of Household Substances*, National Academy of Science, Washington, D.C., 1977, pp. 41–56.

26. Interagency Regulatory Liaison Group, Testing Standards and Guidelines Work Group, Recommended Guidelines for Acute Eye Irritation Testing, January 1981.

27. J. H. Draize, *Food Drug Cosmet. Law J.*, 10:722 (1955).

28. J. H. Draize and E. A. Kelley, *Proc. Sci. Sect. Toilet Goods Assoc.*, 17:1 (1959).

29. J. H. Draize, G. Woodward, and H. O. Calvery, Methods for the study of irritation and toxicity of substances applied topically to the skin and mucous membranes, *J. Pharmacol. Exp. Ther.*, 83:377 (1944).

30. *Food Drug Cosmet. Law Rep.*, 233:8311, 440:8313, 476:8310.

31. *Federal Register*, 37:8534 (1972).

32. W. R. Markland, *Norda Briefs* No. 470 (1975).
33. H. A. Baldwin, T. O. McDonald, and C. H. Beasley, Slit-lamp examination of experimental animal eyes. II. Grading scales of induced pathological conditions, *J. Soc. Cosmet. Chem.*, 25:181 (1973).
34. N. L. Burstein, Preservative alteration of corneal permeability in humans and rabbits, *Invest. Ophthalmol. Vis. Sci.*, 25:1453–1457 (1984).
35. A. M. Tonjum, Permeability of rabbit corneal epithelium of horse-radish peroxidase after the influence of benzalkonium choride, *Acta Ophthalmol.*, 53(3):335–347 (1975).
36. N. L. Burstein, Preservative cytotoxic threshold for benzalkonium chloride and chlohexidine gluconate in cat and rabbit corneas, *Invest. Ophthalmol. Vis. Sci.*, 7(3):308–313 (1980).
37. R. R. Pfister and N. Burstein, The effects of ophthalmic drugs, vehicles and preservatives on corneal epithelium: A scanning electron microscope study, *Invest. Ophthalmol. Vis. Sci.*, 15:246–259 (1976).
38. A. M. Tonjum, Effects of benzalkonium chloride upon the corneal epithelium studied with scanning electron microscopy, *Acta Ophthalmol.* 53(3):358–366 (1975).
39. H. B. Collin and B. E. Grabsch, The effect of ophthalmic preservatives on the healing rate of the rabbit corneal epithelium after keratectomy, *Am. J. Optom. Physiol. Opt.*, 59(3):215–222 (1982).
40. J. Ubels, Measurement of corneal epithelial healing rates and corneal thickness for evaluation of ocular toxicity of chemical substance, *J. Toxiol.-Cut. Ocular Toxicol.*, 1(2):133–145 (1982).
41. *Federal Register*, 18:351 (1953).
42. The *United States Pharmacopeia*, 23, United States Pharmacopeial Convention, Inc., Rockville, Maryland, 1995.
43. K. Green and J. M. Chapman, Benzalkonium chloride kinetics in young and adult albino and pigmented rabbit eyes, *J. Toxicol.-Cut. Ocular Toxicol.*, 5(2):133–142 (1986).
44. C. Thode and H. Kilp, Alteration of the corneal permeability due to ophthalmic preservatives, *Fortschr. Ophthalmol.*, 79:125–127 (1982).
45. A. R. Gasset, Y. Ishii, H. E. Kaufman, and T. Miller, Cytotoxicity of ophthalamic preservatives, *Am. J. Ophthalmol.*, 78:98–105 (1974).
46. R. M. E. Richards, *Aust. J. Pharm. Sci.*, 48(55):S56, S96 (1967).
47. W. Mullen, W. Shepherd, and J. Labovitz, Ophthalmic preservatives and vehicles, *Survey Ophthal.*, 17:469 (1973).
48. T. O. McDonald, Technical Report 036:7320:75/76, Alcon Laboratories (1975).
49. W. M. Grant, *Toxicology of the Eye*, 3rd ed., Charles C. Thomas, Springfield, Illinois, 1986, p. 264.
50. H. F. Edelhauser, M. E. Stern, and J. W. Hiddemen, Nonmercurial disinfection/preservative systems for contact lenses. *Ophthalmology, 90* (Suppl.):47 (1983).
51. M. E. Stern, H. F. Edelhauser, S. J. Krebs, G. R. Carney, and J. W. Hiddemen, A comparison of corneal epithelial and endothelial toxicity of common preservatives, *Invest. Ophthalmol. Vis. Sci., 24*(Suppl.) (3):156 (1983).
52. N. L. Burstein, Preservative cytotoxicity threshold for benzalkonium chloride and chlorhexidine digluconate in cat and rabbit corneas, *Invest. Ophthalmol. Vis. Sci.*, 19:308 (1980).
53. J. A. Dormans and M. J. Van Logten, The effects of ophthalmic preservatives on corneal epithelium of the rabbit: A scanning electron microscopical study, *Tox. Appl. Pharmacol.*, 62:251 (1982).
54. A. R. Gasset and Y. Ishii, Cytotoxicity of chlorhexidine, *Can. J. Ophthalmol.*, 10:98 (1975).
55. K. Green, V. Livingston, K. Bowman, and D. S. Hull, Chlorhexidine effects on corneal epithelium and endothelium, *Arch. Ophthalmol.*, 19:1273 (1980).
56. C. G. Begley, P. J. Waggoner, G. S. Hafner, T. Tokarski, R. M. Meetz, and W. H. Wheeler, *Opt. Vision Sci.*, 68, 189–197 (1991).
57. K. Green, R. E. Johnson, J. M. Chapman, E. Nelson, and L. Cheeks, *Lens Eye Toxic. Res.*, 6, 37–41 (1989).

58. C. M. Lederer, Jr., and R. E. Harold, Drop size of commercial glaucoma medications, *Am. J. Ophthalmol.,* 101:691–694 (1986).

59. R. H. Brown, M. L. Hotchkiss, and E. B. Davis, Creating smaller eyedrops by reducing eyedropper tip dimensions, *Am. J. Ophthalmol.,* 99:460 (1985).

60. G. Petursson, R. Cole, and C. Hanna, Treatment of glaucoma using mini drops of clonidine, *Arch. Ophthalmol.,* 102:1180 (1984).

61. E. M. Van Buskirk and F. T. Fraunfelder, Ocular beta-blockers and systemic effects, *Am. J. Ophthalmol.,* 98:623 (1984).

62. R. A. Moses, *Adler's Physiology of the Eye,* 5th ed., Mosby, St. Louis, 1970, p. 49.

63. M. P. Kavula, J. G. Strom, S. Yen, K. Reed, Validating ophthalmic residence time in rabbits using a single channel analyzer with NaI probe, *American Pharmaceutical Association Annual Meeting Abstracts,* 141:134 (1994).

64. J. L. Greaves, C. G. Wilson, A. T. Birmingham, Assessment of the precorneal residence of an ophthalmic ointment in healthy subjects, *Br. J. Clin. Pharmacol.,* 35 (2):188–192 (1993).

65. D. I. Weiss and R. N. Schaffer, *Arch. Ophthal.,* 68:727 (1962).

66. R. A. Anderson, *Australian J. Pharm.,* 47(37):S8 (1986).

67. K. J. Himmelstein, I. Guvenir, and T. F. Patton, Preliminary pharmacokinetic model of pilocarpine uptake and distribution in the eye, *J. Pharm. Sci.,* 67:603 (1978).

68. R. D. Schoenwald and R. L. Ward, Relationship between steroid permeability across excised rabbit cornea and octanol-water partition coefficients, *J. Pharm. Sci.,* 67:786 (1978).

69. R. D. Schoenwald and H. S. Huang, Corneal penetration behavior of beta-blocking agents. I: Physiochemical factors, *J. Pharm. Sci.,* 72:1266 (1983).

70. M. G. Elber, *Optimization Model for Corneal Penetration of Ethoxzolomide Analogs,* Thesis, University of Iowa, Iowa City, 1984.

71. D. M. Maurice, and S. Mishima, *Ocular Pharmacokinetics* (M. L. Sears, ed.), Springer-Verlag, New York, 1984, pp. 31–32.

72. G. M. Grass and J. R. Robinson, Mechanisms of corneal drug penetration. I: *In vivo* and *in vitro* kinetics, *J. Pharm. Sci.,* 77:3 (1988).

73. G. M. Grass and J. R. Robinson, Mechanisms of corneal drug penetration. II: Ultrastructural analysis of potential pathways for drug movement, *J. Pharm. Sci.,* 77:15 (1988).

74. G. M. Grass, E. R. Cooper, and J. R. Robinson, Mechanisms of corneal drug penetration. III: Modeling of molecular transport, *J. Pharm. Sci.,* 77:24 (1988).

75. M. G. Eller, Thesis, University of Iowa, Iowa City, 1984.

76. K. Kishida and T. Otori, *Jpn. J. Ophthalmol.,* 24:251 (1980).

77. R. W. Baker and H. K. Lonsdale, *Controlled Release: Mechanisms and Rates* (A. C. Tanquary and R. E. Lacy, eds.), Plenum Press, New York, 1974, pp. 15–71.

78. D. D. S. Tang-Liu, J. B. Richman, R. J. Weinkam, H. Takruri, Effects of four penetration enhancers on corneal permability of drugs *in vitro,* *J. Pharm. Sci.,* 83(1):85–90 (1994).

79. M. L. Freidberg, U. Pleyer, B. J. Mondino, Device drug delivery to the eye. Collagen shields, iontophoresis, and pumps, *Ophthalmology,* 98(5):725–32 (1991).

80. H. E. Kaufman, T. L. Steinemann, E. Lehman, H. W. Thompson, E. D. Varnell, J. T. Jacob-LaBarre, B. M. Gebhardt, Collagen-based drug delivery and artificial tears, *J. Ocul. Pharmacol.,* 10, 17–27, 1994.

81. R. Jani, O. Gan, Y. Ali, R. Rodstrom, S. Hancock, Ion-exchange resins for ophthalmic delivery, *J. Ocul. Pharmacol.,* 10 (1):57–67 (1994).

82. D. Meisner, J. Pringle, M. Mezei, Liposomal ophthalmic drug delivery. Part 3. Pharmacodynamic and biodisposition studies of atropine, *Int. J. Pharm.,* 55:105–113 (1989).

83. R. F. Barber and P. N. Shek, Tear-induced release of liposome-entrapped agents, *Int. J. Pharm.,* 60:219–227 (1990).

84. A. M. Durrani, N. M. Davies, M. Thomas, I. W. Kellaway, Pilocarpine bioavailability from a mucoadhesive liposomal ophthalmic drug delivery system, *Int. J. Pharm.,* 88:409–415 (1992).

85. A. Joshi, Microparticulates for ophthalmic drug delivery, *J. Ocul. Pharmacol.*, 10:29–45 (1994).

86. S. E. Leucuta, Kinetics of in-vitro release and the pharmacokinetics of miotic response in rabbits of gelatin and albumin microspheres with pilocarpine, *Int. J. Pharm.*, 54:71–78 (1989).

87. A. Komatsu, K. Ohashi, H. Oba, T. Kakehashi, Y. Mizushima, E. Shirasawa, M. Horiuchi, Application of lipid microsphere drug delivery system to steroidal ophthalmic preparation, *Jpn. J. Ophthalmol.*, 32:41–43 (1988).

88. M. A. Attia, M. A. Kassem, S. M. Safwat, *In vivo* performance of ^{3}H-Dexamethasone ophthalmic film delivery system in the rabbit eye, *Int. J. Pharm.*, 47:21–30 (1988).

89. R. J. Harwood and J. B. Schwartz, Drug release from compression molded films: preliminary studies with pilocarpine, *Drug Dev. Ind. Pharm.*, 8:663–682 (1982).

90. M. F. Saettone, M. T. Torracca, A. Pagano, B. Giannaccini, M. Cini, Controlled release of pilocarpine from coated polymeric ophthalmic inserts prepared by extrusion, *Int. J. Pharm.*, 86:159–166 (1992).

91. M. Diestelhorst, G. K. Krieglstein, Ocular tolerability of a new ophthalmic drug delivery system (NODS), *Int. Ophthalmol.*, 18(1):1–4 (1994).

92. Y. D. Sanzgiri, S. Maschi, V. Crescenzi, E. M. Topp, V. J. Stella, Gellan-based systems for ophthalmic sustained delivery of methylprednisolone, *J. Controlled Release*, 26:195–201 (1993).

93. S. R. Nadkarni, S. H. Yalkowsky, Controlled delivery of pilocarpine. 1. In vitro characterization of Gelfoam matrices, *Pharm. Res.*, 10:109–112 (1993).

94. S. Suzuki and J. K. Lim, PEG-PVA hydrogels as ocular inserts for gentamicin, *Abstracts, American Pharmaceutical Association Annual Meeting*, 141:1 (1994).

95. S. Kumar, B. O. Haglund, K. J. Himmelstein, In-situ-forming gels for ophthalmic drug delivery, *J. Ocul. Pharmacol.*, 10:47–56 (1994).

96. H. Sasaki, Y. Igarashi, K. Nishida, J. Nakamura, Ocular delivery of the beta-blocker, tilisolol, through the prodrug approach, *Int. J. Pharm.*, 93:49–60, 1993.

97. M. F. Saettone, D. Monti, M. T. Torracca, P. Chetoni, Mucoadhesive ophthalmic vehicles: evaluation of polymeric low-viscosity formulations, *J. Ocul. Pharmacol.*, 10:83–92 (1994).

98. N. Bodor, Designing safer ophthalmic drugs by soft drug approaches, *J. Ocul. Pharmacol.*, 10:3–15 (1994).

99. W. H. Havener, *Ocular Pharmacology*, 5th ed., Mosby, St. Louis (1983).

100. B. Smith, *Handbook of Ocular Pharmacology*, Publ. Sciences Group, Acton, MA (1974).

101. P. Ellis and D. L. Smith, *Ocular Therapeutics and Pharmacology*, 3rd ed., Mosby, St. Louis (1969).

102. S. Riegelman and D. G. Vaughn, *J. Am Pharm. Assoc. Pract. Pharm. Ed.* 19:474 (1958).

103. S. M. Blaugh and A. T. Canada, *Am. J. Hosp. Pharm.*, 22:662 (1965).

104. M. L. Linn and L. T. Jones, *Am. J. Ophthalmol.*, 65:76 (1968).

105. S. S. Chrai and J. R. Robinson, *J. Pharm. Sci.*, 63:1218 (1974).

106. C. A. Adler, D. M. Maurice, and M. E. Patterson, *Exp. Eye. Res.*, 11:34 (1971).

107. N. Unlu, A. Ludwig, M. Van Ooteghen, A. A. Hincal, Comparative rheological study on carbopol viscous solutions and the evaluation of their suitability as ophthalmic vehicles and artificial tears, *Pharm. Acta Helv.*, 67:5–10 (1992).

108. F. P. Siegel, Tonicity, osmoticity, osmolality, and osmolarity. In: *Remington's Pharmaceutical Sciences*, 17th ed., Mack Publishing Co., Easton, PA, 1985, pp. 1455–1472.

109. A. Martin, J. Swarbrick, and A. Cammarata, Buffered isotonic solutions. In: *Physical Pharmacy*, 3rd ed., Lea & Febiger, Philadelphia, 1983, pp. 222–224.

110. P. P. DeLuca and J. C. Boylan, Formulation of small volume parenterals, *Pharmaceutical Dosage Forms: Parenteral Medications*, Vol. 1, Marcel Dekker, New York, 1984, pp. 139–201.

111. Federal Standard No. 209, Clean room and Work Station Requirements, Controlled Environment, Secs. 1–5, Office of Technical Services, U. S. Department of Commerce, Washington, D.C., December 16, 1963.

112. P. R. Austin and S. W. Timmerman, *Design and Operation of Clean Rooms,* Business New Publ., Detroit, 1970.

113. P. R. Austin, *Clean Rooms of the World,* Ann Arbor Science Publ., Ann Arbor, MI, 1967.

114. K. R. Goddard, *Air Filtration of Microbial Particles,* U. S. Government Printing Office, Washington, D.C., 1967.

115. K. R. Goodard, Designing a parenteral manufacturing facility, *Bull. Parenteral Drug Assoc.,* 23:69 (1969).

116. *Federal Register* 41, No. 106 (1976).

117. T. L. Grimes, D. E. Fonner, J. C. Griffin, and L. R. Rathbun, Electropolish finishing of stainless steel in pharmaceutical processing equipment, *Bull. Parenter. Drug Assoc.,* 29:64 (1975).

118. E-3A Accepted Practices for Permanently Installed Sanitary Product Pipeline and Cleaning Systems, Serial No. E-60500, U. S. Public Health Service, Washington, D.C.

119. S. Motola and S. Agharkar, Preformulation research of parenteral medications, *Pharmaceutical Dosage Forms: Parenteral Medications*, Vol. 1, Marcel Dekker, New York, 1984, pp. 89–138.

10

Gels

Joel L. Zatz

Rutgers—The State University of New Jersey, Piscataway, New Jersey

Gregory P. Kushla

Knoll Pharmaceutical Company, Whippany, New Jersey

I. CHARACTERISTICS OF GELS

A. Definitions

The term "gels" is broad, encompassing semisolids of a wide range of characteristics—from fairly rigid gelatin slabs, to suspensions of colloidal clays, to certain greases. Gels can be looked on as being composed of two interpenetrating phases.

The United States Pharmacopeia (USP) defines gels as semisolids, being either suspensions of small inorganic particles or large organic molecules interpenetrated with liquid [1]. In the first case, the inorganic particles, such as bentonite, form a three-dimensional "house of cards" structure throughout the gel. This is a true two-phase system, as the inorganic particles are not soluble but merely dispersed throughout the continuous phase.

Large organic molecules tend to exist in solution as randomly coiled flexible chains. These molecules, either natural or synthetic polymers, tend to entangle with each other because of their random motion [2]. Systems such as this are actually single-phase in the macro sense—the organic molecule is dissolved in the continuous phase. However, the unique behavior of long molecules in solution, leading to fairly high viscosity and gel formation, makes it possible to consider such a system as two-phase on the micro level—the colloidal polymer molecule and the solvent.

It is the interaction between the units of the colloidal phase, inorganic or organic, that sets up the "structural viscosity" immobilizing the liquid continuous phase [3]. Thus, gels exhibit characteristics intermediate to those of liquids and solids [4].

B. Uses

The uses of gels and gelling agents are quite widespread, but discussion here is limited to the pharmaceutical and cosmetic fields only.

Gels find use as delivery systems for oral administration as gels proper or as capsule shells made from gelatin; for topical drugs applied directly to the skin, mucous membranes, or eye; and for long-acting forms of drugs injected intramuscularly or implanted into the body.

Gelling agents are useful as binders in tablet granulations, protective colloids in suspensions, thickeners in oral liquids, and suppository bases.

Cosmetically, gels have been employed in a wide variety of products, including shampoos, fragrance products, dentifrices, and skin- and hair-care preparations [5].

C. Classification

The classification of a gel is undertaken by considering some characteristic of either of the two phases. Gels are divided into inorganic and organic gels on the basis of the nature of the colloidal phase. Bentonite magma is an example of an inorganic gel. Organic gels typically contain polymers as the gel former. These are further subdivided according to the chemical nature of the dispersed organic molecules [5]. Most natural gums, such as acacia, carrageenan, and xanthan gum, are anionic polysaccharides [6]. A number of cellulose derivatives have been synthesized and are effective gellants; among them are sodium carboxymethylcellulose, hydroxyethyl cellulose, hydroxypropyl cellulose, and hydroxypropylmethyl cellulose [7,8]. Polyethylene and its copolymers [9] and metallic stearates [10–14] have been useful in gelling oils. Polypeptides (gelatin) and synthetic block copolymers, like poloxamers [15,16], are two additional chemical classes.

The nature of the solvent is also useful in classifying gels. Aqueous gels are, of course, water based. The term hydrogel has evolved to refer specifically to aqueous gels containing an insoluble polymer. Organogels contain a nonaqueous solvent as the continuous phase. Examples of organogels are Plastibase (low molecular weight polyethylene dissolved in mineral oil and shock cooled) [17] and dispersions of metallic stearates in oils.

Solid gels with low solvent concentration are known as xerogels. Xerogels are often produced by evaporation of the solvent, leaving the gel framework behind. They can be returned to the gel state by introduction of an agent that, on imbibition, swells the gel matrix. Examples of xerogels include dry gelatin, tragacanth ribbons and acacia tears [18], and dry cellulose and polystyrene [19].

D. Characteristics

Ideally, gelling agents for pharmaceutical and cosmetic use should be inert, safe, and nonreactive with other formulation components [9]. A potential incompatibility is illustrated by the combination of a cationic drug, preservative, or surfactant with an anionic gel former. Inactivation or precipitation of the cationic substance is possible. Sodium alginate has been shown to reduce the concentration of cationic preservatives in solution [20], as well as complex with chlorpheniramine, reducing the drug-release rate from gelled formulations [21]. Polyethers have been shown to interact with phenols and carboxylic acids, leading to loss of potency [22–24].

The inclusion of a gelling agent in a liquid formulation should provide a reasonable solidlike matrix during storage that can be broken easily when subjected to the shear forces generated in shaking a bottle or squeezing a tube, or during topical application. Cost considerations require a low concentration of gellant to produce the desired characteristics.

The gel should exhibit little viscosity change under the temperature variations of normal use and storage. For example, Plastibase exhibits a lesser decrease in consistency than petrolatum over the same temperature range [9]. This minimizes unacceptable changes in the product's characteristics.

Many gels, particularly those of a polysaccharide nature, are susceptible to microbial degradation. Incorporation of a suitable preservative should prevent contamination and subsequent loss of gel characteristics due to microbial attack.

The gel characteristics should match the intended use. A topical gel should not be tacky. Too high a concentration of gel former or the use of an excessive molecular weight may produce a gel difficult to dispense or apply. An ophthalmic gel must be sterile. Consumers tend to prefer gel products with high optical clarity [25]. The aim is to produce a stable, elegant, economical gel product adequately suited for its intended use.

1. Swelling

Gels can swell, absorbing liquid with an increase in volume. This can be looked on as the initial phase of dissolution [19]. Solvent penetrates the gel matrix so that gel-gel interactions are replaced by gel-solvent interactions. Limited swelling is usually the result of some degree of cross-linking in the gel matrix that prevents total dissolution. Such gels swell considerably when the solvent mixture possesses a solubility parameter comparable to that of the gellant [26].

2. Syneresis

Many gel systems undergo contraction upon standing. The interstitial liquid is expressed, collecting at the surface of the gel. This process, referred to as syneresis, is not limited to organic hydrogels, but has been seen in organogels and inorganic hydrogels as well [19]. Typically, syneresis becomes more pronounced as the concentration of polymer decreases.

The mechanism of contraction has been related to the relaxation of elastic stresses developed during the setting of the gel [27]. As these stresses are relieved, the interstitial space available for solvent is reduced, forcing the expression of fluid. Osmotic effects have been implicated, as both pH and electrolyte concentration influence syneresis from gels composed of the ionic gel formers gelatin or psyllium seed gum [27,28].

3. Structure

Inorganic particles are capable of gelling a vehicle because of the formation of a "house of cards" structure. Clays, such as bentonite or kaolin, possess a lamellar structure that can be extensively hydrated. The flat surfaces of bentonite particles are negatively charged, while the edges are positively charged [29]. The attraction of face to edge of these colloidal lamellae creates a three-dimensional network of particles throughout the liquid, immobilizing the solvent. The interactions between the particles are fairly weak, being broken by stirring or shaking.

The long chains of organic gel formers are extended in good solvents, as would be the case in aqueous gels as the result of hydrogen bond formation between water and hydroxyl groups of the gelling agent. In a poor solvent, the gel molecule would be more tightly coiled, preferring self-interaction to interaction with the solvent [30]. Each segment of the dissolved molecules is in constant random motion, buffeted by the movement of solvent molecules through the bulk of the liquid. This random motion serves to entangle polymer strands. Molecular entanglement is responsible for the viscosity and structure of organic gels.

The organic polymers used in hydrogels tend to be sheathed with an envelope of water of hydration [31]. This enables the polymer molecules to slip past each other at low concentrations because of the lubricity of the intervening water molecules. If the degree of hydration is low, then intermolecular attractive forces such as hydrogen bonding and van der Waals forces form weak secondary bonds between polymer strands. At sufficiently high concentration, a continuous network of weakly interacting chains can be formed. The association may proceed far enough to produce small local regions of crystalline nature dispersed through a bed of randomly entangled polymer strands.

Salts may attract part of the water of hydration of the polymer, allowing the formation of more intermolecular secondary bonds, leading to gelation and precipitation. This is known as salting out. Multivalent cations have a strong effect on the solutions of anionic polymers. Bridging of the polymers by di- or trivalent cations, as in the addition of copper to solutions of sodium carboxymethyl cellulose or calcium to sodium alginate, leads to gel formation.

Alcohols have a similar effect. In addition, alcohols alter the solvent's characteristics, changing the solubility parameter. The addition of alcohol often brings about coacervation rather than gelation. Coacervation is the production of a viscous, solvated, polymer-rich phase, leaving behind a phase that is mostly solvent and, therefore, poor in polymer [2].

The effect of temperature depends on the chemistry of the polymer and its mechanism of interaction with the medium. Many gel formers are more soluble in hot than cold water. If the temperature is reduced once the gel is in solution, the degree of hydration is reduced and gelation occurs. Some polymers exhibit thermal gelation. These polymers are more soluble in cold water; solutions of these materials gel on heating. Examples include methylcellulose and poloxamer [15].

Gelation caused by changes in hydration with changes in temperature tends to be reversible; gels liquefy and set again as the temperature is cycled. Gelation caused by chemical reactions, as in salt bridging or cross-linking, is irreversible. Gels resulting from chemical cross-linking often cannot be liquefied by dilution or temperature changes [31].

Molecular weight is an important consideration in gel formation. Very long polymers can entangle to a greater extent, leading to higher viscosity at a given concentration. Thus, lower concentration of a high molecular weight polymer may be required to gel the solvent. This can be a drawback perceived as difficult spreading of a topical gel due to the high cohesive interactions between the gel strands [9]. Likewise, low molecular weight polymers require a high concentration to build up viscosity and to set to a gel, possibly increasing the cost because of the amount of gellant used and overshadowing the desired properties of the formulation.

4. *Rheology*

Solutions of gelling agents and dispersions of flocculated solids are typically pseudoplastic, exhibiting non-Newtonian flow behavior characterized by decreasing viscosity with increasing shear rate. Such behavior is due to progressive breakdown of the structure of the system [31].

The tenuous structure of inorganic particles dispersed in water is disrupted by an applied shear stress. As shear stress is increased, more and more interparticulate associations are broken, resulting in a greater tendency to flow. Similarly, for macromolecules dispersed in a solvent, the applied shear tends to align the molecules in the direction of flow. The molecules straighten out, becoming less entangled as shear increases, thus lessening the resistance to flow.

It is of note that the microviscosity of a gel product may be significantly different from the bulk viscosity. This can have significant implications for drug release from gels. Despite a very high bulk viscosity, drug diffusion out of the gel may be fairly rapid because of the much lower microviscosity of the solvent medium [32].

Semisolid gels do not exhibit flow at low shear. Rather, they deform elastically in a manner similar to solids. When a critical shear stress, the yield value, is exceeded, the material will begin to flow. Such behavior is termed plastic.

The elastic deformation of inorganic gels is limited, but that of polymer gels may be on the order of 10% to 30% recoverable deformation [31]. Inorganic gels are broken easily to free-flowing liquids when the yield value is exceeded. Organic gels tend to be more resistant. Gels of lower concentration or near the liquefaction temperature tend to flow well when shear stress exceeds the yield value [31].

A more detailed description of the rheological characteristics of viscoelastic systems is found in Chapter 5 of Volume 1 of this book.

E. Stability

The formulation and manufacture of a gel system is not complete without an evaluation of the stability of that system. What is meant by the term stability when referring to gels? Clearly, the chemical integrity of dispersed active ingredients must be assured over the shelf life of the product. But what of the system itself, its physical characteristics?

1. *Definition*

A gel formulation that is unstable or not suitable for marketing under normal circumstances would exhibit some irreversible change in its rheological properties of sufficient magnitude to cause it to be unacceptable in its final use. Examples of unstable gels include gels that "set-up" during storage and can no longer be expressed from a tube, gels that undergo a separation of phases—either of the liquid (as in syneresis) or of the solid (as in particle sedimentation)—and gels that suffer a progressive loss of viscosity or consistency, changing from semisolids to viscous liquids.

It is important to recall that rheological behavior is complex. A change in rheological behavior must be interpreted in the proper frame of reference—the desired properties of the final product. A small decrease in the viscosity of a clear hair dressing may be much less significant than the same change in a topical product with suspended active.

2. *Testing*

Most gels exhibit non-Newtonian rheological behavior and thus cannot be fully characterized by a single viscosity measurement. Nevertheless, apparent viscosity measurements determined at a single shear rate can be useful for comparative purposes, as with different batches or stored samples over time. Single-point measurement gives no clue to the behavior of the material at any other shear rate, and one cannot use the results of a test at one shear rate to extrapolate to behavior at another shear rate. A test is valid if its shear rate duplicates the property being tested. For example, very low shear rates should be used to determine a yield value. Likewise, spreadability tests should use shear rates in the thousands of reciprocal seconds to approximate the high shear experienced by the product when rubbed into the skin [33].

A useful empirical test is the measurement of the force required to extrude the material from a deformable bottle or tube. While not strictly a test of the product's characteristics due to inclusion of the force necessary to deform the container, the method applies shear in the region of the flow curve corresponding to a shear rate exceeding the yield value and exhibiting consequent plug flow. One such apparatus is described in Wood et al. [33].

The yield value of a viscoelastic material can be measured through the use of a penetrometer. Typically, the penetrometer is a metal cone or needle, although dual angle cones consisting of a small angle cone mounted atop a much larger angle cone have also been used. The depth of penetration resulting from the contact of the cone with the product under conditions of known force is measured. The yield value from single angle cone penetrometers can be calculated easily by [34]:

$$S_o = \frac{K_1 mg}{p^n}$$

where: S_o = yield value (dynes/cm^2)
      m = mass of cone and mobile parts (g)
      g = acceleration due to gravity
      p = depth of penetration (cm)
      n = material constant approximated to 2
      $K_1 = \frac{1}{\pi} \cos^2 \alpha \cot \alpha$ (2α is the cone angle)

Yield values within the range 100 to 1000 g/cm^2 are classified as spreadable [35]. Below this range the material is too soft and flowing; above, it is too hard and cannot be spread.

The structure of gels, as previously described, is the result of particle-particle interactions or molecular entanglement. Random motion leads to continual breakage and reformation of bonds. Viscoelastic theory also considers these opposing processes. At low shear the material behaves elastically because of strong bonding. As the applied stress is increased, the structure is modified by undergoing a process of bond breakage and reformation. With sufficient applied force enough bonds are ruptured, the structure is altered, and viscous flow occurs. The inherent elasticity in such a system allows recovery of some, but not all, of the deformation once the stress is released. Creep curves demonstrate graphically this progressive behavior. The primary advantage to characterizing the system in question in this manner is that fundamental characteristics of viscosity and elasticity can be obtained with minimal mechanical stress. Thus, very subtle changes occurring with storage or use can be evaluated and standardized, leading to defined values for acceptable stability [36].

A number of other tests are used to examine semisolid products in general and may be used for gels. These tests explore the product to stressful conditions to determine the range of conditions under which the product will perform well. Freeze-thaw cycling can be used to see whether separation or syneresis will occur. Gel characteristics can be strongly affected by freeze-thaw cycling. Solutions of polyvinyl alcohol condense to rubbery elastic gels after several freeze-thaw cycles [37]. Apparently, the cycling causes physical cross-linking of the polymer molecules. This may be an undesirable phenomenon that should be investigated prior to marketing.

Storage of samples at various temperatures gives good information about the storage requirements for that gel. The elevated temperatures should not be too high, probably not more than 45 to 50°C. The results of elevated storage should be tempered with the knowledge that there may be no correlation with room temperature storage for longer time because of the possibility of phase changes occurring at the higher temperature that are not encountered at room temperature.

A shipping test is useful. Shipping a batch of gel around the country subjects it to the bumps and shocks and temperature variations that the product will experience when marketed. If it arrives and is still a good gel, it has passed an important test.

II. GEL-FORMING COMPOUNDS

A number of polymers are used to provide the structural network that is the essence of a gel system. These include natural gums, cellulose derivatives, and carbomers. Although most of these function in aqueous media, several polymers that can gel nonpolar liquids are also available. Certain colloidal solids behave as gellants as a result of asymmetric flocculation of the particles. High concentrations of some nonionic surfactants can be used to produce clear gels in systems containing up to about 15% mineral oil. These are employed mostly as hair dressings.

A. Natural Polymers

Natural gums have been used in commerce since the beginning of recorded history. Typically, they are branched-chain polysaccharides. Most are anionic (negatively charged in aqueous solution or dispersion), although a few, such as guar gum, are neutral molecules. Differences in proportion of the sugar building blocks that make up these molecules and their arrangement and molecular weight result in significant variations in gum properties. Because of their chemical makeup, natural gums are subject to microbial degradation and support microbial growth. Aqueous systems containing gums should contain a suitable preservative. As mentioned earlier, cationic antimicrobials are not generally compatible with the anionic gums and should usually be avoided. Although many of the most familiar gums are plant exudates or extracts, other sources are also used. Xanthan gum is produced microbiologically. Many derivatives of natural materials, such as cellulose, starch, and algin have been prepared. Several are very important commercially and are considered below. The gums are used widely in food and various industrial products a well as pharmaceuticals. Not all of these applications depend on gelation. Acacia (gum arabic) is an effective emulsifier; gum karaya has remarkable adhesive properties; and xanthan gum is an excellent retardant of sedimentation in suspensions and emulsions in which water is the external phase. Gums employed as gel formers may produce the desired effect as a result of simple dispersion in water (e.g., tragacanth) or through chemical interaction (e.g., sodium alginate and calcium). In any case, the gel exists because of cross-links that tie sections of polysaccharide molecules together while the remainder is solvated.

1. *Alginates*

These polysaccharides, containing varying proportions of D-mannuronic and L-guluronic acids, are derived from brown seaweed in the form of monovalent and divalent salts [38]. Although other alginate salts are available commercially, sodium alginate is by far the most widely used. The National Formulary (NF) [1] defines sodium alginate as "the purified carbohydrate product extracted from brown seaweed . . ." and goes on to say: "It consists chiefly of the sodium salt of alginic acid, a polyuronic acid composed of β-D-mannuronic acid residues linked so that the carboxyl group of each unit is free, while the aldehyde group is shielded by a glycosidic linkage."

Gelation occurs by reduction of pH or reaction with divalent cations. Reduction of pH converts the carboxylate ions to free carboxyl groups [38]. This reduces hydration of polymer segments as well as the repulsion between them. Generally, some calcium must be present; the small amounts contributed by the alginate may be sufficient. The pH at which gelation occurs is inversely related to the amount of calcium in solution. Alginates with low residual calcium begin to gel below a pH of 4. Gel strength is a function of alginate concentration; 0.5% is a practical minimum.

Gels will also form at neutral pH in the presence of polyvalent ions. Calcium is most frequently used commercially; curiously, magnesium is essentially ineffective. Calcium ions react preferentially with the polyguluronate segments to form cross-links that tie polymeric strands together into a three-dimensional network. Gel strength and such characteristics as brittleness and the tendency to undergo syneresis (squeezing out of liquid from a gel) are a function of the chemical makeup of the alginate, which, in turn, depends on its source [39]. Gel properties, as well as the gelation rate, depend on calcium concentration and the temperature. Initially, the interaction is confined to the polymer surface, so that completion of the reaction is rate limited by diffusion of ions through the surface gel. Consequently, development of gel properties is not instantaneous; as diffusion proceeds and further reaction of calcium ions with polymer takes place, gel strength increases.

Although higher calcium concentrations (within limits) result in stronger gels, the rate of structure development can be slower because of tighter surface gelation [40]. A nonuniform gel structure may also result. Slightly soluble calcium salts or sequestrants are frequently used to limit the availability of calcium ions to slow down the reaction [38,39].

2. *Carrageenan*

Carrageenan, the hydrocolloid extracted from red seaweed, is a variable mixture of sodium, potassium, ammonium, calcium, and magnesium sulfate esters of polymerized galactose, and 3,6-anhydrogalactose [1]. The main copolymer types are labeled *kappa-, iota-,* and *lambda*-carrageenan. *Kappa* and *iota* fractions form thermally reversible gels in water [41]. This has been ascribed to a temperature-sensitive molecular rearrangement. At high temperatures, the copolymers exist as random coils; cooling results in formation of double helices that act as cross-links.

All the carrageenans are anionic. Gels of *kappa*-carrageenan, which tend to be brittle, are strongest in the presence of potassium ion; *iota*-carrageenan gels are elastic and remain clear in the presence of calcium [41]. Various commercial grades are available for particular applications, most of which are in the food industry.

3. *Tragacanth*

Tragacanth is defined in the NF [1] as the "dried gummy exudation from *Astragalus gummifer* Labillardière, or other Asiatic species of *Astragalus* (Fam. Leguminosae)." These plants are found in the arid mountains of the Near and Middle East; most commercial tragacanth comes from Iran [42]. With the recent turmoil in that part of the world, the quality of tragacanth has been uneven, and its price has increased considerably.

Tragacanth is a complex material composed chiefly of an acidic polysaccharide (tragacanthic acid) containing calcium, magnesium, and potassium, and a smaller amount of a neutral polysaccharide, tragacanthin. The gum swells in water; concentrations of 2% or above of a "high-quality" gum produce a gel [42]. Hydration takes place over a period of time, so that development of maximum gel strength requires several hours. The rheological properties of tragacanth dispersions depend markedly on the grade used as well as its treatment.

4. *Pectin*

Pectin, the polysaccharide extracted from the inner rind of citrus fruit or apple pomance [1], may be used in pharmaceutical jellies as well as in foods. The gel is formed at an acid pH in aqueous solutions containing calcium and possibly another agent that acts to dehydrate the gum [43]. In foods this agent commonly is sugar, which is often included in the pectin of commerce. Needless to say, the pectin used in drug or cosmetic products should be free of such additives.

Gel formation is more extensive in pectins with a low methoxyl content. Such properties as gel strength depend on a host of factors, which include concentration of additives and pH, in addition to the characteristics of the raw material [43].

5. *Xanthan Gum*

Although xanthan gum is used most frequently as a stabilizer in suspensions and emulsions at concentrations below 0.5%, higher concentrations in aqueous media (1% and above) yield viscid solutions that are jellylike in nature [44]. Xanthan gum is produced by bacterial fermentation, and its availability and quality are not subject to many of the uncertainties that affect other natural products, particularly those that are extracted from plants whose habitat falls within politically unsettled parts of the world. Thermally reversible gels result from combinations of xanthan with guar or locust bean gum [45].

6. *Gellan Gum*

Gellan gum is another polysaccharide produced by fermentation [46] that has FDA clearance for use in foods. Partially acetylated gum forms gels that are thermally reversible with hysteresis. The gels based on material with a lower acetyl content are firmer, similar in consistency to gelatin or agar gels.

Gel strength is a function of gum concentration and ionic content. The gum is highly efficient; as little as 0.05% is required for gel formation [47]. Gels will not form in the absence of free cations. While both monovalent and divalent ions can induce gelation, the divalent ions are required in much lower concentration, roughly 1/25 the concentration of monovalent ions. To produce a uniform gel, the gum is first dissolved in deionized water heated to 70 to 75°C. An electrolyte (typically a calcium salt) is added and the solution cooled. The setting temperature for the gel is usually in the range of 30 to 45°C; however, a much higher temperature is needed to dissolve the gel after it has formed.

The mechanism of gelation has been explored [48]. Modeling suggests that the molecules are random coils at high temperature. Helical conformations develop on cooling, promoting end-to-end association between molecules. Gelation is believed to occur where molecular filaments form crystalline junction zones under the influence of cations.

7. *Guar Gum*

Guar gum is a nonionic polysaccharide derived from seeds. Aqueous guar solutions can be cross-linked by several polyvalent cations to form gels [49]. The mechanism is believed to involve chelate formation between groups in different polymer chains. A disadvantage of these gels is the presence of insoluble plant residue.

8. *Other Gums*

Gelatin is used widely as a bodying agent and gel former in the food industry, and occasionally in pharmaceutical products. Agar can be used to make firm gels; it is most frequently used in culture media.

9. *Chitosan*

Chitosan is a natural biopolymer derived from the outer shell of crutaceans [50]. Chitin is extracted and partially deacetylated to produce chitosan. Unlike most gums, chitosan carries a positive charge (at pH below 6.5) and is thus attracted to a variety of biological tissues and surfaces that are negatively charged. Various derivatives are being explored for specific applications. Concentrated aqueous solutions have a gel-like consistency. Firmer gels result from interaction with polysaccharides, such as alginate.

B. Acrylic Polymers

Carbomer 934P is the official name given to one member of a group of acrylic polymers cross-linked with a polyalkenyl ether [1]. Manufactured under the trade name Carbopol 934P, it is used as a thickening agent in a variety of pharmaceutical and cosmetic products. The suffix "P" identifies a highly purified polymer, suitable for use in orally administered dosage forms, although carbomer 934P is also used widely in topical preparations.

Carbomer forms gels at concentrations as low as 0.5%. In aqueous media, the polymer, which is marketed in the free acid form, is first uniformly dispersed. After entrapped air has been allowed to escape, the gel is produced by neutralization with a suitable base. The introduction of negative charges along the polymer chain causes it to uncoil and expand.

In aqueous systems, a simple inorganic base such as sodium, ammonium, or potassium hydroxide, or a basic salt such as sodium carbonate may be employed. The pH should be adjusted to a neutral value; gel character will be adversely affected by either insufficient neutralization or excessively high pH [51]. Certain amines, such as triethanolamine, are sometimes used in cosmetic products.

By employing organic amines as neutralizing agents, it is possible to gel many semipolar liquids or mixtures of these liquids with water [51]. Compatibility of the polymer with nonaqueous liquids depends on the formation of ion pairs with the amine.

Polyols are capable of hydrogen bonding with the polymer, forming reversible links that augment viscosity. The viscosity of carbomer dispersions is lowered in the presence of ions; the addition of 1% sodium chloride causes more than a 50% drop in Brookfield viscosity (20 rpm) of neutralized carbomer 941, 1%, at neutral pH [51].

A hydrophobic derivative of poly(acrylic acid) has been developed as a polymeric emulsifier [52]. This substance is highly efficient and is required in concentrations below 1%. It can function alone or in combination with low levels of surfactant. Because of the polymer's sensitivity to salts, emulsions based on this polymer break when applied to the skin, depositing an oil film onto the skin surface. The film does not re-emulsify when placed in contact with water and clings to the skin.

Acrylic resins widely used in tablet coating also have the capability of producing gels with polar organic liquids, such as glycerin, propylene glycol, and low molecular weight polyethylene glycols [53]. Gel systems containing various drugs have been suggested as a novel means for rectal administration. A copolymer of methacrylic acid and its methyl ester seemed to function effectively to delivery sustained blood levels of model drugs when unsaturated fatty acids were included in the formulation [53].

C. Cellulose Derivatives

Many useful derivatives are fashioned from cellulose, a natural structural polymer found in plants. Treatment in the presence of various active substances results in breakdown of the cellulose backbone as well as substitution of a portion of its hydroxyl moieties. The major factors affecting rheological properties of the resulting material are the nature of the substituent(s), degree of substitution, and average molecular weight of the resultant polymer.

The cellulose derivatives are subject to enzymatic degradation and should be protected against contact with sources of cellulase. Sterilization of aqueous systems or addition of suitable preservatives is used to prevent viscosity reduction resulting from depolymerization caused by enzyme production by microorganisms.

1. *Carboxymethylcellulose*

Carboxymethylcellulose, also known as sodium carboxymethylcellulose, CMC, and cellulose gum, is an anionic polymer available in a variety of grades that differ in molecular weight and degree of substitution. Gelation requires addition of an electrolyte with a polyvalent cation to a solution of the polymer; aluminum salts are preferred [54,55]. Gel characteristics, such as firmness and elasticity, depend on polymer concentration and molecular weight. Sequestrants are useful in controlling the availability of free cations and preventing polymer precipitation, which can result if the reaction takes place too rapidly.

2. *Methylcellulose*

Methylcellulose is an example of a polymer whose solubility in water decreases as the temperature is raised. If an aqueous solution is heated, viscosity increases markedly at a certain point as the result of formation of gel structure. This property, known as thermal gelation, is a function of polymer chemistry and the presence of additives [56]. The gelation temperature range for Methocel type A (Dow Chemical) is 50 to 55°C. Salts and sugars with a high affinity for water lower the gelation temperature whereas alcohol and propylene glycol have the opposite effect.

3. *Other Cellulose Derivatives*

Hydroxypropyl cellulose is soluble in water as well as many polar organic solvents. Consequently, it is useful as a gelling agent for such liquids and for mixtures of water and various organic liquids, such as alcohol, that adversely affect the rheological properties of gums and certain other hydrophilic agents. High molecular grades of hydroxypropyl cellulose and hydroxyethyl cellulose can be used in the formation of viscid, jellylike aqueous solutions. The solutions, though highly viscous, behave as fluids and do not exhibit a yield value.

D. Polyethylene

Various forms of polyethylene and its copolymers are used to gel hydrophobic liquids. The result is a soft, easily spreadable semisolid that forms a water-resistant film on the skin surface.

Polyethylene itself is a suitable gellant for simple aliphatic hydrocarbon liquids but may lack compatibility with many other oils found in personal care products. For these, copolymers with vinyl acetate and acrylic acid may be used, perhaps with the aid of a cosolvent [57]. To form the gels, it is necessary to disperse the polymer in the oil at elevated temperature (above 80°C) and then shock cool to precipitate fine crystals that make up the matrix.

E. Colloidally Dispersed Solids

Certain finely divided solids can function efficiently as thickening agents in various liquid media. Gel formation depends on establishment of a network in which colloidal particles of the solid are connected in an asymmetric fashion. This requires mutual attraction of the particles (flocculation) and partial wetting by the liquid.

1. *Microcrystalline Silica*

Microcrystalline silica can function as a gellant in a wide range of liquids. Network formation results from attraction of the particles by polar forces, principally hydrogen bonding [58]. Silica with high surface area (small particle size) is most efficient in producing the "chicken-wire" structure to encapsulate liquid. Low concentrations are required in nonpolar liquids; in highly polar liquids, competition of the medium for hydrogen bonding sites weakens particle–particle interactions and thus much higher silica concentrations are required to produce a gel. Glycols may be used to augment structure formation in nonpolar liquids.

An important commercial application of silica is its use in dentifrices [59]. Microcrystalline silica acts as a bonding agent that provides thixotropy to the formulation; at the same time, the required concentration of polishing agents is reduced.

2. *Clays*

Montmorillonite clays are capable of swelling in water as the result of hydration of exchangeable cations and electrostatic repulsion between the negatively charged faces [60]. At high concentrations in water, thixotropic gels form because the particles combine in a flocculated structure in which the face of one particle is attracted to the edge of another (house of cards). The gels are highly thixotropic, tending to liquefy on agitation. Because of the importance of electrostatic forces in flocculation, it is not surprising that rheological properties of clay dispersions are sensitive to salts.

Reaction with certain organic molecules converts the clay particle surface to one that is more hydrophobic, making such derivatives compatible with organic liquids [61]. The addition of the correct amount of a polar additive, such as an alcohol, assists in delaminating the clay platelets, thus augmenting the thickening effect. If the polar liquid content is too low, there will be insufficient clay platelet separation; too high a concentration interferes with interparticle attraction.

3. *Microcrystalline Cellulose*

Microcrystalline cellulose is another solid used as a stabilizer and thickener in aqueous systems. Several commercial products contain a hydrophilic polymer, such as sodium carboxymethylcellulose, to aid in dispersion of the colloidal particles and protect them from electrolytes [62]. The characteristics of gels based on any of these solid particles depends on the method of preparation. High shear is usually required to break down the powdered raw material into primary particles (and individual platelets in the case of the clays) so as to produce the most extensively bonded network.

F. Surfactants

Clear gels can be produced by combinations of mineral oil, water, and high concentrations (typically 20% to 40%) of certain nonionic surfactants [63]. These combinations result in the formation of microemulsions; the semisolid rheology encountered is due to the existence of liquid crystalline phases. Gel characteristics can be varied by adjusting the proportion and concentration of the ingredients. Many commercial applications of this type of gel have been in hair-grooming products.

Poloxamer 407 is a polyoxyethylene/polyoxypropylene block copolymer that functions as a surfactant. A 25% solution is liquid at refrigerator temperature, but a gel at room temperature [64]. Drug solutions can easily be prepared at temperatures below the gelation point. Drug release from gels of poloxamer 407 was inversely related to gellant concentration and lipophilicity within a group of related solutes [64].

G. Other Gellants

Various waxy materials are employed as gellants in nonpolar media. Examples are beeswax, carnauba wax, and cetyl esters wax. Aluminum stearate, a hydrophobic soap, has been employed as a bodying agent in oils for many years. These gelling agents are generally incorporated by fusion.

High molecular weight poly(ethylene oxide), cross-linked by high energy irradiation, can form hydrogels at concentrations of about 5% [65]. Applications include use as culture media and treatment of burned skin.

III. APPLICATIONS AND REQUIREMENTS

A. Bioadhesives

Interest in formulations that would adhere to mucosa arose out of attempts to treat lesions of the oral mucosa. Treatment was only partly successful because traditional formulations were rapidly removed from the site of application. Several gel-forming polymers, notably sodium carboxymethyl cellulose and carbomer, have been found to interact with mucus, swelling and adhering to mucosal tissue when applied topically.

1. Definition

Bioadhesion is defined as the interfacial attraction and adherence of two surfaces, at least one of which is biological in origin [66]. More specifically, bioadhesives of pharmaceutical interest are mucoadhesives. This implies that the substrate for adhesion is the mucus layer itself. Many of the "alternate" routes of administration (buccal, ophthalmic, nasal, vaginal, etc.) lend themselves to the use of bioadhesives because of the presence of mucosal tissue.

2. Mechanism

The process of bioadhesion generally occurs as a two-step process [67]: first the polymer must achieve intimate contact with the mucus, then must interpenetrate with the mucus to be retained at the site of application. The most successful mucoadhesives are able to swell in the presence of water. Favorable surface energy effects lead to wetting of the substate by the polymer and spreading over the surface [68]. Once the surfaces are in intimate contact, the adhesive polymer and the mucin glycoproteins can interdiffuse. Chain entanglement and bond formation (electrostatic, hydrophobic interactions, and van der Waals forces) lead to retention at the site of application.

3. Requirements

Several physicochemical properties of polymer molecules have been identified as promoting the development of mucoadhesion.

   a. *Charge.*   The presence of charged groups on a polymer favors mucoadhesion. Polyanions, particularly polycarboxylates, are preferred to polycations [69,70]. Carboxyl, hydroxyl, amide, and sulfate groups [67] all appear able to interact with mucin glycoproteins to form strong adhesive bonds.

   b. *Solubility/Swelling.*   The best mucoadhesives are those with low water solubility [70]. Mucoadhesives swell on contact with moisture, increasing the mobility of the polymer molecules at the interface and exposing more sites for bond formation. As hydration progresses, the more soluble hydrogels swell to form a fluid mucilage and run off the surface of application. More insoluble polymers swell without dissolving, maintaining contact with the mucosa for a longer time.

   c. *Molecular Weight/Spatial Configuration.*   Higher molecular weight or longer chain length favors chain entanglement and interaction after the polymer and mucin have interpenetrated. This is illustrated with polyethylene glycols, which are not strong mucoadhesives. As molecular weight increases up to 4,000,000 daltons, adhesive properties also increase [71]. However, highly coiled polymers, such as high molecular weight dextrans, are incapable of interpenetration with mucin and make poor bioadhesives [71].

   d. *Molecular Mobility and Viscosity.*   If the polymer is too stiff or the formulation too viscous, little interpretation of the adhesive with the mucin will occur, reducing mucoadhesion [67].

   e. *Concentration.*   Bioadhesives exhibit an optimal concentration for maximal bioadhesion. Low concentrations are incapable of forming enough adhesive bonds to perform well. In concentrated solution, though, the molecules compete for limited solvent and are less hydrated. This translates into a decrease in available chain length for interfacial penetration and a corresponding decrease in adhesive strength [72].

4. *Polymers*

Several polymers have been shown to be effective bioadhesives by a variety of in vitro, in situ, and in vivo test methods. Of the natural gums, tragacanth, sodium alginate, gelatin, and karaya gum exhibit satisfactory to excellent mucoadhesive characteristics [67]. Pectin, although useful in combination with other mucoadhesives, is considered a poor adhesive alone. Chitosan, a polyaminosaccharide, was found an effective mucoadhesive under certain test conditions [73]. Acrylic polymers as a group contain some of the strongest mucoadhesives, polycarbophil and carbomer [67]. Many cellulose derivatives are also effective mucoadhesives, including sodium carboxymethylcellulose, methylcellulose, hydroxypropyl methylcellulose, methylethylcellulose, and hydroxyethyl cellulose [67,74].

5. *Applications*

Bioadhesives have found novel applications that take advantage of a number of nontraditional routes of administration, including buccal, nasal, ophthalmic, vaginal, and rectal. They have also been used for oral dosage forms to prolong the residence time in the gastrointestinal tract [75]. Further details on specific applications and experimental results can be found in several comprehensive reviews [67,76].

B. Hydrogels

Hydrogels are gel systems in which water is immobilized by insoluble polymers. One reason for the interest in hydrogels as components of drug delivery systems and implantable devices is their relatively good compatibility with biological tissues. This is particularly true for polymers whose building blocks are endogenous or biodegradable compounds. Certain polymers used in hydrogels hydrolyze slowly, gradually releasing encapsulated drug. Many polymers addressed to this purpose have been synthesized; an extensive review of fundamentals, functional polymers, and applications as of the mid-1980s has been published [77]. Synthesis of newer agents is a continuing process.

1. *Definition*

The elements of hydrogels are water and a polymeric substance that is hydrophilic, but not water-soluble. When exposed to water, the dry polymer swells and absorbs liquid. The polymer strands are cross-linked either chemically or by physical forces. For convenience, hydrogels may be defined by the type of polymer employed and/or the cross-linking mechanism. One classification divides them into neutral, ionic, and swollen interpenetrating networks (IPNs) [78].

2. *Structure*

The polymer structures underlying most hydrogels for biomedical use are amorphous or semicrystalline [78]. Only a small fraction of the polymer strands need be joined to render the molecule insoluble and permit swelling in the presence of water. Many of the important structural properties may be understood from measurement of $\overline{M}_c$, the average molecular weight between adjacent cross-links [79]. This parameter is inversely related to the molar ratio of cross-links. The degree of swelling is directly related to $\overline{M}_c$, while gel strength moves in the opposite direction.

Another important parameter is the mesh size, which may be thought of as the average space available to each entrapped drug molecule. Mesh size correlates with $\overline{M}_c$. The effective drug diffusion coefficient within the hydrogel is a function of molecular size, the viscosity of the liquid medium, and the mesh size. A small mesh size limits molecular transport, reducing the effective diffusion coefficient.

Many applications of hydrogels depend on the content of water, which functions as a plasticizer as well as a solvent [80]. The equilibrium water content, expressed as a weight/weight percentage, is thus an important characteristic. Some of the water is tightly bound to the polymer network by hydrogen bonding; the remainder is "free" and has the characteristics of bulk water. In a copolymer containing both hydrophilic and hydrophobic monomeric units, equilibrium water content increases with an increase in the hydrophilic component. Addition of cross-linking agents reduces flexibility of the polymer chains and tends to reduce equilibrium water content [80].

3. Polymers and Applications

Synthetic materials used to form hydrogels for biological application include copolymers of poly(2-hydroxyethyl methacrylate), known as PHEMA, polyvinyl alcohol, polyethylene oxides, polyvinylpyrrolidone, polyacrylamide and polymethylacrylamide [81]. PHEMA hydrogels are chemically and mechanically stable [82]. Equilibrium water content depends on the monomers present as well as polymerization conditions, but values reported in the literature range from about 30% to 40% [82].

Diffusion through hydrogels and subsequent release into an aqueous sink occurs principally by two mechanisms. One is diffusion through fluctuating pores within the bulk water phase [81]. This route is used by both hydrophilic and hydrophobic solutes. The latter also partition into bound water and diffuse along polymer segments.

Polyethylene glycols and poly(ethylene oxides) are polymers whose repeating unit is $-CH_2-CH_2-O-$. The same structure is found in most nonionic surfactants. Hydrogels can be formed through a variety of techniques, including radiation, chemical cross-linking, formation of a block copolymer, or complexation with polyacrylic acid [83]. Several commercially available bandages used to cover small skin burns consist of a poly(ethylene oxide) hydrogel whose water content is approximately 96%.

A variety of current and potential future applications for hydrogels have been described [77,84,85]. These include soft contact lenses, wound dressings, implants for prolonged drug delivery, and artificial tendons and other body parts. Toxicity is a major concern; the makeup of the repeating units and cross-linking agents is of obvious importance. In addition, initiators, stabilizers, and other chemicals needed for polymerization or gel formation may be present in small quantities, even after extensive purification. These may leach out over an extended period of time. Preparative methods that exclude such materials are to be preferred.

C. Topical Formulations

1. Ophthalmic

Treatment of ophthalmic conditions often requires frequent application of a drug product. The normal lachrymal turnover causes rapid clearance of solution and suspension dosage forms. Ointments have been used as ophthalmic vehicles, but they distort vision after application and have been reported to interfere with the healing of corneal lesions. Aqueous gels offer several advantages [86]: good tolerability, formation of a protective film over the cornea, and protection from conjunctival adhesions. In addition, retention time is increased compared to solutions. In many cases, activity of the drug substance is prolonged, leading to decreased frequency of administration. Of course, all the normal prerequisites for ophthalmic formulations (sterile, nonirritating, imperceptible particles, etc.) apply to ophthalmic gels.

A wide variety of gel-forming polymers have been successfully incorporated into ophthalmic semisolids, including carbomer, polyvinyl alcohol, cellulose derivatives, poloxamer, polyacrylamide, hyaluronic acid, gellan gum, and pectin [86]. As an example, a 25% poloxamer 407 gel doubled the activity of pilocarpine nitrate in rabbits compared to an aqueous solution [87]. Methazolamide, ineffective as an ophthalmic solution, has been incorporated into carbomer and poloxamer gels for the treatment of glaucoma [88].

Many of the gel formers used in ophthalmics are also bioadhesives, enabling the formulation to adhere strongly to the conjunctiva and prolong the contact of the formulation. Mucoadhesive formulations containing polyacrylic acid or carbomer increased the ocular bioavailability of progesterone [89], timolol [90], and pilocarpine nitrate [91].

2. *Epidermal*

The topical use of gels is well established in the cosmetic and personal care markets. Interest in pharmaceutical uses has been revived by efforts to reduce systemic exposure to drugs through the use of local therapy. Several nonsteroidal anti-inflammatory drugs (felbinac [92,93], piroxicam [94], and ketoprofen [95]) have been incorporated into gels for topical therapy. These products, containing carbomer or poloxamer as the gel former, have been shown to provide adequate tissue levels at the site of application, avoiding common G.I. side effects after oral administration.

Gels may also offer the potential for preparing a topical product when other dosage forms fail. Hydrocortisone-17-valerate is not stable in traditional emulsion or cream systems but was successfully incorporated into hydroxypropyl cellulose gels with sulconazole nitrate for the treatment of fungal infections [96].

IV. FORMULATIONS

Following are examples of gel formulating from various sources. Several are prototype formulas that can be modified to produce gels with somewhat different rheological properties

A. Mineral Oil Gel

	% by weight
Polyethylene (A-C 617, Allied Chemical)	10
Mineral oil, 75 s.s.	90

Directions: With simple agitation, gradually heat the mixture to 90°C and mix until homogeneous. Cool quickly with agitation. (From Ref. 57.)

B. Ephedrine Sulfate Jelly

Ephedrine sulfate	10 g
Tragacanth	10 g
Methyl salicylate	0.1 g
Eucalyptol	1 mL
Pine needle oil	0.1 mL
Glycerin	150 g
Purified water	830 mL

Directions: Dissolve the ephedrine sulfate in the purified water, and add the glycerin, tragacanth, and then the remaining ingredients. Mix well and keep in a closed container for one week, with occasional mixing. (From Ref. 97.)

C. Clear Gel

	% by weight
Mineral oil	10.0
Polyoxyethylene 10 oleyl ether (Brij 97)	20.7
Polyoxyethylene fatty glyceride (Arlatone G)	10.3
Propylene glycol	8.6
Sorbitol	6.9
Water	43.5

Directions: Heat all the ingredients except the water to 90°C, and heat the water separately to about 95°C. Add the water to the other ingredients with moderate agitation. Pour at about 60°C. (From Ref. 63.)

D. Zinc Oxide Gel

	% by weight
Water	76.0
Carbomer 934P (Carbopol 934P)	0.8
Sodium hydroxide, 10% solution	3.2
Zinc oxide	20.0

Directions: Disperse the carbomer in the water. Then add the sodium hydroxide with slow agitation to prevent inclusion of air. Add the zinc oxide in the same manner and mix until homogeneous. (From Ref. 98.)

E. Sunscreening Gel

	% by weight
Ethanol (SD-40)	53.0
Carbomer 940 (Carbopol 940)	1.0
Glyceryl-*p*-amino benzoate	3.0
Monoisopropanolamine	0.09
Water	52.91

Directions: Disperse the carbomer 940 in the alcohol and dissolve the glyceryl-*p*-amino benzoate in the solution. Slowly add the monoisopropanolamine. Slowly add the water and stir carefully to avoid air entrapment; the solution will clear up and gel. (From Ref. 99.)

F. Hydrogen Peroxide Gel

	% by weight
Poloxamer P-127 (Pluronic F-127)	25
Hydrogen peroxide, 30% solution	10
Purified water	65

Directions: Cool the water to 40 to 50°F and place it in a mixing container. Add the poloxamer F-127 slowly with good agitation and continue agitating until solution is complete, maintaining the temperature below 50°F. Add cool hydrogen peroxide solution slowly with gentle mixing. Immediately transfer to containers and allow to warm slowly to room temperature, whereupon the liquid becomes a clear "ringing" gel. (From Ref. 99.)

G. Clear Jelly Base

Sodium alginate (Kelgin MV)	3.0 g
Methylparaben	0.2 g
Sodium hexametaphosphate	0.5 g
Glycerin	10.0 g
Purified water	100.0 g
	113.7 g

Directions: Dissolve the methylparaben in glycerin with the aid of heat. Add the water to the warm glycerin with rapid stirring and dissolve the sodium hexametaphosphate in this solution. Add the sodium alginate with rapid continuous stirring until completely dissolved. (From Ref. 100.)

H. Antifungal/Corticosteroid Topical Gel

	% by weight
Sulconazole nitrate	1.0
Hydrocortisone 17-valerate	0.2
Ethanol	50.0
Propylene glycol	33.0
Isopropyl myristate	5.0
Water	5.0
PPG-5-ceteth-20	4.2
Hydroxypropyl cellulose	0.9
Salicylic acid	0.5
Ascorbyl palmitate	0.2
NaOH 1N to adjust pH to 4.0	qs

Directions: Combine the ethanol, propylene glycol, and isopropyl myristate in a suitable mixing vessel. With rapid mixing, add the PPG-5-ceteth-20 and mix until uniform. With rapid mixing, slowly add the ascorbyl palmitate, sulconazole nitrate, and salicylic acid and continue mixing until all solids are dissolved. Prepare the NaOH solution in a separate vessel (0.079 kg for a 100 kg batch). Add 80% of the water and the NaOH solution to the main mixing vessel and mix until uniform. Add the remainder of the water followed by the hydrocortisone 17-valerate. Mix rapidly for 15 minutes, then add the hydroxypropyl cellulose with rapid mixing and mix for about 2 hours to obtain the desired gel. (From Ref. 96.)

I. Lidocaine Hydrochloride Topical Gel

	% by weight
Lidocaine hydrochloride	1.0 g
Chitosan F	4.0 g
Lactic acid	1.9 mL
Methylparaben	0.1 g
Disodium EDTA	0.2 g
Water qs to make	100.0 g

Directions: Dissolve the lidocaine hydrochloride, methylparaben, and disodium EDTA. Add the Chitosan F in water and mix followed by the lactic acid. Mix for 5 minutes at 5000 rpm in a homomixer. (From Ref. 101.)

Many other examples appear in the scientific and patent literature. Some of the references for this chapter contain a number of additional formulations.

REFERENCES

1. United States Pharmacopeia (USP 23)—National Formulary (NF 18), USP Convention, Rockville, MD.
2. H. Morawetz, ed., *Macromolecules in Solution,* 2nd ed., Wiley, New York, 1975, p. 78.
3. P. Mannheim, *Soap Perfum. Cosmet.,* 37:442 (1964).
4. I. Schmolka, *Cosmet. Toilet.,* 99(11):69 (1984).
5. C. Fox, *Cosmet. Toilet.,* 99(11):19 (1984).
6. G. Meer, *Cosmet. Toilet.,* 99(6):61 (1984).
7. R. G. Rufe, *Cosmet. Perfum.,* 90(3):93 (1975).
8. J. T. Teng, J. M. Lucas, and B. L. Scallet, *Cosmet. Perfum.,* 90(10):32 (1975).
9. I. B. Chang, *Cosmet. Toilet.,* 92(7):25 (1977).
10. J. C. Morrison and J. S. Stephens, *Am. Perfum. Cosmet.,* 82(11) (1967).
11. J. Korbar-Smid and M. Bozic, *Cosmet. Toilet.,* 93(6):33 (1978).
12. M. Bozic, J. Korbar-Smid, and A. Lavric, *Cosmet. Toilet.,* 95(6) (1980).
13. M. Bozic and J. Korbar-Smid, *Cosmet. Toilet.,* 95(6):29 (1980).
14. P. D. Reed, *Am. Perfum. Cosmet.,* 77(10):105 (1962).
15. P. C. Chen-Chow and S. G. Frank, *Int. J. Pharm.,* 8:89 (1981).
16. P. C. Chen-Chow and S. G. Frank, *Acta Pharm. Suec.,* 18:239 (1981).
17. M. N. Nutimer, C. Riffkin, J. A. Hill, M. E. Glockman, and G. N. Cyr, *J. Am. Pharm. Assoc., Sci. Ed.,* 45:212 (1956).
18. A. Martin, J. Swarbrick, and A. Cammarata, *Physical Pharmacy,* Lea & Febiger, Philadelphia, 1983, p. 566.
19. P. H. Hermans. In: *Colloid Science. II. Reversible Systems* (H. R. Kruyt, ed.), Elsevier, New York, 1949, pp. 483–651.
20. G. Richardson and R. Woodford, *Pharm. J.,* 192:52 (1964).
21. A. F. Stockwell, S. S. Davis, and S. E. Walker, *J. Control. Release,* 3:167 (1986).
22. T. Higuchi and J. L. Lach, *J. Am. Pharm. Assoc., Sci. Ed.,* 43:465 (1954).
23. T. Higuchi and R. Kuramoto, *J. Am. Pharm. Assoc., Sci. Ed.,* 43:393 (1954).

24. A. D. Marcus, E. Wetstein, and M. Ruderman, *J. Am. Pharm. Assoc., Pract. Pharm. Ed.*, 17:453 (1956).

25. L. E. Pena, *Drugs Pharm. Sci.*, 42:381 (1990).

26. H. Burrell, *Interchem. Rev.*, 14:3 (1955).

27. J. H. Northrup and M. Kunitz, *J. Phys. Chem.*, 35:162 (1931).

28. A. G. Mattha, *Pharm. Acta Helv.*, 52:233 (1977).

29. H. Schott. In: *Physical Pharmacy* (A. Martin, J. Swarbrick, and A. Cammarata, eds.), Lea & Febiger, Philadelphia, 1983, pp. 592–638.

30. P. C. Hiemenz, *Principles of Colloid and Surface Chemistry*, Marcel Dekker, New York, 1977, p. 118.

31. H. Schott. In: *Remington's Pharmaceutical Sciences, 18th ed.* (A. Gennaro, ed.), Mack Publishing Co., Easton, PA, 1990, pp. 310–326.

32. K. I. Al-Khamis, S. S. Davis, and J. Hadgraft, *Pharm. Res.*, 3:214 (1986).

33. J. H. Wood, W. H. Giles, and G. Catacalos, *J. Soc. Cosmet. Chem.* 15:564 (1964).

34. P. Sherman, *J. Soc. Cosmet. Chem.*, 17:439 (1966).

35. A. J. Haighton, *J. Am. Oil Chemists Soc.*, 36:345 (1959).

36. G. Zografi, *J. Soc. Cosmet. Chem.*, 33:345 (1982).

37. N. A. Peppas and S. R. Stauffer, *J. Control. Release*, 16:305 (1991).

38. A. H. King, Brown seaweed extracts (alginates). In: *Food Hydrocolloids*, Vol. II (M. Glicksman, ed.), CRC Press, New York, 1983, pp. 115–118.

39. *Kelco Algin*, 2nd ed., Kelco Division of Merck & Co., Inc., San Diego.

40. T. N. Julian, G. W. Radebaugh, S. A. Wisniewski, and E. Roche, *Pharm. Res.*, 3:41S (1986).

41. M. Glicksman, Red seaweed extracts. In: *Food Hydrocolloids*, Vol. II (M. Glicksman, ed.), CRC Press, New York, 1983, pp. 73–113.

42. M. Glicksman, Gum tragacanth. In: *Food Hydrocolloids*, Vol. II (M. Glicksman, ed.), CRC Press, New York, 1983, pp. 49–60.

43. G. A. Towle and O. Christensen, Pectin. In: *Industrial Gums* (R. L. Whistler, ed.), Academic Press, New York, 1973, pp. 429–461.

44. J. L. Zatz and S. Knapp, *J. Pharm. Sci.*, 73:468 (1984).

45. *Xanthan Gum*, 5th ed., Kelco Division of Merck & Co., Inc., San Diego.

46. G. R. Sanderson and R. C. Clark, *Food Technology*, 63 (4):63 (1983).

47. *The Preparation of Kelcogel Gellan Gum Gels*, Kelco Division of Merck & Co., Inc., San Diego, 1989.

48. V. J. Morris, Gelation of exocellular polysaccharides. In: *Frontiers of Carbohydrate Research—2* (R. Chandrasekaran, ed.), Elsevier, New York, 1992, pp. 191–207.

49. G. L. Brode, J. P. Stanley, E. M. Partain, and R. L. Kreeger, Glycol modified polysaccharides. In: *Industrial Polysaccharides: Genetic Engineering, Structure/Property Relations and Applications* (M. Yalpani, ed.), Elsevier, New York, 1987, pp. 129–138.

50. P. A. Sandford, High purity chitosan and alginate. In: *Frontiers of Carbohydrate Research—2* (R. Chandrasekaran, ed.), Elsevier, New York, 1992, pp. 250–269.

51. *Carbopol Water Soluble Resins*, B. F. Goodrich Co., Cleveland, OH.

52. R. Y. Lochhead, *Cosmet. Toilet.*, 109(5):93 (1994).

53. S. Goto, M. Kawata, T. Suzuki, N.-S. Kim, and C. Ito, *J. Pharm. Sci.*, 80:958 (1991).

54. J. B. Batdorf, and J. M. Rossman, Sodium carboxymethylcellulose. In: *Industrial Gums* (R. L. Whistler, ed.), Academic Press, New York, 1973, pp. 695–729.

55. *Sodium Carboxymethylcellulose, Physical and Chemical Properties*, Aqualon, Wilmington, DE, 1993.

56. *Methocel Handbook*, Dow Chemical Company, Midland, MI.

57. *Gels of Ethylene Copolymers*, Allied Corp., Morristown, NJ.

58. *How to Thicken Liquids with Cab-O-Sil*, Cabot Corporation, Tuscola, IL.

59. *Aerosil® for Toothpastes*, Degussa Corporation, Ridgefield Park, NJ.

60. H. Van Olphen, *An Introduction to Clay Colloid Chemistry*, Wiley-Interscience, New York, 1963.
61. *NL Rheology Handbook*, NL Chemicals, Hightstown, New Jersey.
62. E. P. Stevens and C. R. Steuernagel, *Drug Cosmet. Ind.*, June (1978).
63. *Clear Gels*, ICI Americas, Inc., Wilmington, Delaware.
64. J. C. Gilbert, J. Hadgraft, A. Bye, and L. G. Brookes, *Int. J. Pharm.*, 32:223 (1986).
65. F. E. Bailey, Jr., and J. V. Koleske, *Alkylene Oxides and Their Polymers*, Marcel Dekker, New York, 1991, p. 215.
66. R. J. Good, *J. Adhesion*, 8:1 (1976).
67. H. E. Junginger, *Pharm. Ind.*, 53:1056 (1991).
68. N. A. Peppas, and P. A. Buri, *J. Control. Release*, 2:257 (1985).
69. M. A. Longer and J. R. Robinson, *Pharmacy Int.*, 7:114 (1986).
70. K. Park, and J. R. Robinson, *Int. J. Pharm.*, 19:107 (1984).
71. J. L. Chen and G. N. Cyr, Compositions producing adhesion through hydration. In: *Adhesion in Biological Systems* (R. S. Manly, ed.), Academic Press, New York, 1970, Chapter 10.
72. R. Gurny, J. M. Meyer, and N. A. Peppas, *Biomaterials*, 5:336 (1984).
73. C-M. Lehr, J. A. Bouwstra, E. H. Schacht, and H. E. Junginger, *Int. J. Pharm.* 78:43 (1992).
74. J. D. Smart, I. W. Kellaway, and H. E. C. Worthington, *J. Pharm. Pharmacol.*, 36:295 (1984).
75. M. A. Longer, H. S. Ch'ng, and J. R. Robinson, *J. Pharm. Sci.*, 74:406 (1985).
76. R. Jiménez-Castellanos, H. Zia, and C. T. Rhodes, *Drug Dev. Ind. Pharm.*, 19:143 (1993).
77. N. A. Peppas, ed., *Hydrogels in Medicine and Pharmacy* (3 vols.), CRC Press, New York, 1986, 1987.
78. N. A. Peppas and A. G. Mikos, Preparation methods and structure of hydrogels. In: *Hydrogels in Medicine and Pharmacy*, Vol. 1 (N. A. Peppas, ed.), CRC Press, New York, 1986, pp. 1–25.
79. N. A. Peppas and B. D. Barr-Howell Characterization of the cross-linked structure of hydrogels. In: *Hydrogels in Medicine and Pharmacy*, Vol. 1 (N. A. Peppas, ed.), CRC Press, New York, 1986, pp. 27–56.
80. I. Piirma, *Polymeric Surfactants*, Marcel Dekker, New York, 1992, pp. 256–265.
81. E. J. Mack, T. Okano, and S. W. Kim, Biomedical applications of poly(2-hydroxyethyl methacrylate) and its copolymers. In: *Hydrogels in Medicine and Pharmacy*, Vol. 2 (N. A. Peppas, ed.), CRC Press, New York, 1987, pp. 65–93.
82. N. A. Peppas and H. J. Moynihan, Structure and physical properties of poly(2-hydroxyethyl methacrylate) hydrogels. In: *Hyrdogels in Medicine and Pharmacy*, Vol. 2 (N. A. Peppas, ed.), CRC Press, New York, 1987, pp. 49–64.
83. N. B. Graham, Poly(ethylene oxide) and related hydrogels. In: *Hydrogels in Medicine and Pharmacy*, Vol. 2 (N. A. Peppas, ed.), CRC Press, New York, 1987, pp. 95–113.
84. A. G. Mikos et al., eds. *Biomaterials for Drug and Cell Delivery* Materials Research Society, Pittsburgh, PA, 1994.
85. C. G. Gebelein, T. C. Cheng, and V. C. Yang, eds. *Cosmetic and Pharmaceutical Applications of Polymers*, Plenum, New York, 1991.
86. B. Giannaccini and C. Alderigi, *Boll. Chim. Farmaceutico*, 128:257 (1989).
87. S. C. Miller and M. D. Donovan, *Int. J. Pharm.*, 12:147 (1982).
88. A. C. Potts, (American Cyanamid Company), UK Patent GB 2,223,166B, March 18, 1992.
89. H-W. Hui, and J. R. Robinson, *Int. J. Pharm.*, 26:203 (1985).
90. F. Thermes, A. Rozier, B. Plazonnet, and J. Grove, *Int. J. Pharm.*, 81:59 (1992).
91. N. M. Davies, S. J. Farr, J. Hadgraft, and I. W. Kellaway, *Pharm. Res.*, 8:1039 (1991).
92. M. Dawson, C. M. McGee, J. H. Vine, P. Nash, T. R. Watson, and P. M. Brooks, *Eur. J. Clin. Pharmacol.*, 33:639 (1988).

93. G. R. McLatchie, M. McDonald, G. F. Lawrence, D. Rogmans, P. Lisai, and M. Hibberd, *Br. J. Clin. Practice*, 43:277 (1989).

94. Anon., *Drug Ther. Bull.*, 28:27 (1990).

95. S.-C. Chi, and H. W. Jun, *J. Pharm. Sci.* 79:974 (1990).

96. J. Wang, B. Patel, T. Au, and H. Shah (Bristol-Myers Squibb Company), US Patent 5,002,938, March 26, 1991.

97. National Formulary, 12th ed., American Pharmaceutical Association, Washington, D.C., 1965.

98. *Personal Care Products: Carbopol Resins,* B. F. Goodrich, Cleveland, OH.

99. M. Ash and I. Ash, *Formulary of Cosmetic Preparations,* Chemical Publishing Co., New York, 1977.

100. *Better Pharmaceutical Gels with Algin,* Kelco Division of Merck & Co. Inc., San Diego.

101. J. Knapczyk, *Int. J. Pharm.,* 93:233 (1993).

11

Toothpastes

David Garlen

Cosmetech Laboratories, Inc., Fairfield, New Jersey

I. INTRODUCTION

Historically the need and desirability of cleaning the teeth paralleled the recognition of the necessity to maintain bodily cleanliness. Early writings attest to a variety of methods and devices for oral hygiene. Many of the materials used and recipes suggested, however, contained materials capable of damaging the teeth and gums. As society developed and diets changed to more and more processed foods, the opportunity for tooth decay became greater. The modern world therefore had a real social, medical, and aesthetic need for well-formulated, safe, and effective dentifrices [1].

II. CHARACTERISTICS OF TOOTHPASTES

A. Function

Cleaning of the surface of the teeth is the primary function of a dentifrice when used with a toothbrush. A dentifrice helps in the removal of food particles, reduction of superficial plaque or stains, polishing of tooth surfaces, and refreshing mouth breath. A therapeutic dentifrice based on the use of a suitable fluoride can reduce dental caries by hardening external tooth surfaces [2]. Other therapeutic and cosmetic functions may be desired, such as whitening, bleaching, desensitizing, inhibition of plaque formation, and protection against periodontal problems.

B. Form and Physical Characteristics

Dentifrices are disperse systems. They consist of water and water-soluble liquids, oils, and both soluble and insoluble solids. As such they are dispersions of solids in a liquid vehicle.

What do dentifrices look like? They may be opaque pastes, clear gels, pastes with colored stripes, part gel/part paste, powders, or liquids. The vast majority of currently marketed dentifrices today are either pastes or gels.

Important characteristics of toothpastes are consistency, abrasiveness, appearance, foaming, taste, stability and safety.

1. *Consistency*

Consistency describes the rheology of a paste. A toothpaste is a semisolid that is normally extruded from a tube. The force required to extrude is related to the viscosity, density, and cohesiveness of the formula. The ideal consistency of a paste is soft enough to be squeezed easily from the tube, yet firm enough to hold its shape and not sag into the bristles of the brush. A paste must have sufficient body to cover the teeth well without spattering during the brushing process. The properties that can be examined and measured involving consistency are density, viscosity, cohesiveness, extrudability, and sag. The consistency of a dentifrice may vary with aging, and it is important in formulating that the ideal consistency achieved remain virtually unchanged during the shelf life of the product.

a. *Density.* Toothpaste density is measured using an aluminum cup pyknometer. This device holds a precise volume of paste and the weight of contents divided by the weight of an equal volume of water yields the specific gravity, which is equal to density. The density is a function of the abrasive identity and the abrasive concentration as well as the humectant and water content. Silica-based pastes have a typical density of approximately 1.3; calcium phosphate–and chalk-based pastes, usually about 1.5 to 1.6. Once the density of a formula is established, the value is useful for determining whether excessive aeration has occurred in manufacture as well as helping to verify that the formulation was correctly prepared.

b. *Viscosity.* Toothpaste viscosities are most easily determined with a Brookfield Viscometer using T bar spindles and a helipath stand. This configuration allows the spindle to spiral down through the paste assuring consistent readings. Toothpaste viscosities generally range from 150,000 to 300,000 centipoise. In addition to being a valuable quality control parameter, tracking viscosity over time yields important information on when equilibrium consistency is achieved.

c. *Cohesiveness.* Although there is no industry standard for measuring cohesiveness, the following technique has proved useful in the laboratory. A known weight of toothpaste is extruded on a metal screen and subjected to a constant water stream. The longer the time required for all the paste to disappear from the screen, the greater the cohesiveness. This evaluation is performed on a comparative basis. An experimental paste is tested along with a control paste with accepted satisfactory cohesiveness. As long as equal weights of the two pastes are used and the water stream is of constant flow rate and pressure, the time to dissolution will give a reasonably reproducible measure.

d. *Extrudability.* Extrudability is measured by the force required to force the toothpaste out of its tube. It is controlled by a combination of the paste consistency and the tube diameter. The lowest force consistent with maintaining other desirable characteristics is to be preferred. To perform this test place an open tube of toothpaste on a paper towel. Place a weighing pan on top of the horizontal tube and add weights in 100 gram increments until the paste is extruded.

e. *Sag.* A toothpaste should hold its form as it emerges from the tube. When applied to the brush it should not sag between the bristles. This property can be visually evaluated by extruding a ribbon of paste onto a brush or piece of paper. The resulting cylinder should show minimal flattening after standing for one minute. Experimental pastes are compared to commercially acceptable samples.

2. Abrasiveness

Abrasiveness is the ability of the dentifrice to mildly abrade or scour the tooth surface. Dentifrices can be formulated in a wide range of abrasiveness. Ideally a dentifrice must be abrasive enough to clean well, remove food particles and remove superficial stains, and polish the tooth surface. It must have a low enough abrasive value so that it will not excessively wear the enamel or the softer dentin that is exposed at the junction of tooth and gum. Abrasivity can be measured by a variety of in vitro techniques. In *Cosmetics: Science and Technology* [2], Gershon and Pader describe the various methods that have been employed and their correlation to measurements made on human teeth. Most commonly used today is a method described as radioactive dentin abrasion or radioactive enamel abrasion in which irradiated teeth are mounted with either the enamel or exposed dentin under the brush. The teeth are brushed under standard conditions. Wear is measured by the level of radioactivity found in the toothpaste slurry [3]. In 1968 Stookey and Muhler [4] studied the enamel and dentin abrasion properties as well as the cleaning and polishing characteristics of common dental polishing agents. In the same study they examined these properties in many of the leading dentifrices then available. They found a high correlation between the results of the radioactive abrasion scores and abrasivity as measured by weight loss. They also found large differences in abrasivity among the toothpastes studied. Although none of the brands tested showed enamel abrasion scores high enough to cause concern, the dentin scores of some brands were so high as to suggest they might be harmful to users with exposed dentin. Publication of this study led to reexamination of abrasive levels by a number of manufacturers and a trend to lower abrasivity that has continued to this day. Factors affecting the abrasiveness of dentifrices include the chemical structure of the abrasive; its hardness, crystal shape, and particle size; and, to a lesser degree, its concentration in the toothpaste. As a guide to abrasive selection one can estimate the expected radioactive dentin abrasion scores in a typical toothpaste formula as related to the abrasives used. Calcium pyrophosphate is used a standard, with a value of 100 in a test slurry. The scores are expressed as a number between 0 and 500 relative to the standard. The estimates that follow (Table 1) are for finished dentifrice formulations using an abrasive concentration that is typical for each abrasive:

Combinations of abrasives of approximately the same crystal structure can usually be blended to achieve any desired abrasive score between their individual values. Typically dicalcium phosphate dihydrate is used with minor additions of dicalcium phosphate, anhydrous, to improve its cleaning ability. Blends of silica with anhydrous dicalcium phosphate are less predictable, because of the differences in their hardness and crystal

Table 1 Estimated RDA Scores of Selected Abrasives

Abrasive	Concentration	Expected RDA score range
Alumina	20–40%	150–500
Dicalcium phosphate, anhydrous	30–50%	250–400
Insoluble sodium metaphosphate	40–50%	175–150
Calcium pyrophosphate	40–50%	100
Calcium carbonate	40–50%	50–400
Hydrated silica	15–30%	30–120
Dicalcium phosphate, dihydrate	40–50%	30–60

structure. There is no maximum standard established for either radioactive dentin abrasion or radioactive enamel abrasion; however, excessive enamel abrasion is not normally encountered, because of the hard structure of enamel. Calcium pyrophosphate is used as a standard and given the value of 100. Pastes with scores more than four times this value are considered too abrasive. Because high dentin abrasion can cause damage when gum recession has caused dentin to be exposed, most companies would not market products today with scores over 200 and consider 150 to be the safe upper limit.

3. *Cleaning and Polishing*

Cleaning is the removal of pellicle, stain, food particles, and other surface debris. It is accomplished by the abrasive action of the paste and brush. If abrasive particles are too hard or large, they may in the course of removing stain create fine scratches in the enamel surface that dull the surface. In contrast, uniform small particles help provide a polished reflective surface on the tooth.

The cleaning ability of a toothpaste is based largely on its abrasivity. Pastes with higher abrasive scores generally clean better than those that are less abrasive. However, a curve of cleaning effectiveness plotted against abrasivity flattens out at a dentin abrasive score of approximately 125. There is therefore little justification for formulating pastes much above this level.

Polishing, on the other hand, appears to be more a function of characteristics of the polishing agent used—its particle size, hardness, and crystal structure. Abrasives with relatively high abrasiveness may or may not be good polishing agents. For example, calcium carbonate varies widely in abrasivity and purity; grades with high levels of impurities of irregular size and shape are among the poorest polishing agents.

4. *Appearance*

A desirable dentifrice should be smooth, uniform, and glossy. It must be free from air entrapment and should exhibit an attractive color.

5. *Foaming*

Foaming agents are used in dentifrices to help suspend and foam away food particles loosened by the brushing process. The concentration of the foaming agent must be sufficient to accomplish these tasks. At the same time the foam must rinse away quickly. Excessive foaming may interfere with the abrasive contact with the tooth surfaces.

6. *Taste*

Dentifrice taste and aroma are probably the most noticeable aspects to the consumer and the most important characteristic in determining whether a consumer will repurchase the product. The perceived taste is a combination of specific flavor and concentrations, level of sweeteners, and mouthfeel.

7. *Stability*

A dentifrice formulation must be stable over its entire shelf life, which may be up to 3 years. It must not separate, it must maintain its viscosity, it must maintain its pH, and it must maintain the desired level of any active therapeutic agents. Formulations must be subjected to a stability test protocol that includes both real-time and accelerated conditions. The requirements for such a protocol will be discussed in detail later in this chapter.

III. COMMONLY USED MATERIALS

Dentifrice ingredients fall into the following classifications: abrasive, binders, surface-active agents, humectant, sweeteners, flavors, colors, preservatives, active therapeutic agents, and other additives [5]. They perform the following functions:

A. Abrasive

Abrasives are insoluble solids that provide cleaning and polishing of the teeth when used with a toothbrush. They generally constitute from 20% to 50% of the total formulation. They fall into a variety of chemical groups and specific abrasives are chosen from this group based on the inherent abrasive level, stability in the presence of other ingredients, and effect on the overall consistency of the paste. Commonly used abrasives are listed below together with their advantages and disadvantages:

1. *Chalk or Precipitated Calcium Carbonate*

Calcium carbonate is inexpensive and readily available in a number of density grades ranging from light to extra dense. As a result of impurities, mainly silica, and of the variability in abrasivity, even among different lots of the same grade and among different sources of supply, the popularity of calcium carbonate is declining.

2. *Calcium Phosphates*

There are a variety of insoluble calcium phosphates that are extremely popular and effective in dentifrice formulations.

    a. *Dicalcium Phosphate, Dihydrate.* This is a material of choice because it is relatively low in abrasion but offers good polishing properties. However, it is incompatible with sodium fluoride because of the formation of insoluble divalent fluoride salts. For dentifrice use it should contain a stabilizer to prevent grittiness, caking, or hardening of the paste on aging. Stauffer Chemical Co. has used magnesium phosphates, magnesium stearate, or magnesium sulfate for this purpose; Monsanto uses tetrasodium pyrophosphate.

    b. *Dicalcium Phosphate, Anhydrous.* This compound is very abrasive and generally used in low concentrations to increase the total abrasivity of the paste. It is also incompatible with some fluorides. A range of abrasiveness from very mild to very abrasive can be achieved by blending different proportions of dicalcium phosphate, anhydrous, with dicalcium phosphate, dihydrate.

    c. *Tetracalcium Pyrophosphate.* This compound was used widely in stannous fluoride–containing pastes. It has declined in popularity because it is incompatible with sodium fluoride, which is now used in most fluoride pastes.

3. *Insoluble Sodium Metaphosphate*

Insoluble sodium metaphosphate is moderately abrasive and compatible with fluorides but relatively costly. Recently, the major supplier of this material withdrew it from manufacture as the result of declining sales, because one of the major users had switched to silica-based formulas.

4. Silicas

Hydrated silicas have become increasingly popular choices as dental abrasive. They fall into two categories:

a. *Abrasive Silicas.*   These are dense, relatively nonabsorbent, odorless, and tasteless powders. Those manufactured by the Davison division of W.R. Grace under the trademark Siloids are prepared under specific manufacturing conditions and are referred to as "xerogels" because their structure is free of voids or air spaces. Hydrated silicas manufactured by Huber Chemical Co. (trademarked Zeodents) provide similar properties. They possess good abrasive characteristics at low concentrations and have minimal effect on the consistency of the finished paste. Their crystalline particles are relatively large and hard. They may be tailored to desired pH ranges and abrasive levels to provide optimum properties in a given formulation.

b. *Thickening Silica.*   These are extremely small sized particles with very large surface areas; they have the capability of swelling and of thickening the resulting pastes. Those manufactured by Davison are called "aerogels," referring to their expanded physical structure and large percentage of air spaces, which are capable of absorbing and holding liquids. Used in combination with the abrasive silicas they are the basis for the typical clear gel pastes: they appear to become transparent when mixed with liquid ingredients that have substantially the same index of refraction. Because of their relatively low cost, silicas are also finding increased utility in opaque dentifrices. They are nonreactive and usually compatible with fluorides and can frequently be used at low concentrations.

5. Hydrated Aluminas

Considerable interest is shown in hydrated aluminas because of their low cost and stability with fluorides. The aluminas are not as effective thickeners as the silicas but are finding increasing applications.

6. Sodium Bicarbonate

The growing popularity of "baking soda" toothpastes is due in no small part to the work of Dr. Paul Keyes, who popularized a periodontal treatment regimen that included brushing the teeth with a paste made by wetting sodium bicarbonate with hydrogen peroxide solution. Sodium bicarbonate becomes useful as a dentifrice abrasive when used in concentrations above its water solubility, which is approximately 8%. Advantages include mild abrasive action and ease of rinsing. Disadvantages include a somewhat granular texture and a salty taste that is difficult to flavor. Sodium bicarbonate is offered in five grades of varying particle size. While the larger particle sizes feel grittier, they also taste less salty, leading to the conclusion that particles size distribution must be chosen with both performance and esthetics considerations. Formulating with sodium bicarbonate also involves negotiating a difficult path through the many patents that have been issued, which cover not only sodium bicarbonate as the sole or principal abrasive, but combinations with other abrasives as well.

B. Binders

Binders are natural or synthetic gums, resins, or other hydrocolloids used in dentifrice formulations to maintain the liquid and solid constituents in the form of a smooth paste. They increase the viscosity of the liquid phase as well as the body of the final formulation, preventing liquid bleeding from the paste. Binders are generally used in concentrations of 0.9% to 2.0% of the formulation. The most popular binder is sodium carboxymethylcellulose, known as CMC. This material is available in a variety of viscosity grades. Carrageenan, gum tragacanth, gum karaya, irish moss, sodium alginate, carbomer resins, and magnesium aluminum silicates are also used. Special care must be taken when formulating pastes designed to be used in tropical climates. An unusual cellulase enzyme is often found in carton dust and can destroy the viscosity of toothpastes formulated with CMC. Development of successful binder systems requires considerable art. The final texture must combine easy extrusion and ability to hold form when dispensed from a tube without sagging on the brush with softness and ease of rinsing. Selection of the right grade or grades of binder as well as the right concentration play a major role in achieving these properties.

C. Surface-Active Agents

Surface-active materials are foaming agents employed at levels of 0.5% to 2.0% to provide desired foaming action. The most popular is sodium lauryl sulfate. The dentifrice grades are high-purity powders that are selected for their foaming properties, safety, and low taste. Care should be taken to keep the concentration below the irritation level, which is about 2% or even less for some individuals. Other surfactants that may be used include sodium *N*-lauroylsarcosinate, sodium laurylsulfoacetate, or sodium dioctyl sulfosuccinate.

D. Humectants

Humectants are incorporated to prevent moisture loss and drying of dentifrices, as well as to contribute to pleasant mouthfeel. In opaque pastes they are generally employed in concentrations of 20% to 40%. Clear gels are formulated with as much as 80%. Most frequently used are sorbitol, glycerin, and propylene glycol.

1. *Sorbitol*

Sorbitol, 70% solution, contributes a feeling of coolness and moderate sweetness. Because sorbitol is less expensive than glycerin, it generally makes up the largest part of the humectant phase.

2. *Glycerin*

Glycerin is popular but contributes a sensation of warmth to the mouthfeel and is more expensive than either sorbitol or propylene glycol. It is typically used at levels of from 5% to 10%.

3. *Propylene Glycol*

Propylene glycol contributes excellent solvent properties, but its low viscosity and bitterness limit its utility.

E. Sweeteners

Most dentifrice flavors are quite bitter and require the use of artificial sweeteners to make them palatable. In the United States sodium saccharin is the only acceptable artificial sweetener and it is generally incorporated at 0.05% to 0.25%. On the other hand, until quite recently, Canada did not permit the use of saccharin but now does permit cyclamates as well as saccharin.

F. Flavors

Dentifrice flavors are generally employed at levels of 0.2% to 2.0%. However, care must be used to avoid potential irritation at the higher concentrations. Oils such as peppermint, spearmint, wintergreen, sassafras, and anise are the most popular. Typically, flavor specialty manufacturers will compound flavors consisting of a relatively large number of components. Tests must be conducted to assure that no undesirable interactions occur between a proposed flavor and the rest of the formulation.

G. Water

Water is present in most dentifrice formulas as both a solvent for soluble salts and as a diluent to decrease raw material costs. Concentrations exceeding 5% to 10% may impair the clarity of clear gel products. Should this occur, a rebalancing of the glycerin/sorbitol/water ratios may correct the problem. Because most dentifrices are manufactured at room temperature, water purity and absence of bacterial contamination is especially important. Only bacteria-free deionized water of high purity should be used. Water levels above 20% carry with them greater need for good preservation of formulas.

H. Preservatives

Generally the water, humectant, and natural gums in dentifrice formulations are capable of sustaining microbial growth; therefore, preservatives such as methyl- and propylparaben or sodium benzoate are usually required at levels of 0.05% to 0.2%.

I. Other Ingredients

Therapeutic ingredients, including sodium fluoride, stannous fluoride, or sodium monofluorophosphate, are generally considered safe and effective anticaries agents. Dentifrices designed for sensitive teeth are available on the market and contain one or more of the following materials that have been promoted as desensitizing agents: formaldehyde, sodium citrate, strontium chloride hexahydrate, and potassium nitrate. The Food and Drug Administration regulates dentifrices containing fluorides, desensitizing agents, and other therapeutic ingredients as drugs. These products must conform to the monograph approved for over-the-counter drug products. A newer development is the introduction of dentifrice formulations designed to reduce bacterial plaque. Among the active agents suggested are chlorhexidine gluconate, sodium borate, sanguinaria or "bloodroot" extract, sodium pyrophosphate, zinc citrate, triclosan, and a variety of essential oils. Buffer salts such as the various sodium phosphates may be used to maintain the pH at the desired levels, and certified colors may be employed. Formulations containing peroxides to release active oxygen to the oral cavity are now on the market with claims suggesting effectiveness in preventing or treating periodontal disease. Whether these claims will withstand FDA scrutiny remains to be seen. Capitalizing on the recent practice of some dentists to bleach the teeth with strong hydrogen peroxide solutions, a number of dental products have come on the market to help whiten teeth with milder peroxide treatments. Clear gels containing 3% hydrogen peroxide have been introduced as part of three-part systems that contain (a) citric acid rinse designed to prepare tooth surfaces for bleaching by mild etching action, (b) the peroxide bleach, and (c) a polishing cream to clean and polish. Other marketers have offered only the bleach gel; still others have introduced toothpastes containing alkaline metallic peroxides such as calcium peroxide and magnesium peroxide, which release active oxygen in the mouth. Dentifrices have been patented and marketed to try to provide the "Keyes" therapy for periodontal disease in a single toothpaste. [6–9]. Because hydrogen peroxide releases active oxygen in alkaline aqueous solution, development of toothpastes containing both peroxide and sodium bicarbonate required special approaches. Schaeffer [6] separated the hydrogen peroxide and sodium bicarbonate into two separate pastes that were codispensed through a single nozzle. Rudy [7] provided a nonaqueous base in which the sodium bicarbonate and/or peroxide is coated with a water-soluble coating to maintain stability. Winston [8] describes a polyethylene glycol paste containing sodium bicarbonate and sodium percarbonate. The sodium percarbonate dissociates in the oral cavity to release hydrogen peroxide. Gordon [9] uses microencapsulated calcium peroxide as the oxygen source with sodium bicarbonate and urea.

IV. TYPICAL FORMULAS

A. Formulation Criteria

When one begins to formulate a dentifrice one should first establish the form and primary functional objective. For example, should the paste be opaque or a clear gel; should the paste be designed as a cosmetic high-cleaning formulation, or should the paste be a fluoride anticaries formulation? These decisions dictate the choice of abrasives. Clear gel formulations generally are built around silicas, which have refractive indices close to that of the humectant/water portion and thus appear clear in the final product. High-cleaning formulas are usually built around combinations of dicalcium phosphate, dihydrate, and dicalcium phosphate, anhydrous.

Fluoride pastes must be formulated with compatible abrasives that contain no soluble calcium salts that may interact with and reduce the concentration of available fluoride ions. Sodium fluoride and stannous fluoride pastes may be formulated with insoluble sodium metaphosphate, silicas, or aluminas. Sodium monofluorophosphate is less susceptible to reaction with soluble calcium salts and a wider choice of abrasive may be successfully used. Humectant choice and concentration are dependent on factors previously mentioned. Most typically, combinations of glycerin and sorbitol are employed. The two most frequently used binders are carrageenan and CMC, although good results have also been obtained using combinations of magnesium aluminum silicate and sodium carboxymethylcellulose (CMC).

After selection of the abrasive, humectant, and binders, experimental formulations are prepared to establish optimum levels for each ingredient group. Viscosity can be increased by increasing binder concentrations or increasing abrasive concentrations. Viscosity can also be varied by varying the viscosity grade of a binder, such as CMC. In silica-based formulas, the concentration of the aerogel or thickening silica may be varied to modify consistency.

Selection of the flavor is critical if consumer acceptance is to be achieved. A well-rounded and compatible combination of essential oils and flavors must be compounded. This task is frequently left to flavor specialists who offer proprietary blends for consideration. The formulator must evaluate these submissions and arrive at an optimum concentration that imparts pleasant taste and a "wake-up" or refreshing feeling in the mouth without burning and irritation. In conjunction with flavor selection, the level of sweetener must be established. Formulators should note that the taste buds of the mouth are less sensitive in the morning after awakening, and that flavors that may seem too strong when tested in the middle of the day may actually taste too weak to a "morning mouth."

Although there is some disagreement on the necessity of preservatives in toothpaste, most formulations contain either 0.1% sodium benzoate or 0.1% to 0.2% methylparaben plus 0.05% to 0.1% propylparaben. The need for preservatives is considered minimal when the total water content of the formulation (including water introduced through sorbitol or other ingredients) is below 20%. However, it is becoming more common to formulate with relatively low levels of silica, resulting in higher water contents. Therefore, attention to preservation requirements becomes more important. In any event, suitable preservative challenge tests should be performed to establish that the preservative system is adequate. Active drug ingredients in dentifrices require special attention in formulating. Anticaries agents, particularly fluorides, are regulated by the Food and Drug Administration under the proposed monograph for safe and effective anticaries agents. Under this monograph the concentration of fluoride ion in dentifrices is limited to a maximum of 1100 parts per million in freshly prepared pastes and may not fall below 600 ppm within the shelf life of the dentifrice. Expiration dating is required on the package unless it can be established that the minimum fluoride concentration is still present after 3 years. The stabilities of the various fluoride salts differ from each other and are greatly affected by the other ingredients in the formula. Sodium and stannous fluoride are unstable in formulas based on dicalcium phosphates, and are most stable in formulations based on insoluble sodium metaphosphate, alumina, or hydrated silicas. Sodium monofluorophosphate has a wider latitude of compatibility and more variety in the abrasive used and amount that is possible. In formulating with sodium monofluorophosphate, one must monitor both the free fluoride and the monofluorophosphate ion over time to make certain that within the shelf life of the product, at least one half of the fluoride is present as monofluorophosphate. In a similar manner, the incorporation of other active ingredients as desensitizers or antiplaque agents must be done with a knowledge of their chemical properties and potential chemical or physical interactions.

B. Patent Considerations

The patent literature on toothpastes is extensive and must be taken into consideration when formulating. Some of the relevant patents are cited in this text, and more are to be found in the suggested reading at the end of this chapter. Expired patents serve as an excellent source for specific formulation concepts and details. Many earlier patents covered surface-active agents as replacements for soap and described specific abrasives in combination with fluorides as well as the first clear gels. Current patents are more likely to be devoted to dentifrices containing both clear gels and opaque pastes in the same tube or delivering a multiple-striped paste, as well as many other concepts. The formulator should conduct complete patent searches, since he or she bears the responsibility for determining that the new formulation does not violate any current patents.

C. Case Histories

Rather than simply citing examples of good formulations for the various types of dentifrices without regard to the experimental steps that were taken to achieve them, we have chosen a series of case histories to present this information. In each case, the starting formulas, which were created on the basis of principles previously discussed, will be examined. This shortcomings will be evaluated, and the step-by-step modifications that were required to achieve a satisfactory formula will be described.

1.   *Case History No. 1*

The development of a sodium fluoride–containing toothpaste similar to the market leader.

   This problem first required a number of preliminary decisions. To achieve 1000 ppm of fluoride ion, sodium fluoride must be used at 0.22% (a 10% overage to allow for loss raises the concentration to 0.24%). A silica abrasive and thickener system was chosen as most compatible with sodium fluoride (Zeo 49 abrasive and Zeosyl 200 thickening silica, manufactured by Huber Chemical Co., are typical examples). The binders were selected xanthan gum (Kelzan or Keltrol, manufactured by Kelco) and carbomer 940 (Carbopol 940, manufactured by Goodrich Chemical Co.), because these were used in the market leader product. The following formula represents the first trial. Close evaluation of the resulting paste will help decide on modifications required for the next experiment. If the viscosity is too low, the level of thickening silica or binder may be increased. Poor cohesion usually requires binder modification. In this manner the physical properties are evaluated and changes made. The formulas are shown in Table 2.

   Examination of the resulting paste (Table 2, formula 1) showed very close correlation in all physical characteristics to those of the market leader except that the viscosity was too low. This suggested, as the next step, a modification in the ratio between the abrasive and thickening silicas as well as an increase in the concentration of the binder ingredients. The second formulation was prepared (Table 2, formula 2).

   These changes resulted in a satisfactory viscosity. The final formula, 3, illustrates a number of modifications that actually required several additional experiments. Glycerin was reduced from 10% to 8% for economy when it was found that no drying of the paste in an open tube occurred. Sorbitol was increased, and the phosphates were rebalanced for better buffering action. At the same time, there was a readjustment of the xanthan/carbomer concentration along with the abrasive silica/thickening silica ratio in order to achieved better texture. Carbomer 940 and titanium dioxide were reduced.

   Flavor and foaming levels were adjusted, and a color adjustment was made. This became the final formula (Table 2, formula 3). This formulation met the design parameters and was shelf life. Initial fluoride assays were conducted to measure any loss in available fluoride during aging. Samples were tested for radioactive dentin abrasion and compared to the target paste.

   Had these results indicated a significant variance from the target, it would have been necessary to reexamine the source, grade, and concentration of the polishing agent. There are a number of acceptable grades with differing abrasivities.

2.   *Case History No. 2*

The development of a dentifrice containing sodium monofluorophosphate.

   This project allows more freedom in the choice of abrasive as there is less incompatibility between this more stable salt and the abrasive. In this project, dicalcium phosphate dihydrate was chosen as the abrasive, because it is economical, exhibits moderate abrasivity, and provides good polishing and consistent quality. Inclusion in the following formulas of tetrasodium pyrophosphate as a soluble stabilizer was required to prevent hardening of the toothpaste in its tube on aging. This is a condition that may occur with dicalcium phosphate. Radioactive dentin abrasion (RDA) studies have shown

Table 2 Sodium Fluoride Toothpastes

No.	Phase	Ingredient	Percent by Weight		
			Formula 1	Formula 2	Formula 3
1	A	Glycerin 96%	10.00	10.00	8.00
2	A	Xanthan gum	.25	.30	.50
3	B	Sorbitol 70%	27.75	27.75	32.75
4	C	Carbomer 940	.25	.30	0.00
5	C	Carbomer 94 (2%)	0.00	0.00	12.50
5	D	Deionized water	29.60	29.85	14.50
6	D	Monosodium phosphate	.70	.70	.55
7	D	Trisodium phosphate	1.25	1.25	1.35
8	D	Sodium saccharin	.20	.15	.25
9	D	Sodium fluoride	.24	.24	.24
10	E	Abrasive silica	15.00	14.00	18.00
11	E	Thickening silica	7.00	8.00	3.50
12	E	Titanium dioxide	.50	0.5	.02
13	F	Sodium lauryl sulfate	1.20	1.20	1.25
14	F	Flavor	1.00	.70	1.00
15	F	Sorbitol 70%	5.00	5.00	5.00
16	F	FD&C Blue #1 (1%)	.06	.06	.55
17	F	FD&C Yellow #5 (1%)	0.00	0.00	.04
		TOTAL	100.00	100.00	100.00
		pH:	6.7	6.5	8.9
		Viscosity in cps:	56M	70M	78M

Brookfield Viscometer Model RVT
Spindle F @ 5 rpm, Helipath Stand.

Manufacturing Instructions: Sprinkle xanthan into glycerin in a beaker with motor-driven propeller type agitation (Phase A). Once uniform add Phase B with agitation. In a separate vessel sprinkle carbomer 940 into rapidly agitating cold Phase C water. Once uniform, add to batch with agitation. Combine Phase D with agitation. Add to batch with agitation. Transfer to bowl of vacuum mixer.[a] Add ingredients of Phase E one at a time with agitation. Seal unit with cover and apply 28 or more inches of vacuum for 30 to 45 minutes with continuous agitation. Combine Phase F with agitation; once uniform, add to batch with agitation. Mix under vacuum for 5 minutes.

---

[a]The vacuum mixer may be a laboratory-scale version of a production vessel such as an Abbe Mixer or a Nauta Mixer or (as in my laboratory) a KitchenAid (Hobart) mixer enclosed in a sealed vessel that can be evacuated with a laboratory vacuum pump.

that when a single abrasive is used, such as dicalcium phosphate, dihydrate, the concentration in the formula has minimal effect on the abrasivity. The concentration (40% to 60%) is therefore selected to optimize the paste texture and form. The experimental formulas prepared leading up to an acceptable product are shown in Table 3.

The results of the first experiment (Table 3, formula 1) revealed a paste very similar to the leading white sodium monofluorophosphate paste. The viscosity was somewhat low, but the cost was too high because of its high glycerin content. To correct this the following revision was then made in the second experiment. Twelve percent of the glycerin was replaced by sorbitol solution (70%) and the binder CMC was increased to

Table 3 Sodium Monofluorophosphate Toothpaste

			Percent by Weight	
No.	Phase	Ingredient	Formula 1	Formula 2
1	A	Glycerin 96%	22.00	10.00
2	A	CMC-9M31XF (Hercules)	.65	.85
3	B	Sorbitol	0.00	12.00
3	B	Deionized water	25.01	24.81
4	B	Tetrasodium pyrophosphate anhydrous	.25	.25
5	B	Sodium saccharin	.20	.20
6	B	Sodium benzoate	.10	.10
7	B	Sodium monofluorophosphate	.84	.84
8	C	Sodium hydroxide (50%)	.05	.05
9	D	Dicalcium phosphate, dihydrate	48.70	48.70
10	E	Flavor	1.00	1.00
11	F	Sodium lauryl sulfate	1.20	1.20
		TOTAL	100.00	100.00
		pH:	7.2	7.2
		Viscosity:	79M cps	136M cps

Brookfield Viscometer Model RVT
Spindle F @ 5 rpm, Helipath Stand.

Manufacturing Procedure: Add glycerin to vacuum mixer. Slowly sprinkle in CMC with rapid agitation. In a separate vessel dissolve ingredients of Phase B in Phase B water. Add to batch. Add Phase C, cover, and mix under 27 to 29 inches of vacuum for 5 to 10 minutes. Add Phase D. Mix under vacuum for 30 minutes. Add E and F, mix under vacuum for 5 minutes.

0.85% to increase viscosity. This formulation (Table 3, formula 2) closely duplicated the market leader and was judged satisfactory for final testing and approval.

3. *Case History No. 3*

Development of a smokers' toothpaste.

Smokers' toothpastes are designed to help remove superficial stains caused by tobacco tar depositing on the pellicle of the teeth. Studies have consistently demonstrated that there is a relation between the abrasivity of a toothpaste and its ability to remove stains. Increasing abrasiveness increases the removal of stained plaque and discoloration up to a point. Above a given level of abrasivity, stain removal is not improved. While even high abrasive formulations do not appear to abrade dental enamel significantly because of the toughness of the enamel structure, such formulas may damage exposed dentin at the gum line of individuals who have receding gums due to age or periodontal disease. Therefore, the necessity exists to develop smokers' toothpaste formulas at an abrasive level high enough to assure good stain removal yet safe even for users with exposed dentin. As previously noted, a radioactive dentin abrasion score of 140 to 150 on a scale on which calcium pyrophosphate in a standard slurry is 100 achieves the best cleaning and stain removal and is considered within the upper limits for safety.

The formulations tested are shown in Table 4. The first formula (Table 4, formula 1) illustrates the use of the combination of dicalcium phosphate, anhydrous, with di-

Table 4 Product: Smokers' Toothpaste

No.	Phase	Ingredient	Percent by Weight				
			(#1)	(#2)	(#3)	(#4)	(#5)
1	A	Glycerin 96%	5.00	5.00	10.00	10.00	10.00
2	A	CMC 9M31XF	1.00	1.00	1.00	.60	1.00
3	B	Sorbitol 70%	24.00	24.00	19.00	22.00	18.00
4	C	Deionized water	16.95	16.95	16.95	21.10	16.95
5	C	Sodium benzoate	.10	.10	.10	.10	.10
6	C	Sodium saccharin	.20	.20	.20	.02	.20
7	C	Trisodium phosphate	.25	.25	.25	.25	.25
8	D	Abrasive silica	0.00	0.00	0.00	24.00	8.00
9	D	Calcium pyrophosphate	0.00	0.00	0.00	0.00	10.00
8	D	Dicalcium phosphate, dihydrate	35.00	30.00	30.00	0.00	0.00
9	D	Dicalcium phosphate anhydrous	10.00	15.00	15.00	12.00	24.00
10	D	Thickening silica	0.00	0.00	0.00	.75	4.00
11	D	Kaolin	0.00	0.00	0.00	.50	0.00
12	D	Alumina	0.00	0.00	0.00	.50	0.00
13	E	Sodium lauryl sulfate	1.50	1.50	1.50	1.50	1.50
14	E	Flavor	1.00	1.00	1.00	1.00	1.00
15	E	Sorbitol 70%	5.00	5.00	5.00	5.00	5.00
		Total	100.00	100.00	100.00	100.00	100.00
		pH:	7.0	7.1	7.1	7.2	7.2

Viscosity: Brookfield Model RVT, Helipath stand
Initial: 300,000 cps (Spindle #TG@5 rpm.)
After 48 hrs: 500,000 cps
Radioactive Dentin Abrasion Score: 95   115   115   95   130

Manufacturing Instructions: In the bowl of a KitchenAid blender equipped for vacuum blending, sprinkle CMC into glycerin with agitation (Phase A). Add Phase B to Phase A. Add ingredients of Phase C to Phase C water with mixing, heat if necessary to dissolve, and add to batch. Add ingredients of Phase D one at a time with mixing to batch. Vacuum mix 30 minutes. Premix Phase E and add to batch.

calcium phosphate, dihydrate, to increase abrasivity and cleaning ability. While superior to ordinary pastes as a stain remover, this formulation was only moderately abrasive, yielding a score of 95. In formula 2 (Table 4) the ratio of anhydrous salt to dihydrate was increased and the resulting product met the cleaning and stain removal objectives but tended to dry out in the tube if the cap was left off. This was overcome by an increase in the glycerin content of the toothpaste as shown in formula 3 (Table 4).

This formula was satisfactory and was well accepted by the consumer until competitive pressures required further improvement in its cleaning score. Formula 4 (Table 4) introduced hydrated silicas as both polishing agent and auxiliary thickeners. In addition, low levels of alumina and Kaopolite SAF, a specially treated form of kaolin clay manufactured by the Kaopolite Corp., were added to enhance the polishing action.

The results of this experiment were disappointing in that the modified abrasive system yielded a lower than expected abrasive level and, as a consequence, diminished rather than improved cleaning. Dicalcium phosphate blends generally yield an abrasive score that is close to the weighted average of the abrasivities of the individual abrasive. Blends of dicalcium phosphate anhydrous with hydrated silica are more dependent on other factors, such as bulk density, particle size, and particle hardness. This interferes with the predictability of the abrasivity of these combinations. In formula 5 (Table 4) calcium pyrophosphate was added as an abrasive, the alumina and kaolin were dropped, and the abrasives were rebalanced. This formula met all objectives.

4. Case History No. 4

Development of a clear fluoride toothpaste.

Clear toothpastes depend for their clarity on the principle that a solid appears transparent when suspended in a liquid of equal refractive index [10]. This principle can be applied to toothpaste formulation when using hydrated silicas both as abrasive and also as thickeners. Suitable blends of glycerin, sorbitol, and water can be found to match the refractive index of silica. Clarity also depends on the total absence of dispersed air and, therefore, vacuum deaeration is especially important. Polyethyleneglycol-32 is included to reduce stringiness and promote a "short" texture. The formulas prepared are shown in Table 5.

Table 5 Product: Clear Toothpaste

No.	Phase	Ingredient	(#1)	(#2)	(#3)	(#4)
1	A	Glycerin 96%	14.00	14.00	14.00	14.00
2	A	CMC 9M31XF	.40	.30	.30	.30
3	B	Sorbitol 70%	41.25	41.85	42.10	41.56
4	C	Sodium saccharin	.20	.20	.20	.20
5	C	Sodium benzoate	.08	.08	.08	.08
6	C	Sodium fluoride	.22	.22	.22	0.00
7	C	Sodium monofluorophosphate	0.00	0.00	0.00	.76
8	C	Deionized water	5.00	5.00	5.00	5.00
9	D	Polyethylene glycol-32	5.00	5.00	5.00	5.00
10	E	Abrasive silica	14.00	14.00	14.00	14.00
11	E	Thickening silica	8.00	7.50	7.50	7.50
12	F	Glycerin 96%	5.50	5.50	5.50	5.50
13	F	Sodium lauryl sulfate	1.00	1.00	1.25	1.25
14	F	Polysorbate-20	2.00	2.00	2.00	2.00
15	F	FD&C Blue #1 (1%)	.05	.05	.05	.05
16	F	FD&C Yellow #5 (1%)	.10	.10	.10	.10
17	F	Flavor	1.20	1.20	.70	.70
18	F	Alcohol SD38B	2.00	2.00	2.00	2.00
		Total	100.00	100.00	100.00	100.00

Manufacturing Instructions: Add glycerin to vacuum mixer. Slowly sprinkle in CMC with agitation to prepare Phase A. Add Phase B. Dissolve Phase C ingredients in Phase C water and add to mixer. Add Phase D and E ingredients with agitation. Close cover and mix under 26 to 30 inches of vacuum for 20 minutes. Premix and add Phase F, mix under vacuum for 10 more minutes.

Formula 1 (Table 5) tries to take advantage of these principles. This experiment resulted in a clear paste that was too heavy in consistency. Not only was the viscosity somewhat high, but the paste was too cohesive and did not rinse well. Therefore, reductions in both the carboxymethylcellulose, which affects both viscosity and cohesiveness, and the thickening silica, which contributes to viscosity, were indicated. The viscosity of formula 2 was soft and acceptable and, in addition, the rinsability was improved. Foam was judged to be too low, and formula 3 was prepared by increasing the sodium lauryl sulfate content. The resulting formula met all specifications and was accepted. Formula 4 illustrates a modification employing sodium monofluorophosphate.

5. *Case History No. 5*

Development of a sodium bicarbonate "baking soda" toothpaste.

This project first required the study of the large body of patent literature covering various aspects of baking soda toothpastes. On first examination, all avenues appear to have already been covered by patents. Several old approaches that predated these patents were found, but the resulting toothpastes were inferior. It was therefore decided to take advantage of the recent expiration (on February 10, 1993) of a series of patents [11–15] issued to Thomas Delaney et al. and assigned to the Colgate-Palmolive Co. This

Table 6 Sodium Bicarbonate Toothpaste

			Percent by Weight			
No.	Phase	Ingredient	(#1)	(#2)	(#3)	(#4)
1	A	Glycerin 96%	24.60	20.50	20.50	20.50
2	A	CMC 9M31XF	1.25	1.10	1.10	1.10
3	B	Deionized water	18.62	23.17	28.72	27.84
4	B	Sodium saccharin	0.25	0.25	0.25	0.25
5	B	Sodium benzoate	0.10	0.10	0.10	0.10
6	B	Sodium monofluorophosphate	0.00	0.00	0.00	0.88
7	C	Sodium bicarbonate USP #1	30.00	30.00	26.00	26.00
8	C	Abrasive silica	15.00	15.00	13.50	13.50
9	C	Titanium dioxide #3328	0.40	0.40	0.35	0.35
10	D	Sodium–Lauroyl sarcosinate	2.30	2.00	2.00	2.00
11	D	Glycerin 96%	5.60	5.60	5.60	5.60
12	D	Sodium lauryl sulfate	0.98	0.98	0.98	0.98
13	D	Peppermint flavor	0.90	0.90	0.90	0.90
		TOTAL	100.00	100.00	100.00	100.00
		pH:	8.90	8.90	8.90	8.90
		Specific gravity:	1.444	1.444	1.444	1.444
		Viscosity:	750M	660M	420M	420M

Brookfield RVT Model
Helipath Stand, Spindle TF @ 5 rpm

Manufacturing Instructions: Add glycerin to vacuum mixer. Slowly sprinkle in CMC with agitation to prepare Phase A. Dissolve Phase B ingredients in Phase B water and add to mixer. Add Phase C ingredients with agitation. Close cover and mix under 26 to 30 inches of vacuum for 20 minutes. Premix and add Phase D, mix under vacuum for 10 more minutes.

allowed the formulator to work with sodium bicarbonate levels up to 60% and allowed combinations of sodium bicarbonate with other suitable abrasives. The formulations prepared are shown in Table 6. Formula 1 produced a generally satisfactory product in terms of cleaning ability and abrasive level. The ratio of two parts of sodium bicarbonate to one part of silica produced a paste that retained more body in the mouth than did sodium bicarbonate without silica. Viscosity was too high, however, and texture was too cohesive. Formula 2 addressed these problems. Reduction of glycerin and CMC levels improved viscosity but not enough. Formula 3 further reduced abrasive level to reduce viscosity to 420,000 cps; it met all design parameters and was considered successful. A final version (formula 4) was prepared by adding sodium monofluorophosphate to provide cavity control.

V. EQUIPMENT AND PREPARATION TECHNIQUES

A. Equipment

Successful toothpaste preparation—even in the laboratory—requires a means of excluding or removing entrapped air. This is best accomplished by conducting the entire manufacturing operation under vacuum. In a production setting commercial equipment is available, such as the Day-Nauta vacuum mixer (manufactured by the J. H. Day Co. of Cincinnati, Ohio). This is a large conical mixing vessel with a swing arm and helical screw mixer supplemented by high-speed grinding mills inserted at the base. Another piece of equipment, the Abbe mill, uses a paddle mixer plus high-speed milling capability. Both of these units are operated under a vacuum of 28 inches of mercury or greater.

Where vacuum equipment is unavailable or as a supplement, a unit called the "Versator" (manufactured by Cornell Manufacturing Co. of Springfield, New Jersey), may be employed. This consists of a rapidly spinning disk enclosed in a vacuum chamber. The paste is drawn into the chamber under vacuum and dispersed as a thin layer on the rapidly revolving disk. It becomes instantly deaerated during its passage. A system found most useful in the laboratory is to enclose a KitchenAid Mixer (manufactured by Hobart Manufacturing Co.) in a small stainless steel tank fitted with an airtight cover and connected to a laboratory vacuum pump. A sealed electric outlet is provided inside the tank to connect the mixer. This device simulates the Day-Nauta or Abbe and can prepare good reproducible laboratory samples of as little as one kilogram.

B. Preparation Methods

There are a number of acceptable procedures that may be used to combine dentifrice ingredients. The following three methods have proved effective in the laboratory.

1. *A Cold Method*

The paste is prepared as follows: the humectant, such as glycerin or sorbitol, is added to the bowl of the mixer. Binder is sprinkled in under agitation so that the particles are dispersed in the absence of water, preventing swelling at this point. A separate liquid phase is prepared, which includes the available water, sweetener, preservatives, and any therapeutic additives. This solution is then added to the humectant/binder mixture. The mixture is placed under vacuum for about 5 minutes to deaerate the thick gelatinous liquid phase. The vacuum is opened, and the abrasives are added with mixing until they are sufficiently moistened by the binder so that they will not dust when vacuum is applied. Vacuum is reapplied, and the paste is mixed for at least 30 minutes under 28 inches or more of vacuum. In the meantime the surface-active agents and flavors are dispersed in about 5% of the available humectant. At the conclusion of the 30-minute time, the vacuum is again opened, and the flavor mixture is added. Five minutes of additional mixing under vacuum should produce a smooth air-free paste.

2.   *Heated Liquid Phase Method*

A variation of this method, recommended by some suppliers, involves the use of a hot liquid phase. In this method the abrasive, binder, and preservative are premixed as dry powders in the mixer. A hot solution of glycerin, sorbitol, water, and sweetener is then slowly added with mixing to the dry powders. The resulting mass is mixed under vacuum for 30 minutes after which the solution of flavor, surfactant, glycerin, or sorbitol is added for a final 5 minutes of vacuum mixing.

3.   *Multiple Liquid Phase Method*

The third method is particularly adaptable to formulations using an aluminum magnesium silicate/carboxymethylcellulose (CMC) binder system. Magnesium aluminum silicate is added to hot water in the mixing vessel followed by the sweetener. A separate phase is prepared consisting of the bulk of the humectant, the binder, the flavor and preservative. This solution is added to the mixer followed by the balance of the humectant. Five minutes of vacuum mixing follows to deaerate the liquid mixture. Abrasives are added and again mixed for 30 minutes under vacuum. After this the surfactant is added in dry form followed by another 5 minutes of vacuum mixing.

Similar methods may be used to prepare clear gel dentifrices. In this case the cold vacuum procedure described previously is most effective. However, when the abrasive system consists of both an abrasive silica and a thickening silica, the abrasive silica should be added first, followed by the incremental addition of the thickening silica and additional vacuum steps.

C.   Other Considerations

1.   *Evaluation*

Experimental pastes should be evaluated to assure that they meet the established characteristics. Samples in tubes should be placed under stability testing at various temperatures, not only to ensure the stability of the formulation, but also to assure compatibility with the tubes chosen for marketing of the product.

Final formulations must also be evaluated for safety before the product is ready for consumer use. This involves knowledgeable selection of raw materials with regard to their physiological properties as well as comprehensive testing of the finished formula. Radioactive dentin and enamel abrasion tests determine the relative abrasivity of the formulation with regard to objectives and to competitive products. In vitro animal safety screening, including oral toxicity and mucosal irritation, should be performed before human tests are conducted. Human tests include use tests to determine both product satisfaction and any possible adverse reactions, as well as clinical evaluations consisting of controlled use by a volunteer panel supervised by a dentist designed to detect allergic response, irritation, or other oral problems, while at the same time documenting effectiveness in meeting formulation objectives.

2. *Stability*

As with other dosage forms, stability is the ability of a toothpaste to retain its important characteristics essentially unchanged throughout its expected shelf life. Tests must assess the physical stability of the paste as well as the chemical stability of its ingredients.

In addition to visual comparisons of freshly prepared and aged samples, physical characteristics that can be quantitatively determined should be used for evaluation. Specifications should be established for appearance, color, uniformity, flavor, net weight, pH, viscosity, and specific gravity, and these parameters should be recorded for each stability storage condition at each time interval.

In the case of therapeutic toothpastes, which are considered drugs, the stability of the active ingredients must be established and be reflected in the expiration date on the package.

Stability evaluation must be conducted in conjunction with package development. Final stability tests are always performed on product packed in its commercial container.

Ideally, stability studies should reflect the storage conditions that will occur during the expected lifetime of the product. Therefore, evaluation at temperatures from freezing to 120°F over the shelf life of the product are necessary.

Insight into long-term stability can often be attained through the use of accelerated stability studies during which increased temperatures may simulate the behavior of the product over a long period in a relatively short time. This is based on the fact that reactions that adversely affect stability are temperature dependent and occur more rapidly at elevated temperatures. In this manner, a 90-day study at 45°C is considered the equivalent of 12 to 18 months at room temperature. Similarly, cycling a sample between the frozen state and 45°C for three cycles multiplies the stress of freezing and thawing.

A formal stability program for toothpaste consists of placing samples that have been weighed, chemically analyzed, and measured for physical properties in storage at room temperature, 5°C, 37°C, and 45°C. Samples are withdrawn at intervals and reevaluated. Recommended evaluation intervals are 1 week, 1 month, 3 months, and 6 months at elevated and reduced temperatures and continuing room temperature studies for 1, 2, and 3 years. In addition, samples should pass three cycles of freezer (–20°C)/oven (45°C) without separation or major changes in specifications.

Initial expiration dates for drug-containing toothpastes may be based on accelerated test data but should be modified as real-time data become available. Pastes that still retain their original specifications after 3 months at 45° C may carry an estimated expiration date of 2 years after manufacture. The first three commercial batches of a new formula are subjected to the same test conditions, and the expiration date may be extended if supported by real-time studies.

3. *Packaging*

Traditionally toothpaste has been packaged in collapsible tubes. Metal tubes have been produced from lead, tin, or aluminum. Interior linings may be wax or epoxy lacquer. Wax-lined lead tubes are used for many industrial purposes but are not considered suitable for toothpaste because of the oral toxicity of lead. Tin tubes are safe and sufficiently strong and flexible but are costwise not competitive with aluminum. Aluminum tubes, either uncoated or expoxy lined, are suitable for most pastes, but may be reactive with some active ingredients. Comparability studies must be conducted to assure that there are no chemical interactions between the tube and the toothpaste formula. Because some unstabilized fluoride pastes react with aluminum, a laminated plastic, aluminum foil, and paper tube with a polyethylene neck has been developed and manufactured by the American Can Co. under the tradename Glaminate. Glaminate tubes are induction heat sealed on special equipment and then clipped at the sealed end. Glaminate tubes are lightweight, economical, and resistant to most toothpaste ingredients. Their disadvantages are that when deformed or squeezed they still retain some memory for their original shape and may suck in some air. If a toothpaste is sensitive to oxidation, this type of tube may create a stability problem.

Low-density polyethylene tubes are not satisfactory for toothpaste both because of their shape memory and because most flavors permeate the walls of the tubes. In the past 2 years, high-density polyethylene has been successfully used by several manufacturers in stand-up tubes that rest vertically on their caps. Some years ago semiliquid pastes were sold in inverted polyethylene bottles. These had limited success and were followed by pressurized aerosol containers, dispensing paste through a dip tube and foam style valve. These pastes were pressurized with nitrogen. They failed in the marketplace for several reasons. As the paste was dispensed the remaining paste in the container tended to cavitate, eventually discharging the nitrogen, inactivating the container, and wasting the balance of the product. Accidental misuse caused loss of the nitrogen propellant and was responsible for many failures. Furthermore, the low viscosity that was required caused the paste to sag between the bristles.

The modern equivalent to these "aerosol" toothpastes is the "pump." The pump is a rigid plastic sleeve, with a soft plastic pump top and a carefully designed spring device in the base. Actuating the pump causes the spring device to "walk up" the interior of the sleeve and thus force toothpaste out of the spout.

4. *Commercial Manufacturing*

The formulator must be aware of manufacturing techniques so he or she can fine-tune formulations to achieve the most efficient commercial production method, as well as to assist in the solving of product-based production problems.

Bulk toothpaste, manufactured in vacuum mixing kettles as previously described, is pumped to storage or holding tanks to await filling. Pumps, piping, storage tanks, and all surfaces that come in contact with product must be constructed of nonreactive material, such as stainless steel. Pumps must be capable of moving high-viscosity and high-density pastes without aeration. Paste is pumped to the hoppers of tube-filling machines. Empty tubes are then positioned in the filling machines either manually or automatically. An orientation mark on the tube is read by an electric eye to position the label panels. Tubes are automatically filled and sealed. Metal tubes are closed by folding the open end and crimping the fold. Glaminate tubes are sealed by ultrasonically heating the inner plastic surfaces of the open end, pressing the end closed to seal it, and clipping off the excess.

Filled tubes pass on a conveyor belt to an automatic cartoner. The cartoner is fed with folded individual cartons; these are opened, the tube is inserted, and the cartons are closed. Cartoned tubes are either cellophane bundled or packed into shipping cartons.

Because the production line has been set up and designed for specific formulations, failure of a paste to meet its design specifications not only may result in substandard paste but may interfere with the proper functioning of the production line. Quality control inspection of samples taken at all stages of the production process is required to assure efficient manufacturing and the production of high-quality product.

REFERENCES

1. Dr. I. I. Lubowe and F. V. Wells, *Cosmetics and the Skin*, Reinhold Publishing Corp., New York, 1964, pp. 235–247.
2. S. D. Gershon and M. Pader, Dentifrices. In: *Cosmetics: Science and Technology*, Vol. I, 2nd ed. (M. S. Balsam and E. Sagarin, eds.), Interscience, New York, 1972, pp. 423–531.
3. R. J. Grabenstetler, R. W. Broge, F. L. Jackson, A. W. Radike, The measurement of the abrasion of human teeth by dentifrice abrasion: A test utilizing radioactive teeth, *J. Dent. Res.*, 37:1060 (1958).
4. G. K. Stookey and J. C. Muhler, Laboratory studies concerning enamel and dentin abrasion properties of common dentifrice polishing agents, *J. Dent. Res.* 47:524–532 (1968).
5. W. A. Poucher, *Perfumes, Cosmetics and Soaps*, Vol. III., (revised by G. M. Howard), Chapman and Hall, London, 1974, pp. 54–77.
6. H. Schaeffer, U.S. Patent 4,983,379, Dental Preparation, Article and Method for Storage and Delivery Thereof, January 8, 1991.
7. J. Rudy et al., Peroxydent Group, Livingston, N.J., U.S. Patent 4,837,008, Periodontal Composition and Method, June 6, 1989.
8. A. Winston, Church & Dwight Co., Inc., Princeton, N.J., U.S. Patent 4,891,211, Stable Hydrogen Peroxide–Releasing Dentifrice, January 2, 1990.
9. N. Gordon, U.S. Patent 4,980,154, Toothpaste and Gum Dentifrice, Composition and Method of Making Same, December 25, 1990.
10. M. Pader, W. Weisner, Lever Bros., New York, U.S. Patent 3,538,230, Oral Compositions Containing Silica Zerogels as Cleaning and Polishing Agents, November 3, 1970.
11. T. Delaney, W. Pierson, Colgate-Palmolive Co., New York, U.S. Patent 3,937,804, Toothpaste, February 10, 1976.
12. T. Delaney, W. Pierson, Colgate-Palmolive Co., New York, U.S. Patent 3,937,803, Flavored Dental Creams, February 10, 1976.
13. T. Delaney, W. Pierson, Colgate-Palmolive Co., New York, U.S. Patent 3,937,321, Toothpaste, February 10, 1976.
14. T. Delaney, W. Pierson, Colgate-Palmolive Co., New York, U.S. Patent 3,943,240, Toothpaste, March 9, 1976.
15. T. Delaney, W. Pierson, Colgate-Palmolive Co., New York, U.S. Patent 3,935,305, Toothpaste, January 27, 1976.

SUGGESTED READING

D. Aldcroft et al. (Unilever Patent Holdings), U.S. Patent 4,992,251, An amorphous silica for toothpaste is disclosed.

A. Baderstein and J. Engleberg, Plaque removing effects of brushing with a dentifrice. Tandlak., 64 (23), 770; *Oral Res.* Abst., 9, 1531 (1974).

J. B. Barth (Colgate-Palmolive Co.), U.S. Patent 4,180,467, A denture soak product includes sodium bicarbonate.

J. B. Barth (Colgate-Palmolive Co), U.S. Patent 4,132,770, Aqueous oral product contains sodium chloride in a deionized water.

J. D. Blue, U.S. Patent 4,978,521, A dentifrice preparation comprises sodium bicarbonate. British Standards Institute, Specifications for Toothpastes, BS 136 (1974).

A. Cabardo, Jr., U.S. Patent 4,276,287, A periodontal powder comprises sodium bicarbonate powder.

A. M. Cabardo Jr., U.S. Patent 4,414,203, A powder mixture for treatment of periodontal disorders comprises a mixture of sodium bicarbonate and aluminum bicarbonate.

F. E. Cocherell et al., U.S. Patent 4,812,306, A toothpaste composition comprises sodium bicarbonate, peppermint, glycerin, saccharin, sodium lauryl sulfate.

F. E. Cocherell et al., U.S. Patent 5,004,596, A toothpaste comprises a sodium bicarbonate, a flavoring oil, glycerin and vegetable oil.

W. B. Davis and D. A. Rees, A parametric test to measure the cleaning power of toothpaste. *J. Soc. Cosmet. Chem.* 26:217 (1975).

P. F. DePaola, Clinical studies of monofluorophosphate dentifrices, *Caries Res.,* 17(Suppl. 1): 119–135 (1983).

J. E. Eastoe and A. E. W. Miles, *Structural and Chemical Organization of Teeth*, Vol. II, Academic Press, New York and London, 1975.

M. E. Foulk and E. Pickering, A history of dentifrices, *J. Am. Pharm. Assoc.* 24:975 (1935).

M. C. Gaffar (Colgate Palmolive Co.), U.S. Patent 4,143,126, A dental paste comprises an abrasive, a humectant and gelatin.

P. O. Gerdin, Studies in dentifrices. I. Abrasiveness of dentifrices and removal of discoloured stains. S.T.T., 63:275 (1970).

W. M. Glandorf et al., (The Procter & Gamble Co.), U.S. Patent 4,849,212 Dentifrice composition includes from about 0.01 to about 0.50% of non-toxic pearlescent particles of titanium dioxide coated mica.

N. Gordon, U.S. Patent 4,522,805, A dentifrice comprises a sodium bicarbonate.

H. Harth et al. (Blendax-Werke R. Schneider GmbH), U.S. Patent 4,209,504, A toothpaste contains a silica polishing agent such as Zeolite A.

K. Harvey et al. (Colgate-Palmolive Co.), U.S. Patent 4,374,823, A dentifrice composition utilizes a sorbitol and a gelling agent.

J. R. Heath and H. J. Wilson, Classification of toothpaste stiffness by a dynamic method. *Br. Dent. J.,* 130:59 (1971).

J. J. Hefferen, How abrasive should a toothpaste be?, *Pharmacy Times*, July, pp 50–52 (1974).

J. I. Jacobson, U.S. Patent 4,367,218, An oral rinse composition includes a combination of alkali metal bicarbonates and alkali metal carbonates.

R. M. Katilainen, (Suomen Calcusan Oy-Finska Calaissan A.B.), U.S. Patent 4,885,156, A mouth wash solution contains water-soluble alkali metal salts of amino (carboxylic) acids such as EDTA.

K. Y. Kim (Monsanto Co.), U.S. Patent 4,007,260, An opaque dentifrice composition containing a silica polishing agent is claimed.

D. K. Kiozpeoplou (Colgate-Palmolive Co.), A toothpaste contains sodium bicarbonate, a polishing agent, gelling agents.

T. Malyama (Lion Corp.), U.S. Patent 4,618,488, A toothpaste contains abrasive silica or silicate.

S. Mazzanobile et al. (Beecham Inc.), U.S. Patent 4,108,978, A dentifrice gel consists of a silica polishing agent, sorbitol, sodium lauryl sulfate, sweetening, thickening and flavoring agents.

S. T. Melsheimer (Design & Funding, Inc.), U.S. Patent 4,312,889, A concentrate comprises sodium bicarbonate.

K. M. Muller (Degussa AG), U.S. Patent 4,705,679, A dental care toothpaste composition comprises water and an abrasive agent such as a silica.

K. M. Muller (Degussa AG), U.S. Patent 4,753,791, A toothpaste comprises a precipitated silica.

K. M. Muller et al. (Degussa AG), U.S. Patent 4,664,907, A toothpaste composition comprises a thickener and an abrasive.

M. Oyote et al. (Lion Corp.), U.S. Patent 4,612,189, A silica-containing dentifrice composition is claimed.

J. Peterson, L. Williamson, and R. Cassad, Caries inhibition with MTP–calcium carbonate dentifrice fluoridated area. A.I.D.R. Conference, London (1975).

J. J. Pollock et al. (The Research Foundation of State University of New York), U.S. Patents 4,618,489 & 4,861,582, A composition comprises from about 0.08% to about 1.6% bicarbonate ion.

F. Reiff et al. (Merck Patent Gesellschaft Mit Beschrankter Haftung), U.S. Patent 4,605,794, Sorbitol, process for its preparation, and use thereof, August 12, 1986.

M. W. Rosenthal (Jeffrey Martin, Inc.), U.S. Patent 4,863,722, Dentifrice compositions, September 5, 1989.

E. K. Seybert, U.S. Patent 4,153,680, Discloses the use of silica gels in dentifrice formulations.

A. M. Slee, E. Cimijotti, S. I. Rothstein, The effect of daily treatments with an Octenidine dentifrice formulation on gingival health in cynomolgus monkeys, *J. Periodontal Res.*, 20(5):542–549.

M. L. Tainter, C. E. Alford, E. T. Hinkel, F. C. Nachod, and M. Priznar, A quantitative method for measuring polish produced by dentifrices, *Proc. Toilet Goods Assoc.*, 7:38 (1974).

N. J. Van Abbe, A. J. Bridge, J. W. Ribbons, P. M. Dean, and J. A. Lazarou, The efect of dentifrices on extrinsic tooth stains, *J. Soc. Cosmet. Chem.*, 22:457 (1971).

S. K. Wason (J. M. Huber Corp.), U.S. Patent 4,144,321, A toothpaste composition comprises a silica polishing agent.

S. K. Wason (J. M. Huber Corp.), U.S. Patent 4,122,161, A toothpaste contains silica.

C. A. Watson (Lever Brothers Co.), U.S. Patent 3,864,470, A toothpaste contains a synthetic hydrated precipitated silica.

J. B. Wilkinson and B. R. Pugh, Toothpastes—cleaning and abrasion, *J. Soc. Cosmet. Chem.*, 21:595 (1970).

M. E. Wingall et al. (W. R. Grace & Co.), U.S. Patent 4,631,184, A dentifrice composition contains a particulate dialytic silica.

A. Winston et al. (Church & Dwight Co.), U.S. Patent 4,812,308 & 4,891,211, Sodium bicarbonate and sodium percarbonate containing tooth powder.

A. Winston et al. (Church & Dwight Co.), U.S. Patent 4,547,362, Sodium bicarbonate containing tooth powder, October 15, 1985.

A. Winston et al (Church & Dwight Co.), U.S. Patent 4,663,153, A tooth powder contains sodium bicarbonate particles.

12

Suppository Development and Production

Marion Gold

Centerchem, Inc., Stamford, Connecticut

Murti VePuri

Able Labs, South Plainfield, New Jersey

Lawrence H. Block

Duquesne University, Pittsburgh, Pennsylvania

I. INTRODUCTION

Suppositories are the neglected dosage form of medicine. Despite much work that has been done in recent years, especially in Europe and in a few progressive research centers in the United States and elsewhere, there continues to be a general rejection of rectal delivery as a routinely used route of administration. Pharmacology textbooks generally relegate rectal dosage either to situations in which the patient is comatose, nauseous or vomiting, or elderly or extremely young, or for local therapeutic effect.

There are—as will be shown later—important reasons to consider suppositories as a preferred route of administration in many situations. In addition to their obvious advantages when used in the above circumstances, use of rectal (and vaginal) anatomy and physiology for drug delivery can offer advantages that may overcome limitations inherent in alternative, more widely utilized pathways (See Table 1).

Physicians in northern European and Anglo-Saxon countries, where social conventions preclude greater use of rectal delivery, generally do not prescribe suppositories. In direct contrast, Latin Americans and Mediterranean Europeans use suppositories far more routinely. Yet rectal—as well as urethral and vaginal—delivery of drugs via suppositories makes excellent therapeutic sense, and in fact their use can be traced as far back as the Old Testament and in the writings of Hippocrates [1].

This surprising (perhaps) lack of acceptability of suppositories is certainly evident. Pharmaceutical companies in the United States, for example, report poor sales of drugs manufactured as suppositories (approximately 1% are so formulated); in Germany the figure is five times greater. In fact, one research group investigating rectal administration of insulin relates that, in an informal study among its "enlightened" research sci-

Table 1 Use of Suppositories by Therapeutic Application[a]

For Local Effect	
Antihemorrhoidal	16.4%
Gynecological, contraceptive	6.0
For Systemic Effect	
Analgesics	15.4%
Antiasthmatics, broncholytics, expectorants	11.9
Antiemetics	4.6
Antirheumatics	7.9
Cardiovascular	6.0
Influenza	8.3
Sedatives, antipsychotics	5.5
Miscellaneous	2.5

[a]The table represents a breakdown of 456 suppository products listed in the "Rote Liste" of drugs in Germany (1975).

entists, the vast majority would opt for subcutaneous injection versus rectal suppository insulin administration were they to develop diabetes. Clearly, despite the merits of suppositories, there is unfortunately a substantial resistance to their more widespread use, even within the medical community.

II. SUPPOSITORY CHARACTERISTICS

A. Definition

Suppositories can be defined in a number of ways, depending on the point of reference. Functionally, they may perhaps best be described as solid or semisolid dosage forms used for rectal, vaginal, or urethal administration of therapeutic agents. They typically consist of a dispersion of the active ingredient in an inert matrix generally composed of a rigid or semi-rigid base. Ideally, this dispersion is one that does not entail any chemical interactions between the active and the excipient, in order to avoid any alteration either of the active or its release from the suppository. Within limits, the dispersed phase can be incorporated into the suppository as a solid (e.g., powder) or a liquid (either aqueous, alcoholic, or glycolic solutions, oils, extracts, etc.) The material for the base, which can be either naturally or synthetically derived, is selected on the basis of its ability to soften, melt, or dissolve at approximately the temperature of the vagina or rectal ampulla and thereby release the incorporated medicament to either local or systemic targets. Finished suppositories are manufactured in a variety of shapes and sizes to best suit the treatment requirements (nature of the active ingredient, site of administration, age and condition of the patient, desired release pattern, etc.) and are available in a range of physical forms (e.g., molded or compressed, foil or plastic wrapped, or gelatin encapsulated).

Although some formulators might not view suppositories as disperse systems, particularly when the active ingredient(s) is dissolved rather than dispersed in the suppository base, one must nonetheless consider that drugs are dissolved, suspended, or dispersed in a vehicle that in itself comprises a disperse system. The lipoidal or polymeric components of the vehicle are present as heterogeneous admixtures in a multiphasic system.

B. Applications

Traditionally, suppositories are chosen either for local use or in cases where alternative routes of administration are unavailable, and a wide range of drugs has been incorporated into this dosage form. For example, Compazine suppositories are prescribed to control severe nausea and vomiting because oral ingestion for this indication could well be ineffective. Local anesthetics, laxatives, analgesics, and the like are also good candidates for rectal administration using suppositories; local antibiotic treatment is responsive to treatment by vaginal and urethral suppositories.

Suppositories are becoming increasingly important for systemic delivery as well. A number of anti-inflammatory agents are now being sold in suppository form, as are analgesics, antipyretics, and sedatives and hypnotics. And even more avenues for future rectal dosage are being explored: as stated above, ongoing work is being directed at insulin therapy in suppository form, and early results are promising (at least from a pharmacological point of view) [2].

C. Advantages

Suppositories *do* offer a number of advantages that make them worthy of far more intensive research and eventual employment [3]. Perhaps most importantly, rectal dosage of medicaments can be used effectively to substantially reduce hepatic first-pass elimination and to enhance drug bioavailability. This results from physiological differences in the venous drainage of the rectum; blood flow from the lower portion of the rectum, in contrast to that of the upper segment, does not immediately pass into the portal circulation (and subsequently into the liver for enzymatic degradation). Instead, drugs absorbed from the lower rectum pass directly into the general circulation, and experiments have shown that increases in bioavailability of as great as 100% over oral delivery are seen following rectal administration [4]. Alcoholic and aqueous solutions can be rapidly absorbed, and this is used to considerable advantage, for example, to administer diazepam in the treatment of acute convulsive attacks.

There is, in addition, a wide range of therapeutic agents that for any one of a number of reasons are efficaciously administered through the rectal mucosa. This is due either to their intrinsic physicochemical nature (which enables them to be efficiently taken up from the rectum), or to the manner in which they are handled by the body (which makes them ineffectively assimilated through other routes).

D. Comparison with Oral Delivery

Many studies have attempted to compare the efficacy of drugs administered rectally versus orally, but results are quite often inconclusive. Much depends on which parameters are being considered, the experimental conditions, and finally the choice of excipient. Moreover, certain active ingredients are just not well suited for suppository dosage.

For example, investigations have been inconclusive in determining the relative superiority of absorption of indomethacin [5,6] and aspirin [7,8] when given by either of the two routes; diazepam (administered as an alcoholic solution [9]) and propranolol [10] *have* been shown to exhibit greater bioavailability when administered rectally (for propanolol this is probably the consequence of significant hepatic metabolism following oral dosage). Bioequivalence to oral administration by theophylline suppositories was found only when microcrystalline drug was used [11], and not with standard suppository formulation [12]. Others report approximate bioequivalence between oral and rectal delivery with pentobarbital [13] despite its slower rectal absorption.

Not surprisingly, perhaps, some researchers propose that limited drug uptake with this route is more a function of formulation inadequacies than an inherent limitation of rectal dosage. They note that in cases where there is no first-pass metabolism, it has been shown that rectal administration of drugs *in solution* can provide bioavailability equivalent to that seen with oral administration. In fact, it may even be higher [14].

Rectal administration has not been immune to the significant ongoing research directed at development of sustained-release dosage forms. Suppositories composed of controlled-release pellets containing ketoprofen and disopyramide and other drugs have been administered rectally and evaluated. Release of the drugs (selected because they are not metabolized by first-pass metabolism) has shown good correlation with earlier in vitro studies indicating constant release for many hours at pH 6.9. Such work has led to the inference that 24-hour continual release from suppositories is indeed achievable, and that insertion of a new suppository following defecation would not cause drug overdosing.

It should be quickly apparent that knowledge of rectal administration is at a relatively early stage, with much need for continued investigation to fully realize its potential advantages. With the increasing necessity to develop better targeting of pharmaceutical agents—and the simultaneous desire to reduce unwanted side effects of increasingly potent drugs—research in this area is expanding rapidly, with good prospects for future improvements in the art.

E. Physiological Considerations

When one anticipates drug behavior subsequent to rectal administration, a primary element to keep in mind is the nature of the uptake process in the rectum. There, unlike in the upper colon, absorption of materials is via passive diffusion; no carrier-assisted means take part in the passage of drug through the lipid membrane. Thus, success or failure of therapeutic delivery is a function of liposolubility of the agent *as well as its vehicle*, because the partition coefficient of the drug between the suppository base and the lumen contents influences the latter's release into the bowel and eventually the active's passage through the wall of the intestine. Enhancement agents that affect the mucous membrane similarly affect absorption and are useful for "boosting" delivery of poorly absorbed agents such as antibiotics and high molecular weight materials [15,16].

III. FORMULATION

A. Choice of Drug

What makes a particular drug a candidate for administration in the form of a suppository? First, it must be sufficiently absorbed through the rectal mucosa to permit therapeutic blood levels to be reached. In some cases, such absorption can be realized only in the presence of a "promotion adjuvant," an auxiliary agent used to promote improved uptake of the drug from the rectum when absorption is otherwise insufficient.

Other possibilities for rectal administration include drugs that are poorly absorbed after oral dosage or that cause irritation to the gastrointestinal mucosa; also, certain antibiotics cause detrimental changes to the balance of intestinal flora, and these would be better given so as to bypass this portion of the gut. Similarly, dosage of small polypeptides—normally subject to the enzymatic activity of the upper gastrointestinal tract—can often be better administered via the rectum, where such activity is substantially nonexistent. Sometimes, the pH of the upper gastrointestinal tract causes inadequate or otherwise undesirable uptake, and the possibility of avoiding this problem by using lower colorectal introduction is highly desirable. And, of course, therapy of local conditions is readily achieved using a suitable suppository formulation.

In summary, then, any pharmacological agent that is either disadvantageously administered using other routes or that treats disorders of the lowest bowel (or vagina) should be considered for administration via suppository.

1. Nature of the Active

As is the case with any dosage form, the physical nature of the active together with its chemical behavior largely governs many aspects of product development. Three principal factors that define formulation requirements are the active's physical state under ambient conditions, its solubility characteristics, and finally its physicochemical activity with regard to potential excipients.

a. *Physical State.* For suppository formulation, actives can be either liquid, pasty, or solid in nature. Because suppository manufacture is normally carried out by making a dispersion or solution of the active in a melt of the base (excipient), different considerations are mandated in the case when the active is liquid or pasty than when it is a solid. In the latter case, granulometry is of prime relevance, as it considerably influences a range of therapeutic and physical parameters of the finished product: a reduced particle size can positively affect drug bioavailability (through increased surface area) and with it, the kinetics of dissolution in the rectal ampulla. At the same time, it can adversely affect the product by thickening the active/excipient mix. This is detrimental because it hinders flow during filling of the suppository into molds, and it also retards resorption of the active later on. Finally, the presence of the active as coarse crystals (whether due to the state of the active when added to the base, or to any ensuing crystal formation) can be a source of irritation to sensitive rectal mucosal surfaces.

b. *Bulk Density.* Specific gravity (bulk density) of the active is another important formulating consideration. If there is a significant difference in the densities of the active and the excipient, maintaining product homogeneity will require special effort. This potential problem can be overcome relatively easily by reducing the particle size, or by increasing product viscosity. This last task can be as simple as either using a thickening agent or alternatively by reducing the temperature of the mixture in order to bring it closer to its solidification point and thus to lower its fluidity.

c. *Solubility.* The degree (if any) to which the active ingredient is soluble in the excipient influences manufacture in several ways. For example, increased solubility of the active in the suppository base helps to improve product homogeneity, but at the same time it diminishes the release of the active if there is *too* great a propensity for it to remain in the excipient. This can be used advantageously, within limits: one function of a suppository is to maintain a drug at its target site, and a controlled affinity of the active for the excipient can be governed by the degree of miscibility of the two suppository components. From a formulator's point of view, solubility of the active in the base represents a rather straightforward situation: the principal point to consider is that the melting point of the base will be lowered after addition of the active, so that a base with a higher melting point should be used. However, suppository crystallinity (and subsequently hardening and product cohesion) is affected, and should be assessed during formulating trials. In any case, chemical interactions between the active and the excipient are to be avoided, and they in fact occur only rarely (usually only in instances of saponification—with sodium soaps, for example—or hydrolysis).

On the other hand, insolubility of the active in the excipient necessitates treatment of the mix as an emulsion or suspension; that is, handling as a dispersion, a more difficult problem. In this situation, it is necessary to maintain product homogeneity of two phases within the product melt. A number of standard approaches to emulsification can be used; all however, must be reviewed in light of their potential irritation to the rectal mucosa. Thus, certain surfactants entirely acceptable for other uses cannot be considered for this application. Usually, these problems can be readily resolved with the addition of appropriate emulsifying agents (such as polysorbate) to the suppository base, and indeed, some manufacturers provide bases preformulated with these materials. As a further assurance of product homogeneity, continuous agitation of the melted active/ base blend should be maintained from the point of introduction of the solution into the base just to the point of pouring into the mold.

B. Choice of Base

Suppository bases serve two primary roles:

> They enable a selected active to be fabricated in a manner appropriate to both its physicochemical characteristics and the requirements of the manufacturer, and
> They are used to control delivery of the medication at its site of absorption.

Excipients exert considerable influence on the incorporation and subsequent release of the active ingredient from the suppository mass. For this reason, manufacturers of suppository bases offer a wide selection of raw materials in order to anticipate a correspondingly broad range of product needs. Selection criteria are based on a variety of factors, including nature of the active, manufacturing capabilities, and desired release characteristics. Also, as with any pharmaceutical carrier, there must be chemical nonreactivity with the active, and the base must be nontoxic and nonirritating and stable when formulated.

1. *General Remarks*

Rather than simply being inert vehicles, suppository bases serve several functions during different phases of suppository manufacture and distribution, and selection of the appropriate base must encompass the following considerations. At each stage of a suppository's "life," the inherent characteristics of the base determine relative success or failure of the finished product.

a. *During Production.*

Contraction.   Slight contraction upon cooling of the suppository volume is desirable in order to facilitate removal from the mold.

Inertness.   Obviously, there must be no chemical interaction between the base and the active ingredients.

Solidification.   The interval between melting and solidification must be optimal: If too short, rapid solidification of the melt will interfere with pouring into the mold; too long, and slow solidification will cause a decreased rate of production.

Viscosity. If the viscosity is insufficient, the dispersed components of the blend will form a sediment, compromising the integrity of the final product.

b. *During Storage.*

Impurity. Bacterial/fungal contamination should be minimized by selecting a non-nutritive base with minimal water content.

Softening. The suppository should be formulated so that it does not soften or melt under anticipated transportation and storage conditions.

Stability. The selected materials cannot oxidize when exposed to air, humidity, or light.

c. *During Use.*

Release. Choice of the proper base provides optimal delivery of the dispersed active into the target site.

Tolerance. The finished suppository should have minimal (if any) toxicity and not be irritating to sensitive rectal mucosal tissue.

From the point of view of composition, suppository bases can be described as falling into one of three categories: naturally derived, synthetic, or "semisynthetic."

2. *Natural Bases*

Virtually all naturally derived suppository bases in use today are produced from cocoa butter, a fatty material composed of a mixture of C16 to C18 saturated and unsaturated fatty acid triglycerides obtained from the roasted seed of *Theobroma cacao* Linn [17]. Approximately 97% of the fatty acids are unsaturated, primarily oleic (mostly oleopalmitostearic—more than 50%), and oleodistearic (about 25%). Because cocoa butter is formed exclusively from triglycerides, there is no hydroxyl index, and the presence of ethylene bonds confers an iodine value of about 35.

Cocoa butter was perhaps the first modern base used, and although well tolerated it presents several problems when formulated in suppositories. For example, while it readily liquefies at body temperature, its unique melting point prohibits the incorporation of materials that would cause a significant increase or decrease in the melting point of the final suppository mass. Moreover, its slow rate of crystallization (which reflects how fast a melted base solidifies and then stabilizes) makes it quite difficult to adapt a formulation that has been used for a particular production system to another. From a more practical viewpoint, the vagaries of the market are such that pricing and availability can be erratic: natural events can affect harvest of the raw material, and the needs of the food industry, which utilizes enormous quantities of cocoa butter, often have priority over those of the pharmaceutical industry.

In addition to cocoa butter, other natural materials such as gelatin, agar, and waxes have been employed as suppository bases. However, their utilization has been limited and often relegated to special applications because special problems are encountered with their use. For the majority of applications, though, cocoa butter is the most often used of the naturally derived materials.

a. *Advantages.* Cocoa butter, as stated, is exceptionally nonirritating and can in fact be used beneficially to treat local irritations, as in the case of antihemorrhoidal preparations. Use of this excipient allows a rapid release—by melting—of active ingredi-

454   *Gold et al.*

ents dispersed in it. It is also widely available and has a long history of experience and safe use.

     b.   *Disadvantages.*   In addition to the drawbacks previously discussed, cocoa butter is immiscible in body fluids. Thus, release of lipophilic agents from cocoa butter–containing suppositories is hampered. Also, cocoa butter has a relative high tendency to oxidize. This is due to its 30% unsaturated fatty acid content, which can lead to significant rancidity.

     Because of its low solidification point and a resulting tendency of denser active ingredients to sediment, cocoa butter cannot be used in direct casting equipment for high-speed manufacture. In the case of active ingredients used in suspension, it is not possible to obtain a homogeneous suppository. This is due in part to cocoa butter's inherent polymorphism (discussed below), which causes alterations in crystal structure over time. Because these different crystalline forms have unique melting temperatures, solidification is affected, increasing the risk of sedimentation of the active ingredients in the base.

     Avoiding this problem entails heating the cocoa butter to between 40° and 50°C, cooling just to the point at which a paste is formed, and then reheating only until a sufficient fluidity is obtained to allow pouring. At that point, the active ingredients are added under continuous stirring during cooling.

     Another drawback to the use of this material as a suppository base stems from the lack of hydrophilicity because of the exclusive presence of triglycerides in its makeup, which can be overcome only partially by the inclusion in the formula of water-in-oil (W/O) emulsifiers.

     For these reasons, the use of cocoa butter as a suppository base is becoming increasingly less attractive, particularly in light of the availability of more modern alternatives.

3.   *Synthetic Bases*

As a result of the deficiencies of cocoa butter, newer bases with improved characteristics have been developed. Principally derived from petrochemical derivatives of fractionated fatty alcohols, synthetic bases overcome many of the disadvantages of those made from completely natural origins. Of chief importance in this group are bases composed of mixtures of polyethylene glycols (PEGs) selected from among those with melting temperatures greater than that of the body cavity. Chemically, they are formed by an addition polymerization of water and ethylene oxide to yield $H(OCH_2CH_2)_nOH$, where n denotes the average number of oxyethylene groups.

     a.   *Advantages.*   Release of active ingredients from these bases is a function of the suppository base's *dissolution*, rather than its *melting*. For this reason, problems of manufacture, shipping, and storage stemming from elevated ambient temperatures can be effectively reduced. In addition, investigations have shown that the hydrophilic nature of these excipients can serve to promote absorption for a range of materials including such compounds as heparin, gentamicin, and insulin [18].

     b.   *Disadvantages.*   The higher melting point ranges of these bases must be considered when heat-sensitive materials are incorporated into them. This problem can sometimes be circumvented using direct compression (i.e., tableting) techniques to produce the suppositories, but this approach introduces new problems (one example is the need for ancillary agents such as lubricants); furthermore, the means for doing this are not generally available in most suppository production facilities.

Another problem with synthetic bases is the potential delaying effect they can have on the release of the active ingredient. This is especially true with elevated levels of high molecular weight PEGs, which can cause problems with drug retention. Because dissolution is the basis for their drug-release properties, any time there is a dryness in the rectal ampulla (as is often seen in the elderly, for example) special care must be taken to ensure that the active will properly leave the base. Actually, it is sometimes recommended that suppositories manufactured from these bases be moistened with water prior to introduction into the rectum. This is also related to the tendency of such bases to cause local irritation [19]. In fact, one of the major drawbacks of PEG-based suppositories inherent with their use is the risk of traumatizing sensitive tissue. This is thought to be due to alterations to the intestinal epithelium, and in at least one animal study ulceration has been observed [20].

The chemical activity of these materials also causes problems for the formulator. Because of the chemical reactivity of these materials, their elevated hydroxyl index, and their water content, the capacity for chemical reaction between the active and the base is always present. For this reason, for example, it is impossible to make aspirin suppositories using PEG-based suppository bases (because of the potential for inter-esterification between the active and the base). Also, the potency of antibiotics such as penicillin and chloramphenicol is greatly compromised as a result of the oxidative instability of these bases.

Finally, storage conditions can sometimes adversely affect the quality of finished suppositories: excessive humidity in the air can cause moisture uptake into the product.

4. *Semisynthetic Bases*

These excipients are produced from vegetable fats and oils that are chemically modified during their manufacture. Such reactions yield a range of products with controllable characteristics making them suitable for incorporation into suppositories. Chemically, they are usually derivatives of fatty acids that undergo chemical alterations (e.g., transesterification) to enhance their use for this application. For example, hydrogenation is typically carried out to substantially improve stability (e.g., enhanced resistance to oxidation) and to increase chemical inertness. Melting point ranges can be more precisely tailored to specific requirements, as can the relative oil-water solubility.

Examples of semisynthetic suppository bases are the Novata, Suppocire, Wecobee, and Witepsol types [21].

a. *Advantages.*   Manufacture of semisynthetic suppository bases by transesterification results in the retention in the final base of more short and medium chain fatty acids (i.e., C_6 to C_{10}, which are liquid at normal ambient temperature) than is seen with semisynthetic bases manufactured by means of esterification, and thus the final products are more supple. This facilitates manufacture (because the suppositories are softer and do not readily fissure after production), but perhaps more importantly it serves to improve patient acceptance and compliance because the more brittle suppositories prepared from other bases can be more rigid and thus harder to introduce rectally. Stability is also improved because postproduction hardening phenomena are substantially reduced. Semi-synthetic bases obtained from the transesterification of vegetable fats and oils can also be less irritating (chemically) and damaging (mechanically) to sensitive rectal mucosa. Their use can, in fact, confer intrinsic lubricating properties to the suppository.

b. *Disadvantages.*   As is the case with cocoa butter, release of active ingredients results from the melting of the suppository base. For this reason, a fairly low melting temperature is required, mandating that precautions be taken to prevent damage to finished products during transport and storage. In addition, polymorphism (a characteristic of all fatty materials that affects crystallization during aging of finished products) must be taken into consideration when formulating and also when designing stability evaluation protocols.

5. *Hydrogels*

Currently, an alternative vehicle for rectal delivery is being actively investigated (and will be only briefly mentioned here). Hydrogels [22] may be defined as macromolecular networks that swell, but do not dissolve, in water. The swelling of hydrogels, i.e., the absorption of water, is a consequence of the presence of hydrophilic functional groups attached to the polymeric network. The aqueous insolubility of hydrogels results from the cross-links between adjacent macromolecules. The use of a hydrogel matrix for drug delivery involves the dispersal of the drug in the matrix, followed by drying of the system and concomitant immobilization of the drug. When the hydrogel delivery system is placed in an aqueous environment, e.g., the rectum, the hydrogel swells, and drug is then able to diffuse out of the macromolecular network. Hydrogels employed for rectal drug administration have been prepared from such polymers as polyvinyl alcohol, hydroxyethyl methacrylate, polyacrylic acid, and polyoxyethylene. The rate and extent of drug release from these hydrogel matrices are dependent on the dynamic processes of water migration into the matrix and drug diffusion out of the swollen matrix.

Although hydrogel-based drug delivery systems have yet to appear in suppository or insert form commercially, research efforts in this direction are increasing. The achievement of controlled drug delivery with hydrogel matrices, the potential of these hydrogels for bioadhesion and retention at the site of administration, and their biocompatibility make these bases very attractive to formulators. Indomethacin, β-adrenergic blocking agents such as propranolol and atenolol, bacampacilin, morphine sulfate, and pentoxifylline have all been the focus of recent studies of the preparation and evaluation of hydrogel delivery systems.

6. *Selection Criteria*

In order to choose the base most appropriate for the formulation, the excipients must be evaluated on the basis of their physicochemical characteristics. These parameters affect the chemical stability of the final product as well as the release from the base and subsequent bioavailability of the active ingredient. Of prime importance are melting temperature, iodine value, and hydroxyl index. These measurements are widely used in the pharmaceutical industry for a range of applications, and the discussion here will be limited to their significance to suppository base selection.

a. *Melting Temperature Range.*   Specifications for the melting temperature of suppository bases (especially of the fatty types) define a melting temperature *range* rather than a single point. This practice is not due to inadequate controls but rather to the range of temperatures between the stable and unstable forms, a result of the polymorphism (existence in several crystalline states) of these materials [details of this phenomenon are discussed later on]. When a base is selected on the basis of its melting temperature, one should keep in mind that the range offered by a manufacturer has been designed to provide flexibility for working within a particular active ingredient/therapeutic requirement framework. For example, the incorporation of a liquid agent into a base will generally tend to *decrease* the final melting temperature of the finished suppository, so that selection of a higher melting temperature base is advised. Similarly, inclusion of large quantities of fine powders will bring about an increase in product viscosity, requiring a base with a lower melting temperature.

     b. *Iodine Value.* Rancidification (oxidation) of suppository bases can be more of a problem than with other dosage forms. Because of the sensitivity of rectal mucosal tissue, and the possibility of its extended exposure to the melted suppository base, potentially irritating antioxidants are generally not advised for incorporation into suppositories. To avoid their use, bases with iodine values less than 3 (and preferably less than 1) should be employed exclusively.

     c. *Hydroxyl Index.* The determination of the hydroxyl index reveals the presence of mono- and diglycerides in a particular substance and indicates its relative rate of crystallization. In general, a lower value permits a faster rate of suppository manufacture. Materials possessing a low hydroxyl index also provide better stability in cases where the active ingredient is sensitive to the presence of the hydroxyl group.

7. *Ratio of Components*

Once the correct excipient has been selected, the proper proportion of the components needs to be established. Generally, it is expedient to use a relatively high excipient:active ratio to improve the dispersion of the active ingredient in the suppository and to facilitate transfer of the active ingredient following suppository administration.

     One important aspect to consider in suppository formulation is that of displacement. Suppositories generally weigh between 1 and 4 grams, and displacement of the excipient by the active ingredient must be calculated when the product is formulated. Simply, this step takes into account the volume of suppository base that will be displaced by an insoluble drug dispersed into it. This is necessitated by the practice of placing *weighed* quantities of suppository ingredients into molds whose contents are measured volumetrically.

     The amount of excipient to be used can be determined using the following formula:

$$M = F - (f*S)$$

where: M = the quantity (weight) of suppository base needed
       F = the total capacity of the suppository mold
       f = the displacement factor of the active ingredient
      S = the quantity of the active ingredient per suppository

The displacement factor "f" is itself a calculated value, and specific for the drug/excipient system being used. The calculation for the displacement factor is:

$$f = \frac{\text{weight of active ingredient}}{\text{weight of excipient displaced}}$$

Fortunately, suppository excipient densities are quite uniform (i.e., .97) so that the weight of excipient displaced per weight of active is constant for a vast range of excipients. For this reason, tables of standard displacement factors are available (see Table 2).

Table 2 Displacement Factors of Selected Materials

Acetylmorphine hydrochloride	0.71
Acetylsalicylic acid	0.63
Beeswax	1.00
Benzocaine	0.68
Bismuth subgallate	0.37
Bismuth subnitrate	0.33
Codeine phosphate	0.80
Glycerine	0.78
Phenacetin	0.60
Phenobarbital	0.84
Phenobarbital, sodium	0.62
Procaine	0.80
Quinine chlorohydrate	0.83
Sulfamide	0.60
Theophylline	0.63
Zinc oxide	0.20

C. Choice of Adjuvants

The addition of selected ancillary materials can improve many aspects of suppository development and production. Properly chosen, they can enhance homogeneity of the finished product, increase solubilization of the active ingredients in the selected excipient, alleviate handling of difficult actives, facilitate production, and so forth.

Adjuvants are selected:

1. *To Improve Incorporation of Powdered Actives*

Elevated levels of powdered active ingredients can compromise the integrity of the suppository by causing an excessive increase in the viscosity of the melt, thereby hindering its flow into the mold. A number of agents are available that can help to overcome this, some already incorporated into the bases themselves. Among them are:

a. *Magnesium Carbonate.* This material is used to ease incorporation of glycerine into the manufacture of lipidic suppository bases; it can also be used effectively to incorporate dry extracts, particularly those that are hygroscopic.

b. *Neutral Oils.* These are low-viscosity saturated C_8 to C_{12} fatty acid glycerides (Labrafac Lipo, Labrafac Hydro, Neobee, Miglyol, and Syndermin [23]) that are used at levels of about 10% of the weight of the suppository. The active ingredient should first be softened by mixing in the oil. The use of these oils can also modify the suppository's melting temperature and viscosity.

c. *Water.* The formulation of 1% to 2% water (depending on the absorptive capacity of the base) into the suppository augments the introduction of certain dry powders. Care must be taken, however, to avoid problems of hydrolysis, microbial growth, and diminution of bioavailability.

2. *To Improve Hydrophilicity*

Care must be taken with the use of adjuvants affecting hydrophilicity. Incorporation of selected agents such as those below can be used to accelerate dissolution of the product in the rectum. However, they can also adversely affect the uptake of the active. In general, *when used in low concentrations,* they increase absorption. When used at greater levels, they decrease it. A final precaution. Some researchers believe these agents capable of causing some local irritation.

One way to avoid the need for these additives is to employ special bases specifically designed to have an intrinsically enhanced hydrophilicity. For example, the increased hydrophilicity of Suppocire P [23] is due to its amphiphilic chemical structure, and it can often be used advantageously when rapid and significant release of active ingredients from a suppository is desired.

Examples of these additives are:

a. *Anionic Surfactants.* Bile salts, calcium oleate, cetylstearyl alcohol plus 10% sodium alkyl sulfate (Lanette SX [24]), sodium dioctylsulfosuccinate, sodium lauryl sulfate (1%), sodium stearate (1%), and triethanolamine stearate (3% to 5%).

b. *Nonionic and Amphoteric Surfactants.* Fatty acid esters of sorbitan (Span Arlacel), fatty acid esters of ethoxylated sorbitan (Tween), ethoxylated esters and ethers (polyethyleneglycol 400 myristate, polyethyleneglycol 400 stearate [Myrj], polyethyleneglycol ethers of fatty alcohols), modified oils (polyoxyethylenated hydrogenated palm oil [Labrafil M2273], ethoxylated castor oil [Cremophor EL] [25], lecithin, cholesterol).

c. *Partial Glycerides.* Mono- and diglycerides (Atmul 84 [26], glycerine monostearate and glycerine monooleate, stearic and palmitic acid mono- and diglycerides).

3. *To Improve Viscosity*

Controlling viscosity of the suppository melt during cooling can be critical for avoiding sedimentation. Although most applicable for use with cocoa butter, viscosity-increasing materials also find considerable use with the semisynthetic bases. In addition to affecting the viscosity, they can also change both the melting temperature and the range over which the melting temperature occurs—factors to be considered when they are used.

a. *Fatty Acids and Derivatives.* Aluminum monostearate, glyceryl monostearate, stearic acid.

b. *Fatty Alcohols.* Cetyl, myristyl, and stearyl alcohols.

c. *Inert Powders.* Bentonite, colloidal silica.

4. *To Alter Melting Temperature*

It is sometimes desirable to modify the melting point of a suppository mixture, to improve either its handling during manufacture or its behavior in the rectal ampulla. For example, a number of active ingredients, such as procaine base, phenols, chloral, and essential oils, decrease the melting temperature to the point at which risk of product damage during storage and transportation is considerably increased. Melting temperature modulators are used, for the most part, in formulations based on cocoa butter.

Adjuvants used to remedy these conditions, however, can themselves introduce difficulties, and for this reason their cautious use is advised. Specifically, most of the agents listed below possess an intrinsic crystallinity quite different from that of the glycerides often seen in suppositories, causing the appearance of surface anomalies in the finished suppository. Furthermore, the effectiveness of these materials can be dependent on the amounts used in the formula.

For this reason, if a change in melting temperature of the base is desired, the simplest solution is often to use a semisynthetic base with a higher or lower melting temperature.

Auxiliary agents used are fatty acids and fatty acid derivatives (glycerol stearate and stearic acid), fatty alcohols (cetyl alcohol and cetylstearic alcohol), hydrocarbons (paraffin), and waxes (beeswax and carnauba wax).

5. *To Improve Mechanical Strength*

Breaking of suppositories is a particular problem when synthetic bases are used (cocoa butter and semisynthetic bases are less fragile, and thus less prone to fracture and thereby irritate the rectal mucosa). In order to overcome this problem, a number of agents can be added to the synthetic bases. Among these are polysorbates, castor oil, fatty acid monoglycerides, glycerine, and propylene glycol.

6. *To Change Appearance*

Although not always desirable, colorants can be used for a wide range of functions when making suppository bases. They can be added for psychological reasons (to mask undesirable features or to disguise placebos), or for practical purposes (such as assuring color uniformity from lot to lot). Color coding of different products is often important, especially in hospital pharmacies, and colorants can also be used to conceal faults in manufacture, such as surface exudation or crystallization. Hydrosoluble, liposoluble, and insoluble materials can all be used effectively to tint suppositories.

7. *To Protect Against Degradation*

Antimicrobial and antifungal agents are particularly important when suppositories contain plant-derived materials or (more commonly) water. Either sorbic acid or its salts are indicated when the pH of the aqueous solution of the active is less than 6. Parahydroxybenzoates can be used as is or as sodium salts when the pH is lowered. However, the potential of these materials to cause rectal irritation must be considered.

Antioxidants such as BHT, BHA, and ascorbic acid are also used advantageously to prolong suppository life when rancidity presents a problem during the formulation of cocoa butter suppositories.

Finally, sequestering agents such as citric acid and combinations of antioxidants have been used to complex metals that catalyze redox reactions. For example, a mixture of three parts each BHT, BHA, and propylgallate with one part citric acid has been found to yield satisfactory results when used at .01%.

8. *To Modify Absorption*

In cases where a drug has the disadvantage of limited rectal absorption, means are sometimes available to enhance the drug's uptake. A number of such promoters—and many new ones now under investigation—have been proposed as means to enhance bioavailability of active ingredients incorporated into suppositories. For example, the incorporation of depolymerizing enzymes (mucopolysaccharidases) has been studied to accelerate penetration of selected active ingredients [27].

IV. MANUFACTURE

A. Polymorphism

Before any discussion of manufacture of suppositories can begin, the subject of polymorphism must be broached. Common to all fatty-based excipients, polymorphism is a characteristic of these materials which exist in different crystalline states as a function of natural aging process. This attribute becomes problematic only when it is not properly considered as a normal component of product stabilization following manufacture. In fact, it must always be evaluated when suppositories are formulated. Polymorphic behavior and changes can be demonstrated using differential scanning calorimetry, or DSC.

Semisynthetic and natural glycerides exhibit a complex thermal behavior. This is a function of both the traits of each component glyceride in the blend, as well as of the relatively large number of glycerides used. It is manifested as an increase in the melting temperature of the material during storage. This rise in melting temperature increases with the temperature of storage up to the point at which the suppository completely resoftens, at which point it can effectively be considered to have been "re-manufactured." The process then starts over again, as though the product had been freshly prepared [28]. It appears that this increase is also greater as the initial melting time of the base increases.

In addition to increased melting temperature, increased hardness of the suppository mass is also seen as aging occurs. This effect, thought to be the result of several possible causes (including changes in polymorphic phase or crystallinity), can sometimes be avoided by the addition of an additive such as soy lecithin.

This phenomenon is the consequence of changes of the fatty material constituents as they go from an unstable to a stable crystalline state. The rate at which it occurs is a direct function of the temperature at which the material is kept following manufacture—the more elevated the storage temperature (and consequently the closer to its melting point), the faster the transition speed will be.

The metamorphosis occurs in three stages. Alternately, it can be stated that each glyceride constituent of the blend can exist in three crystalline forms. These are known as α, β' and β. Some glycerides can exist in an additional metastable crystalline form, the γ polymorph. The existence of these crystalline forms can be demonstrated by any one of a variety of analytical means, including X-ray diffraction, differential thermal analysis, dilatometry, and nuclear magnetic resonance. Again, all semisynthetic glyceride-type suppository excipients undergo these polymorphic modifications, and the progression of transformation is always in the same direction, toward an increased melting temperature resulting from a more stable crystalline structure:

$$\alpha \quad \rightarrow \quad \beta' \quad \rightarrow \quad \beta$$

Unstable form   Stable form

As the suppository reaches its melting temperature and returns to its liquid form, it reverts back to its unstable (α) state. As previously mentioned, when finished products are stored at or near their melting temperature, they completely soften (i.e., melt) and recommence the aging process.

What makes this knowledge relevant (and vital) to the manufacture of suppositories is its bearing on the production steps of suppository manufacture. Traditionally, suppositories are fabricated by melting of the active/excipient blend, pouring of the blend into an appropriate mold, and then cooling. To put it another way, suppository manufacture first yields an unstable product.

As with any production process, the goal is to have a stable finished product. In the present case, this can be achieved by accelerating the rate of polymorphic transformation via storage of the suppository at about 3°C below its theoretical melting point. This rapidly transforms suppositories to a more stable state. It additionally defines the maximum melting point. Such accelerated aging, or "tempering" as it is also known, is essential in the development of a suppository dosage form, provided that a nondestructive method of measuring the melting point (such as a U-tube, described later on) has been used.

A number of faults of manufacture, too, can be explained by polymorphism: most notably fat bloom and whitening. Fat bloom is seen as a dullness on the surface of the suppository that, upon microscopic examination, is found to be an exudation of certain fatty chains. It appears as crystallization proceeds and increases with storage temperature. Whitening, on the other hand, is caused by the migration of *active* ingredients, which are often insoluble in the excipient, to the suppository surface.

Melting point variation measurements during storage permit an assessment of the influence of active ingredients on the base. These influences can—depending on the active's relative solubility (or insolubility) in the excipient—aggravate or attenuate polymorphic changes. However, when polymorphic effects are studied, it is important not to melt the sample before measurement of melting point variations. Melting will obviously renew the polymorphic transmutations and prevent any accurate evaluation. Generally, it is recommended that a U-tube be used.

B. Theoretical Considerations of Suppository Manufacture

In order to maximize the efficiency of suppository scale-up and manufacture, it is obvious that much is to be gained by avoiding pitfalls to the greatest extent possible. Many of the potential problems that may be encountered can be at least minimized by a good understanding of some of the physical principles involved in production. The processes of particular concern for suppository manufacture include melting, mixing or blending, flow and/or mass transfer, and congealing.

1. *Melting*

By and large, suppository manufacture requires the melting of most, if not all, of the formulation components. Rate equations for the melting of a solid in contact with its own melt have been derived by simultaneous consideration of both mass and heat transfer in a biphasic system. The change in size or linear dimension, and correspondingly, the change in the cube root of the weight of a solid of a given geometric shape, during steady state melting, is linear with time. Thus

$$L = -m\Theta + L_0$$

and,

$$W^{1/3} = -m'\Theta + W_0^{1/3}$$

in which W_0 and L_0 represent the initial weight and size of the solid, respectively, Θ is time, and m and m' are slopes of the linear equations. Extension of these relationships to the melting of a number of particles, N, allows the total weight and area of the particles to be represented as W and A, respectively:

$$W = N\rho\mathbf{b}L^3$$

$$A = NeL^2$$

(where ρ is density [g cm^{-3}], **b** is a shape factor related to volume, and **e** is a shape factor related to area), and

$$[W/N]^{1/3} = -m\Theta + [W_0/N]^{1/3}$$

When melting is complete, W and L are zero; hence, melting time can be obtained from the above equations. From a practical standpoint, however, the heterogeneity—in size and shape—of the solids normally processed minimizes the utility of these approximations.

On the other hand, while this characterization of the melting of a solid in its own melt as a one-step process may be helpful as far as the PEGs are concerned, for natural and semisynthetic lipoidal excipients, melting is not a simple one-step process. The multiple melting behavior of acylglycerides was reported over 140 years ago and ascribed to different crystalline forms or polymorphs almost 50 years ago. Polymorphism (as previously mentioned) is commonly encountered with acylglycerides. Furthermore, formulation additives and processing variations abound, all of which have an effect on the melting behavior of the suppository matrix. One additional potential problem, that of polytypism, which has been viewed as one-dimensional polymorphism, has hardly been addressed in the pharmaceutical literature. Its pharmaceutical influence is uncertain as yet. (Polytypism can be differentiated from polymorphism in that the latter concerns the structural differences within one molecular layer or in the unit cell structure arising from different molecular conformations and molecular packings, whereas the former involves differences in the stacking mode of the molecular layers in the crystalline solid.)

> If melting of excipient results in a marked decrease in η, significant leakage around seals, nozzles, or mold cavity seams can result.
> A final issue: even with the use of fully jacketed kettles or tanks to optimize temperature control and melt uniformity, the temperature within a melting kettle or mixing tank can still vary sufficiently to affect melt composition.

Heat flow q into an agitated vessel is determined principally by the heat transfer coefficient, U, the heat transfer area, A, and the temperature difference $(\Theta_0-\Theta_i)$ between the melt and the heat-transfer fluid, i.e. the fluid film immediately adjacent to the heat-transfer surface:

$$q = UA(\Theta_0-\Theta_i)$$

The heat transfer coefficient is influenced by geometric and operating parameters. The heat transfer area, A, in contact with the melt depends on the geometry of the heat transfer surface, and the temperature difference is controlled primarily by process conditions. The heat transfer coefficient, U, can be described in terms of three heat transfer processes: the first, h_i, the inside-film coefficient, involves the efficiency of heat transfer through the fluid film on the melt side of the tank or kettle wall; the second concerns conduction through the walls; and the third reflects the efficiency of heat transfer from the outer wall of the vessel. The inside-film coefficient, h_i, lumps together the convective and conductive effects in the melt immediately adjacent to the heat transfer surface. It is usually the limiting resistance and is affected by the agitation intensity within the tank. In practice, the unavoidable presence of a stagnant layer of melt at the tank wall hinders heat transfer. This can be minimized by the use of scrapers that can effectively double the heat transfer coefficient, although at the cost of increased power consumption.

Dimensional analysis of the temperature distribution, Θ^*, within an agitated, jacketed tank has been shown to be a function of the Reynolds and Prandtl numbers, i.e. $\Theta^* = f(N_{Re}, N_{Pr})$. In effect, the temperature distribution within the tank is a function of the relative diffusivity of heat and momentum. Taking into consideration the longer processing times necessary for larger batches, scale-up poses additional problems in terms of time-dependent thermally induced transitions in molecular order.

Given the problems inherent in the diverse physical and chemical composition of commercial excipients—the presence of polymorphs, variations in the degree of crystallinity, polytypism, broad versus narrow molecular weight ranges, and so on—and the interdependence of time and temperature effects, it is amazing that suppository scale-up problems are not encountered more often than they are.

2. *Mixing or Blending*

The objective of the mixing or blending process is to achieve and maintain uniformity of the mix. Among the determinations to be made is whether the melt behaves in a Newtonian or non-Newtonian manner—i.e., is it time-dependent?

Non-Newtonian systems may be particularly troublesome insofar as maintaining mixing tank uniformity, particularly in the presence of solids. The agitation intensity or impeller speed required to achieve complete uniformity throughout the tank and complete "off-bottom suspension" for any particulates increases exponentially with the viscosity of the suppository melt. Thus, if swirling or vortexing occurs in the course of the mixing or blending process, incomplete mixing and/or air entrapment may occur with consequences for melt uniformity, decreased oxidative stability and so on.

For the same melt viscosity, there is a greater tendency for swirling to occur in large tanks than in small ones. The more viscous the melt, the less tendency there is for vortexing and swirling. Also, swirling or vortexing is more apt to occur in unbaffled tanks than in baffled tanks. Because pilot plant equipment is often unbaffled, suppository scale-up may require the installation of baffles to ensure mix uniformity and minimal air entrainment.

The presence of particulates in the suppository melt can complicate the picture considerably. For turbine impellers, suspension uniformity varies in accordance with $(D/T)^{1.5}$, where D is the diameter of the impeller and T is the diameter of the tank: thus, relatively large impellers can significantly improve process results. Etchells et al. [29] analyzed scale-up issues for Bingham plastics and found an excellent scale-up correlation between impeller tip speed, impeller diameter, and flow. Their contention is that as long as geometrically similar equipment is being used with comparable matériel (albeit on a smaller scale) the results can be quite satisfactory.

Further complications can arise from centrifugal effects near the impeller in a mixing tank along with complex impeller-induced flow patterns that result in the impeller "not seeing" the viscosity and density of the melt in its immediate vicinity. Finally, lack of homogeneity can give rise to temperature variations, which can give rise to further changes in density or composition: scale-up estimates or simulations that do not consider the changes in processing or holding time may be misleading.

3. *Mass Transfer*

The transfer of the suppository melt from mixing tanks or holding tanks to the filling line or to the injector, or from the injector into the mold, is especially perturbing when the melt is non-Newtonian. Engineers occasionally need to determine the optimal pipe size for given flow requirements for liquids. Guidelines have long been readily available for time-independent Newtonian liquids but not for non-Newtonians. However, algorithms have been published relatively recently that facilitate the calculation of fluid flow and the pressure drop-pipe diameter relationship for time-independent non-Newtonian fluids.

Time-dependency can be dealt with but it must first be recognized. Consider the effect of capillary or injection-filling nozzle length and diameter on the flow curve for a *thixotropic* material: increased fluidity can be expected with longer and narrower capillaries or filling nozzles. Non-Newtonian rheology is becoming increasingly relevant, too: a recent U.S. patent (U.S. Patent 5,004,601) on injection-molded dosage forms touts the advantages of a PEG formulation that softens and becomes thixotropic at body temperature but that retains its shape on handling and at temperature extremes encountered in commerce.

Keep in mind that the presence of suspended particulates, whether of drug or of suppository base, can markedly complicate the rheological behavior and transport properties of the suppository melt. This stems from particle-particle or particle-melt interactions. Extensive interactions or hindered settling may hamper the transport of these formulations, e.g., from mixing tank to dosing pump, or from dosing pump to mold. On the other hand, suspension formulations in which the base interferes only minimally with settling are at risk for variations in content uniformity.

Among other considerations that may play a role in production success (or failure):

Power per unit volume is a function of particle size and solids concentration, but the exact relationship needs to be determined on a case-by-case basis. Failure to do so can lead to problems during manufacturing scale-up.

Flow projections based on isothermal rheological studies are inadequate: because temperature-sensitive substances are frequently employed, rheological behavior should be evaluated as a function of both time and temperature.

One other phenomenon, strain-induced crystallization or SIC, has been described in the polymer literature and may well be encountered with polymeric excipients for suppositories. For linear polymers, the rate of SIC increases with shear rate and decreases with temperature, in accordance with an Arrhenius-type relationship. Under a given shearing condition, the nucleation rate may increase dramatically with molecular weight leading to molecular fractionation during SIC [30].

When considering velocity profiles for Newtonian fluids, Bingham plastics, and non-Newtonian fluids in capillaries: Newtonian fluids display a parabolic velocity profile; Bingham plastics, a parabolic velocity profile with a plug-flow region; and non-Newtonian fluids, a velocity profile in accordance with a power law relationship.

An additional concern for suppository scale-up is the increased opportunity—with melts behaving rheologically as either Bingham bodies or non-Newtonian fluids— for nonuniformity, abetted by nonuniform temperatures within the capillary, nozzle, or pipe.

4. Congealing

In years past, pharmacists were generally aware of a negative aspect of polymorphism exhibited by cocoa butter: when heated to about 40°C, all polymorphic forms are melted.

Rapid cooling in suppository molds of the poured melt below 15°C results in the melt's crystallization in the γ form (with a melting point [m.p.] of 15°C). The gradual warming of the mold to room temperature results in successive transformations of the γ polymorph to the α form, with a 22°C m.p.; the β' form, with a 28°C m.p.; and the stable β form, with a 34.5°C m.p. The suppositories thus formed consist of unstable mixtures of polymorphs that melt at room temperature. Had the melt been cooled more slowly, the γ polymorph formed would have reverted to the stable β form and suppository integrity maintained at room temperature. This classic example of the importance of polymorphism in the use of fatty suppository bases is really an example of the impact, not only of temperature, but of cooling rate, on crystalline form.

A formal consideration of the process of congealing begins with an examination of heat transfer from a fluid to a solid surface. The rate of heat flow across the solid-fluid interface would be expected to depend on the temperature difference between the two phases and the interfacial area:

$$q = -hA\Delta\Theta$$

where q is the heat transfer rate across area A, Θ is the temperature difference between the two phases, and h is the proportionality constant referred to as the heat-transfer coefficient. This relationship is sometimes known as *Newton's law of cooling*.

Specific formulation requirements for congealing time, temperature, and rate need to be determined early on. Simulations of the temperature distribution in injection molding cavities for non-Newtonian fluid certainly convey the impression that such estimates should be made in the course of scale-up.

C. Suppository Production Methods

Manufacture of most suppositories employs one of the following techniques.

1. *Melting*

The preferred method for suppository manufacture is to place the active into a melt of the base and then to cool the mixture. This is generally carried out by heating the excipient to 45° to 50°C within a thermostatically controlled melting vessel. The relatively low melting temperature is used in order to preserve as much of the base as possible in its stable β form. An additional benefit is that it also permits the introduction of active ingredients under less destructive conditions.

Once the mixture has been made and homogenized, it can then be poured into molds of selected size and form. Importantly, this pouring must be carried out at a temperature—established during formulation studies—that is optimally based on the particular viscosity of the mixture as well as on the type of excipient used.

The melt can be poured into special precooled metal alloy molds. Once hardened, the molds are scraped to remove excess material, and the suppository is then removed and packed into individual alveoli. Alternatively, preshaped packs made of plastic, aluminum, composite, or other materials can be used directly to receive, harden, and package suppositories for eventual shipping, storage, and sale.

For the laboratory, small-batch metal molds are sold that enable manual or pump-filling for formulating trials: The melt is poured or pumped into the cavities of the mold, allowed to cool, and then removed for stability and/or other studies (Fig. 1).

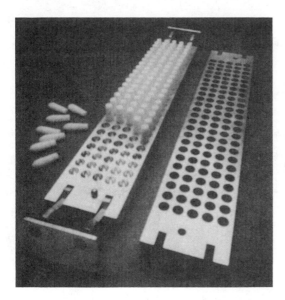

Fig. 1 Suppository mold used in formulating trials. The components of the mold are shown in an open position, allowing removal of the finished hard suppositories after cooling.

In today's modern suppository production facility, automated machinery can handle a multitude of tasks, from receiving the unmelted raw materials to stamping and dating the sealed, finished suppositories (Fig. 2). In principle, this equipment mimics the lab bench process in a rapid and highly efficient manner, using the same basic steps in a highly precise fashion. Importantly, the batching procedure must assure that the active drug is uniformly mixed throughout the batch and that the drug and the base are not adversely affected by the batching process. Such adverse effects might include decomposition of the drug substance or base, precipitation of base components, physical instability of the base (particularly of concern when cocoa butter is a component).

a. *Temperature Controls.* Careful control of temperature is important throughout the process, because temperature can affect the physical structure of the suppository, as well as hasten oxidation or cause other detrimental chemical effects on the active drug substance. Temperature ranges must be selected for each stage of the procedure to enable the process to proceed at a reasonable speed, while maintaining the physical properties of the molten mass within a controlled range of viscosity. This prevents sedimentation of insoluble components and efficient solidification after the filling/molding stage.

Premelting of the base. The suppository base generally constitutes the largest component in the batch and often makes up 90% or more of the suppository weight. Premelting of the base in preparation for batching takes the greatest portion of time required to prepare a batch for filling/molding. Batching does not begin until the base is in a molten condition, ready for the addition of the other components of the product. A temperature range for melting must be selected that is high enough to melt the entire quantity of base in an appropriate time and yet at the same time is not so high as to risk degradation or other adverse effects on the base material.

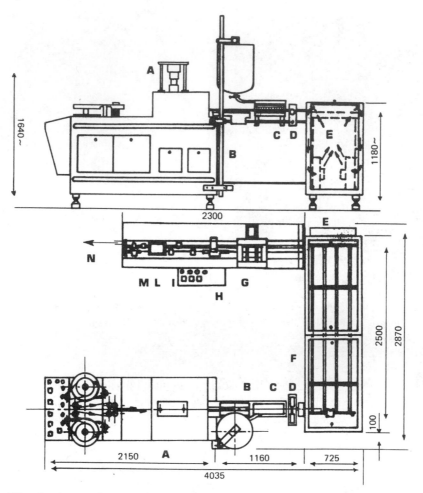

Fig. 2 Automatic suppository manufacturing equipment. This machine produces finished suppositories packaged in aluminum or plastic strips. The packaging materials (rolls of aluminum or plastic ribbons) are prepared at (A) by being shaped over molds and welded together. The bottom of the ribbon is then trimmed at (B) just before volumetric filling at (C). The continuous band is cut into 28–30 unit lengths at (D), which then passes into cooling tunnel (E) for hardening. The strips are then weighed (and if necessary ejected) at (F) and then sealed at (G). At (H) the top of the strips is trimmed. Perforation occurs at (I) and the strip is then coded at (L). A second cutting into 5–10 unit strips takes place at (M), after which the suppositories can pass automatically to packaging equipment at (N).

The starting point in determining a melting temperature is the defined melting range of the base. Most bases melt over a narrow temperature range of a few degrees. The temperature for melting the base in production conditions is generally set higher than the melting temperature of the base. This enables melting to occur more quickly. It also has the advantage of hastening the production process and reducing the holding time of the base material while melting takes place.

Some suppository bases, such as cocoa butter (which exist in a number of unstable crystalline states), perform best when melted gently at temperatures near their defined melting range. Because slow melting can tie up production equipment for an extended period of time (up to several days), the base is often premelted in a separate vessel and transferred to the batching equipment when batching is set to take place.

Mixing temperature. Once the base is melted and in the batching tank, the temperature of the base may require adjustment in order to permit the addition of the drug and other components. A suitable temperature is determined by several factors, including the melting temperature of inactive components, the solubility of the drug, and the physical stability of the base. Mixing is generally performed by a homogenizer, which stirs the mass rapidly with a high-speed rotor. The friction and shearing action of the homogenizer contributes heat to the mass and may require the removal of heat from the batch tank in order to maintain the proper batching temperature.

Higher temperatures may be required when soluble components are added to the batch. The temperature elevation can be minimized by ensuring that the components are finely powdered and added slowly to the batch. Some components, such as waxes, are best incorporated when added as a melt. However, if the base is not raised to a sufficiently high temperature prior to addition of these components, they can rapidly solidify into large particles and precipitate out of the mass. Elevating the temperature of the batch prior to addition of a soluble drug substance must be done with caution, and only if the stability of the drug at these temperatures has been ensured. When higher batching temperatures are needed for the incorporation of certain components, these components should be added early in the batching procedure, so that the temperature can be gradually lowered for addition of the active drug substance and subsequent filling and molding of the suppositories.

Lower temperatures may be required when insoluble components are added to the batch. These temperatures maintain the mass at a higher viscosity and help to prevent the insoluble components from rapidly settling to the bottom of the batch tank before they can be effectively mixed by the homogenizer. The insoluble components should have a small particle size (micronized) to assist in the mixing and help maintain them in suspension in the mass.

Lower temperatures are required when an unstable polymorphic base such as cocoa butter is used. Ideally, the batch should be maintained at the melting temperature of the finished suppository. If the batch temperature must be raised to incorporate certain components, this must be performed early in the procedure, so that the temperature can be gradually lowered to bring the base into a stable crystalline form. The return to a stable form can be assisted by the addition of a small quantity of fresh base to form seed crystals around which the stable recrystallization can occur. The quantity of seeding material required is small, less than one part in a thousand of the total mass. After seeding, the mass will require at least four hours to stabilize.

Filling temperature. The injection of the molten suppository mass should be carried out as closely as possible to the solidification temperature of the suppository. This minimizes the amount of heat that must be removed during cooling. In this manner, solidification can occur quickly to prevent sedimentation of insoluble components. When the molten suppository mass tends to be viscous, the injectors do not operate efficiently, and excessive weight variation from suppository to suppository can occur. In this case, the filling temperature must be raised sufficiently to reduce the viscosity and to ensure proper flow through the fillers. Subsequent cooling of the suppositories will require lower temperatures to remove the additional heat and can lead to fractures and surface irregularities.

When the suppository is formulated with an unstable polymorphic base, the filling temperature should be maintained as low as possible. This low temperature should extend to the holding tank and piping system as well, because excessive heat at any point in the system can lead to physical instability of the base. This results in a granulated suppository. The suppository mass does not solidify into a solid structure, but rather forms small granules that cause the suppository to crumble easily and that are unsuitable in a finished dosage form. If instability is a particular problem with a formulation, the temperature can be maintained slightly below the solidification temperature of the mass, provided the mass is kept in constant motion with stirring and recirculation throughout the delivery system.

2. *Compression*

The second manufacturing method is compression. It is used far less commonly than fusion (melting) and will be touched on only briefly. This technique requires finely powdered excipients (often difficult to maintain in this form) and special machines that allow high production speeds. Although not widely used, this refined technique is particularly appropriate for the manufacture of suppositories containing heat-sensitive actives [31].

While there are problems with this technique (such as the handling problem mentioned above), advantages offered by direct compression of suppositories using rotary presses include:

Use of same equipment as for tablet manufacture
No problems of sedimentation following filling
Increased rate of production
Elimination of temperature change–related problems
Fewer difficulties arising from incompatibility

3. *Injection*

A recently devised technique for suppository production involves the modification of injection-molding equipment employed in the plastics industry for the production of pharmaceutical dosage forms.

As proposed, a typical injection-molding production process involving PEGs as the base might proceed as follows [32,33]: the PEGs are first melted and mixed in a vessel equipped with a stirrer and a heating device (e.g. heating mantle or steam jacket) at about 60° to 80°C. Additional viscosity- and plasticity-adjusting ingredients, auxiliary ingredients, and active(s) are added while stirring. Once blending is complete, the melt is extruded into precision-machined multicavity molds. Rapid solidification of the melt is followed by ejection of the molded units from the mold cavities.

The claimed advantage that this method offers is the precise metering and molding coupled with high production capacity and a potential for a great range of suppository shapes and sizes.

V. BATCHING PROCEDURES

A. Setup for Filling and Molding

The filling and molding operation requires a properly executed and documented setup procedure to ensure that the resulting suppositories are properly formed at a specific weight and enclosed in a fully closed shell. After the proper molding dies are installed, two parallel strips of shell material (usually aluminum or plastic) are fed through the molding section and the filling section. This is usually performed manually, or while jogging the machine by operating it intermittently. The shell material is coated on one side with polyethylene. The polyethylene-coated sides on each strip must be facing each other.

The sealing, filling, and cooling sections should be brought to within the specific temperature range. The molding stage may require a temperature setting as well. For aluminum shell material, the molding stage does not require a temperature control. Plastic shell material is usually heated as it is molded.

With the molding and sealing stations enabled and the filling and cooling stations disabled, the machine is started. The shell material should pass through the molding and sealing stations smoothly. The molding station will form cavities into each of two parallel strips of shell material. The cavities should be examined for tears, cracks and other imperfections. After molding, the two strips are fused together at the sealing station. The sealing is accomplished by heat applied to the shell material, which causes the polyethylene coating to melt and form a bond between the two strips of shell material. The cavities formed in each strip at the molding station are joined together to form a suppository shell. The shell is still open at one end and will act as a mold into which the molten suppository mass is injected. The formed shell should be examined to ensure that the seal is complete. This can usually be accomplished by visual examination. However, a pull test or other appropriate means may be employed to measure seal integrity.

When the molding and sealing stations are functioning properly, the hopper is filled with suppository mass and the filling station enabled. At this point, the fillers are adjusted to ensure that the target weight of the suppository mass is injected into each shell. The coarse adjustment is performed by filling a number of shells in a strip (e.g., 10 shells or a number equal to the number of fillers). Using a comparable strip of empty shells as tare weight, the net weight of the suppositories can be determined to set the filler. After each adjustment performed on the filler, an additional set of shells is filled and weighed until the net weight is within specifications. Fine adjustment is performed by allowing the suppositories to solidify and weighing each suppository individually. Filling nozzles can be adjusted individually to bring individual suppository weight to within specification.

Once the filling station is properly adjusted, the cooling station is enabled and the strip of formed suppositories is fed in. Once the machine is started, the molten suppositories pass through a cooling gradient and into the final sealing station where the open end of the shells is sealed shut. The cooling temperatures should remain within a specified range and the solidified suppositories checked for cracking and surface defects that may indicate improper cooling. The finished suppositories should be hermetically sealed. Seal integrity can be readily determined with a standard vacuum dye leak test.

At some point in this process, a die embosses coding information into the shell material, usually a lot number and expiration date. The movable type in this die should be verified before installing the die in the machine and again on the finished suppository strips at the end of the process. Verification before installation is essential, because type is clear and easier to read than imprint on the shell material.

B. Specifications

Specifications must be determined for all machine parameters applicable to each product. This is particularly important for hopper temperatures, filling temperatures, and cooling temperatures. Sealing temperatures are related to the type of shell material used and are generally similar from product to product. Machine speed (cycle time) should be specified, because it affects the dwell time in the sealing sections and the rate of cooling. Sealing temperatures are related to the type of shell material used and are generally similar from product to product.

Product weight ranges must be established to ensure that product dosing meets applicable standards. The filling weights should conform to a tight range around the target weight. Modern filling equipment should be able to maintain fill weights within 4% to 6% of the target weight.

C. In-Process Controls

Proper monitoring of product physical characteristics is necessary to ensure that the production process remains under control throughout filling, which may last from a few hours to several days.

1. *Visual Examination*

A periodic examination for physical defects of finished suppositories provides valuable information for process monitoring. Color variations, chips, cracks, depressions, and surface irregularities are evidence of problems that require attention. Generally, these difficulties can be solved by machine adjustments.

2. *Weight Checks*

Periodic weighing of individual suppositories will reveal problems in the filling operation. The number of sequential suppositories weighed should correspond to the number of filling nozzles. Individual weights are preferred over averages, so that damage, obstructions, and misadjustment in individual filling units are apparent.

3. *Leak Test*

The quality of the seal is a parameter that can affect the stability of the product. The seal integrity is easily determined by a leak test, such as the classic vacuum dye method. A properly operating system should have no leakers.

VI. SUPPOSITORY QUALITY CONTROL

Subsequent to suppository development and manufacture, the finished product must undergo a number of simple tests in order to ascertain quality. Ideally, these tests should be repeated periodically during storage as well.

A. Physical Analysis

1. *Visual Evaluation*

Surface appearance and color can be verified visually to assess

    Absence of fissuring
    Absence of pitting
    Absence of fat blooming
    Absence of exudation
    Absence of migration of the active ingredients

This last test is best accomplished by taking a longitudinal section of the suppository to verify the homogeneity of the active ingredient(s) within the mass.

2. *Melting Point*

The melting point is a critical factor in the determination of the release rate of the active ingredient(s) from the suppository. It must be evaluated periodically using a non-destructive method, such as a U-tube (see below for description). No technique that causes the suppository to melt before measurement can be used, because this transforms the suppository constituents into a metastable state. In any case, the melting point of the finished suppository should generally not be greater than 37°C.

3. *Liquefaction Time*

This important element indicates the physical behavior of a suppository subjected to its maximum functional temperature (37°C). Krowczynski's method is well suited for this type of study, which is complementary to, and directly related to, the determination of melting point (Fig. 3). It measures the time necessary for a suppository to liquefy under pressures similar to those found in the rectum (e.g., 30 grams) in the presence of water at body temperature. A rule of thumb is that liquefaction time should be no longer than 30 minutes.

4. *Mechnical Strength*

This is the determination of the mechanical force necessary to break a suppository, and it indicates whether a suppository is brittle or elastic. The Erweka method (Fig. 4.) is used for this test, and it measures the mass (in kilograms) that a selected suppository can bear without breaking: for satisfactory results, the mechanical strength should in no case be less than 1.8 to 2 kg.

5. *Melting and Solidification*

The release of the active ingredient(s) from a semisynthetic or cocoa butter–based suppository is to a large degree a function of its melting temperature (and is influenced by solubility in the vehicle). Obviously, suppositories go through two distinct phases during manufacture, regardless of the excipient selected: melting (or fusion), and solidification. Therefore, for ideal therapeutic efficacy, an understanding of those factors influencing these two parameters is critical in determining the bioavailability to be obtained from the final dosage form.

A number of well-known and acceptable methods exist for the analysis of melting behavior. A problem arises when determining melting point, however, when comparing results obtained using different techniques. This stems from the fact that these methods all act to "freeze" chronometrically what is actually a complex, continuous, and successive melting of the different triglyceride components in the excipient to the point of liquefaction.

The most commonly used methods are:

Open capillary tube
U-tube
Drop point

These methods, while similar in principle, differ somewhat in their methodologies. All require the introduction of a sample into a specified place in the apparatus, after which

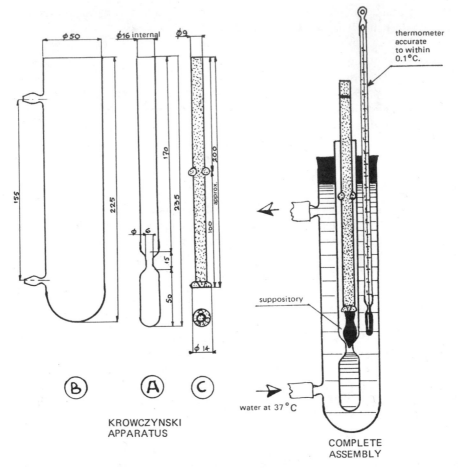

Fig. 3 Determination of liquefaction time. A tube with a stricture (A) is filled with distilled water to just below the stricture and heated in a water bath (B) to a temperature of 37°C ±0.1. The sample suppository is introduced into the top of the tube and carefully pushed down its length until it rests on top of the stricture. A glass rod (C) of specified weight is placed into the tube so that it rests on top of the suppository. The time that it takes the weight resting on the suppository to reach the stricture (due to the melting of the suppository) is measured. The liquefaction time is the average of three determinations of this time interval.

heat is applied in a controlled manner. Means are provided for the determination of the point at which the test material undergoes a change in physical state (i.e., melts). The methods are illustrated in Figs. 5, 6, and 7, respectively.

Solidification as well is not a simple process, and difficulties can arise when comparing results obtained by using different methods of determination. The technique that is most commonly employed is Shukoff's method, a procedure for ascertaining the point at which solidification of a cooling suppository mass occurs [34]. This method utilizes an evacuated flask into which the melt is placed, and the temperature of cooling noted. After the liquid is shaken until turbid, the temperature is recorded at which a transitory rise in temperature occurs during cooling. This is known as the solidification point.

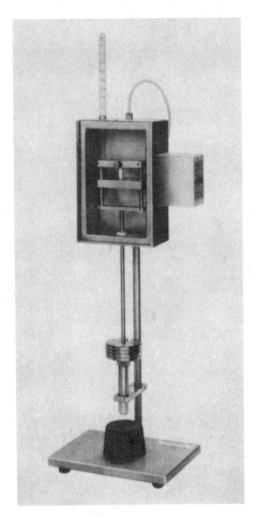

Fig. 4 Determination of mechanical strength. The apparatus consists of a stand-mounted chamber into which the suppository is placed, and a hanging rod attached to the suppository by means of a cap that rests on top of the suppository. Weights are suspended from the hanging rod and increased incrementally until the suppository breaks. Temperature control of the chamber environment is possible by means of a thermostat.

Crystallization, too, can affect solidification, especially when mono- and diglycerides are present. Because glycerolysis during the formation of glycerides causes the formation of free hydroxyl moieties, chemical incompatibility between the excipient and certain actives can occur. Thus, it is preferable to use excipients with a very low hydroxyl index, especially when high production rates demand a rapid crystallization of the molten mixture.

The influence of the hydroxyl index on solidification can be seen in the curves of solidification, known as Pichard curves (Fig. 8). These graphs plot solidification time against temperature, and demonstrate the effect of the free hydroxyl content of a given material. The heat of crystallization is indicated by a slight shoulder on the curve dur-

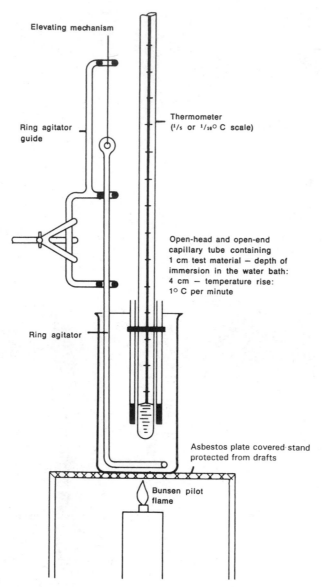

Fig. 5 Open capillary tube determination of melting temperature. The open capillary tube is most useful for verifying the melting point of excipients used in suppository manufacture. The method consists of filling two capillary tubes (open at both ends) with a melt of the test material, and then allowing it to slowly solidify. The tubes are then attached to a thermometer at the level of the mercury bulb, and then immersed into a water bath that is uniformly heated. The melting point is the mean of several observations of the point at which the sample in the column moves upward.

ing cooling. Generally, with a lower hydroxyl index, this heat of crystallization becomes more significant, and has a greater effect during cooling of the excipient.

For a better understanding of the phenomena of melting and solidification, modern analytical techniques offer significant potential. In particular, the examination of liquid

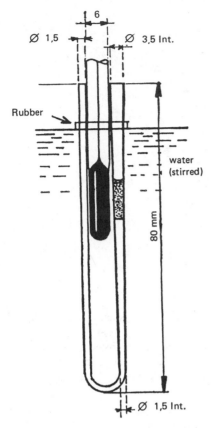

Fig. 6 U-tube determination of melting temperature. The U-tube method is similar to the capillary tube method, except instead of using two open-ended capillary tubes, a single U-shaped tube is employed. Because of the shape of the tube, the sample can be introduced without melting it, and it is therefore effective for the evaluation of finished suppositories. The sample is placed into one end of the tube, which is then attached to the thermometer so that the sample is as close as possible to the mercury. The average of several measurements of the temperature at which the sample begins to slip in the tube is the melting temperature.

and solid contents at different melting temperatures can be obtained by dilatometry, differential thermal analysis, NMR, or differential scanning calorimetry.

B. Chemical Testing

1. *Analytical Testing*

A careful assessment of product quality with reference to batch-to-batch uniformity is—among other things—an analytical issue. It depends, to a good degree, upon the caliber of the methods applied in the specification testing. Furthermore, routine quality control testing of suppository products is associated with unique problems specific for this dosage form. While ample information is available on testing of other dosage forms, investigations of the determination of assay, content uniformity and dissolution parameters of suppository formulations are (unfortunately) limited.

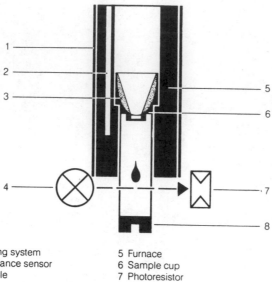

1 Heating system   5 Furnace
2 Resistance sensor   6 Sample cup
3 Sample   7 Photoresistor
4 Lamp   8 Collector

Fig. 7 Drop point determination of melting temperature. The drop point gives results similar to those obtained with the U-tube (as long as the sample is not melted before analysis), but it offers the advantage of automation. The sample to be measured is placed into a cup inside a small furnace. When the test material is heated, an opening at the bottom of the cup allows the escape of melted liquid. The first drop to fall interrupts a beam of light striking a photocell, and the temperature at that point is recorded as the drop point.

a.   *Assay.*   There are generally four steps involved in the analysis of active ingredients in unit dose formulations. They are as follows:

Preparation of a uniform composite
Extraction of the drug from the excipients
Separation of the excipient from the mixture
Analysis that selectively quantitates the active component(s)

For a general discussion of these methods, one can refer to any of numerous discussions found in the literature [35]. This chapter, however, will address problems specifically associated with the analysis of active ingredients in suppository formulations.

Conventionally, most of the unit dose formulations are analyzed after preparation of the analytical sample as follows: at least 5 to 20 unit doses (a requirement in most compendial methods) are weighed and composited by an appropriate method and an accurately weighed analytical sample (generally one unit dose weight) is taken for the assay. The error introduced at this step in the analysis of suppository formulation, however, can be significant. For example, it can be dependent on the nature of the active drug substances versus the excipients, or whether the active drug substance is soluble, partially soluble, or insoluble in the excipient mixture. Ease of preparation of the composite increases with the increasing solubility of the active drug substance in the excipients in disperse dosage systems including suppositories.

Preparation of a uniform composite.   To prepare the suppository composite, the following method has been found to be successful: About 20 to 30 suppositories are

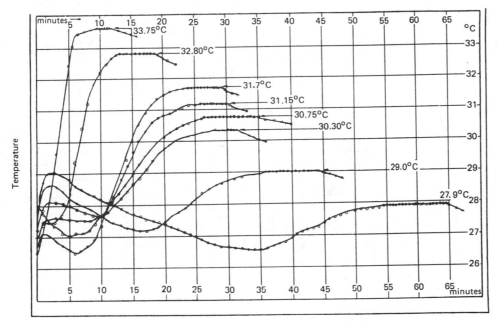

Fig. 8 Solidification point—effect of hydroxyl index. These Pichard curves illustrate the effect that hydroxyl index has on solidification. Next to each curve is given the hydroxyl index ("I.OH") of each material tested. As the index increases, the less marked is the "shoulder" of the curve, indicating a reduced heat of crystallization.

placed into a beaker and completely melted on a hot water bath. The molten mass is mixed with an electric mixer (approximately 100 rpm), and kept in an ice water bath and rapidly solidified as it is being mixed. The beaker is covered with Parafilm and kept at 0° to 4°C for an additional 30 minutes in order to achieve complete solidification. Three individual samples, each equivalent to one suppository weight, are taken from the composite and weighed for analysis. Methods described in the compendium for the preparation of suppository composite use a glass rod to mix the molten mass during solidification. This method is effective for most suppository formulations, but it is somewhat less precise when a water-soluble drug substance is present in a fatty base, or vice versa. Segregation of the drug substance and the base can occur when the suppositories are melted. Mixing with a glass rod may not be sufficient to obtain a good composite. To overcome this, an electric mixer can be used.

Extraction of the active drug substance from the suppository. Many extraction procedures have been used to separate active drug substances from suppository bases, depending on the nature of the ingredients. There are nearly 15 different suppository formulations that have been the subject of compendial monographs [36]. Extraction procedures adopted in these monographs for separating the active drug substances from the suppository bases range from simple methanolic–dilute tartaric acid extraction used for ergotamine tartrate and caffeine suppositories, to extensive partitioning of the drug and hydrophobic excipients between hexane, pentane, chloroform, or ether and aqueous media. Table 3 shows the solubility characteristics of the active drug substances in

Table 3 Suppository Active Ingredient Solubility Characteristics

Suppository	Solubility	Compendial method
Acetaminophen	Boiling water (s.) MeOH (s.) EtOH (f.s.)	Partition between hexane and water RP-HPLC-UV
Aminophylline	Water (f.s.) Alcohol (i.s.) Ether (i.s.)	Partition between ether and dilute HNO_3 Titration
Aspirin	Water (sl.s.) Chloroform (s.) EtOH (f.s.) Absolute ether (sp.s.)	Extract with chloroform Purification on column UV absorption at 280 nm
Bisacodyl	Water (i.s.) Chloroform (s.) MeOH, EtOH (sp.s.) Ether (sl.s.)	Partition between hexane and acetonitrile RP-HPLC-UV
Chlorpromazine	Water (i.s.) EtOH (f.s.) Benzene (f.s.) Chloroform (f.s.) Ether (f.s.)	Partition between ether and 0.1 N·HCl UV difference between 254 nm and 277 nm
Ergotamine tartrate and caffeine	EtOH (sl.s.) Tartaric acid (s.) Water (sp.s.) EtOH (sp.s.)	Extract with methanol and 1% tartaric acid RP-HPLC-UV and FD
Glycerin	Water (s.) EtOH (s.)	Titration
Hydrocortisone acetate	Water (i.s.) EtOH (sp.s) Chloroform (sp.s)	None

Drug	Solubility	Assay method
Indomethacin	Water (i.s.) EtOH (sp.s.) Chloroform (sp.s.) Ether (sp.s.)	Partition between ether and water UV at 320 nm
Miconazole nitrate	Water (v.sl.s.) EtOH (sl.s.) MeOH (sp.s.) Chloroform (sl.s.)	Extraction of excipients with pentane GC with internal standard
Nystatin	Water (v.sl.s) EtOH (sp.s) Chloroform (i.s.)	Extraction with dimethylformamide Microbial assay
Oxymorphone hydrochloride	Water (f.s.) EtOH (sp.s.) MeOH (sp.s.)	Partition between chloroform and 0.01 N HCl RP-HPLC-UV
Prochlorperazine	Water (v.sl.s.) Ether (f.s.) EtOH (f.s.) Chloroform (f.s.)	Partition between ether and 1% acid UV difference between 254 nm and 278 nm
Promethazine hydrochloride	Water (v.s.) Hot dehydrated EtOH (v.s.) Chloroform (v.s.) Ether (i.s.)	Partition between hexane and 0.05 N HCl Vis. at 450 nm after oxidation
Triethylperazine maleate	Water (s.)	Partition with ether and tartaric acid and then extraction with chloroform and MeOH UV at 263 nm
Trimethobenzamide HCl and benzocaine	MeOH (s.) Water (s.) Warm EtOH (s.) Ether (i.s.) Water (v.sl.s) EtOH (f.s.) Ether (f.s.)	None

KEY: v.s., very soluble; f.s., freely soluble; s., soluble; sp.s., sparingly soluble; sls, slightly soluble; v.sl.s., very slightly soluble; i.s., insoluble; FD, fluorescence detector; RP-HPLC-UV, reverse phase HPLC with UV detection; MeOH, methanol; EtOH, ethanol the suppositories of USP monographs and a few others, and the extraction solvents used in the analytical procedure. Nearly 10 of these procedures require multiple extraction of the fatty suppository bases with organic solvents. The methods are time-consuming and can be prone to imprecision.

Some of these methods can be simplified with an innocuous single extraction with a solvent to accomplish excellent precision and accuracy. The single extraction procedures similar to the method described for ergotamine and caffeine suppositories [36] reduce significant errors that may be introduced by partitioning between organic and aqueous solutions with an associated emulsion formation. Furthermore, an increased number of steps in an analytical procedure invariably increases analytical error in addition to being time consuming. The imprecision of some methods can result from a slight solubility of the drug substance in the solvents used for removing the suppository bases. As an example, ether is used for the extraction of excipients from acetaminophen [37]. However, acetaminophen is slightly soluble in ether, which may adversely affect the excipient recovery. Inclusion of structural analogues of the drug substances as internal standards for the extraction steps will improve precision and accuracy in many of these methods. Furthermore, inclusion of internal standards precludes the requirement for multiple extractions [38]. Suppository formulation with water-soluble bases poses fewer problems in the analysis of drug substances [39]. In the present regulatory environment, it is very important to have reproducible, robust analytical methods.

Separation of the excipients from the mixture. Excipients, when not separated from drug substances, can interfere with analytical methodology. When methanol or acetonitrile is used for extraction of the drug substance from fatty suppositories, separation of fatty excipients from the solution is accomplished by a simple filtration using membrane filters. It is essential to reduce the temperature below ambient temperature during filtration, so that some of the dissolved fatty excipient will not precipitate at a later time and clog the high-pressure liquid chromatography (HPLC) system. This is one of the reasons for developing elaborate extraction procedures with nonpolar solvents such as ether, chloroform, hexane, and pentane in many laboratories.

Analytical methods for quantitation. Once the drug substance is separated from the excipient(s), any of the many analytical procedures can be used for quantitation of the drug [40,41]. The use of HPLC in pharmaceutical analysis has become a method of choice. Compared to other analytical methods (GC, UV/Vis, titrations, etc.) the suitability of HPLC (especially as a stability-indicating method) has provided the basis for its popularity with both manufacturing firms and regulatory agencies. Although compendial methods do not claim to be stability-indicating, out of the 15 suppository monographs, four of the assays are by HPLC. Except for glycerin, all the other drug substances in the 15 suppository formulations can be analyzed by HPLC.

The extent of purification of the drug substance from the suppository bases will have an effect on HPLC column properties. While elaborate purification before chromatography will properly maintain HPLC columns, the accuracy of the method will suffer. The drawback of extraction by methanol and acetonitrile before chromatography is that the solution will have some of the dissolved hydrophobic fatty excipients. Chromatography of these solutions may lead to rapid deterioration of the HPLC columns due to adsorption of the fatty excipients on the reverse phase packing material. This problem can be successfully resolved by working with dilute extracts at higher sensitivity settings in the instrument and regeneration of the deteriorated columns, by successive washing with methanol, methylene chloride, hexane, methylene chloride, and methanol to wash off adsorbed hydrophobic excipients. Where the active component is also partially or completely hydrophobic, normal phase chromatography has provided an excellent solution for improved precision and accuracy and reducing the chromatographic problems [42].

Content uniformity. While the average specification for a dosage form can be met with the assay of the dosage form from a composite made from five to 20 suppositories, it is desirable to go beyond this and analyze randomly selected suppositories individually, which will provide information on dose-to-dose variation in a manufactured lot. The USP specification for the content uniformity of tablet and capsule dosage forms has been in effect for some time. Recently, the Pharmaceutical Manufacturing Association Quality Control Section, upon a request from the USP, evaluated the available data on content uniformity from six pharmaceutical companies [43]. Based on the findings, the specification for the tablets has been found to be applicable to suppository formulations as well and has been made official [44].

2. Dissolution Testing

Dissolution testing is one of the most important quality control tools available for the in vitro assessment of product efficacy. Under FDA guidelines, dissolution testing is also a requirement for suppositories to test for hardening and polymorphic transformation of drug substances and suppository bases in both control and stability testing.

While dissolution testing of tablet and capsule dosage forms is well established, dissolution testing of suppository formulation still lacks standardized test methodology. In an attempt to compensate for this situation, numerous attempts have been made to investigate drug release from suppository formulations and to correlate these in vitro results with in vivo bioavailability. These methods have been recently reviewed [45].

Dissolution testing of suppositories can be considered to be similar to that of solid oral dosage forms with these exceptions:

A problem is seen in cases where the vehicle containing the drug is immiscible in the aqueous solution in which the testing is being carried out: a partitioning occurs between the suppository base and the solution. Thus, an *equilibrium* rather than a *dissolution* is observed.

Membranes that serve as filtration means (to obtain clear solutions for improved analytical ease) can also introduce an artificial element of transport. This risks causing an apparent decrease in the rate of release of the active that can cause erroneous results—it can effectively alter actual differences between different formulations.

Variations in density—even changes during the test—between the suppository and the receiving fluid must be considered as a test parameter.

Release kinetics must be made as similar as possible to the in vivo situation, as with other test methods. Here, however, such mimicking of release from the melted suppository mass requires a sufficiently large and/or agitated surface area.

For these reasons, flow-through rather than standard dissolution techniques are considered advantageous, as they can overcome the above limitations. Studies using this approach have shown good early correlation with in vivo behavior [46].

a. *Methods of Dissolution Testing.*

Basket method.   This method utilizes the conventional USP Method I dissolution apparatus [47–53]. Problems encountered using the wire-mesh baskets stemming from clogging with fatty base can be partially eliminated by using a basket designed by Palmier [54,55]. This basket is commercially available and has slots instead of wire mesh. Reproducible data are obtained for dissolution of aspirin suppositories [54]. The advantage of the basket method is that fatty suppositories that generally float can be held in position.

Paddle method.   The paddle method utilizes the conventional USP Method II for tablets and capsules. Here, the suppository is allowed to sink into the bottom of the apparatus with steel spirals locked over the suppository. Increased rotational speed can enhance the release of drugs [56,57].

Beaker method.   This method was used in some of the earliest studies in which a suppository was allowed to sink into a medium in a beaker [58–61]. A modification of this includes mixing with a stirring element [58].

Membrane diffusion method.   The apparatus used here consists of a sample chamber separated from the dissolution liquid by a membrane [63–73]. An apparatus similar to this was developed by Muranishi [74], which is available commercially from Toyoma Sangyo Co., Ltd. (Osaka, Japan). It comprises a glass cylinder with a wire mesh at the bottom, wherein the suppository is placed. The device also consists of a metallic rotating shaft, a magnetic stirring bar, and a thermostatic arrangement for heating the fluid. This method has been used quite often with considerable success to determine suppository dissolution.

Dialysis method.   In this method a suppository is placed in a dialysis bag in which all liquid has been removed. This mass is held in position within the dissolution fluid by a heavy clamp or other weight within a beaker containing a stirring element [75–87]. A modification of this procedure uses the USP Method II paddle arrangement [56]. As the suppository melts, it spreads in a thin film. This approach probably most closely mimics the situation found in the in vivo system.

Continuous flow method.   In this method, medium is allowed to flow through the sample placed on wire mesh [85,86] or in the middle of glass beads [87,88]. The advantage claimed for the glass-beaded system is that when a suppository softens and eventually melts, it will spread on the bead to provide a large area in which dissolution may occur.

VII. PRODUCTION TROUBLESHOOTING

A. Overview

A general overview of problems that can be encountered in suppository manufacture is provided in Table 4 (below). Additional details and suggested resolutions follow.

B. Mixing Problems

1. *Nonuniformity of Mix*

Nonuniformity of a suppository mass can result from a number of conditions attributable to both operating procedures and equipment.

Table 4 Trouble-Shooting Guide

Problem	Causes	Solution
Splitting, pitting, and cracking	Excipient contracts strongly	Use an excipient that crystallizes more slowly
	Too great a difference between the temperatures of pouring and cooling	Reduce the differential by either dropping the pouring temperature (if possible) or increasing the cooling temperature, or both
Sticking to mold	Improper molds or alveoli	Use appropriate equipment
	Premature removal from mold	Prolong molding period
	Excipient contracts weakly	Use an excipient that crystallizes more rapidly
	Insufficient cooling	Reduce cooling temperature
Thickening prior to pouring	Solid active ingredients that partially solubilize hot in the excipient with time; high proportion of finely powdered active ingredients	Use a mass containing an anti-crystallizing agent
Poor product homogeneity	Insufficient stirring	Improve technique
	Pouring temperature too high	Reduce if possible
	Cooling too slow or too weak	Increase if possible
Product insufficiently solid	Inclusion of air	Check the stirring level and type
	Improper excipient	Use an excipient having a high mechanical resistance
Surface anomalies (fat bloom, whitening)	Excipient melting at more than 60°C	Reduce melting temperature; check behavior of active ingredient
Exudation	Incorrect excipient/active ratio	Reformulate aqueous solutions; use an excipient containing an emulsifier

a.   *Inadequate Mixing Time.*   This is often a primary cause of nonuniformity. Mixing time may *appear* to be adequate and may be validated, but nevertheless, on occasion, yield a batch with poor uniformity. For this reason, it is important that sufficient effort be devoted during process development to determine the optimum time range required to produce a uniform mix.

b.   *Mixing Equipment.*   Mixers can lose efficiency over time or suffer damage that can produce a poor mix. The speed of the mixer should be checked and compared against appropriate specifications and against the speed of the mixer observed at the time of validation. The mixing blade or rotor should be examined for wear or damage and, in the case of a homogenizer, the distance between rotor and stator measured for comparison with manufacturer's specifications. In fact, experienced operators can often tell if there is a mixer problem by a change in sound or by a change in the vortex created by the mixer in the mixing tank.

c.   *Temperature.*   A change in temperature can cause viscosity changes in the suppository base that may affect the quality of mix. Temperature can also change the physical state of an excipient. This may bind up the active drug before it is properly dispersed. The batch temperatures should be measured and the temperature controller should be checked for accuracy and recalibrated, if necessary. Quarterly recalibration of temperature gauges will prevent batch failures.

d.   *Operator Error.*   Failure to follow the manufacturing procedures and batching technique can readily lead to mix uniformity problems. The components may be added in the wrong order or in the wrong manner. This can occur if the operator is inexperienced or inattentive. It can also result when batching carries over a shift change due to miscommunication or poor documentation. Often this results in deviations from the established manufacturing procedures. Nonuniformity can be seen if the components, particularly the active drug, are added to the batch too quickly to cause agglomeration or precipitation and prevent adequate mixing.

2.   *Precipitation of Components*

Precipitation can result from some of the same conditions that cause nonuniformity in a mix, because precipitation of components would be a direct cause of nonuniformity.

a.   *Temperature.*   Components that are melted before being added to the batch may solidify and precipitate out if the material in the batch tank is at a temperature significantly below that of the melting point of the added material. This problem can apply to both soluble and insoluble components with a high melting point. Remedies to be taken are the same as those given above.

b.   *Mixing Equipment.*   Insoluble components may require extremely efficient mixing in order to maintain them in suspension in the base. A decline in mixing efficiency due to wear or damage in the mixing equipment can allow insoluble components to settle out of the mix. Here, too, the above solutions can be followed.

c.   *Operator error.*   Many low-density components must be added to the batch slowly so that the particles become "wetted." This prevents the material from being thrown out of the tank and creating a loss of active ingredients (if the material is the active) and/or creating a safety hazard for actives such as bisacodyl. It also prevents the material from floating on the surface and agglomerating. Denser materials must be added slowly to prevent them from settling rapidly to the bottom of the tank before the mixer can adequately disperse them. A lack of care on the part of the operator or undue haste in the batching process can lead to an inadequate suspension of insoluble components.

3. *Decomposition of Components*

Exposure to adverse conditions in the batching process can result in decomposition of the components.

a. *Temperature.* Although a low temperature may lead to nonuniformity or agglomeration or precipitation as described above, an excessively *elevated* temperature can decompose materials that are sensitive to heat. If the batch temperature must be raised to accommodate the addition of a particular component, the temperature should be lowered to a set range before addition of heat-sensitive components, particularly the active drug. Heat-sensitive material should be added at the end of batching by lowering the temperature and before final mixing. Generally, this is less of a problem with hydrogenated vegetable oil or cocoa butter bases, which are batched at temperatures below 45°C.

b. *Mixing Equipment.* The shearing forces produced by a homogenizer can have a detrimental effect on a sensitive drug, stemming from both physical degradation and frictional heat. Decomposition problems can occur when a mixer is rebuilt, a new mixer is installed, or a larger mixer is installed. A component that held up well with the older or smaller mixer may show evidence of degradation after the equipment change.

c. *Batching Time.* The time during which product components are exposed to the elevated temperatures of batching can affect the stability of the product. An extended batching process that lasts longer than usual can lead to decomposition. It is important to specify a maximum time interval for the various steps needed for suppository production.

d. *Melting Temperature Time of Base.* The melting temperature of a cocoa butter base has a significant effect on a suppository's appearance. Higher melting temperatures can cause gravitation of the suppository. Optimum temperature for melting of a cocoa butter base is 30° to 35°C. Holding the melted base within the optimum melting temperature range for extended periods of up to 10 days has no effect on the quality of the product. Solidification of the base and remelting also have no effect on quality.

C. Molding Problems

1. *Tearing and Splitting*

The suppository shell can tear and/or split during the molding step if the thickness of the foil varies excessively. Tolerances in the molding process, particularly for aluminum foil, are very narrow. Even variations in the thickness of the ink printed onto the foil can lead to problems in molding. Another cause of damage to the foil is mistiming of the molding stage in the machine. Generally, timing problems result in significant damage to the foil, such as ripping and shredding. However, excessive wear in a critical bearing, for example, can lead to small defects that are perplexing and difficult to correct.

2. *Improper Sealing*

Bad sealing is usually seen with low sealing temperatures or high machine speeds. The sealing temperature should be high enough to assure proper fusion of the two halves of the suppository shell, while minimizing heat carryover into the filling stage. If the temperature is set close to the minimum needed for an effective seal, increasing the machine speed may produce an inadequate fusion by reducing the dwell time.

D. Filling Problems

1. *Surface Defects*

Surface defects are often caused by either temperature or cooling problems. The filling temperature and/or the temperature of the shell that is either too high or too low for the product can cause surface imperfections as the material contacts the inner surface of the shell. Raising or lowering the filling temperature may solve this problem. The foil or plastic shell should be checked for excessive heat carryover from the sealing section. This heat carryover can be reduced by slowing down the machine or by use of fans to cool the webbing prior to filling. Rapid cooling after filling can also cause surface imperfections, especially in products with a cocoa butter base. Increasing the temperature of the initial cooling stage or slowing down the machine may help this situation.

2. *Structural Defects*

Like surface defects, structural defects are often due to temperature or cooling problems.

   a. *Soft suppositories.*   Soft suppositories are usually caused by inadequate cooling. This problem can be solved by reducing the cooling temperature or by slowing the machine so that the suppositories spend more time in the cooling section.

   b. *Suppository cracking.*   Cracking of suppositories is often caused by cooling that is too rapid. This can be addressed by changes in temperature settings or machine speed to create a more gradual cooling gradient.

   c. *Granulation.*   Granulation of the suppository matrix is a problem usually associated with cocoa butter–based products. It is manifested as a suppository, composed of large granules, that crumbles easily. Often the granulation does not appear until 12 to 24 hours after filling. Usually, however, a suppository that is destined to granulate will appear "wet" on the surface after cooling or will melt quickly when handled. This is caused by the formation of an unstable crystal structure within the suppository base and is usually due to excessively high temperature in batching, the storage tank, hopper, or filler or heat carryover in the webbing from the sealing stage. Shock cooling can also lead to this problem, but cracking of the suppository is more likely to result from excessively low cooling temperatures than from granulation. Generally, lowering the temperature of the problem vessel and waiting 8 to 12 hours for the material to stabilize will end the problem of granulation. The stabilization can be sped up by "seeding" the batch with a small quantity of fresh base. The material can stabilize in as little as 2 to 4 hours after seeding.

3. *Weight Variation*

This is usually a mechanical problem with the filler. This can be caused by a single filling piston being out of alignment or improper adjustment of the filling section. Another cause can be obstruction of one or more filling nozzles from suspended particles or solidification of the suppository mass in an area of low temperature. If readjustment of the filler weight settings does not help, applying gentle heat to the filling block to melt any occluding material can be tried. If these procedures still do not solve the problem, the filler should be dismantled and examined for obstructions and damaged seals.

   To assure homogeneity of the active-excipient combination, the chemical characteristics, solubilities, and behavior of the suppository components when heated must also

Table 5 Problems Due to Solubility Conditions

Physical State of Active: Solubility in Excipient:	Solid		Liquid	
	Soluble	Insoluble	Soluble	Insoluble
Potential Problems	Increased melting point Recrystallization	Thickening of mixture Migration	Decreased melting point Glyceride crystallization changes	Aqueous solution Glycerin, glycol, PEG
	Glyceride crystallization	Difficult particle size		Alcohol extract
				Possible nonaqueous exudation

be taken into consideration. Table 5 describes some of the problems that may be encountered under a range of solubility conditions.

VIII. FORMULARY

The following formulary provides examples of stable formulations for a selection of pharmaceutical actives. These illustrations are certainly not the only way to formulate these active ingredients, nor do they necessarily represent the preferred formulation. Rather, they are offered to show acceptable approaches to typical formulating requirements. All formulas yield one suppository.

A. Analgesic, Antipyretic

1. *Formula 1*

Aspirin	500 mg
Novata B	1500

Melt the excipient to 50°C, and add the active ingredient at about 45°C while stirring rapidly for 5 minutes. Follow by slower stirring to maintain a good suspension. Pour into mold between 36° and 38°C, and let cool.

2. *Formula 2*

Paracetamol	200 mg
Codeine phosphate	20
Aspirin	150
Witepsol H35	ad 2000

Pulverize all actives and mix well. Add small quantity of molten suppository base that has been cooled to between 38° and 40°C. Add the remaining base while stirring vigorously until homogeneous and pour into mold. Let cool.

B. Bronchopulmonary, Antitussive, etc.

1. *Formula 3*

Propythenazone	1250 mg
Theophylline	310
Caffeine	625
Ephedrine hydrochloride	310
Atropine methylbromide	1
Witepsol H15	ad 2000

Pulverize all actives and mix well. Add small quantity of molten suppository base that has been cooled to between 38° and 40°C. Add the remaining base while stirring vigorously until homogeneous and pour into mold. Let cool.

2. *Formula 4*

Theophylline	400 mg
Phenobarbital	20
Suppocire AML	1580

Melt the excipient to 50°C, and add the active ingredient at about 45°C while stirring rapidly for 5 minutes. Follow by slower stirring to maintain a good suspension. Pour into mold between 36° and 38°C and let cool.

3. *Formula 5 [92]*

Theophylline	50 mg
Glycerin	120
Distilled water	30
Castor oil	6
Tween 60	30
Macrogol 1540	13
Macrogol 4000	1186
Macrogol 6000	64

Disperse theophylline in an emulsion prepared by admixing the Tween, castor oil, water, and glycerin. The dispersion is then incorporated uniformly in the molten blend of the Macrogols and poured into molds.

C. Antibiotic

1. *Formula 6*

Terramycin	200 mg
Suppocire M	1800

Melt the excipient to 50°C, and add the active ingredient at about 40°C while stirring rapidly for 5 minutes. Follow by slower stirring to maintain a good suspension. Pour into mold between 36° and 38°C and let cool.

2. *Formula 7 (Urethral Nitrofurazone Suppository) [93]*

Nitrofurazone	2.6 mg per insert
Lidocaine	1.0%
in a base comprising	
Glyceryl laurate	10.0%
Polyethylene sorbitan monostearate	90.0%

The base is prepared by melting glyceryl laurate and polyethylene sorbitan monostearate on a water bath, adding the requisite amount of drug, and stirring until the dispersion is homogeneous. Urethral molds are then filled while the dispersion is stirred and allowed to cool.

D. Cardiovascular

1. *Formula 8*

Powdered digitalis leaf	50 mg
Theobromine sodium salicylate	250
Witepsol S55	ad 2000

Pulverize all actives and mix well. Add small quantity of molten suppository base that has been cooled to between 38° and 40°C. Add the remaining base while stirring vigorously until homogeneous and pour into mold. Let cool.

2. *Formula 9*

Phenylethylbarbituric acid	50 mg
Belladonna extract	40
Lactose	40
Glycerol 78%	80
Witepsol S55	ad 2000

Pulverize belladonna extract together with lactose, add glycerol, and heat the mixture on a water bath until the extract is completely dissolved. Add a portion of the suppository base and blend until the mixture is homogeneous. Mix phenylethylbarbituric acid with a second portion of the base at 38°C and add to the first blend. Stir vigorously and add the remaining suppository base. Pour into mold and let cool.

E. Antihemorrhoidal

1. *Formula 10*

Benzocaine	50 mg
Menthol	20
Resorcin	10
Zinc oxide	300
Hamamelis (liquid extract)	50
Witepsol S55	ad 2000

Mix all powdered ingredients and add to melted suppository base at 38°C. Add hamamelis extract and pour into mold. Let cool.

2. *Formula 11*

Anhydrous bismuth oxide	23 mg
Resorcinol	23
Bismuth subgallate	53
Bismuth oxyiodide	1
Zinc oxide	278
Boric acid	477
Peruvian balsam	46
Suppocire BM	1899

Pulverize all actives and mix well. Add small quantity of molten suppository base that has been cooled to between 38°C and 40°C. Add the remaining base while stirring vigorously until homogeneous and pour into mold. Let cool.

F. Hypoglycemic (U.S. Patent 4,164,573)

Formula 12

Myrj 45	105 mg
Myrj 51	53
Synthetic lecithin	3
Suppository base	163
Protamine zinc insulin suspension	26

Note: Insulin suspension is 381 units/mL insulin, 1.25 mg/100 units protamine.

Dissolve surfactants (Myrj's) and suppository base in ether in warm water bath. Mix the lecithin dispersion with the insulin suspension and add cooled suppository base dispersion. Flash evaporate the mixture, and then evaporate under reduced pressure (0.5 mm Hg). Dry for at least 30 minutes. Weigh suppository mass, and reconstitute the water content with distilled water to formula strength.

APPENDIX

Product Trade Names and Their Manufacturers

Cremaphor	BASF Wyandotte Corporation (Parsippany, NJ)
Suppocire, Labrafil, Labrafac	Gattefossé Etablissements (St.-Priest, France)
Novata, Lanette, Syndermin	Henkel International (Dusseldorf, Germany; Hoboken, NJ)
Arlacel, Myrj, Span, Tween, Atmul	ICI Americas (Wilmington, DE)
Witepsol, Miglyol	Kay-Fries, Inc. (Rockleigh, NJ)
Wecobee, Neobee	PVO International, Inc. (New York, NY)

REFERENCES

1. R. de Rosemont, *Histoire de la Pharmacie a Traverse les Ages*, Vol. 1, Peyronnet et Cie., Paris, 1931, p. 15.
2. W. A. Ritschel and G. B. Ritschel, Rectal administration of insulin. In: *Rectal Therapy* (B. Glas and C. J. de Blaey, eds.), J.R. Prous, 1984, p. 67.
3. A. G. de Boer, F. Moolenaar, L. G. J. de Leede, and D. D. Breimer, Rectal drug administration: Clinical pharmacokinetic considerations, *Clin. Pharmacokinet.*, 7:285 (1982).

4. A. G. de Boer, D. D. Breimer, H. Mattie, J. Pronk, and J. M. Gubbens-Stibbe, Rectal bioavailability of lidocaine in man: Partial avoidance of first-pass metabolism, *Clin. Pharmacol. Ther., 26:701* (1979).

5. G. Fredj, R. Farinotti, F. Hakkow, A. Astier, and L. Palmer, Biodisponsibilité de l'indométacine par voie orale et par voie rectale, *J. Pharm. Belg., 38:105* (1983).

6. G. Alvan, M. Orme, L. Bertilsson, R. Ekstrand, and L. Palmer, Pharmacokinetics of indomethacin, *Clin. Pharmacol. Ther., 18:364* (1975).

7. M. Gibaldi and B. Grundhofer, Bioavailability of aspirin from commercial suppositories, *J. Pharm. Sci., 64:1064* (1975).

8. E. L. Parrot, Salicylate absorption from rectal suppositories, *J. Pharm. Sci., 60:867* (1971).

9. F. Moolenar, S. Bakker, J. Visser, and T. Huizinga, Comparative biopharmaceutics of diazepam after single rectal, oral, intramuscular, and intravenous administration in man, *Int. J. Pharm., 5:127* (1980).

10. D. D. Breimer, L. G. J. De Leede, A. G. De Boer, *New Drug Delivery Systems as Tools in Clinical Pharmacology*, Proc. Sec. World Conf. Clin. Pharmacol. Ther., Washington, D.C. (1983).

11. T. B. Tjandramaga, R. Verbesselt, A. Van Hecken, and P. J. de Shepper, *Curr. Med. Res. Opin.* 6(Suppl. 6):142 (1979).

12. J. F. Thiercelin, L. Sansom, J. R. Powell, and S. Riegelman, Bioavailability of aminophylline suppositories—clinical implications. In: *Proc. of First Eur. Cong. Biopharm. Pharmacokin.* (Clermont-Ferrand) Part I: 389 (1981).

13. J. T. Doluisio, R. B. Smith, A. H. Chun, and L. W. Dittert, Pentobarbital absorption from capsules and suppositories in humans, *J. Pharm. Sci., 67:1586* (1978).

14. A. Beckett, Bioavailability following rectal absorption, *Bulletin Technique* (Gattefossé Report), 1983; p. 21

15. S. Muranishi, Y. Tokunaga, K. Taniguchi, H. Sezaki, Potential absorption of heparin from the small intestine and the large intestine in the presence of monoolein mixed micelles, *Chem. Pharm. Bull.* (Tokyo) 25(5):1159–1161 (1977).

16. N. Muranushi, M. Kinugawa, Y. Nakajima, S. Muranishi, and H. Sezaki, Mechanism for the inducement of the intestinal absorption of poorly absorbed drugs by mixed micelles. I. Effects of various lipid-bile salt mixed micelles on the intestinal absorption of streptomycin in rat, *Int. J. Pharm., 4:271* (1980).

17. United States Pharmacopeia XXIII and National Formulary XVI, United States Pharmacopeial Convention, Rockville, MD

18. E. Touitou, M. Donbrow, and E. Azaz, New hydrophilic vehicles enabling rectal and vaginal absorption of insulin, heparin, phenol red and gentamicin, *J. Pharm. Pharmacol., 30:662* (1978).

19. N. Senior, Rectal administration of drugs, *Adv. Pharm. Sci., 4:363* (1974).

20. E. M. Holyhead, N. W. Thomas, C. G. Wilson, The regeneration of rectal epithelium in the rat following wounding with suppositories of polyoxyethylene (23) lauryl ether. *Br. J. Exp. Pathol.* 64(4):456–461 (1983).

21. Trademarks: Novata, Henkel International (Dusseldorf, Germany); Suppocire, Gattefossé Etablissements (St.-Priest, France); Wecobee, PVO International, Inc. (New York); Witepsol, Dynamit Nobel (Troisdorf-Oberlar, Germany).

22. A. B. Scranton and N. A. Peppas, eds., Theme: Modern hydrogel delivery systems, *Adv. Drug Del. Rev.,* 11(1,2): i–viii, 1–191 (1993).

23. Trademarks: Labrafac, Gattefossé Etablissements (St.-Priest, France); Miglyol, Dynamit Nobel (Troisdorf-Oberlar, Germany); Neobee, PVO International (New York); Syndermin, Henkel International (Dusseldorf, Germany)

24. Trademark: Lanette, Henkel International (Dusseldorf, Germany).

25. Trademarks: Arlacel, Myrj, Span, Tween, ICI Americas, Inc. (Wilmington, DE); Cremophor,

BASF Wyandotte Corporation (Parsippany, NJ); Labrafil, Gattefossé Etablissements (St.-Priest, France).

26. Trademark: Atmul, ICI Americas Inc. (Wilmington, DE).

27. V. Brustier, M. Podesta, S. Bellan, A. Amselem, L. S. Nang, [On the activity of mucopolysaccharidases administered rectally] Sur l'activite des mucopolysaccharidases administrees par voie rectale. *Farmaco [Prat]* 24(4):203–214 (1969).

28. K. Thoma, Stability problems of availability. In: *Rectal Therapy* (B. Glas and C. J. de Blaey, eds.), J. R. Prous, 1984, p. 27.

29. W. A. Etchells, W. N. Ford, and D. G. R. Short, Mixing of Bingham plastics on an industrial scale. In: *Fluid Mixing III,* Institution of Chemical Engineers, Symposium Series No. 108, Hemisphere Publ. Corp., Bradford, 1987, pp. 271–285.

30. K.-Z. Hong, Strain-induced crystallization of polymers, Ph.D. Dissertation, University of Michigan, 1981.

31. A Riva, M. Surer, Manufacture of suppositories using compression, *Bulletin Technique* (Gattefossé Report) 1983: p. 25.

32. A. D. Keith, W. C. Snipes, Buccal drug dosage form, U.S. patent 4,764,378 (August 16, 1988), assigned to Zetachron, Inc., State College, PA.

33. W. C. Snipes, Low melting moldable pharmaceutical excipient and dosage forms prepared therewith, U.S. patent 5,004,601 (April 2, 1991), assigned to Zetachron, Inc., State College, PA.

34. L. Waginaire, Excipient pour suppositoires. Point de solidification selon Shukoff. Etude critique de la méthode. *Bulletin Technique Gattefossé,* 70:43–50 (1977).

35. T. D. Wilson, Liquid chromatographic methods validation for pharmaceutical products. *J. Pharm. Biomed. Anal.,* 8:389–400 (1990).

36. The United States Pharmacopeia, XXII, The United States Pharmacopeial Convention, Inc., Rockville, MD, 1990.

37. Norlyn Tymes, Compendial monograph evaluation and development—Acetaminophen, *Pharmacopeial Forum,* Jan-Feb., 1480–1484 (1990).

38. M. S. Bergren, M. M. Battle, G. W. Halstead, and D. L. Theis, Investigation of the relationship between melting-related parameters and in vitro drug release from vaginal Suppositories, *J. Pharm. Biomed. Anal.,* 7(5):549–561 (1989).

39. G. Lootvoet, E. Beyssac, T. G. K. Shiu, J. M. Aiachi, and W. A. Ritschel, Study on the release of indomethacin from suppositories, *Int. J. Pharm.* 85:113–120 (1992).

40. J. W. Munson, ed., Pharmaceutical Analysis, Modern Methods, Part A and Part B, 1981.

41. J. W. Munson, Analytical techniques in dissolution testing and bioavailability studies, *J. Pharm. Biomed. Anal.,* 4(6):717–724 (1986).

42. A. R. Lea, J. M. Kennedy, and G. K.-C. Low, Analysis of hydrocortisone acetate ointments and creams by high-performance liquid chromatography, *J. Chrom.,* 198:41–47 (1980).

43. J. Sanabia, M. Hardy, E. Liberator, L. Pasteelnick, T. A. Scheponik, C. Stern, and P. E. Manni, Dose uniformity for suppositories, *Pharmacopeial Forum,* Sept.-Oct., 2424–2426 (1991).

44. The United States Pharmacopeia, XXII, The United States Pharmacopeial Convention, Inc., Rockville, MD, 1990, p. 2938.

45. U. V. Banakar. In: *Pharmaceutical Dissolution Testing* (U.V. Banakar, ed.), Marcel Dekker, New York, 1991, pp. 280–285.

46. F. Langenbucher, Suppository dissolution testing, *Bulletin Technique* (Gattefossé Report) 1983, p. 23.

47. C. J. deBlaey and J. J. Rutten-Kingma, Biopharmaceutics of aminophylline suppositories II. In vitro release rate during storage, *Pharm. Acta Helv.,* 52:11–14 (1977).

48. I. W. Kellaway and C. Marriott, Correlations between physical and drug release characteristics of polyethylene glycol suppositories, *J. Pharm. Sci.,* 64:1162–1166 (1975).

49. V. E. Krogerus, and M. Tolvi, Uber die Wirkung von Suppositoriengrundmassen auf die Rektalresorption von Arzneimitteln, *Acta Pharm. Suec,* 2:327–344 (1965).

50. E. L. Parrott, Influence of particle size on rectal absorption of aspirin, *J. Pharm. Sci.*, 64:878–880 (1975).

51. L. Roller, Formulation, dissolution and bioavailability of paracetamol suppositories, *Aust. J. Hosp. Pharm.*, 7:97–101 (1977).

52. S. E. Leucuta, L. Popa, M. Ariesan, L. Popa, R. D. Pop, M. Kory, and S. Toader, Bioavailability of phenobarbital from different pharmaceutical dosage forms, *Pharm. Acta Helv.*, 52:261–266 (1977).

53. A. Peck, Y. Lasserre, and M. Jacob, In vitro kinetic release of active principles from suppositories. Part 1. Study of new apparatus, *Trav. Soc. Pharm. Montpellier*, 37:165–172 (1977).

54. A. Palmieri, Suppository dissolution testing: Apparatus design and release of aspirin, *Drug Dev. Ind. Pharm.*, 7:247–259 (1981).

55. A. Palmieri, Dissolution of suppositories and acetaminophen release, *Pharm. Technol.*, 6(6), 70–80 (1982).

56. N. Aoyagi, N. Kaniwa, Y. Takeda, M. Uchiyama, F. Takamura, and Y. Kido, Release rates of indomethacin from commercial Witepsol suppositories and the bioavailabilities in rabbits and pigs, *Chem. Pharm. Bull.*, 36(12):4933–4940 (1988).

57. Vepuri, Able Laboratories, Inc. Personal communications.

58. C. W. Whitworth, and J. P. LaRocca, A Study of the effect of some emulsifying agents on drug release from suppository bases, *J. Am. Pharm. Assoc. Sci. Ed.*, 48:353–355 (1959).

59. A. J. M. Schoonen, F. Moolenaar, C. Haverschmidt, and T. Huizinga, The Interphase Transport of Drugs from Fatty Suppository Bases, *Pharm. Weekbl.*, 3:585–589 (1976).

60. H. M. Gross, and C. H. Becker, A study of suppositories bases. II. A colorimetric method for measuring medicinal release from suppository bases, *J. Am. Pharm. Assoc., Sci. Ed.*, 42:96–100 (1953).

61. S. N. Pagay, R. I. Poust, and J. L. Colaizzi, Influence of vehicle dielectric properties on acetaminophen bioavailability from polyethylene glycol suppositories, *J. Pharm. Sci.*, 63:44–47 (1974).

62. B. W. Mueller, Significance of the particle size distribution for the manufacture in suspension suppositories, *Pharm. Ind.*, 36(12):943–946 (1974).

63. L. Bardet and J. Cemeli, Study with radioisotope tracers of the effectiveness of some suppository excipients, *Trav. Soc. Pharm. Montpellier.*, 16:200–206 (1956).

64. V. P. Bhavnagri and P. Speiser, *In vitro* kinetics of drug release from oral dosage forms, lyophilized and conventional rectal suppositories, *Pharm. Acta Helv.*, 51:10–18 (1976).

65. M. A. Ghafoor and C. L. Huyck, The *in vitro* activity of chloramphenicol in several suppository bases. *Am. J. Pharm.*, 134:63 (1962).

66. A. A. Kassem, E. Nour El-Din, A. Abd El-Bary, and H. M. Fadel, *In vitro* Release of chloramphenicol from different suppository bases, *Pharmazie*, 30,472–475 (1975).

67. L. Krowczynski, Time of complete deformation of suppositories and ability to liberate drugs as criteria for evaluation of modern bases. II. *In vitro* investigation of liberation of substances from fat vehicles, *Acta Pol. Pharm*, 19,127–142 (1962).

68. Z. Kubiak and L. Szczurek-Moskal, Attempts of obtaining "sink" conditions in drug release study from lipophilic vaginal suppositories, *Farm. Pol.* 37(7):383–387 (1981).

69. V. H. Muhlemann and R. H. Neuenschwander, Ober die Eignung Moderner Grundlagen als Suppositorienmassen, *Pharm. Acta Helv.*, 31:305–329 (1956).

70. M. Kapas, G. Kedvessy, G. Regdon, E. Minker, and A. Magyariaki, Biopharmaceutical testing of suppositories containing salicylic acid derivatives. *In vitro* membrane diffusion methods, *Acta Pharm. Hung.* 51(4):161–167 (1981).

71. G. Regdon, A. Magiarlaki, G. Kedvessy, E. Minker, and E. Regdon, Biopharmaceutical study of sulfadimidine-containing suppositories, *Pharmazie*, 33:67–69 (1978).

72. R. Voigt and G. Falk, Water solubility of drugs as a criterion for drug liberation from fatty galenic bases (cetylium phthalicum, Lasupol G) with regard to viscosity-increasing adjuvants, *Pharmazie*, 23:709–714 (1968).

73. G. B. Carp, D. Brossard, C. Chemtob, and J. C. Chaumeil, The control of active principle release in vitro from suppositories, *Sci. Tech. Pharm.*, 7:159 (1978).

74. S. Muranishi, Y. Okubo, and H. Sezaki, Manufacture and examination of apparatus for drug release from suppositories, *Yakuzaigaku*. 39:1–7 (1979).

75. J. M. Plaxco, Jr., C. B. Free, Jr., and C. R. Rowland, Effect of some nonionic surfactants on the rate of release of drugs from suppositories, *J. Pharm. Sci.*, 56:809–814 (1967).

76. W. H. Thomas and R. McCormack, The drug release characteristics of various rectal suppositories as determined by specific ion electrodes, *J. Pharm. Pharmacol.*, 23:490–494 (1971).

77. T. Stozek, The study of the bioavailability of coated acetylsalicyclic acid in suppositories after rectal administration, *Pol. J. Pharmacol. Pharm.*, 27:227–233 (1975).

78. L. Turakka and V. E. Krogenus, Effect of some nonionic surface-active agents on the rate of release of drugs from suppositories. I. Effect of concentration of surface-active agents, *Farm. Aikak.*, 83:59–70 (1974).

79. L. Turakka and V. E. Krogenus, Effect of some nonionic surface-active agents on the rate of release of drugs from suppositories. I. Effect of the HLB [hydrophile-lipophile balance] value of the surface-active agent, *Farm. Aikak,* 83,105 (1974).

80. J. W. Ayres, D. Lorskulsint, A. Lock, L. Kuhl, and P. A. Laskar, Absorption and distribution of radioactivity from suppositories containing 3H-benzocaine in Rats. *J. Pharm. Sci.*, 65(6): 832–838 (1976).

81. C. G. Hartman, The permeability of the vaginal mucosa, *Ann. N.Y. Acad. Sci.*, 83:318–327 (1959).

82. H. P. M. Kerckhoffs and T. Huizinga, Vergelijkend Onderzoek Over de Opname Van Geneesmiddelen na Toediening Langs Orale, Rectale en Parenterale Weg. I. Theofyllinepreparaten, *Weekbl.*, 102:1255–1268 (1967).

83. C. F. Peterson, and A. J. Guida, Suppository bases. I. An evaluation of the rate of release of theophylline, *J. Am. Pharm. Assoc. Sci. Ed.*, 42:537–540 (1953).

84. H. Piasecka and Z. Zakrewski, Studies on aminophenazone and phenobarbital release from suppositories prepared on different bases. *Pol. J. Pharmacol. Pharm.*, 28:199–203 (1976).

85. W. A. Ritschel and M. Banarer, Correlation between in vitro release of proxyphylline from suppositories and in vivo data obtained from cumulative urinary excretion studies, *Arzneimittelforschung* 23:1031–1035 (1973).

86. S. Tsuchiya, M. Hiura, and H. Matsumaru, Studies of absorption of suppositories. VIII. Effect of the amount of base on absorption of sulfonamides from rabbit rectum, *Chem. Pharm. Bull.*, 25:667–674 (1977).

87. S. Itoh, N. Morishita, M. Yamazaki, A. Suginaka, K. Tanabe, and M. Sawanoi, Biopharmaceutical characteristics of suppository base containing poly(oxyethylene)-poly(oxypropylene copolymer, Unilube. 1. Effects of a suppository base containing Unilube 70DP-950B on release and rectal absorption of aminopyrine in rabbit, *J. Pharmacobio-Dyn.*, 10:173–179 (1987).

88. M. R. Baichwal, and T. V. Lohit, Medicament release from fatty suppository bases, *J. Pharm. Pharmacol.*, 22:427–432 (1970).

89. H. W. Puffer, and W. J. Crowell, Salicylate release characteristics of selected polyethylene glysol suppositories, *J. Pharm. Sci.*, 62:242–645 (1973).

90. T. J. Roseman, G. R. Derr, K. G. Nelson, B. L. Lieberman, and S. S. Butler, Continuous flow bead-bed dissolution apparatus for suppositories, *J. Pharm. Sci.*, 70:646–651 (1981).

91. J. C. McElnay and A. C. Nicol, The comparison of a novel continuous-flow dissolution apparatus for suppositories with the rotating basket technique, *Int. J. Pharm.*, 19:89–96 (1984).

Index